PIGMENTARY DISORDERS
A Comprehensive Compendium

PIGMENTARY DISORDERS
A Comprehensive Compendium

Editors

Koushik Lahiri MBBS DVD (Cal) FIAD FAAD FFAADV MRCPS (Glasgow)
Senior Consultant Dermatologist
Apollo Gleneagles Hospitals
Nightingale Hospitals
WIZDERM
Kolkata, West Bengal, India

Col Manas Chatterjee MD DNB
Senior Advisor
Professor and Head
Department of Dermatology
Command Hospital (Eastern Command)
Kolkata, West Bengal, India

Rashmi Sarkar MD MNAMS
Professor
Department of Dermatology
Maulana Azad Medical College and
Associated Lok Nayak Hospital
New Delhi, India

Foreword

James J Nordlund

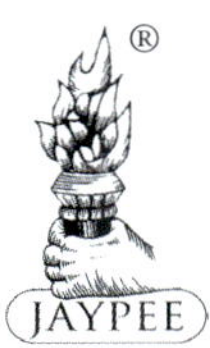

JAYPEE BROTHERS MEDICAL PUBLISHERS (P) LTD

New Delhi • London • Philadelphia • Panama

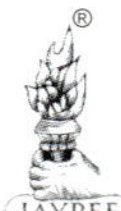

Jaypee Brothers Medical Publishers (P) Ltd.

Headquarters

Jaypee Brothers Medical Publishers (P) Ltd.
4838/24, Ansari Road, Daryaganj
New Delhi 110 002, India
Phone: +91-11-43574357
Fax: +91-11-43574314
Email: jaypee@jaypeebrothers.com

Overseas Offices

J.P. Medical Ltd.
83, Victoria Street, London
SW1H 0HW (UK)
Phone: +44-2031708910
Fax: +02-03-0086180
Email: info@jpmedpub.com

Jaypee-Highlights Medical Publishers Inc.
City of Knowledge, Bld. 237, Clayton
Panama City, Panama
Phone: +1 507-301-0496
Fax: +1 507-301-0499
Email: cservice@jphmedical.com

Jaypee Medical Inc.
The Bourse
111, South Independence Mall East
Suite 835, Philadelphia
PA 19106, USA
Phone: +1 267-519-9789
Email: joe.rusko@jaypeebrothers.com

Jaypee Brothers Medical Publishers (P) Ltd.
17/1-B, Babar Road, Block-B
Shaymali, Mohammadpur
Dhaka-1207, Bangladesh
Mobile: +08801912003485
Email: jaypeedhaka@gmail.com

Jaypee Brothers Medical Publishers (P) Ltd.
Bhotahity, Kathmandu, Nepal
Phone: +977-9741283608
Email: kathmandu@jaypeebrothers.com

Website: www.jaypeebrothers.com
Website: www.jaypeedigital.com

Pigmentary Disorders: A Comprehensive Compendium

First Edition: **2014**

ISBN 978-93-5090-658-3

Printed at Replika Press Pvt. Ltd.

Dedicated to

My parents, partner, progenies
and
patients

Koushik Lahiri

My parents, wife Dr Mrs Vibhu Chatterjee
and
daughter Miss Puja Chatterjee

Manas Chatterjee

My late father, Dr AK Sarkar; my mother, Mrs Chhobi Sarkar
my husband, Dr Srikanta Basu
and
my son, Abhik Sarkar Basu

Rashmi Sarkar

Contributors

Keshavmurthy A Adya MD
Assistant Professor
Department of Dermatology, Venereology and Leprosy
Shri BM Patil Medical College
Hospital and Research Center
BLDE University
Bijapur, Karnataka, India

Shweta Agarwal MD
Assistant Professor
Dr DY Patil Medical College and Hospital
Navi Mumbai, Maharashtra, India

Latika Arya MD
LA Skin Centre
New Delhi, India

Raghubir Banerjee MD
Associate Professor
Department of Dermatology
Vivekananda Institute of Medical Sciences
Kolkata, West Bengal, India

Shivani Bansal MD
Senior Resident
Department of Dermatology
Maulana Azad Medical College
New Delhi, India

Maria I Barona MD
Centro Medico Imbanaco
Centro Dermatologico de Cali
Board of Directors
Calle 5B3 # 38-44
Cali, Colombia

Shyamanta Barua MD
Assistant Professor
Department of Dermatology
Assam Medical College and Hospital
Dibrugarh, Assam, India

Meenakshi Batrani MD (Pathology)
Consultant Dermatopathologist
Delhi Dermpath Laboratory
New Delhi, India

Shashikumar BM MD
Associate Professor
Department of Dermatology
Mandya Institute of Medical Sciences (MIMS)
Bengaluru, Karnataka, India

Valerie D Callender MD
Associate Professor
Department of Dermatology
Howard University College of Medicine
Washington, DC, USA
Medical Director
Callender Dermatology and Cosmetic Center
Glenn Dale, MD, USA

Manas Chatterjee MD DNB
Senior Advisor
Professor and Head
Department of Dermatology
Command Hospital (Eastern Command)
Kolkata, West Bengal, India

Namrata Chhabra MD
Senior Resident
Department of Dermatology and STD
University College of Medical Sciences and GTB Hospital
University of Delhi
New Delhi, India

Angelo Massimiliano D'Erme MD
Division of Dermatology
Department of Surgery and Translational Medicine
University of Florence
Florence, Italy

Paschal D'Souza MD
Consultant Dermatologist
Siliguri, West Bengal, India

Bhavesh Shantilal Devani MD
Drashti Cosmetic Laser Center
Morbi, Gujarat, India

Sandipan Dhar MBBS MD DNB
Professor and Head
Department of Pediatric Dermatology
Institute of Child Health
Kolkata, West Bengal, India

Sunil Dogra MD DNB MNAMS FRCP (London)
Associate Professor
Department of Dermatology Venereology and Leprology
Postgraduate Institute of Medical Education and Research
Chandigarh, India

Rafael Falabella MD
Professor
Centro Dermatologico de Cali
President of the Board of Directors
Centero Internacional de Entrenamientoe Investigaciones Medicas (CIDEIM)
Institute for Research and Training for Tropical Diseases
Board of Directors
Calle 5B3 # 38-44
Cali, Colombia

Sanjay Ghosh MD
Professor
Department of Dermatology
Mata Gujri Memorial (MGM) Medical College and LSK Hospital
Kishanganj, Bihar, India

Kiran Godse MD DVD FRCP
Associate Professor
Dr DY Patil Medical College and Hospital, Navi Mumbai
Maharashtra, India

Narendra Gokhale MD
Consultant Dermatologist
Indore, Madhya Pradesh, India

Somesh Gupta MD
Professor
Department of Dermatology and Venereology
All India Institute of Medical Sciences
New Delhi, India

Vishal Gupta MBBS
Junior Resident
Department of Dermatology
and Venereology
All India Institute of Medical Sciences
New Delhi, India

Rebat M Halder MD
Professor and Chairman
Department of Dermatology
Howard University College of Medicine
and Hospital
Washington, DC, USA

Iltefat Hamzavi MD FAAD
Multicultural Dermatology Center
Department of Dermatology
Henry Ford Hospital
Detroit, MI, USA
3031 West Grand Blvd, Suite 800

Iffat Hassan MBBS MD
Professor and Head
Postgraduate Department of Dermatology,
Sexually Transmitted Diseases and Leprosy
Government Medical College
Srinagar, Jammu and Kashmir, India

Daniel Hewitt MBBS FACD
Consultant Dermatologist
Burswood Dermatology
Victoria Park, WA, Australia

Ahmad Reza Hossani-Madani MD MS
Chief Resident
Department of Dermatology
Howard University Hospital
Washington, DC, USA

Arun C Inamadar MD
Professor and Head
Department of Dermatology, Venereology
and Leprosy
Shri BM Patil Medical College, Hospital and
Research Center
Bijapur Liberal Development Education
(BLDE) University
Bijapur, Karnataka, India

Prescilia N Isedeh MD
Multicultural Dermatology Center
Department of Dermatology
Henry Ford Hospital, Detroit, MI, USA
3031 West Grand Blvd, Suite 800

Hee Young Kang MD PhD
Professor
Department of Dermatology
Ajou University School of Medicine
Suwon, Korea

Amrinder Jit Kanwar MD
Professor and Head
Department of Dermatology
Postgraduate Institute of Medical
Education and Research
Chandigarh, India

Sushruta Kathuria MD
Specialist
Department of Dermatology and STD
Vardhman Mahavir Medical College and
Safdarjung Hospital, New Delhi, India

Binod K Khaitan MD MNAMS
Additional Professor
Department of Dermatology and
Venereology
All India Institute of Medical
Sciences, New Delhi, India

Rehan Khan MD
Department of Biochemistry
All India Institute of Medical Sciences
New Delhi, India

Asha Kubba
Diplomate
American Board of Pathology
Diplomate
American Board of Pathology in
Dermatopathology
Consultant Dermatopathologist
Delhi Dermpath Laboratory
New Delhi, India

Ravinder Kumar PhD
Department of Dermatology
Postgraduate Institute of Medical
Education and Research
Chandigarh, India

M Sendhil Kumaran MD
Assistant Professor
Department of Dermatology
Postgraduate Institute of Medical
Education and Research
Chandigarh, india

Prasad Kumarasinghe
MBBS MD FCCP FAMS FACD
Clinical Associate Professor
Royal Perth Hospital/University of Western
Australia, Perth, WA, Australia

Saurav Kundu MD
Assistant Professor
Department of Dermatology
MGM Medical College and LSK Hospital
Kishanganj, Bihar, India

Koushik Lahiri MBBS DVD (Cal) FIAD
FAAD FFAADV MRCPS (Glasgow)
Senior Consultant Dermatologist
Apollo Gleneagles Hospitals
Nightingale Hospitals, WIZDERM
Kolkata, West Bengal, India

Torello Lotti MD
Professor and Chairman
Department of Dermatology
and Venereology
University of Rome "G Marconi"
Rome, Italy

Khushboo Goel Mahajan MD
Senior Resident
Department of Dermatology
Maulana Azad Medical College
New Delhi, India

Rahul Mahajan MD
Department of Dermatology, Venereology
and Leprology
Postgraduate Institute of Medical
Education and Research
Chandigarh, India

Imran Majid MD
Associate Professor
Department of Dermatology
Government Medical College, Srinagar
Director
Cutis Skin and Laser Institute
Srinagar, Jammu and Kashmir, India

Rajib Malakar MD
Clinical Tutor
Department of Pediatric Dermatology
Institute of Child Health, Kolkata
West Bengal, India

Subrata Malakar MD
Director
Rita Skin Foundation
Kolkata, West Bengal, India

Amiya Kumar Mukhopadhyay MD PhD
DNB (Derm) DNB (Derm and Vener) MNAMS
Consultant Dermatologist and
Independent Researcher on the History
of Dermatology and Medicine
Asansol, West Bengal, India

Tarun Narang MD
Assistant Professor
Department of Dermatology
Postgraduate Institute of Medical
Education and Research
Chandigarh, India

Vic A Narurkar MD FAAD
Chairman
Department of Dermatology California Pacific Medical Center
Associate Clinical Professor
Dermatology
University of California Davis Medical School
Director and Founder
Bay Area Laser Institute
San Francisco, CA, USA

Sudhir Nayak UK MD DDVL
Assistant Professor
Department of Dermatology and Venereology
Kasturba Medical College and Hospital
Manipal, Karnataka, India

Jean-Paul Ortonne MD
Professor and Chairman
Department of Dermatology
University of Nice-Sophia Antipolis
Nice, France

Saumya Panda MD
Associate Professor
Department of Dermatology
KPC Medical College
Kolkata, West Bengal, India

Davinder Parsad MD
Additional Professor
Department of Dermatology
Postgraduate Institute of Medical Education and Research
Chandigarh, India

Smitha Prabhu MD DVD
Associate Professor
Department of Dermatology and Venereology
Kasturba Medical College and Hospital
Manipal, Karnataka, India

Priyanka MBBS
Academic Junior Resident
Department of Dermatology and Venereology
All India Institute of Medical Sciences
New Delhi, India

Reena Rai MD
Professor
Department of Dermatology
PSG Institute of Medical Sciences and Research
Coimbatore, Tamil Nadu, India

M Ramam MD
Professor
Department of Dermatology and Venereology
All India Institute of Medical Sciences
New Delhi, India

Parvaiz Rather MD
Senior Resident
Postgraduate Department of Dermatology, Sexually Transmitted Diseases and Leprosy
Government Medical College
Srinagar, Jammu and Kashmir, India

Sanjay K Rathi MD
Professor and Head
Department of Dermatology
Employees State Insurance Postgraduate Institute of Medical Science and Research (ESIC-PGIMSR), New Delhi, India

Raghunatha Reddy R MD DNB FRGUHS
Professor and Head
Department of DVL
PES Institute of Medical Sciences and Research (PESIMSR)
Kuppam, Andhra Pradesh, India
Consultant Dermatologist and Dermatosurgeon
Mathapitha Polyclinic
Bengaluru, Karnataka, India

Vineet Relhan MD
Assistant Professor
Department of Dermatology
Maulana Azad Medical College
New Delhi, India

T Salim MD
Medical Director
Cutis Institute of Advanced Dermatology and Esthetic Sciences, Calicut, Kerala, India

Rashmi Sarkar MD MNAMS
Professor
Department of Dermatology
Maulana Azad Medical College and Associated Lok Nayak Hospital
New Delhi, India

Nilendu Sarma MD
Assistant Professor
Department of Dermatology
NRS Medical College
Kolkata, West Bengal, India

Alpana Sharma MD
Department of Biochemistry
All India Institute of Medical Sciences
New Delhi, India

Shrutakirthi D Shenoi MD DVD
Professor and Head
Department of Dermatology and Venereology
Kasturba Medical College and Hospital, Manipal, Karnataka, India

Archana Singal MD MNAMS
Professor
Department of Dermatology and Sexually Transmitted Diseases
University College of Medical Sciences and Guru Teg Bahadur Hospital
University of Delhi, New Delhi, India

Gautam Kumar Singh MD MUHS
Graded Specialist
Department of Dermatology Venereology and Leprosy
Command Hospital (EC)
Kolkata, West Bengal, India

Sidharth Sonthalia MD
Consultant Dermatologist and Dermatosurgeon
Skinnocence—The Skin Clinic
Gurgaon, Haryana, India

CR Srinivas MD
Professor and Head
Department of Dermatology
PSG Institute of Medical Sciences and Research
Coimbatore, Tamil Nadu, India

SK Tan MD, FAAD, MBA
Senior Medical Director
The IDS Clinic, Singapore

Manoj Kumar Tembhre MD
Department of Dermatology and Venereology
All India Institute of Medical Sciences
New Delhi, India

Steven Thng MRCP(UK) FAMS FRCP(Edin)
Adjunct Assistant Professor
Consultant Dermatologist
National Skin Center, Singapore

Annyce Treherne MD
2207 Executive Drive Suite A
Hampton, VA 23666, USA

Biju Vasudevan MD
Assistant Professor
Armed Forces Medical College and Command Hospital
Pune, Maharashtra, India

Ruby Venugopal MD
Resident
Armed Forces Medical College and
Command Hospital
Pune, Maharashtra, India

Rajesh Verma MD DNB
Professor and Head
Department of Dermatology
Armed Forces Medical College and
Command Hospital
Pune, Maharashtra, India

Vijay Zawar MD DNB DVD FAAD
Professor, Consultant Dermatologist
Skin Diseases Center
Nashik, Maharashtra, India

Foreword

Most physicians probably do not recognize that the skin is one of the few organs essential for life. They consider the skin more or less an inert type of plastic wrap that separates us from the world. But, in fact, the skin is our interface with the environment and helps us by many different processes to adapt to the vagaries of our world, i.e. the sun, the heat, cold, wet and humid, the dry, the chemicals and all the many microorganisms. It is the job of the epidermis in particular to help us respond to these potential threats so we can survive and live better.

The epidermis has just three cell types—keratinocytes, Langerhans cells and melanocytes. Keratinocytes form the mechanical barrier between us and the world, Langerhans cells are an immune barrier, and melanocytes compose a biochemical interface involved in inflammation, in prevention of injury and response to and repair of damaging elements like sunlight, i.e. they produce tanning that minimizes subsequent sun damage. The color of skin is so very important for both normal skin color and the disfigurement caused by its disorders. Parts of our environment are the friends, family and neighbors around us, and our skin color and appearance, often denigrated as just cosmetic issues, in fact, are of great importance.

The science of pigmentation has grown exponentially over the last 50 years beginning with the work of two dermatological giants—Aaron B Lerner from Yale University and Thomas Fitzpatrick from Harvard University, USA. Hundreds of other scientists have subsequently contributed to the understanding of the pigmentary system. Unfortunately, not all of that valuable information have been translated into clinical applications that help the clinician diagnose and treat pigmentary disorders.

So, it is always an exciting step forward when a new, updated book, prepared by many experts is published, its purpose to help consultant dermatologists, dermatologists in training, and family physicians to appreciate and evaluate skin color, diagnose its disorders and to offer the best therapies available worldwide. This new volume *Pigmentary Disorders: A Comprehensive Compendium* does just that. The editors have reached out to more than 50 best experts from both hemispheres to write sections of the book on topics for which they have special understanding. The book is comprehensive about the biology of pigmentation and all its disorders. It emphasizes two particular disorders—vitiligo and melasma, opposite problems but of great concern especially for those with dark skin. The book is richly illustrated with photographs from the extensive library of clinical pictures available to the editors and contributors.

Every dermatologist, dermatology student, general doctor, and other medical personnel caring for patients with any and all forms of skin disease, most of which cause pigmentary abnormalities, will find the pigmentary disorders a very helpful, indeed necessary, addition to their personal libraries.

James J Nordlund MD
Professor
Department of Dermatology
Wright State Boonshoft School of Medicine
Dayton, Ohio
Group Health Associates
Cincinnati, Ohio, USA

Preface

It happened one day when one of us was earnestly approached by one of the biggest medical publishing houses requesting to take up editing a book on "*Pigmentary Disorders*".

Looking back, it is indeed surprising that in spite of pigmentary disorders comprising one of the top five dermatological conditions seen by us in our practice, a treatise covering the subject in its entirety has been missing from our subcontinent! There are textbooks on the subject of vitiligo but a book covering both hypo- and hyperpigmentary disorders is definitely what the doctor ordered, we felt.

In order to give shape to this eclectic vision, the three of us got together to put in our collaborative efforts to bring out the book and rope in the best global experts as well as young upcoming authors on this topic.

Interestingly, although we never thought of it in that way but the three of us, share a common mother tongue, Bengali, besides our common passion for researching and writing on pigmentary disorders. Although Dr Koushik Lahiri has lived in Kolkata, West Bengal, India, Dr Manas Chatterjee in different parts of India, and Dr Rashmi Sarkar in Chandigarh and Delhi, India, perhaps, the book was waiting to bring the three of us even closer together! While Dr Koushik Lahiri has been the voice and the brain, Dr Manas Chatterjee has been the heart, and Dr Rashmi Sarkar, the energetic spirit of this exciting project.

An attempt has been made to elucidate common and uncommon pigmentary disorders over multiple face-to-face discussions, e-mails, telephonic conversations, several cups of tea/coffee and liaisons with our international friends. Knowing some of the authors helped us draw on their personal experience as well as scientific evidence in these chapters.

The final result is a never-before compilation on this subject from this part of the globe authored by fifty top thought leaders in the field.

This is an astonishing treatise; a collective wisdom of key academic opinion leaders bejeweled with rich illustration from the extensive and priceless clinical arsenal of the authors.

We hope this comprehensive compendium will be of value to all dermatologists whether postgraduate students, senior practitioners or academicians in India, Asia and the globe.

This is our sincere and humble effort to bridge the gaps in the subject while presenting the latest advances to our fellow dermatologists. We know the road ahead is still long but a beginning was necessary.

We look forward to your feedback.

Koushik Lahiri
Col Manas Chatterjee
Rashmi Sarkar

Acknowledgments

We were little apprehensive and skittish when we first agreed to take up this project.

It was surprising that in spite of our obsession with disorders of pigmentation, unfortunate and unbelievable social stigma attached to most of the pigmentary disorders, no compendium of this magnitude on this topic was ever conceived before from this part of the globe. Notwithstanding, the existence of astonishingly rich clinical material and experience in dealing with these disorders.

Our trepidation and edginess turned into pleasure and enthusiasm when almost all the esteemed contributors whom we approached responded in a very positive way and that too in a timebound manner. They are virtually the topmost key opinion leaders in these topics in our country and abroad. We would like to personally thank each and every author who came forward to contribute high-quality chapters for this project.

All the credit of the book goes to all these brilliant editors and contributors only.

Astonishing polymath Professor (Dr) S Premalatha, *Dermamom*, as she is fondly known in India, helped us divide the chapters and topics. We sincerely appreciate her invaluable contribution.

We must thank M/s Jaypee Brothers Medical Publishers (P) Ltd, New Delhi, India, one of the most reputed, respected and one of the largest medical publishing houses in the world, to suggest us the title and for giving us the opportunity.

Shri Jitendar P Vij (Group Chairman) took personal care of this project. We owe a lot to him. Dr Madhu Choudhary (Senior Editor) was there with us from day one with her untiring zeal to excel. She is a thorough professional and a pure perfectionist.

All the contributors of the book are special but some are icons in their respective fields. Professors JP Ortonne, Rafael Falabella, Torello Lotti, and Rebat M Halder were among these luminaries. We have no words to express our gratitude to these giants.

The icing on the cake was the foreword from a real living legend, Professor James J Nordlund. His priceless foreword has certainly augmented the credibility and added value and recognition to our humble effort.

Contents

1

History and Evolution of Pigmentary Disorders in Human

Amiya Kumar Mukhopadhyay

"Those about to study Medicine, and the younger Physicians, Should light their torches at the fires of the Ancients"
— Rokitansky

Key Features

- Historically the idea and concentration of pigmentary disorders mostly revolved around white-spot (or patch) diseases. These white-spot diseases could range from vitiligo to leprosy, psoriasis and many other similar or dissimilar disorders of modern phraseology.
- Almost all major ancient and religious texts throughout the world mention about skin diseases, of which leprosy and/or vitiligo had gained the most importance. Rituals regarding "clean" and "unclean" from disease were prevalent in all major communities.
- Most of the pigmentary disorders of present day have been described in last 200–300 years after the discovery of pigment cell and its biology.

INTRODUCTION

The study of the history is an integral part of the process of going into the deeper and broader aspect of any subject as far as the evolution, present status and the foretelling (depending on the past experience and sense of logic) of that subject is concerned. This is true in the study of pigmentary disorders too.

As the early ancestors of the human race moved out of Africa about 100,000 years ago, the diversity of skin color appeared due to various reasons. This lead to the idea of "normal" color of people living in a common condition, and any variation beyond a certain limit was considered abnormal giving rise to the entities of various pigmentary disorders. The impact of pigmentary disorders on the social system was so prominent that it could be seen in almost all the major religious and ancient texts across the globe. The stigma and the morbidity of these disorders had prompted the physicians and health scientists from the early days to search for the root and remedy of these problems.

The pigmentary disorders, for the purpose of discussion from the historical point of view, may be broadly grouped into:

- Disorders of de- and/or hypopigmentation
- Disorders of hyperpigmentation
- Disorders of aberrant pigmentations
- Man-made pigmentary disorders, e.g. tattoos.

Also the topics will be discussed in two shades of time frame:

1. From early historical period till 18–19th century AD.
2. From 18–19th century AD (the beginning of modern dermatology) till present time.

Disorders of De- and/or Hypopigmentation in Ancient Literatures of the East

Any partial or complete loss of skin color has attracted attention of the community from time immemorial. From the ancient days till last 200–300 years back any hypopigmented (or even scaly!) diseases of the skin were lumped into a common entity: white spot or vitiligo. Of the various de-/hypopigmentary diseases leukoderma (vitiligo) received the lion's share of the dialogue and attention from the ancient time. The exact period of beginning of the history of vitiligo is really difficult due to the imprecision of translation of archaic literatures in the light of modern views and also because of the conceptual and nosological confusions that existed regarding the exact and scientifically defined nature of the

A brief pigmentary disorder timeline	
2200 BC:	First known description of vitiligo
1550 BC:	Ebers papyrus describes pigmentary disorders among other skin diseases
1500 BC:	***Atharva Veda*** mentions about white-spot disease and its remedy
1200 BC:	Shinto prayer book ***Makato minoharai*** mentions ***shira bito***—a disorder of hypo-/depigmentation
800–500 BC:	Indian ***Ayurvedic*** texts like ***CS*** and ***SS*** describes about the etiology, classification, management and prognosis of different pigmentary disorders
449 BC:	Greek scholar Herodotus wrote about white-skin disease
250 BC:	Translation of Hebrew Bible to Greek took place. Controversy regarding the exact meaning of ***zara'at*** begins
25 BC–50 AD:	Period of Celsus. First to introduce the term vitiligo
700–800 AD:	***Aṣṭanga hṛdaya*** of Vagbhatt mentions a condition called ***jatumani***—a reddish birth mark (portwine stain or other vascular nevi)
980–1037 AD:	Period of Arabic physician Avicenna. Describes about various pigmentary disorders in his ***al Qanun***.
17th century AD:	Malpighi publishes first scientific paper on skin color
18th century AD:	Hunter dissected pigment layer from the skin
1917 AD:	Bruno Bloch mentions dopa–reaction to stain melanin
1948 AD:	Mason classified melanin
1988 AD:	Fitzpatrick classified the skin into six sun-reactive types.

disease. With the advent of modern laboratory techniques various disease entities with the features of diminution or loss of color is emerging in the scientific literature in recent time. In this situation the condition that in the following section will be viewed upon as vitiligo, may be any disease that might or might not be the vitiligo of modern day definition, even in some cases it could be leprosy, psoriasis and other diseases of patchy and discolored configuration.

The first historical description of vitiligo is found during the period of *Ausooryan* (c. 2200 BC) as has been discussed in *Tareekh-i-tibb-i-iran*.[1,2] In the winter of 1872, the German Egyptologist George Ebers purchased a 110-page, about 20 meter long scroll at Luxor, which contained an amazing scenario of medicine of the ancient civilization of Egypt. Though these papyri were dated to a period of c. 1550 BC, but the subjects were a compilation of practice that were prevailing since last few hundred to thousands of years.[3] Among the various skin diseases and tumors mentioned, the interesting description of a skin condition could be that of vitiligo.[4]

Vedas are the ancient scriptures of the Indo-Iranian Aryans whose antiquity is yet to be ascertained, though most authorities believed the period of compilation to be 1500–1000 BC or much earlier.[5] Among the four *Vedas* the *Atharva Veda* is more concerned with diseases than the others. The mention of a condition *kilāsa* most probably describes leukoderma (vitiligo) which is very much apparent in the following hymn:

> *"naktaṃ jatsyouṣadhe rame kṛṣne asikni ca*
> *idaṃ rajani rajaya kilāsaṃ palitaṃ ca ya't"*
> —*Atharva Veda I.23.1.*

"Night-born art thou, O herb, O dark, black (and) dusky one; O colorer, do thou color this hypopigmented (?) spot and which is pale."

The two charms I.23 and I.24 of the *Atharva Veda* specifically deal with the white spots and their remedies. In the hymns I.24.3–4 prayers have been offered to the herb for the restitution of the normal hue on the affected skin.[6] The use of some black seeds along with other herbs like *Bhringaraja*, *Indravaruni* and turmeric is also mentioned as a treatment.[7]

Avesta is another sacred scripture of the Indo-Iranian Aryans. It also mentioned about vitiligo.[8,9]

In the later Vedic period, particularly during the period of early Buddhism the prevalence of leukoderma is evident in major text like *Mahavagga* (1.39, 1.76.1) of the *Vinay Pitaka* (624–544 BC).[10]

In the process of evolution of medical system that started from the early Vedic era or even earlier, *Āyurveda*—the science of life, appeared as a special subject dealing exclusively with disease and remedies. The pigmentary disorders were dealt in detail in major texts like *Caraka Saṃhitā* (*CS*), *Suśruta Saṃhitā* (*SS*), *Bhela Saṃhitā* (*BS*) and others.

In the *CS* (c. 800–600 BC), the word *svitra* stands for some hypo-/depigmentation and have been further subdivided in to three varieties: (1) *dārūṇa*, (2) *arūna* and (3) *kilāsa* and it also mentioned that when the perturbed *doṣa* (humor) affects the *meda* (fatty tissue), the color of the disease becomes white. The white spots may merge with one another and leukotrichia and extensive involvement of skin was considered bad prognostic signs and also considered difficult to treat (*CS Cikitsā Sthānam* 7).[11]

In *SS* (c. 500 BC), the word *kilāsa* was used for leukoderma and it had been differentiated from leprosy by the fact that *kilāsa* was never a discharging condition whereas, *kuṣṭha* (leprosy) could be a discharging disease. This treatise also specifically mentioned that white spots affecting palms, soles, anal orifice and those developed as a result of burn is difficult to cure:

> *"...tesu sambandhamandalamante jātaṃ raktaroma ca sādhyamagnidagdhaṃca"*
> —(*SS Nidānasthānam 5:12*)[12]

The ancient Hindu law book *Manu-smriti* (c. 200 BC) bore references of leukoderma (*svitra*) and said that a stealer of clothes would suffer from the disease as a result of his misdeed in the earlier live (XI.51). It forbade marriage with a subject or the family affected with *svitra* (III.7) and also prescribed that in a religious and social occasion even a Brahmin affected with *svitra* should not be invited (III.161).[13]

The Bower manuscript (compilation *c.* 450 AD) in the leaf I verse 5-9 also mentions *vajraka tailam*—a medicated application for the treatment of *svitra*.[14] the ancient Saṃskṛt book of lexicon *Amarakoṣa* (AD 600) described *svitra* as leukoderma.[15]

Other famous texts of ancient Saṃskṛt literature like *Aṣṭāṅga-hṛdaya-Saṃhitā* (c. 7-8th century AD), *Mādhava-Nidān* (c. AD 700), *Cakradattā* (c. 11th century AD), *Śārandhar Saṃhitā* (c.13th century AD) have elaborately mentioned about the white spot diseases and its remedies.[16-19]

The mention and description of vitiligo is prevalent in the old literatures of the other Eastern nations like China, Japan and Korea. In *Makatominoharai,* a Shinto prayer book (c. 1200 BC) the word *Shira-bito* stands for leukoderma.[20,20a] The first description of vitiligo and other hypopigmentary conditions in Chinese literature is found during Sui dynasty (618-626 AD). The classification of vitiligo into localized and generalized was done during the Sung dynasty (960-1279 AD).

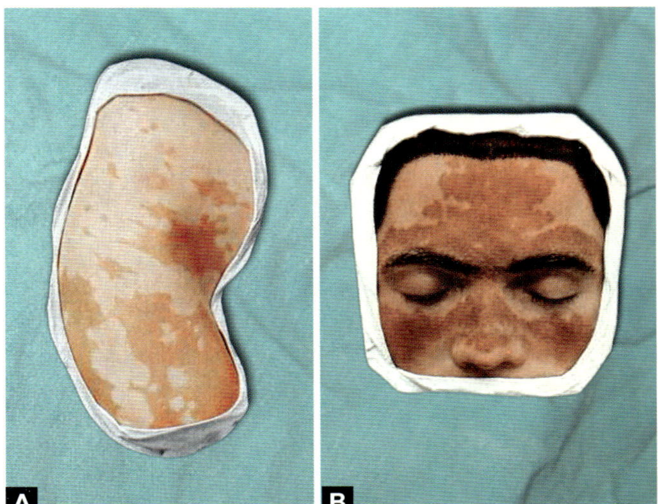

Figs 1A and B: Vitiligo and chloasma. [*Source:* Jerome Kingsbury's Portfolio of Dermachrome (1921)]

The early description of hypopigmentary disorder is found in *Dongey Bogam*—an early 17th century Korean medical book. The 18th century paintings showing the nobles afflicted with vitiligo have been published in the literature.[21]

In the Siddha system—an ancient Tamil medical system (c. 400 AD or even earlier) there is mention of white skin diseases and its remedy.[22]

In the holy book of Islam *Al'Quor'ān* some verses like verse 49 of *Al-'Imran* (Chapter 3) and verse 110 of *Al-ma'idah* (Chapter 5) there is mention about a disease resembling leukoderma.[23]

In the famous medical text of the Greco-Arabic medicine *al-Qanun fi-al-tibb* (11th century AD), *Alī al-Husayn ibn 'abd Allāh ibn Sinā* (980-1037), popularly known as *Avicenna* in the Western world has given description of leukoderma (*Bahaq* and *Baras*).[24]

Disorders of De- and/or Hypopigmentation in Ancient Literatures of the Western World

The analyses of medical system of the Western world showed that the idea about the hypopigmentary disorders was developing since the early period of the history. The famous Greek scholars Herodotus (484-425 BC) in the First Book *"Clio"* composed in 449 BC wrote that a native with white sickness should not be allowed to enter the city and a foreigner afflicted with this be driven away from the country.[25] Other great scholars like Hippocrates (460-370 BC) and Aristotle (384-324 BC) also mentioned about this disease in their literatures.[26,27]

The Illustrious Latin medical author Aulus Cornelius Celsus (25 BC-50 AD) of Rome first used the term *vitiligo* and wrote about it in the Chapter 28 of his fifth book *"De Medicina"* and divided the entity into: *Alphos, Melas* and *Leuce*. Of these *Leuce* probably represented vitiligo.[28]

The most discussed topic about leprosy-vitiligo is centered on the Biblical reference about the disease. The mention of white spot(?leukoderma, ?leprosy) can be found in *Exodus* 4:6, *Leviticus* 13,14,21, numbers 5:2,12:10, *Deuteronomy* 24:4S II *Samuel* 3:29,II *Kings* 5:27II *Chronicles* 26-19:23 of the *Old Testament and Matthew* 8:2-3,,10:8,11:5, *Mark* 1:40,14:3, *Luke* 4:27,17:12-19 of the *New Testament*.[29] The Biblical controversy of leprosy-vitiligo started in 250 BC during the period of Ptolemy II, the Septuagint translation of Hebrew Bible into Greek took place. It translated the Hebrew word *Zara'at* (*Leviticus* 13) to lepra. Most authorities believe that the entity was not leprosy but some other skin disease(s)—one possibility could be vitiligo.[25,30]

The controversy went on for centuries and it has been opined that some of the "leper knights" of the order of St. Lazarus fighting the Crusade in 13th century were not actually lepers but were suffering from vitiligo.[31]

Hieronymus Mercurialis (1530-1606) in his *"De Morbis Cutaneis et Omnibus Corporis Humani excrementis Tractaus"*—the first ever book on skin diseases written in

Latin in 1572 mentioned about different varieties of white patches and told about their remedies.[32]

These confusion and debate continued till the beginning of modern day dermatology when the classification of diseases and contributions from great authorities like Plenck, Willan, Batemen, Alibert, Hebra and others lead to the clearing of the cloud. This will be discussed in other section of this chapter.

Disorders of Hyperpigmentation

The issue of hyperpigmentation has, surprisingly been attracted much less attention of the ancient medical men both in the East as well as West. As some conditions like melasma, birth marks (e.g. melanocytic nevi), postinflammatory hyperpigmentation are quite prevalent in all societies, so these conditions were probably considered *normal* and hence did not attract much attention.

There is mention of various *kṣhetriya* (hereditary and/or congenital) disorders in the *Atharva Veda* (V.II.8.1–8, II.10.1–8, etc.). Whether some of them were associated with any pigmentary manifestation is not very clear. The very clear description of hyperpigmentary condition is available in major Āyurvedic texts like *Caraka Saṃhita, Suśruta Saṃhita, Aṣṭangahṛdaya, Mādhavanidān* and others.

Melasma has been described as *vyanga* in *Caraka Saṃhita, Suśruta Saṃhita, Aṣṭanga hṛdaya, Śarangdhara* and others.[33-37]

The astute physicians of the ancient India also noted the darkening of the lips and areolae of breasts from the third month of pregnancy (*Caraka Saṃhita, Śarīrasthānam* 14).[38]

The change of skin color and its prognostic importance in various diseases have also been described in the *Indriyasthānam* section of the *Caraka Saṃhita*. It has been said in the same section of the book that sudden appearance of melanocytic nevi (? pigmented seborrheic keratoses), melasma should considered as ominous sign.[39]

In the Greco-Arabic medicine similar observations have been made. Various sections of the Avicenna's *al-Qanun fi-al-tibb* (11th century AD) describes about various changes in skin color and their significance.[40]

Disorders of Aberrant Pigmentations

Apart from the classical leukoderma or *vitiligo* like pigmentary disorders, the various aberrations of the common normal skin color have received attention from the ancient time. Among them birth marks, moles and nevi, change of color in diseases (if we consider the change in skin color in a broader sense of pigmentary anomaly) and many other conditions were described in different literatures.

The Book I of the *Atharva Veda* mentions a condition called *harimān* and its remedy in verses 22.1–4 which stands for the yellowness of the body or jaundice in modern sense.[41] Similar mention is also found in the Buddhist text of *Mahavagga* where a drink made of cow's urine and yellow *myrobalan* was used as treatment (*Mahavagga* 6.14.6).[42]

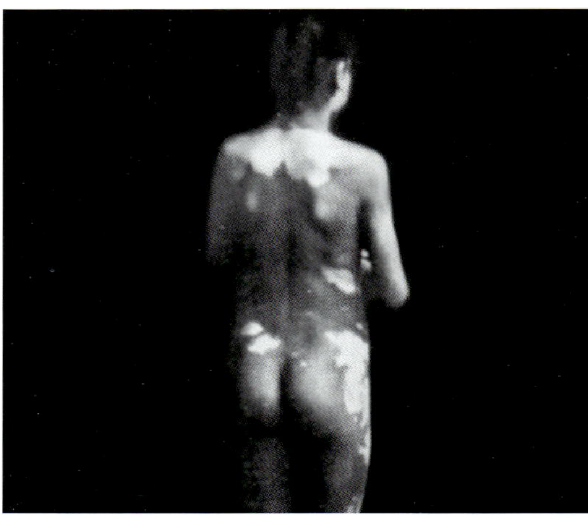

Fig. 2: Vitiligo or leukoderma. [*Source:* Norman Walker's An Introduction to Dermatology (1904)]

The later *Vedic* literatures like treatises of *Caraka, Suśruta, Vagbhatt* and others also enumerated different pigmentary changes. In *CS* the word *halīmaka* probably stands for biliary jaundice in which the greenish or blackish discoloration of the body were noted along with other systemic symptoms (*Cikitsāsthānam*16:124–137). Hyperpigmentation of the lips and areola of the breast haven mentioned in *raktagulama* (molar pregnancy) (*CS Nidānasthānam*.3).[43] The *SS* also described change of color in conditions like burn injury (*Sūtrasthānam* 12.13). It mentioned about *tialakālaka* (melanocytic nevi) and nyaccha (nevi and other birth marks that arise *de novo*. (*SS. Nidānasthānam*13.35-36).[44] In another famous text, *Āṣṭānghṛdaya* of *Vagbhata* mentions about melasma, nevi and birthmarks. The mention of a condition named jatumani, a reddish birthmark which was probably port wine stain or some other vascular nevi is interesting. (*Uttarasthāna* XXXI: 24–26).[45]

A number of diseases like Addison's disease, Fanconi's anemia, incontinentia pigmenti and many others are associated with pigmentary changes. Some nevi like Mongolian spots, nevus of Ota, nevos of Ito, Hori's nevus, and *café au lait* macules, etc. are responsible for pigmentary changes. The story of evolution of these conditions are interesting topic of the medical history, but could not discussed due to the want of space.

Man-made Pigmentary Disorders

The pigmentary changes of skin are not always an unwanted entity. Man from the early days of its history started performing tattoos for magical, religious, social, practical and medical reason apart from decorative. Sometimes it act as a totem, sometimes it was believed to protect the man from the demonic influences of harmful invisible satanic forces, but whatever be the reason the art is still in vogue. It has sometimes been used to hide the blemishes of different diseases. The interested reader may consult treatises and articles dealing in detail about the subject.[46-50]

The use of different drugs and chemicals like arsenic, clofazimine, chloroquine, amiodarone, etc. and misuses and side effects of some others like hydroquinone, topical potent and superpotent corticosteroids and many others may give rise to aberrant pigmentation causing some distinct disorders like exogenous ochronosis, Riehl's melanosis, poikiloderma of Civatte and others.

HISTORY AND EVOLUTION OF PIGMENTARY DISORDERS IN MODERN DERMATOLOGY

The medicine related to skin that used to be practiced as a part of surgery and general medicine gradually took the shape of a well-defined specialty during the last quarter of the 18th century.[51] The science and art of skin diseases were not in a systematized state till then, but now got classified by Plenck, Willan, Alibert and others.[52] But the history of pigmentary disorders was witnessing a major change in concept even before that. The first publication of scientific study of the skin color came from Malpighi in 17th century.[53] In the following century John Hunter (1728–1793) dissected the pigment layer from the skin.[54] The famous 18th century German philosopher Kant (1724–1804) believed that the excessive amount of a substance—phlogiston is the cause of dark coloration of the skin.[55] The first evidence of the occurrence of pigment cell in the human dermis came from Baelz in1885.[56] Bruno Bloch in 1917 described the dopa reaction for the identification of melanoblasts. In 1934 Du-Shane first showed that melanoblasts of the axonal system originated in the neural crest and Mason in 1948 classified the melanin into animal, plant and synthetic forms.[53] These whole development lead to the revolution of pigmentary cell biology, diseases associated with it and their remedial methodologies. One after another diseases with pigmentary disorders were described. The research was not confined to the mere variation of colors but the spectrum included the malignant conditions pertaining to pigment and other cells too.[57,58] The treatment protocol that started with the incantations, charms, amulets of the magico or empirico-magical system in the hands of the shamans now entered the most sophisticated laboratories of the pigment cell biologists and photobiologists.[59]

Notes on Transliteration

ā,ī,ū are longer forms of **a,i,u**
ṛ is pronounced as **ri**
c is pronounced as **ch** in *chit*
ṭ, ṇ are pronounced with retroflexion of the tip of the tongue towards the back of the palate
s is pronounced as **sa** in *say*
ṣ is as in shun
ś is pronounced as **sh** in *shall*
ṃ is called *anusvāra* that nasalize the preceding vowel.

CONCLUSION

The disorders of cutaneous pigmentation remained one of the interesting, but enigmatic issues since the very early days of human civilization. Even during the mid-18th century of the present Christian era the confusion was prevailing in the medical world about these disorders. A fascinating (!!) definition of vitiligo may be an amazing example in this regard:[60]

"Vitiligo (vitium) a kind of leprosy or cutaneous eruption consisting of spots, sometimes black, sometimes white, called morphea, alphus, melas, leuce; also in general a cutaneous eruption. Celsus & Pliny". (Lexicon of the Latin language of Facciolati & Forcellini, edited by FP Leverett, Boston; Wilkins & Carter and Little & Brown, 1841).

However, strange this definition appears, the reality is: none of us can guarantee cure of most of the pigmentary disorders with the presently available armamentarium of therapeutics. But this statement will not appear as gloomy as it sounds and the rest part of this compendium will show that the ongoing researches would bring hope and relief for the sufferers and healers alike in coming days.

REFERENCES

1. Prasad PV, Bhatnagar VK. Medico-historical study of "kilasa" (vitiligo/leucoderma): a common skin disorder. Bull Indian Inst Hist Med Hyderabad. 2003;33(2):113-27.
2. Badri SS. Vitiligo. [online]. Available from http://www.clinicalpharmacy.ir/Upload/Modules/Contents/Asset0/vitiligo.pdf. [Accessed on 27.03.2013].
3. Bryan CP. The Papyrus Ebers. London: Geoffrey Bles; 1930. pp. 1-6.
4. Ebbel B. The Papyrus Ebers. Copenhagen: Levin & Munksgaard; 1937. p. 45.
5. Mukhopadhyay AK. Skin Diseases ("Dermatology") in India-History and Evolution. Kolkata: Allied Book Agency; 2011. p. 16.
6. Whitney DW, Lanman CR. *Atharva-Veda-Samhitā*. Delhi: Motilal Banarsidass Publishers Pvt Ltd.; 2001. p. 24.
7. Fitzpatrick TB, Pathak MA. Historical aspects of methoxalen and other furocoumarins. J Invest Dermatol. 1959;32 (2, Part 2):229-31.
8. Darmesteter J, tr. The Zend-Avesta. Max Muller Sacred Books of the East., 23, 31.2005:Vendidad 20.6 and Yasna 9.3-4.
9. Mortazavi H, Dowlati Y, Dowlati B. A brief history of dermatology in Iran. Arch Dermatol. 2001;137(7):936-7.
10. Zysk KG. Asceticism and Healing in Ancient India. Delhi: Motilal Banarsidass Publishers Pvt. Ltd; 1998. p. 99.
11. Sen DN, Sen UN. Charaka Samhita. Calcutta: *Cikitsā Sthānam*; 1897. verse 7.
12. Bhisagratna KL. *Nidānasthānam*. 2nd volume. Calcutta: The *Sushruta Samhita*; 1911. verse-XIV 5:12.
13. Bühler G. The Laws of Manu. Max Muller. Sacred Books of the East. Vol-25.2001:76-106.

14. Hoernle AFR. The Bower Mnuscript. (Part III). India, Calcutta: Office of the Superintendent of Government Printing; 1897. p. 181.
15. Sardesai NG, Padhye DG. Amarakoṣa (Amara's *Nāmalingān-uśāsanam*). Pune: Oriental Book Agency; 1940.verse-56-154.
16. Sen Sharma KK, Bhattacharyya SS. *Aṣṭāṅga-hṛdaya. Nidānasthāna*. Kolkata: Deepayan; 2001. verse-XIV.34-37.
17. Śāstri BS. *Mādhava Nidāna*. Benaras: The Chowkhamba Sanskrit Series Office; 1943. pp. 164-8.
18. Sen Sharma KK, Bhattacharyya SS, *Chakradutta. Kuṣṭhacikitsā*. Kolkata: Deepayan; 1999. verse-1.
19. Sen Sharma KK, Bhattacharyya SS (Eds). *Śarangdhara: Cikitsā Saṃgraha*. Kolkata: Deepayan; 1998. Madhyakhanda verse-II.112 and XII.249-258.
20. Feeny P. The Fight Against Leprosy. London: Elek Books, 1964. In: Nair BK H. Vitiligo: a retrospect. Int J Dermatol. 1978;17(9): 755-7.
21. Hann S, Chung HS. Historic view of vitiligo in Korea. Int J Dermatol. 1997;36(4):313-5.
22. Thas JJ. Siddha Medicine—background and principle and the application for skin diseases. Clin Dermatol. 2008;26(1): 62-78.
23. Ali A. Al-Quor'ān. Delhi: Oxford University Press; 1987. pp. 51-113.
24. Al Sharif. Judham, Baras, Wadah, et al. A study of terms and concepts in "*Al Qanun Fit Tibb*" of Ibn-Sina.JISHIM.[online] Available from www.ishim.net/ishimj/910/JISHIM%20. NO.10%PDF/05.pdf.
25. Goldman L, Moraites RS, Kitzmiller KW. White spots in biblical times. A background for the dermatologist for participation in discussions of current revisions of the bible. Arch Dermatol. 1966;93(6):744-53.
26. Page TE, Capps E, Rouse WHD. Aristotle: Aristotle problem I-XXI. Cambridge: Mass. Harvard University Press; 1936. p. 205.
27. Adams F. Hippocrates: The Genuine Works of Hippocrates. London: The Sydenham Society.1848. p. 269.
28. Verbov J. Celsus and his contributions to Dermatology. Int J Dermatol. 1978;17(6):521-3.
29. Young R.tr. The Holy Bible. Edinburgh: GA Young and Co, Bible Publishers; 1898.
30. Lieber E. Skin diseases: contagion and sin in the Old Testament. Int J Dermatol 1994:33(8):593-5.
31. Millington GWM, Levell NJ. Vitiligo: the historical curse of depigmentation. Int J Dermatol 2007;46(9):990-5.
32. Sutton RL. Diseases of the skin: Mercurialis, 1572. Arch Dermatol. 1966;94(6):763-72.
33. Sen DN, Sen UN. Indriya Sthānam. Calcutta: *Charaka Samhita*; 1897. verse 6.
34. Bhisagratna KL. Nidānasthānam,2nd volume. Calcutta: The *Susruta Samhita*; 1911. verse-13:38.
35. Sen Sharma KK, Bhattacharyya SS. Aṣṭāṅga-hṛdaya. Kolkata: Deepayan; 2001. *Sūtrasthānam* IV: 19-20 and *Uttarasthānam* XI: 27.
36. Ibid. Uttarasthānam XI: 27.
37. Sen Sharma KK, Bhattacharyya SS. *Śarangdhara: Cikitsā Saṃgraha*. Kolkata: Deepayan; 1998. Purvakhanda VII: 84-92.
38. Sen DN, Sen UN. Śarīra Sthānam. Calcutta: *Charaka Samhita*; 1897. verse 14.
39. Sen DN, Sen UN. Indriya Sthānam. Calcutta: *Charaka Samhita*; 1897. verse 6-9.
40. Gruner OC. A treatise on the Canon of medicine of Avicenna. New York: AMS Press Inc.; 1973. Aphorism 221 and 795.
41. Whitney DW. *Atharva-Veda-Samhitā*. Delhi: Motilal Banarsi-dass Publishers Pvt Ltd; 2001. pp. 22-3.
42. Mukhopadhyay AK. Skin Diseases ("Dermatology") in India-History and Evolution. Kolkata: Allied Book Agency; 2011. p. 41.
43. Sen DN, Sen UN. Cikitsāsthānam and Nidānasthānam. Calcutta: *Charaka Samhita*; 1897. pp. 16:124-137 and 3
44. Bhisagratna KL. *Sūtrasthānam* 12.13 and *Nidānasthānam* 13.35-36. Calcutta: The Susruta Samhita.1911.
45. Sen Sharma KK, Bhattacharyya SS. Aṣṭāṅga-hṛdaya. Kolkata: Deepayan; 2001. *Uttarasthānam* XXXI: 24-26.
46. Wikipedia. History of tattoing. [online] Available from http://en.wikipedia.org/wiki/History_of_tattooing. [Accessed on 28.03.2013].
47. Michigan State University. [online] http://www.msu.edu./~kremari1/individual/history/tattoo.html. [Accessed on 28.03.2013].
48. Levy J, Sewell M, Goldstein N. II. A short history of tattooing. J Dermatol Surg Oncol. 1979;5(11):851-6.
49. Gilbert S. The Tattoo History: A Source Book. Brooklyn: PowerHouse Books; 2000.
50. Wolf EK, Laumann AE. The use of blood-type tattoos during the Cold War. J Am Acad Dermatol. 2008;58(3):472-6.
51. Mukhopadhyay AK. Skin Diseases ("Dermatology") in India-History and Evolution. Kolkata: Allied Book Agency; 2011.p. 138.
52. Potter BS. Bibliographic landmarks in the history of dermatology. J Am Acad Dermatol 2003; 48(6):919-32.
53. Klaus SN. Some early scientific studies of skin color. Yale J Biol Med. 1973;46(5):334-6.
54. Nordlund JJ, Abdel-Malek ZA, Boissy R, et al. Pigment cell biology: An historical review. J Invest Dermatol. 1989;92 (4 Suppl):53S-60S.
55. Lovejoy AO. Kant and evolution. In: Glass B, Temkin O, Straus WL (Eds). Forerunners of Darwin: 1745-1859. Baltimore, John Hopkins Press; 1959. pp. 173-206.
56. Garnis-jones S, Jackson R. Origin of nevus cell: a retrospective. Int J Dermatol 1992;31(4):291-4.
57. McLeod GR, Davis NC. Historical overview of melanoma. Clin Dermatol. 1992;10(1):5-7.
58. Bennett LP, Hall P. Moles and melanoma: a history. Ann R Coll Surg Engl. 1994;76(6):373-80.
59. Roelandts R. The history of phototherapy: something new under the sun? J Am Acad Dermatol. 2002;46(6):926-30.
60. Sutton RL. On definition of vitiligo (letter). Arch Dermatol. 1965;91:288.

2

Evolution of Skin Color in Human: An Anthropological Overview

Amiya Kumar Mukhopadhyay

"It has often and confidently been asserted, that man's origin can never be known: but ignorance more frequently begets confidence than does knowledge: it is those who know little, and not those who know much, who so positively assert that this or that problem will never be solved by science. The conclusion that man is the co-descendant with other species of some ancient, lower, and extinct form is not in any degree new."

—Charles Darwin *(The Descent of Man and Selection in Relation to Sex)*

Key Features

- Modern human (*Homo sapiens*) and their ape-like ancestors share a common evolutionary line. Therefore anthropological and genetic history of the ape-like animals provides much useful information about the pigmentary and other developments of human being.
- Variation of color occurred due to the influence of ultraviolet radiation on melanin synthesis, folate and vitamin D metabolism and thermoregulation of the body.
- Sexual selection has also played part in the pigmentary variation between sexes.

INTRODUCTION

The blue planet—our beloved earth is a beautiful portrait of multiple colors in different shades. This different shade of colors is stretched across the whole world of flora and fauna. We, the human being live on this planet with varied hues of skin colors that range from very pale to very dark. The influence of color on the social, political, psychological aspect of history of the human race is so strong that it has determined the course of the history of human civilization and the opportunity of honorable living. Even during this present era of intense technical development and modernized and rational thinking the color of the skin may affect the political scenario and choice of the people in this regard.[1] The concept of race and racism depending on the color is erroneous no doubt, but its role in the making of history of mankind is irrefutable. The differences in various shades of color attracted attention from ancient period. The mention of different skin tones and their social status is cited in Book I (100.18), Book VI (47.21), Book VII (5.3) and many other places of the *Ṛig Veda* (c. 1300 BC or even much earlier)—the most ancient literature of the Aryans.[2-4] The earliest known visual evidence of skin color variation is depicted on the wall of the tomb of the Sethos (c.1300 BC) where different shades of dye were used to portray the people of different races like Libyans, Nubians, Asians and Egyptians.[5] But did this different shades existed from the beginning of the human evolution? To explore the answer we have to consider the facts regarding the evolution of modern human species and anthropological aspect of this evolution.

EVOLUTIONARY TIMELINE OF HUMAN BEING

Circa 4600 million: A huge mass of dust and gases came together and this planet was born. This gradually cooled down and about 3500 million years ago (MYA) first life in the form of single-celled bacteria and blue-green algae appeared on the face of the earth. With the passage of time, the cell and tissue organization became more and more complex and the earth was witnessing the appearance of various organisms in both plant and animal kingdom. The class Mammalia in the course of evolution gave rise to super family Hominoidea which was composed of different apes, ape-like human ancestors and modern human **(Flow chart 1)**. Ultimately,

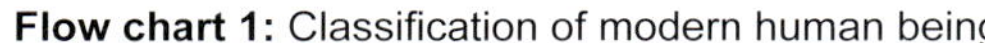

Flow chart 1: Classification of modern human being

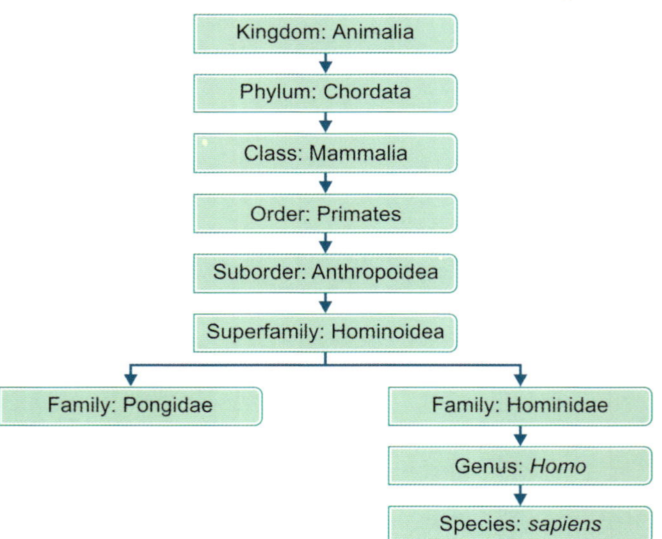

Source: Adapted from Grant PG, Hoff CG. The skin of primates. XLIV Numerical taxonomy of primate skin. Amer J Phys Anthrop. 1975;42:151-66.

Flow chart 2: Relationship, possible era of divergence and emergence among different apes and human ancestors (MYA, million years ago)

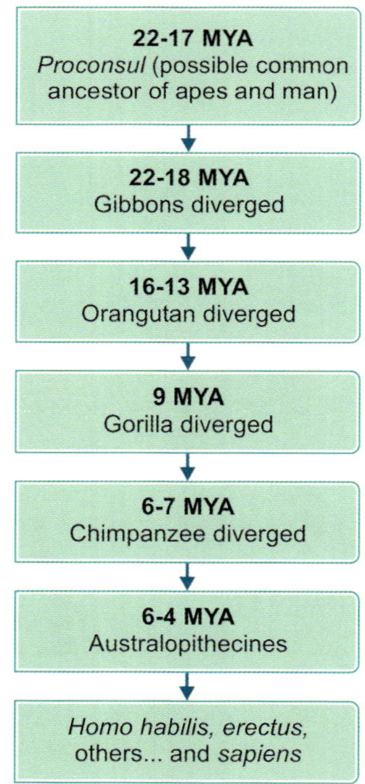

about 5–1.8 MYA, during Pliocene epoch of the tertiary period of the Cenozoic era ape-like human ancestors evolved.[6,7] The *Australopithecus* or "southern ape" as named by Dart to a skull of the earliest human ancestor discovered at Taung in 1925.[8] Further discoveries showed that at least four different species existed on this planet about 4 MYA. In the course of evolution the human genus *Homo*, as named by Linnaeus in 1758 evolved and the genus prominently contained *Homo habilis*, *Homo erectus* and the *Homo sapiens* among some other related species **(Flow chart 2)**. The *Homo sapiens* finally survived and the modern human being are the direct descendant of this species. This transition took place during 2,000,000–200,000 years back and about 90,000 years ago the fully developed modern human evolved.[6] This theory of "single origin" has been supported both by genetic as well as phenotypic studies.[9,10]

EVOLUTION OF VARIOUS COLORS: VARIOUS OPINIONS, VARIOUS THEORIES

Regarding the appearance of different colors of human skin a number of opinions that range from the effect of sun rays on bile to modern genetic research exist.[11,12] The archaic man diverged from its closest relative chimpanzee (*Pan satyrus*) in the process of evolutionary steps about 6 MYA.[13] These chimpanzees have a deoxyribonucleic acid (DNA) homology of about 98% with the modern human. From the evolutionary point of view the examination of the behavior of chimpanzee skin toward the environment and other factors would clarify many of our questions regarding the appearance of different colors in human population. These chimpanzees were born with a universal pale skin, but with time they developed mottling due to the sun exposure and ultimately a uniform dark color developed on the exposed part whereas, rest of the body covered with thick hairs remain pale throughout the life. As very little change happened in chimpanzee from the evolutionary point of view, it has been inferred that our ancestors, who diverged from chimpanzee, as discussed earlier, had also similar pale skin color at the beginning.[14,15]

EFFECT OF CLIMATE AND CHANGE OF LIFESTYLE

Charles Darwin in his famous work "The origin of species by means of natural selection" had opined that climate had profound effect on the color of the skin.[16] Similar effect is true in case of human evolution.

The basic characteristic of the earliest human species was their bipedalism and larger brain size in comparison to other primates. This gave them speed and power (due to two upper limbs available for use like holding and hunting) and intelligence to become more efficient than their contemporaries. During this stage the hominids left forest and came out in the open field of savannahs in search of food and began hunting. They were exposed to the scorching heat of the Sun and their new lifestyle of "hunter and gatherer" led to the higher physical activity with the resultant production of excessive body heat. To adapt with this new change they gradually lost the thick cover of the body hair and developed eccrine sweat glands both in quantity and quality that kept the core temperature at a proper level to avoid dehydration, denaturation of body proteins and brain damage.[17] The nude skin now no more protected and the intense ultraviolet radiation (UVR) of Africa (from where our ancestors are believed to be evolved as shown by fossil evidence) led the melanocytes to generate more melanin pigment causing darkening of the skin which was pale earlier.[15] As UVR can induce cutaneous malignancies, more so in the paler skin, this saved them from cutaneous UVR induced malignancies and also protected the sweat glands from UVR damage.[15,18,19] It has also been suggested that thermoregulation too played part in imparting dark coloration in this prevailing situation.[20]

It is assumed that the early modern man, who lived in the forest area of southern Africa, had a brown skin. In the process of migration these people moved in two directions from their ancestral homeland **(Fig. 1)** and developed two opposite color of the skin: those who moved to open planes of equatorial Africa developed deep dark skin in repose to intense UVR, whereas those migrated to northern Africa and away from Africa to the Asian and European continents developed a paler skin due to low sun rays and other factors.[21]

PIGMENT AND FOLATE METABOLISM

The effect of UVR on folate metabolism played an important role in the evolution and natural selection of man.[22] This B-vitamin is necessary for the production and repair of DNA and proper cell division including spermatogenesis.[23-26] Low level of folate can give rise to decrease in cell division, production of lesser number of spermatozoa and neural tube defect in fetus.[14,21] The UVR has a deleterious effect on the circulating level of folate by photo-deactivation and redirecting the available folate to the UVR-induced photo-damaged DNA repair in the skin and other body parts. This creates lower level of folate and in consequence the production of spermatozoa is reduced affecting reproduction process. As melanocytes are most effective sun protectors, the excessive melanin in the dark skin act as natural shield for the folate in sunny climate like equatorial region.[27,28] Though this hypothesis does not hold good in case of the pale skin color of the native South American, arguments of recent migration, cultural behavior and some genetic influence may explain the cause.[17]

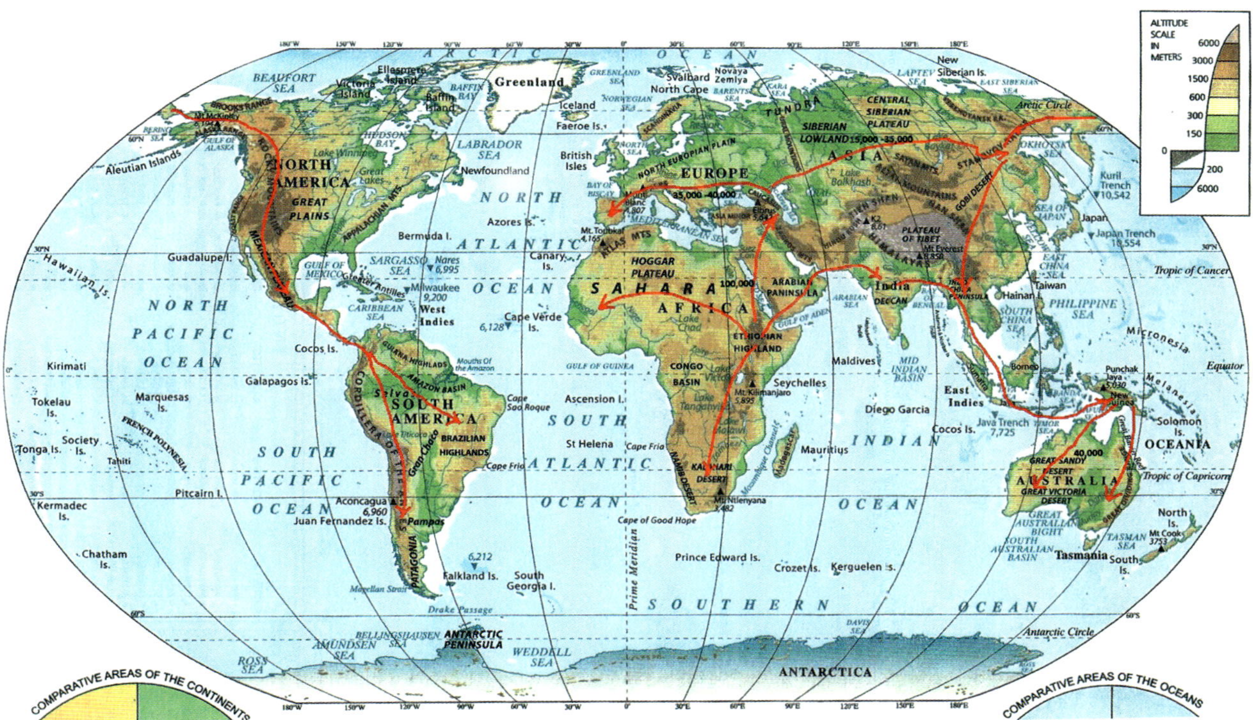

Fig. 1: Possible route of migration of early human from the place of origin. (*Source:* Westerhof W. Evolutionary, biologic, and social aspects of skin color. Dermatol Clin. 2007;25:293-302)

PIGMENT AND VITAMIN D

The story of vitamin D and color of the skin is just the opposite of the folate-pigment relationship. According to the "out of Africa" theory, the modern man started migrating from its original home of Africa to various directions.[29-31] About 100,000–80,000 years ago some of them migrated toward the North polar direction. The intensity of Sun is much less there than their original place of inhabitation. As UVR from the Sun is the most important factor for vitamin D synthesis, the lower availability of sun rays led to the deficiency of vitamin D in the body leading to malformed bone development and defective skeletal architecture. The development of agrarian culture led to the further deficit of vitamin D which is not available in diet that is predominantly dependent on grains. The low level of this vitamin gave rise to defective pelvic architecture in females, leading to difficulty in labor which might cause death of the baby and/or mother in many cases. Vitamin D is essential for healthy immune system as well as cardiovascular system. Hence, a vitamin D deficiency may also cause immune deficiency and cardiovascular morbidity, which in turn may lead to higher morbidity and mortality.[21,32,33] This whole factors led to the selection of a lighter color which could solve all these problems and hence people migrating toward less sunny regions developed lighter shade of color.

FAIR SEX, FAIR COLOR AND SEXUAL SELECTION

The role of the women had remained mostly confined in the indoor activities. Also they need more vitamin D and calcium to avoid defective pelvic architecture to maintain proper health of the bones as discussed above. This could be the reason of paler complexion of females in every race.

The sexual selection, as advocated by numerous authorities may be responsible for the fairer hues of the females. Charles Darwin in his famous work "*The Descent of Man and Selection in Relation to Sex*" had argued in favor of influence of skin color in relation to sexual selection: "...... *We know from many facts already given that the color of the skin is regarded by the men of all races as a highly-important element in their beauty; so that it is a character which would be likely to be modified through selection, as has occurred in innumerable instances with the lower animals*."[34] It is also said that in every society paler complexion is a preferred choice in partner selection.[35-37] The theory of sexual dimorphism has been contested by others.[38] Some other researchers believe that smoothness and fairness of skin is a childlike trait that helped the female to lessen the aggressiveness of the male counterpart.[39]

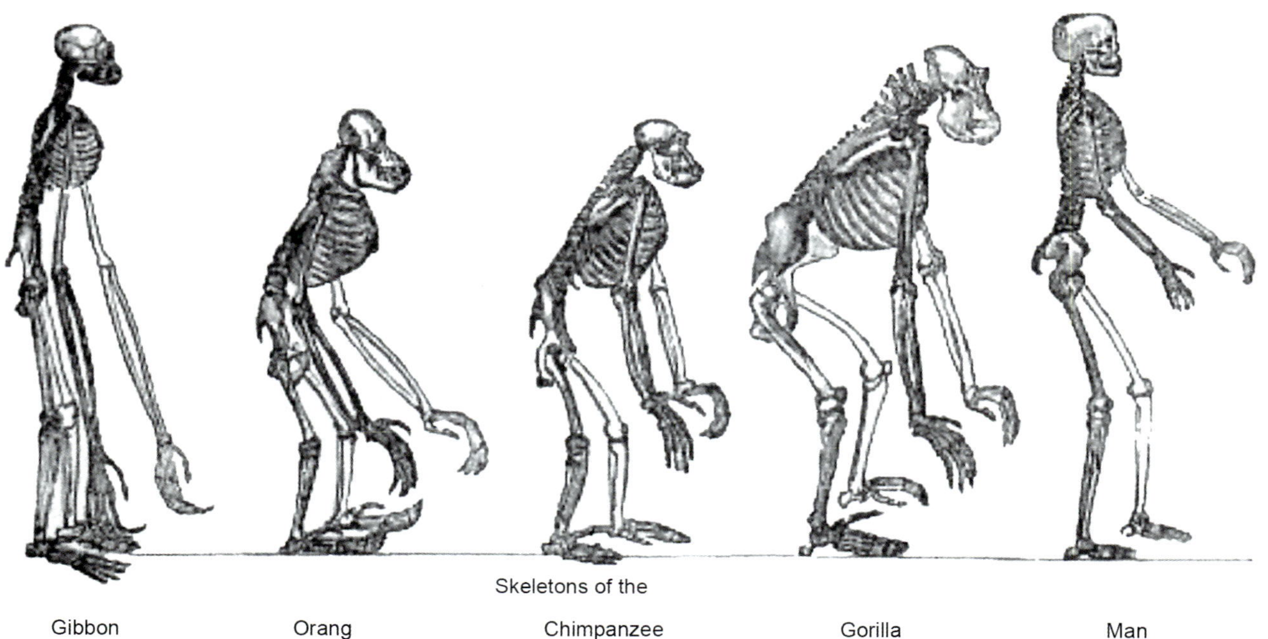

Fig. 2: Evolution of man—from Thomas H Huxley's Evidence as to man's place in nature, 1879. Photographically reduced from diagrams of the natural size (except that of the Gibbon, which was twice as large as nature), drawn by Mr Waterhous Hawkins from specimens in the Museum of the Royal College of Surgeons

SKIN, GENE AND COLOR

The study of genetic architecture has explained many unanswered mysteries and supplied a lot of new information regarding the evolution of colors. It has been shown that about 10% color variation occurs within groups of the human subjects throughout the globe and a variation of about 90% occurs between the groups.[40] Also it has been shown that genetic variation among major continental group is around 10–15% of the total genetic variation only, but the range of color difference is quite significant. This could be the effect of natural selection.[19] The study of the gene on the evolution of different colors has attracted attention of many authorities.

The early work of Davenport and Danielson in 1913 on the West Indian subjects showed that two pairs of gene were responsible for African-European color differences.[41] Later studies revealed further details about the evolution of pigmentation. The color of the skin is mainly imparted by the melanin—a pigment produced by the melanocytes in the epidermis. This melanin influences both constitutive and facultative color and are of two types: eumelanin which is plentiful in dark skin and pheomelanin—responsible for red hairs, freckling of the celtic skin. Interestingly, the number of melanocytes is same in a particular region of the body in both dark as well as light skin individuals.[42] The skin color is the sum total effect of type, distribution and quantity of the melanin in the epidermis of the subject. A number of genes like *MC1R, OCA2, OCA4, SLC24A5, MATP, TYR, ASIP, MYO5A, HPS7,* melanosomal P-protein gene, etc. are responsible for all these affairs including the causation of various pigmentary disorders.[43-46] It is now known that mutations of these genes are responsible for variation in human color. Among all genes the mutation of melanocortin 1 receptor (*MC1R*) gene mainly affects the human color variation though identification of similar *MC1R* haplotype among people with varying phenotypical color expression points toward the role of some other loci.[47,48] Westerhof et al. in an interesting analysis of Westerhof syndrome in three generation of a single family opined that variation of a single gene may be responsible for differences in color.[49] About 65 or more human *MC1R* alleles have been recognized. The role of *MC1R* gene is further supported by a study showing wide distribution variation of *MC1R* haplotypes between African and Eurasian population.[47]

Now, how this *MC1R* affects the pigmentation? Stimulation of receptor leads to escalated cyclic ampicillin concentration inside the cell which leads to altered gene expression resulting in the production of eumelanogenic melanosomes. This causes dark coloration of the skin, on the other hand, absence of signal stimulation results in reduced pigmentation.[21]

INFLUENCE OF CULTURE ON PIGMENTATION

Differences in cultural behavior also have bearing upon the pigmentation of a population. The example of two different population groups on two sides of the Red sea is a vivid example. The tribes living on the western side for the last 6,000 years have a dark skin whereas, the Arabs of European origin living on the eastern side have light skin in the similar environment as those of the dark tribes. This Arab population is living there only for the last 2000 years, but wears protective clothing and stay within tent and shaded area. These cultural dissimilarities are the reason of disparity in color between two populations living in almost identical environmental condition.[14,15]

CONCLUSION

The evolution of different colors occurred as an obligatory process to adapt in the face of diverse natural condition, necessity of survival, sexual selection and many other factors in our ancestors. The availability of fast transportation facility from one end of the globe to the other within a span of hours and migration, mingling and intermarriage of different people of very different cultural and environmental background as well as cultural and behavioral evolution would affect the evolutionary process and in future might lead to further change in pigmentary distribution in human population.

REFERENCES

1. Caruso EM, Mead NL, Balcetis E. Political partnership influences perception of biracial candidates' skin tone. Proc Natl Acad Sci USA. 2009;106(48):20168-73.
2. Mukhopadhyay AK. Skin Diseases ("Dermatology") in India-History and Evolution. Kolkata: Allied Book Agency; 2011. pp. 16-7.
3. Kaegi A. The Rigveda: The Oldest Literature of the Indians (English translation by Arrowsmith R), 2nd edn. Boston: Ginn and Company; 1886. p. 22.
4. Griffith RTH. The Hymns of the Ṛigveda. Delhi: Motilal Banarsidass Publishers Pvt. Ltd.; 1973. pp. 101-336.
5. Holubar K. What is Caucasian? J Invest Dermatol. 1996;106(4):800.
6. Matthews R. Consultant: History Timelines. Essex: Miles Kelly Publishing Ltd; 2011. pp. 14-8.
7. Ash R. Whitaker's World of Facts. New Delhi: Penguin Books India; 2007. p. 52.
8. Dart RA. Australopithecus Africanas: the man-ape of South Africa. Nature. 1925;115:195-9.
9. Prugnolle F, Manica A, Balloux F. Geography predicts neutral genetic diversity of human populations. Curr Biol. 2005;15(5):R159-60.
10. Manica A, Amos W, Balloux F, et al. The effect of ancient population bottlenecks on human phenotypic variation. Nature. 2007;448(7151):346-8.
11. Smith SS. An Essay on the Causes of the Variety of Complexion and Figure in the Human Species. New York: J Simpson and Co. and Williams and Whiting; 1810. pp. 52-9.

12. Myles S, Somel M, Tang K, et al. Identifying genes underlying skin pigmentation differences among human populations. Hum Genet. 2007;120(5):613-21.
13. Jablonski NG. Human skin pigmentation as an example of adaptive evolution. Proc Am Philos Soc. 2012;156(1):45-57.
14. Jablonski NG, Chaplin G. Skin deep. Sci Am. 2002;287(4):74-81.
15. Jablonski NG, Chaplin G. The evolution of human skin coloration. J Hum Evol. 2000;39(1):57-106.
16. Darwin C. The Origin of Species by Means of Natural Selection, 6th edn. London: Watts and Co.; 1929. pp. 100-8.
17. Steindal AH, Moan J. The evolution of different skin colours. In: Espen Bjertness (Ed). Solar Radiation and Human Health. Oslo: The Norwegian Academy of Science and Letters; 2008. pp. 114-22.
18. Suskin RR. Environment and skin. Environ Health Perspect. 1977;20:27-37.
19. Parra EJ. Human pigmentation variation: evolution, genetic basis, and implications for public health. Am J Phys Anthropol. 2007;(Suppl 45):85-105.
20. Ibraimov AI. Evolution of human skin color and thermo-regulation. Int J Genet. 2012; 4:111-5.
21. Westerhof W. Evolutionary, biologic, and social aspects of skin color. Dermatol Clin. 2007;25(3):293-302.
22. Jablonski NG, Chaplin G. Colloquium paper: human skin pigmentation as an adaptation to UV radiation. Proc Natl Acad Sci USA. 2010;107(Suppl 2):8962-8.
23. Mathur U, Datta SL, Mathur BBL. The effect of aminopterin-induced folic acid deficiency on spermatogenesis. Fertil Steril. 1977;28(12):1356-60.
24. Cosentino MJ, Pakyz RE, Fried J. Pyrimethamine: an approach to the development of a male contraceptive. Proc Natl Acad Sci USA. 1990;87(4):1431-5.
25. Wong WY, Merkus HM, Thomas CM, et al. Effects of folic acid and zinc sulfate on male factor subfertility: a double-blind, randomized, placebo-controlled trial Fertil Steril. 2002;77(3):491-8.
26. Ebisch IM, Pierik FH, DE Jong FH, et al. Does folic acid and zinc sulphate intervention affect endocrine parameters and sperm characteristics in men? Int J Androl. 2006;29(2):339-45.
27. Quevedo WC, Szabó G, Virks J. Influence of age and UV on the populations of dopa-positive melanocytes in human skin. J Invest Dermatol. 1969;52(3):287-90.
28. Ortonne JP. Pigmentary changes of the ageing skin. Br J Dermatol. 1990;122(Suppl 35):21-8.
29. Wikipedia (2013) Recent African origin of modern humans. [online] Available from www.en.wikipedia.org/wiki/recent_African_Origin_of_modern_Humans. [Accessed February 2013].
30. Oppenheimer S. Out-of-Africa, the peopling of continents and islands: tracing uniparental gene trees across the map. Philos Trans R Soc Lond B Biol Sci. 2012;367(1590):770-84.
31. Huxley TH. Evidence as to man's place in nature. New York: D. Appleton and Co.; 1879. pp. 9-71.
32. Cantorna, MT, Mahon BD. D-hormone and the immune system. J Rheumatol Suppl. 2005;76:11-20.
33. Norman AW. From vitamin D to hormone D: Fundamentals of the vitamin D endocrine system essential for good health. Am J Clin Nutr. 2008;88(2):491S-499S.
34. Darwin C. The Descent of Man and Selection in Relation to Sex. New York: D. Appleton and Co. 1871. pp. 261-300.
35. Harpending H, Rogers A. Genetic perspective in human origin and differentiation. Annu Rev Genomics Human Genet. 2000;1:361-85.
36. Aoki K. Sexual selection as a cause of human skin colour variation: Darwin's hypothesis revisited. Ann Hum Biol. 2002;6:589-608.
37. Ihara Y, Aoki K. Sexual selection by male choice in monogamous and polygamous human. Theor Popul Biol. 1999;55: 77-93.
38. Frost P. Human Skin-Color Sexual Dimorphism: A Test of the Sexual Selection Hypothesis. Am J Phys Anthropol. 2007; 779-81.
39. Guthrie RD. Evolution of human threat display organs. Evol Biol. 1970;4:257-302.
40. Relethford JH. Apportionment of global human genetic diversity based on craniometrics and skin color. Am J Phys Anthropol. 2002;18:393-98.
41. Harrison GA. Differences in human pigmentation: measurement, geographic variation and causes. J Invest Dermatol. 1973;6(6):418-26.
42. BarshGS. What controls variation in human skin color? PLoS Biol. 2003;1(1):e27.doi:10.1371/journal.pbio.0000027.
43. Norton HL, Kittles RA, Parra E, et al. Genetic evidence for the convergent evolution of light skin in Europeans and East Asians. Mol Biol Evol. 2007;24:710-22.
44. Sturm RA. A golden age of human pigmentation genetics. Trends Genet. 2006;22:464-8.
45. McEvoy B, Beleza S, Shiver M. The genetic architecture of normal variation in human pigmentation: an evolutionary perspective and model. Hum Mol Genet. 2006;15(2): R176-81.
46. Sturm RA, Box NF, Ramsay M. Human pigmentation genetics: difference is only skin deep. BioEssays. 1998;20: 712-21.
47. Harding RM, Healy E, Ray AJ, et al. Evidence for varied selecting pressure at MC1R. Am J Hum GeneT. 2000;66: 1351-61.
48. Rana BK, Hewett-Emmett D, Jin L, et al. High polymorphism at the human melanocortin 1 receptor locus. Genetics. 1999;151(4):1547-57.
49. Westerhof W, Beemer FA, Cormane RH, et al. Hereditary congenital hypopigmented and hyperpigmented macules. Arch dermatol. 1978;114:931-36.

3

Melanocyte

Ravinder Kumar, Davinder Parsad

Key Features

- Melanocytes are specialized skin cell that produces the protective skin-darkening pigment melanin. Melanocytes are originated from neural-crest progenitors that migrate to the skin during embryonic development.
- Epidermal melanocytes have a key role in protecting human skin from the damaging effects of UV radiation and in preventing skin cancer due to the presence of melanin. Melanin are produced in the melanosomes. Melanocytes can absorb ultraviolet radiation (UVR) and survive considerable genotoxic stress.
- Main enzymes and regulatory proteins that are trafficked to the melanosome for the conversion of tyrosine to melanins are tyrosinase gene family, i.e. tyrosinase, tyrosinase-related protein-1, and dopachrome tautomerase/tyrosinase-related protein-2 (Dct/TYRP 2).
- Each melanocyte is estimated to make a contact with 36 keratinocytes in the basal and suprabasal layers and form a epidermal melanin unit. Melanins are polymorphous and multifunctional biopolymers that include eumelanin, pheomelanin and neuromelanin.
- Melanocytes have also been reported to appear in the stria vascularis of the cochlea, in the leptomeninges, substantia nigra and locus coeruleus of the brain and in the heart.

INTRODUCTION

Melanocytes are the cells with dendrites and life-saving pigment called melanin. Because of this melanin pigment melanocytes are dark in color **(Fig. 1)**.

The skin is the largest organ in the human body. Multiple cells and layers of skin perform different functions to protect and regulate the body. The skin is the main barrier to the external environment, and relies on melanocytes for photoprotection and thermoregulation by producing melanin. Epidermal melanocytes are specialized skin cell that produces the protective skin-darkening pigment melanin. Epidermal melanocytes, cells which produce pigment in the skin, lie at the base of the epidermis, while keratinocytes—both squamous cells and basal cells—make up the majority of the top layer of the skin. Melanocytes have also been reported to appear in the striavascularis of the cochlea,[1] in the leptomeninges,[2] substantia nigra and locus coeruleus[3] of the brain, in the heart.[4,5] There are typically between 1,000 and 2,000 melanocytes/mm^2 of skin. Melanocytes comprise of 5–10% of the cells in the basal layer of epidermis. Although their size can vary, melanocytes are typically 7 micrometers in length. Melanocytes are known to produce melanins, the pigments responsible for skin and hair color. Melanocytes are

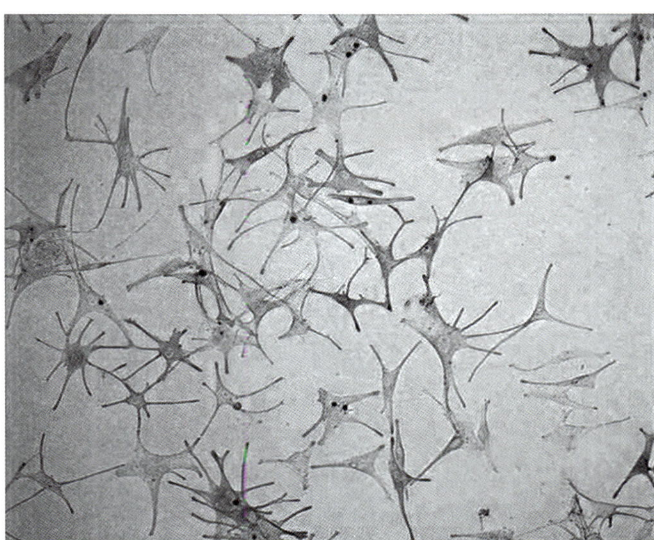

Fig. 1: Cultured melanocytes showing dendrites and melanin

originated from neural-crest progenitors that migrate to the skin during embryonic development. In the skin melanoblasts resides in the basal layer of the epidermis and in the outer root sheath of hair follicles, where they proliferate and then differentiate into melanin-producing cells, melanocytes. Melanocytes are key components of the skin's pigmentary system. Melanocytes have long dendritic processes, with the help of these dendrites each melanocytes makes contact with around 30–40 keratinocytes.

DEVELOPMENT OF MELANOCYTES

During development the neural crest cells differentiate into numerous cell lineages, including neurons, glia, smooth muscle, craniofacial bone, cartilage and melanocytes. The precursors of the melanocytes are known as melanoblasts. Melanoblast starts to migrate from neural crest to peripheral site. Progenitor melanoblasts migrate dorsolaterally between the mesodermal and ectodermal layers to reach their final destinations in the hair follicles and the skin. Melanoblasts migrate along with extracellular matrices and enter the mesenchymal layer. Within the dermal mesenchyme, they migrate to all regions of the developing skin.[6] They reach specific target sites, mainly the dermis, epidermis and hair follicles, the uveal tract of the eye, the striavasculare, the vestibular organ and the endolymphatic sac of the ear, and leptomeninges of the brain. From the dermis, melanoblasts then begin to populate the epidermis, where these proliferate and differentiate to melanocytes. Pigment producing cells can be found in fetal epidermis as early as the 50th day of gestation. Mature melanocytes have been identified using 3,4-dihydroxyphenylalanine (DOPA) reaction and morphologic criteria. Distribution of melanocytes in the adult is appearing to be nonrandom[7] and each melanocyte is attached with 36 keratinocytes through dendrites in epidermal melanin unit. During embryogenesis migration of neural crest-derived cells is highly dependent on interactions between specific receptors on the cell surface and their extracellular ligands. By interacting with their specific cell surface receptors, these molecules induce intracellular and intranuclear signaling to influence gene transcription and protein synthesis.

MELANOCYTE SIGNALING PATHWAYS

Melanoblast migration and differentiation into melanocytes and their functions are controlled by four significant signaling pathways which are influenced by a number of signaling molecules **(Table 1)**. These signaling molecules include Wnt, endothelin-3 (ET-3), stem cell factor (SCF), c-Kit ligand.[8-13] These molecules interact with their specific cell surface receptors; induce intracellular and intranuclear signaling to influence gene transcription and protein synthesis.

Endothelins

Endothelins bind and activate transmembrane G protein-linked receptors endothelin receptor (ENDR) A and B. ET-3 binds to its ENDR B receptor which is very important for melanoblast migration. Endothelin-3 receptors expression is also required for survival, proliferation of melanoblasts. Defects in melanocyte and melanoblasts morphogenesis resulting from disruption in ET-3 and ENDR B signaling are implicated in Hirschsprung disease in human.[14]

Wnt

The Wnt family binds and activates Frizzled, a transmembrane heptahelical G protein-linked receptor,[15] and induce the accumulation of catenin. Binding of Wnt to its receptor Frizzled inhibits enzyme glycogen synthase kinase 3β activity, leading to β-catenin accumulation in the cytosol followed by its translocation to the nucleus. In the nucleus, β-catenin binds specific transcription factors, and induces the transcription of microphthalmia-associated transcription factor (MITF).[13] MITF regulate the transcription of three

Table 1: Melanocyte signaling pathways

Ligand	*Receptors*	*Secondary messenger/ signaling intermediates*	*Transcription factor*	*Target genes*		
				Differentiation	*Proliferation*	*Survival*
Endothelin-3	Endothelin receptor B (EDNRB)	PKC	PAX3, SOX10	MITF, TYR, TRP-1, TRP-2, Mart-1, Aim1, MC-1R, Silver, Dct	P^{16}, P^{21}, CDK-2, Tbx2	Bcl2, Met
Wnt1/3a	Frizzled	β-catenin	MITF/TCF/LEF			
Stem cell factor	C-Kit	MAPK	MITF			
α-MSH	MC-1R	cAMP/PKA	MITF/CREB			

Abbreviations: CREB, cAMP regulatory element-binding protein; cAMP, cyclic adenosine monophosphate; CDK, cyclin dependent kinase; MITF, microphthalmia-associated transcription factor; α-MSH, α-melanocyte-stimulating hormone; PKA, protein kinase A; TRP, tyrosinase-related protein; TYR, tyrosinase enzymes that regulate melanin synthesis: tyrosinase (TYR), tyrosinase-related protein-1 (TRP-1), and DOPA chrome tautomerase (TRP-2).

Stem Cell Factor

Stem cell factor along with its tyrosine kinase transmembrane receptor c-Kit is very important for the early melanoblast development.[16] Stem cell factor is expressed by epidermal keratinocytes, and, as soon as c-Kit is expressed on melanoblasts, they begin their migration to their final destination.[17] The human piebald trait, characterized by patchy pigmentation, is due to the defect in melanocyte morphogenesis resulting in absence of melanocyte in these areas of skin. Mutations in the *KIT* gene decrease the ability of the KIT receptor to be activated by the steel factor and are responsible for at least one type of human piebaldism.[18] Affected individuals display broad depigmented patches, most prominent on the central forehead and trunk.

α-Melanocyte-stimulating Hormone

One of the factors that regulate melanocytes and skin pigmentation is melanocortin peptide α-melanocyte-stimulating hormone (α-MSH). The effects of α-MSH on melanogenesis are mediated via the melanocortin-1 receptor (MC-1R) and TYR. MC1R that regulates the quality and quantity of their melanin production. Binding of α-MSH to its receptor MC-1R increases TYR activity and eumelanin production. MC1R is controlled by the α-MSH agonists[19] which stimulate the melanogenic cascade and thus the synthesis of eumelanin, as well as by the antagonist agouti signaling protein (ASP).[20]

FORMATION OF MELANOSOMES

In humans embryo, neural crest migration process takes place between the 10th and the 12th week of development for the dermis and about 2 weeks later for the epidermis.[21] The production of melanin pigment begins at around 12 weeks based on both electron microscopic studies and DOPA staining.[22] Once the melanocytes get established they start producing specialized organelle called a pigment granule or melanosomes. Melanosomes development is typically divided into four maturation stages (I–IV) determined by their structure and the quantity, quality, and arrangement of the melanin produced[23,24] **(Fig. 2)**. Nascent melanosomes are assembled in the perinuclear region near the Golgi stacks, receiving all enzymatic and structural proteins required for melanogenesis.

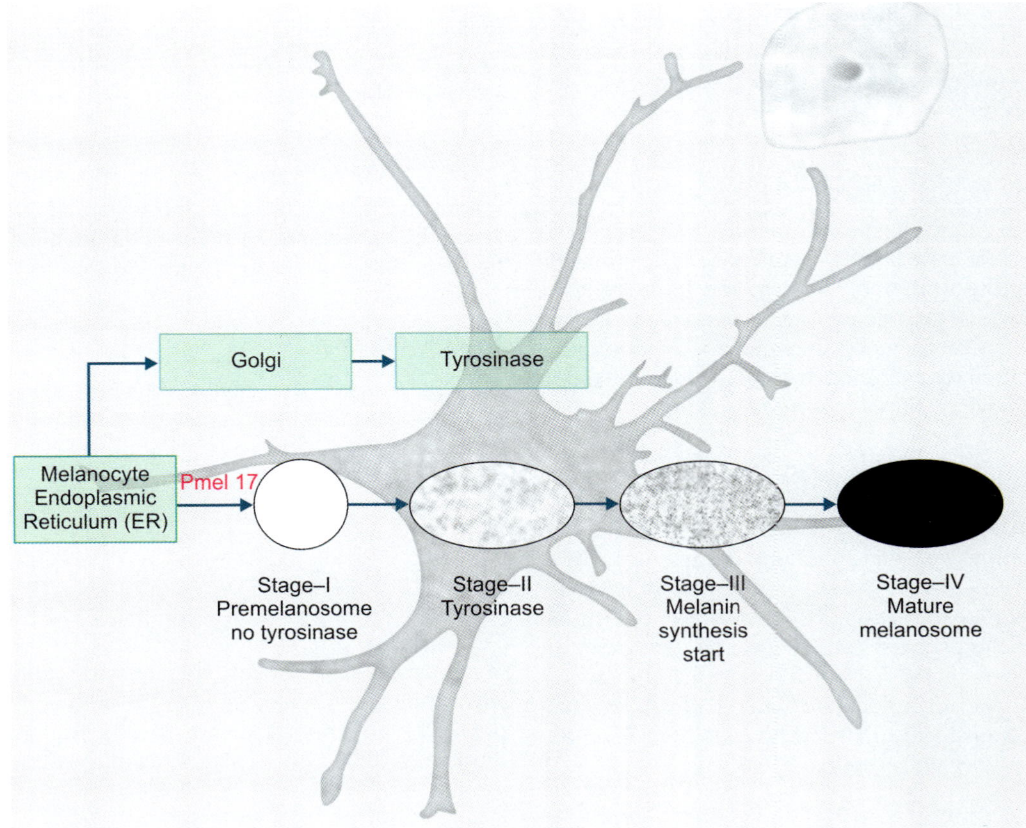

Fig. 2: Different stages of melanosome formation in the melanocyte

- *Stage-I:* At this stage relatively spherical organelle called premelanosomes with matrix material and lacking TYR activity start to assemble without any structural component.
- *Stage-II:* An oval shaped organelle containing organized internal matrix without appearance of melanin. TYR is subsequently trafficked to Stage II melanosomes.
- *Stage-III:* Melanosomes are termed at Stage III when the melanin synthesis starts and the pigment is uniformly deposited on the internal matrix.
- *Stage-IV:* This is the final stage of melanosome development. Organelle completely filled with melanin is termed to be in stage IV. These melanosomes are either elliptical or ellipsoidal, electron-opaque due to complete melanization, and have minimal TYR activity. Besides these, melanosomes contain other melanocyte-specific proteins that have structural functions, e.g. Pmel-17 is involved in regulating the pH within melanosomes, such as P protein- or membrane-associated transporter protein (MATP).

MELANIN-PRODUCING ENZYMES

Main enzymes and regulatory proteins that are trafficked to the melanosome for the conversion of tyrosine to melanins are TYR gene family, i.e. TYR, TRP-1, and dopachrome tautomerase (DCT)/TRP-2. These glycoproteins are transcribed at rough endoplasmic reticulum, undergo carbohydrate maturation in the Golgi apparatus and ultimately transported to the premelanosomes.

Tyrosinase

Tyrosinase is the main enzyme required for the synthesis of melanin in the melanosomes. Tyrosinase is responsible for the rate-limiting initial step of tyrosine hydroxylation, an important step in melanogenesis. Tyrosinase is known to catalyze the conversion of L-tyrosine to dopaquinone. Dopaquinone is then used for the synthesis of both eumelanin and pheomelanin which impart color to the skin.

Tyrosinase-related Protein-1

Tyrosinase-related protein-1 is involved in the production of melanin, although its exact functions are unclear. TRP-1 may stabilize TYR, which is the enzyme responsible for the first step in melanin production. TRP-1 may also determine the shape of melanosomes, which are the structures in melanocytes where melanin is produced and also affects melanocyte proliferation and melanocyte cell death.[25] A small number of mutations in the TRP-1 gene have been found to cause oculocutaneous albinism type 3 (OCA3).

Dopachrome Tautomerase/Tyrosinase-related Protein-2

Dopachrome tautomerase, also known as DCT, is an enzyme that isomerizes the melanogenic intermediate 3,4-dihydroxyphenylalanine-chrome (DOPA-chrome) to 5,6-dihydroxyindole-2-carboxylic acid (DHICA) in the biosynthesis of melanin. Its expression is regulated by the MITF.

MELANIN SYNTHESIS

Melanins are polymorphous and multifunctional bio-polymers that include eumelanin, pheomelanin and neuromelanin. Melanocytes numbers are consistent even in different skin types and ethnic groups therefore the number of melanocytes does not determine the degree of pigmentation. Skin pigmentation is considered to depend upon the level of melanogenic activity. Human melanocytes are known to produce both the brown-black eumelanin and reddish-yellow pheomelanin.[26] Both eumelanin and pheomelanin are involved in binding of cations, anions, drugs and chemicals, etc. and therefore play an important protective role within melanocytes.[27]

Melanin is synthesized in specialized intracellular membrane coated organelles present in the cytoplasm of melanocytes called melanosomes. Tyrosinase and the TRP-1, TRP-2 were synthesized in the melanosomes during their development.

Eumelanin

Eumelanin is the more photoprotective of the two melanins. Eumelanin, on the other hand, is the pigment present in the humans with dark skin and hair **(Flow chart 1)**.

Pheomelanin

Pheomelanin is the major type in red hair and also predominates in the epidermis of skin types I and II[28] **(Flow chart 2)**.

EPIDERMAL MELANIN UNIT

Melanin biosynthesis occurs in membrane-bound organelles called melanosomes which are present in the melanocytes. The process of melanin synthesis is very complex.[29] Melanosomes filled with melanin are transferred to the surrounding keratinocytes with the help of dendrites, where they play an important role in the photoprotection from ultraviolet (UV) light. This association of melanocytes and

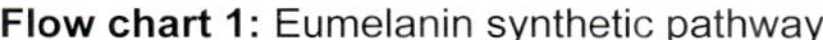

Flow chart 1: Eumelanin synthetic pathway

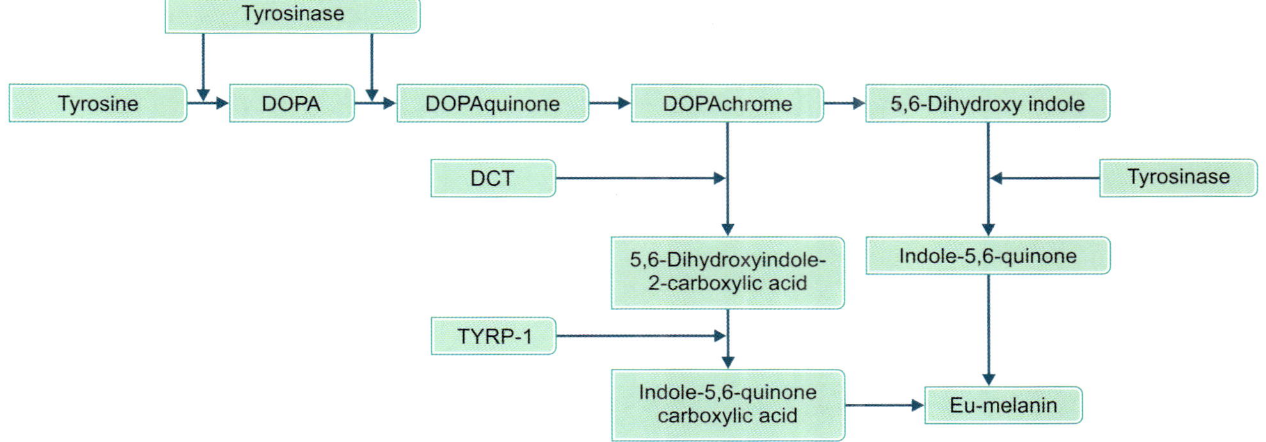

Flow chart 2: Pheomelanin synthetic pathway

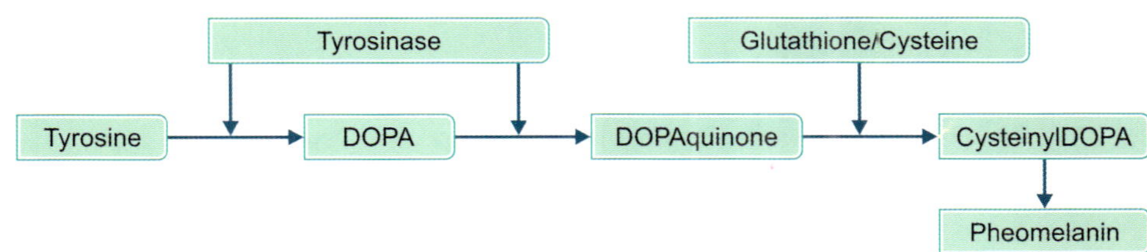

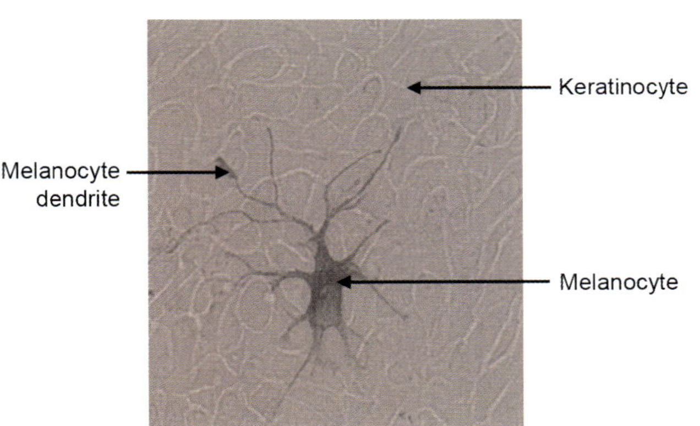

Fig 3: Epidermal melanin unit: In the skin one melanocyte is surrounded by 36 keratinocytes

keratinocytes in the skin is known as epidermal melanin unit. Each melanocyte is estimated to make a contact with 36 keratinocytes in the basal and suprabasal layers[30] **(Fig. 3)**.

MELANOSOME TRANSFER FROM MELANOCYTE TO KERATINOCYTE

Trafficking of melanosomes from melanocyte to keratinocyte is very important for the skin pigmentation. Once melanin is produced the melanosomes are transferred into the neighboring keratinocytes with the help of dendrites. The exact mechanism of melanin transfer from melanocytes to keratinocytes is not known. Association of melanosomes with microtubules and actin filaments via motor proteins, such as kinesin, dynein and myosin V, is important for melanosome migration along the dendrites and for the transfer of melanin to keratinocytes.[31-37] There are three major theories of melanosome transfer from melanocytes to keratinocytes through dendrites (1) a bit of melanosome dendrite is phagocytized by the keratinocyte (2) melanosomes are discharged by the dendrites into the intracellular spaces and then phagocytized by the keratinocytes (3) a cytoplasmic channel is formed by the fusion of plasma membrane of dendrite and keratinocytes through which melanosomes transfer from melanocyte to keratinocyte.[38-40] Protease-activated receptor 2 (PAR-2), which is expressed only on keratinocytes plays a central role in melanin transfer via phagocytosis. What exactly is being phagocytosed—naked melanin, melanosomes or melanocytic cell parts—remains unknown. A recent study showed that activation of the PAR-2 increases melanin transfer to keratinocytes.[41] This process of melanin transfer from melanocytes to keratinocytes is under hormonal control, including the MSH and adrenocorticotropic hormone (ACTH) peptides that are produced from the precursor proopiomelanocortin. In the skin, melanin acts as an optical and chemical photoprotective

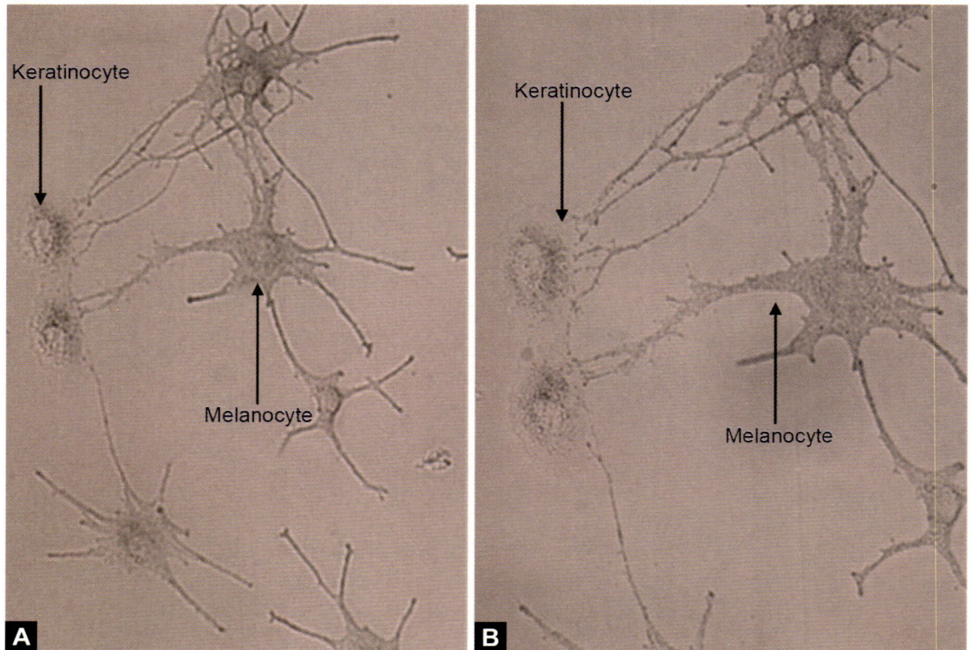

Figs 4A and B: Melanosome transfer from melanocyte to keratinocyte: Melanin is produced in the melanocytes and then transferred to the keratinocyte through dendrites

filter, which reduces the penetration of all wavelengths of light into subepidermal tissues[42,43] **(Figs 4A and B)**.

MELANOCYTE FUNCTIONS

Epidermal melanocytes have a key role in protecting human skin from the damaging effects of UV radiation and in preventing skin cancer. Melanocytes can absorb UV radiation (UVR) and survive considerable genotoxic stress. Absorption of UVRs protects the functional cells such as langerhans cells and basilar keratinocytes.

Keratinocytes secrete factors in response to the UVR that regulate melanocyte survival, differentiation, proliferation and motility. These factors also stimulate melanocytes to produce melanin and resulting in the tanning response. Melanin is a sunscreen. Melanin is produced in the melanocytes and then transferred to the keratinocytes with the help of fine dendrites processes. Therefore those people who lack the functional melanocytes results in pigmentary disorders such as vitiligo and albinism are hypersensitive to UVR. Melanocytes are also the precursors of melanoma, the most deadly form of skin cancer. Skin cancer is the third most common cancer in human. Many skin diseases are caused by the exposure to UV light like lupus erythematosus, porphyria cutanea tarda, xeroderma pigmentosum, pellagra, etc. Melanocytes also play a crucial role during the embryogenesis in early human development for example a number of individuals with OCA1. OCA1 results from the dysfunction of TYR, which leads not only to impaired pigmentation of skin, hair and eyes,[44] but also to misrouting of the optic nerves at the chiasm.[45]

There is increasing evidence that melanocytes are not simply melanin-producing cells but may have a number of functions. It has been proposed that melanin minimizes the photolysis of folic acid.[46,47] Melanocytes are capable of secreting a wide range of signaling molecules and it has been suggested that they could function as regulatory cells in maintaining epidermal homeostasis.[48] Their ability to respond to regulatory peptides such as α-MSH might be an integral part of such a function. Melanocytes can produce many other factors besides melanin. Melanocyte also produce proopiomelanocortin and MSH.[49,50] Melanocytes are also shown to produce and respond to interlukins (IL-1, IL-6 and tumor necrosis factor-α).[51,52] Melanocytes are also capable of synthesizing and responding to prostaglandin E and leukotrienes.[53,54]

EXTRACUTANEOUS MELANOCYTES

Extracutaneous melanocytes found in eye, ear and various internal body parts are unique from epidermal melanocytes as these extracutaneous melanocytes synthesise melanosomes and melanin only during short interval after arriving in their target tissue. These melanocytes also do not transfer their melanosomes to neighboring cell and retain them throughout their life.

Hair Follicle Melanocyte

Melanocytes are also present in the hair follicles but they do not have a protective effect. Melanocytes are located in the proximal hair bulb, and there is a ratio of 1:5 between melanocytes and keratinocytes.[55]

Dermal Melanocytes

Dermal pigmentation results from the presence of melanocytes within dermis. Dermal melanocytes are present in very small number in human adult skin. Dermal melanocytes synthesize melanosomes but do not transfer these to the surrounding cells. Possibly retain, degrade and replace these melanosomes periodically. Classic expression of normal dermal hyperpigmentation is mongolian spot or congenital dermal melanocytosis.[56]

Melanocytes of Eye

The importance of melanin for proper ocular function is demonstrated by the visual abnormalities observed in patients with albinism.[57] Eye contains two types of pigment cells: (1) uveal cells (2) retinal pigment cells (RPE). RPE plays a crucial role in retinal development and functions, therefore controlling visual activity, whereas uveal melanocytes provide the color of the iris. RPE melaocytes are also responsible for the successful embryonic development and organization of neural retina proper. Unlike cutaneous melanocytes, ocular melanocytes are in contact only with each other, and they do not transfer their melanosomes.

Melanocytes of Heart

Melanocytes are found in many locations in heart including valves and septa. The function of cardiac melanocytes remains unclear. They may play role in atrioventricular (AV) valve function. They also contribute to the triggering of arrhythmia by regulating the calcium and ROS levels.

Otic Melanocytes

Melanocytes also play an important role in the hearing process as melanocytes reside in the cochlea and loss of these melanocytes leads to deafness.[58] Melanocytes play a critical role in the maintenance of potassium in the endolymph.[59,60] Loss of melanocytes can lead to deafness, and patients with Waardenburg syndrome type 2 are deaf because of lack of melanocytes in the inner ear.[61,62]

Melanocytes in the Leptomeninges and Neuromelanins

Melanocytes are also present in the human brain specifically the meninges covering the ventrolateral surfaces of the medulla oblongata and the upper cervical cord.[63,64] The pigment of melanocytes in the leptomeninges differ from the dark pigment found in the neurons throughout the brain which is known as neuromelanin and is thought to be auto-oxidative product of dopamine generated by neuronal synthesized tyrosine hydroxylase molecule.[65-67] Leptomeninges melanocyte function is not clear. Brain melanocytes may have a neuroendocrine and detoxification function. During embryonic development, aberrant proliferation of these melanocytes leads to congenital melanocytic neves.[68]

REFERENCES

1. Tachibana M. Sound needs sound melanocytes to be heard. Pigment Cell Res. 1999;12:344-54.
2. Goldgeier MH, Klein LE, Klein-Angerer S, et al. The distribution of melanocytes in the leptomeninges of the human brain. J Invest Dermatol. 1984;82:235-8.
3. Zecca L, Tampellini D, Gatti A, et al. The neuromelanin of human substantia nigra and its interaction with metals. J Neural Transm. 2002;109:663-72.
4. Brito FC, Kos L. Timeline and distribution of melanocyte precursors in the mouse heart. Pigment Cell Melanoma Res. 2008;21:464-70.
5. Yajima I, Larue L. The location of heart melanocytes is specified and the level of pigmentation in the heart may correlate with coat color. Pigment Cell Melanoma Res. 2008;21:471-6.
6. Mayer TC. The migratory pathway of neural crest cells into the skin of mouse embryos. 1973;34:39-46.
7. Holbrook KA, Vogel AM, Underwood RA, et al. Melanocytes in human embryonic and fetal skin: A review and new findings. 1988;(1 Suppl):6-17.
8. Kleber M, Lee HY, Wurdak H, et al. Neural crest stem cell maintenance by combinatorial Wnt and BMP signaling. J Cell Biol. 2005;169(2):309-20.
9. Dunn KJ, Brady M, Ochsenbauer-Jambor C, et al. WNT1 and WNT3a promote expansion of melanocytes through distinct modes of action. Pigment Cell Res. 2005;18(3):167-80.
10. Lee HY, Kléber M, Hari L, et al. Instructive role of Wnt/beta-catenin in sensory fate specification in neural crest stem cells. Science. 2004;303(5660):1020-3.
11. Jin EJ, Erickson CA, Takada S, et al. Wnt and BMP signaling govern lineage segregation of melanocytes in the avian embryo. Dev Biol. 2001;233(1):22-37.
12. Dunn KJ, Williams BO, Li Y, et al. Neural crest-directed gene transfer demonstrates Wnt1 role in melanocyte expansion and differentiation during mouse development. Proc Natl Acad Sci USA. 2000;97(18):10050-5.
13. Grimes CA, Jope RS. The multifaceted roles of glycogen synthase kinase 3 beta in cellular signaling. Prog Neurobiol. 2001;65(4):391-426.
14. McCallion AS, Chakravarti A. EDNRB/EDN3 and Hirschsprung disease type II. Pigment Cell Res. 2001;14:161-9.

15. Liu T, DeCostanzo AJ, Liu X, et al. G protein signaling from activated rat frizzled-1 to the beta-catenin-Lef-Tcf pathway. Science. 2001;292(5522):1718-22.
16. Nishikawa S, Kusakabe M, Yoshinaga K, et al. In utero manipulation of coat color formation by a monoclonal anti-c-kit antibody: Two distinct waves of c-kit-dependency during melanocyte development. EMBO J. 1991;10(8):2111-8.
17. Wehrle-Haller B. The role of Kit-ligand in melanocyte development and epidermal homeostasis. Pigment Cell Res. 2003;16(3):287-96.
18. Bolognia J. Molecular advances in disorders of pigmentation. Adv Dermatol. 1999;15:341-65.
19. Millington GW. Proopiomelanocortin (POMC): the cutaneous roles of its melanocortin products and receptors. Clin Exp Dermatol. 2006;31:407-12.
20. Suzuki I, Tada A, Ollmann MM, et al. Agouti signaling protein inhibits melanogenesis and the response of human melanocytes to α-melanotropin. J Invest Dermatol. 1997; 108:838-42.
21. Haake A, Holbrook K. The structure and development of skin. In: Freedberg IM, Eisen AZ, Wolff K, Austen KF, Goldsmith LA, Katz SI, Fitzpatrick TB (Eds). Fitzpatrick's Dermatology in General Medicine. New York: McGraw-Hill; 1999. pp. 70-114.
22. Zimmerman AA, Becker SW. Precursors of epidermal melanocytes in the Negro fetus. In: Gordon M (Ed). Pigment Cell Biology. New York: Academic Press; 1959. pp. 159-70.
23. Seiji M, Shimao K, Birbeck MS, et al. Subcellular localization of melanin biosynthesis. Ann NY Acad Sci. 1963;100:497-33.
24. Kushimoto T, Basrur V, Valencia J, et al. A model for melanosome biogenesis based on the purification and analysis of early melanosomes. Proc Natl Acad Sci USA. 2001;98:10698-703.
25. Sarangarajan R, Boissy RE. Tyrp1 and oculocutaneous albinism type 3. Pigment Cell Res. 2001;14(6):437-44.
26. Hunt G, Kyne S, Ito S, et al. Eumelanin and phaeomelanin contents of human epidermis and cultured melanocytes. Pigment Cell Res. 1995;8:202-8.
27. Nordlund JJ. The pigmentary system. New interpretation of old data. J Dermatol. 1985;12:105-16.
28. Thody AJ, Higgins EM, Wakamatsu K, et al. Phaeomelanin as well as eumelanin is present in human epidermis. J Invest Dermatol. 1991;97:340-44.
29. Hearing VJ. The regulation of melanin production. In: Hori W (Ed). Drug Discovery Approaches for Developing Cosmeceuticals, Advanced Skin Care and Cosmetic Products. Southborough, Massachusetts: IBC Library Series; 1997. pp. 3.1.1-3.1.21.
30. Fitzpatrick TB, Breathnach AS. The epidermal melanin unit system. Dermatol Wochenschr. 1963;147:481-9.
31. Provance DW, Wei M, Ipe V, et al. Cultured melanocytes from dilute mutant mice exhibit dendritic morphology and altered melanosome distribution. Proc Natl Acad Sci USA. 1996;93:14554-8.
32. Wu X, Bowers B, Rao K, et al. Visualization of melanosome dynamics within wild-type and dilute melanocytes suggests a paradigm for myosin V function *In vivo*. J Cell Biol. 1998;143:1899-1918.
33. Wu X, Bowers B, Wei Q, et al. Myosin V associates with melanosomes in mouse melanocytes: evidence that myosin V is an organelle motor. J Cell Sci. 1997;110:847-59.
34. Lambert J, Onderwater J, Vander Haeghen Y, et al. Myosin V colocalizes with melanosomes and subcortical actin bundles not associated with stress fibers in human epidermal melanocytes. J Invest Dermatol. 1998;111: 835-40.
35. Hara M, Yaar M, Byers HR, et al. Kinesin participates in melanosomal movement along melanocyte dendrites. J Invest Dermatol. 2000;114:438-43.
36. Vancoillie G, Lambert J, Mulder A, et al. Cytoplasmic dynein colocalizes with melanosomes in normal human melanocytes. Br J Dermatol. 2000;143:298-306.
37. Vancoillie G, Lambert J, Mulder A, et al. Kinesin and kinectin can associate with the melanosomal surface and form a link with microtubules in normal human melanocytes. J Invest Dermatol. 2000;114:421-9.
38. Jimbow K, Quevedo Wc, Prota G, et al. Biology of melanocytes In: Freedberg IM, Eisen AZ, Wolff K, Austen KF, Goldsmith LA, Katz SI, Fitzpatrick TB (Eds). Dermatology in General Medicine, 5th edn. New York: McGraw-Hill; 1999. pp. 192-220.
39. Marks M, Seabra MC. The melanosome. Membrane dynamics in black and white. Mol Cell Biol. 2001;2:1-11.
40. Yamamoto O, Bhawan J. Three modes of melanosome transfers in Caucasian facial skin: hypothesis based on an ultrastructural study. Pigment Cell Res. 1994;7:158-69.
41. Seiberg M, Paine C, Sharlow E, et al. The protease-activated receptor 2 regulates pigmentation via keratinocyte-melanocyte interactions. Exp Cell Res. 2000;254:25-32.
42. Daniels F. The physiological effects of sunlight. J Invest Dermatol. 1959;32:147-155.
43. Kaidbey KH, Pohagin P, Sayre RM, et al. Photoprotection by melanin-a comparison of black and Caucasian skin. J Am Acad Dermatol. 1979;1:249-60.
44. Spritz RA. Molecular genetics of oculocutaneous albinism. Hum Mol Genet. 1994;3(Spec No):1469-75.
45. King RA, Hearing VJ, Creel DJ, et al. Albinism. In: Scriver CR, Beaudet AL, Sly WS, Valle D (Eds). The Metabolic and Molecular Bases of Inherited Disease. Vol. II. 8th edn. New York: McGraw-Hill; 2001. pp. 5587-627.
46. Aoki K. Sexual selection as a cause of human skin colour variation: Darwin's hypothesis revisited. Ann Hum Biol. 2002;29:589-608.
47. Jablonski NG, Chaplin G. The evolution of skin coloration. J Hum Evol. 2000;39:57-106.
48. Slominski A, Paus R, Schadendorf D. Melanocytes as "sensory" and regulatory cells in the epidermis. J Theor Biol. 1993;164:103-120.

49. Bhardwaj R, Luger TA. Proopiomelanocortin production by epidermal cells: evidence for an immune neuroendocrine network in the epidermis. Arch Dermatol Res. 1994;287:85-90.
50. Schauer E, Trautinger F, Köck A, et al. Proopiomelanocortin derived peptides are synthesised and released by human keratinocytes. J Clin Invest. 1994;93:2258-62.
51. Swope VB, Sauder DN, McKenzie RC, et al. Synthesis of interleukin-1 alpha and beta by normal human melanocytes. J Invest Dermatol. 1994;102(5):749-53.
52. Swope VB, Abdel-Malek ZA, Sauder DN, et al. A new role for epidermal cell-derived thymocyte activating factor/ IL-1 as an antagonist for distinct epidermal cell function. J Immunol. 1989;142(6):1943-9.
53. Abdel-Malek ZA, Swope VB, Nordlund JJ. The Nature and Biological Effects of Factors Responsible for Proliferation and Differentiation of Melanocytes. Pigment Cell Res. 1990;(3)S2:43-47.
54. Medrano EE, Farooqui JZ, Boissy RE, et al. Chronic growth stimulation of human adult melanocytes by inflammatory mediators *in vitro*: implications for nevus formation and initial steps in melanocyte oncogenesis. Proc Natl Acad Sci USA. 1993:90(5):1790-94.
55. Tobin DJ, Paus R. Graying Geronto biology of the hair follicle pigmentary unit. Exp Gerontol. 2001;36(1):29-54.
56. Mosher DB, Fitzpatrick TB, Ortonne JP, et al. Disorders of pigmentation. In: Dermatology in General Medicine, Section 14. Disorders of Melanocytes, 3rd edn, volume 1, In: Fitzpatrick TB, Eisen AZ, Wolff K, Freedberg IM, Austen KF (Eds). New York: McGraw-Hill; 1987. pp. 794-876.
57. Creel D, O'Donnell FE, Witkop CJ. Visual system anomalies in human ocular albinos. Science. 1978;201(4359):931-3.
58. Tolleson WH. Human melanocyte biology, toxicology, and pathology. J Environ Sci Health. 2005;23(2):105-61.
59. Wangemann P. K+ cycling and the endocochlear potential. Hear Res. 2002;165(1-2):1-9.
60. Ando M, Takeuchi S. Immunological identification of an inward rectifier K+ channel (Kir4.1) in the intermediate cell (melanocyte) of the cochlear stria vascularis of gerbils and rats. Cell Tissue Res. 1999;298(1):179-83.
61. Price ER, Fisher DE. Sensorineural deafness and pigmentation genes: Melanocytes and the MITF transcriptional network. Neuron. 2001;30:15-8.
62. Watanabe K, Takeda K, Yasumoto K, et al. Identification of a distal enhancer for the melanocyte-specific promoter of the MITF gene. Pigment Cell Res. 2002;15(3):201-11.
63. Baader O. Uberdie Pialmelanose. Z Mikrosk Anat Forsch. 1935;22:735.
64. Symmers W. Pigmentation of the pia mater with special reference to the brain of modern Egyptians. J Anat. 1905; 40:25-7.
65. Enochs WS, Nilges MJ, Swartz HM. Purified human neuromelanin, synthetic dopamine melanin as a potential model pigment, and the normal human substantia nigra: characterization by electron paramagnetic resonance spectroscopy. J Neurochem. 1993;61:68-79.
66. Odh G, Carstam R, Paulson J, et al. Neuromelanin of the human substantia nigra: a mixed type melanin. J Neurochem. 1994;62:2030-6.
67. Zecca L, Mecacci C, Seraglia R, et al. The chemical characterization of melanin contained in substantia nigra of human brain. Biochim Biophys Acta. 1992;1138:6-10.
68. Marghoob AA, Dusza S, Oliveria S, et al. Number of satellite nevi as a correlate for neurocutaneous melanocytosis in patients with large congenital melanocytic nevi. Arch Dermatol. 2004;140(2):171-5.

4

Systemic Disorders with Cutaneous Pigmentary Alterations

Keshavmurthy A Adya, Arun C Inamadar

Key Features

- This chapter mainly focuses on various systemic diseases with cutaneous manifestations/associations.
- The mucocutaneous pigmentary manifestations/associations of such systemic diseases are described in detail stressing upon the clinical characteristics and underlying etiopathogenesis of the pigmentary alterations.
- The etiology, systemic features and the nonpigmentary cutaneous features of the conditions/syndromes are briefly highlighted in Tables and Boxes.

Cutaneous pigmentary changes in systemic diseases may be consequent to the internal metabolic derangements or be associated as a part of the disease or syndrome. As the skin is said to be the window to systemic illnesses, such cutaneous pigmentary changes provide useful clues towards the underlying internal defects and in many instances, serve as disease severity and/or prognostic markers as well.

PIGMENTARY DERANGEMENTS IN ENDOCRINE DISORDERS

Pituitary Diseases

Acromegaly

Acromegaly is the result of postpubertal chronic exposure of the body tissues to increased serum levels of human growth hormone (hGH) and insulin-like growth factor 1 (IGF-1), usually due to a somatotrope pituitary adenoma. The hGH directly as well as through the IGF-1 exerts trophic effects on various tissues of the body. Onset of acromegaly is insidious and the mean age of diagnosis is around the fourth decade. Acral bony overgrowth along with soft tissue swelling lead to coarse facies with cutis verticis gyrata, frontal bossing, prognathism with large greasy nose, large hands and feet with heel pad thickening. Other features include a deep hollow voice, macroglossia, skeletal anomalies and visceromegaly affecting the heart and thyroid. Dermatological manifestations include seborrhea, acrochordons, acanthosis nigricans (AN), hyperhidrosis and pigmentary alterations.[1]

The pigmentary changes include hyperpigmentation, mainly over the light-exposed areas, and AN. Cutaneous hyperpigmentation is seen in about half of the cases and is attributed to increased melanocyte-stimulating hormone (MSH).[2,3] Development of AN is mediated through the IGF-1 stimulation of tyrosine kinase growth factor receptor signaling pathways in epidermis.[4] Melanocytic nevi and lentigens may also be seen in increased numbers.

Hypopituitarism

Pituitary insufficiency may be glandular (primary) or consequent to hypothalamic diseases (secondary). Various causes of hypopituitarism[1,3,5] are listed in **Table 1**. The

Table 1: Causes of pituitary insufficiency

Congenital/ developmental defects	Pituitary aplasia, empty sella syndrome, congenital hypothalamic disorders (Prader-Willi syndrome, Laurence-Moon-Biedl syndrome, Kallmann syndrome, Septo-optic dysplasia)
Infections	Tuberculosis, pituitary abscess, encephalitis, histoplasmosis
Infiltrations	Sarcoidosis, hemochromatosis, histiocytosis X
Traumatic	Head injury, iatrogenic (surgery, radiotherapy)
Neoplastic	Adenoma, craniopharyngioma, meningioma
Others	Sheehan syndrome, pituitary apoplexy, chronic systemic illnesses

Table 2: Dermatological manifestations of pituitary insufficiency

Dermatological manifestations	*Associated deficient hormone*
Hypotrichosis with decreased secondary sexual hair	FSH/LH ACTH (decreased axillary and pubic hairs in women)
Ichthyotic and xerotic skin	TSH ACTH
Myxedematous changes	TSH
Abnormal fat deposition over the chest and trunk	Prepubertal hGH deficiency
Pigmentary alterations	*See text and Table 3*

Abbreviations: ACTH, adrenocorticotropic hormone; FSH, follicle-stimulating hormone; hGH, human growth hormone; LH, luteinizing hormone; TSH, thyroid-stimulating hormone

manifestations of pituitary insufficiency depend upon the predominant hormonal deficit. In classical hypopituitarism, all the hormones are affected to some extent.[3]

The dermatological manifestations consequent to the respective hormonal deficiency are outlined in **Table 2**. Cutaneous pigmentary changes predominantly include pallor, the cause for which is multifactorial **(Box 1)**. The hypopigmentation is more conspicuous over the face, genitalia and nipple areolae and unless accompanied by anemia, it is associated with normal mucous membranes. There is also a reduced malar flush and an inability to tan even after prolonged ultraviolet exposure that may lead to sunburn. Yellowish tinge to palms and soles, and the nasolabial folds secondary to hypothyroidism-induced carotenemia, and pigmentary dilution of hair due to α-MSH deficit are the other changes seen in hypopituitarism.[6]

Box 1

Causes of cutaneous pallor in hypopituitarism

- Hypothyroidism associated reflex cutaneous vasoconstriction, hypometabolic state, and mucin deposition in the skin that alters the refraction of light
- Pituitary ACTH deficiency
- α-MSH deficiency
- Associated anemia

Abbreviations: ACTH, adrenocorticotropic hormone; α-MSH: α-melanocyte-stimulating hormone

Adrenal Diseases

Cushing's Syndrome

Chronic exposure to excess glucocorticoids leads to development of a host of cutaneous and systemic derangements. The causes of excess glucocorticoid production **(Table 3)** may be categorized into those due to excess adrenocorticotropic hormone (ACTH) secretion (ACTH-dependent) and those due to excess glucocorticoids (ACTH-independent).[5,7] Cushing's syndrome refers to the various manifestations of glucocorticoid excess due to any cause. When the cause is a pituitary corticotrope adenoma (which accounts for about 70% of endogenous ACTH-dependent glucocorticoid excess), the term Cushing's disease is applied. The most common cause of Cushing's syndrome in clinical practice however is iatrogenic (long-term administration of synthetic glucocorticoids).[5]

The clinical manifestations of Cushing's syndrome are described in **Table 4**. Pigmentary alterations include wide

Table 3: Causes of hypercorticism

ACTH-Dependent	*Endogenous*	*Pituitary ACTH hypersecretion*	*Corticotrope adenoma*
		Ectopic ACTH hypersecretion	Bronchial carcinoid Pancreatic carcinoid Medullary thyroid carcinoma Pheochromocytoma Small cell carcinoma of lung CRH syndrome
	Exogenous	*Iatrogenic*	ACTH therapy
ACTH-independent	*Endogenous*	*Adrenal cortisol hypersecretion*	Adenoma Carcinoma Primary pigmented nodular adrenal disease (PPNAD) ACTH-independent massive adrenal hyperplasia (AIMAH)
		Others	McCune-Albright syndrome
	Exogenous	*Iatrogenic*	Long-term glucocorticoid therapy

Abbreviations: ACTH, adrenocorticotropic hormone; CRH, corticotropin-releasing hormone

Table 4: Clinical manifestations of hypercorticism

General appearance	Moon face, buffalo hump, pot belly and lean lower limbs due to abnormal body fat redistribution
Dermatologic	Acne, hirsutism, wide pigmented striae distensae, telangiectasia, brittle skin with tendency to easy bruising
Cardiovascular	Hypertension, atherosclerosis with increased risk of deep vein thrombosis (DVT)
Central nervous system	Irritability, depression and in severe cases, paranoid psychosis
Musculoskeletal	Proximal myopathy; vertebral fractures due to osteoporosis and osteopenia
Endocrinologic	Amenorrhea, hypogonadism, decreased libido (due to excess cortisol-induced suppression of gonadotrophins); hypothyroidism (due to suppression of hypothalamic-pituitary-thyroid axis and resultant thyroid-stimulating hormone deficiency)
Metabolic	Glucose intolerance, dyslipidemia, protein catabolism
Hematologic	Blood hypercoagulability (adds to the risk of DVT), leukocytosis and eosinopenia
Immunologic	Increased susceptibility to infections, delayed wound healing, extensive dermatophyte and candidal infections

fleshy-pink coloration of the abdominal striae, telangiectasia, and an Addisonian hyperpigmentation (see below) which is rather specific to the cases associated with ectopic ACTH hypersecretion. Unlike the ACTH of pituitary tumors, ectopically secreted ACTH does not exert negative feedback sensitivity to cortisol and hence, in such cases both ACTH and cortisol levels are high. The ACTH, along with associated excess of proopiomelanocortin cleavage products, stimulates the melanocytes with resultant hyperpigmentation.[3,5,7]

Adrenal Insufficiency

Adrenal insufficiency, characterized by decreased production of cortisol and mineralocorticoids, may be primary or secondary **(Table 5)**. Primary adrenal insufficiency is characterized by reduced cortisol and mineralocorticoid secretion by the adrenals, and hence, is associated with increased serum ACTH due to absence of negative feedback control. Secondary adrenal insufficiency, which is much more common than primary, is the result of reduced ACTH secretion due to extra-adrenal causes with a consequent low serum cortisol. Mineralocorticoid production in secondary hypoadrenalism is usually normal as it is regulated by the renin-angiotensin-aldosterone cycle which is intact. The clinical manifestations of adrenal insufficiency are outlined in **Table 6**.[5,7]

The principal dermatological manifestation of hypoadrenalism is pigmentary change which is different in primary and secondary forms. Primary adrenal insufficiency (Addison's disease) is characterized by hyperpigmentation due to excess ACTH and α-MSH that have a stimulatory effect on the melanocortin-1 receptors (MC1R) expressed on the melanocytes. The pattern of pigmentation (Addisonian hyperpigmentation) is typical and preferentially affects certain areas of the body **(Box 2)**. However, in a subset of cases, no pigmentation is present—the so called "white Addison's disease", making the diagnosis difficult and such patients may

Table 5: Causes of adrenal insufficiency

Primary	Congenital	Congenital adrenal hyperplasia
		Congenital adrenal hypoplasia
	Autoimmune	Isolated autoimmune adrenalitis
		Autoimmune polyglandular syndrome 1 and 2
	Familial	Familial glucocorticoid deficiency 1, 2 and 3
	Infections	Tuberculosis
		Histoplasmosis
		Cytomegalovirus
		Cryptococcosis
	Infiltrations	Amyloidosis
		Sarcoidosis
		Hemochromatosis
		Metastases
	Drug-induced	Metyrapone, ketoconazole, aminoglutethimide
	Trauma	Surgical
		Radiotherapy
Secondary	Pituitary tumors	Pituitary adenomas (functional/nonfunctional)
	Parasellar masses	Craniopharyngioma, meningioma, metastases
	Infections	Tuberculosis, encephalitis, histoplasmosis
	Infiltrations	Amyloidosis, sarcoidosis, histiocytosis-X
	Trauma	Head injury, irradiation, surgery
	Iatrogenic	Withdrawal of glucocorticoids

Table 6: Clinical features of adrenal insufficiency

Type	*Hormonal derangement*	*Clinical manifestations*
Primary	Glucocorticoid deficiency	Weakness, anorexia, postural hypotension, hypoglycemia, dilutional hyponatremia, hypercalcemia,
	Mineralocorticoid deficiency	Hypotension, salt craving, hyponatremia, hyperkalemia
	ACTH excess	Pigmentation (see below)
	Adrenal androgen deficiency (in females)	Decreased libido, loss of secondary sexual hair, improvement in acne
Secondary	Glucocorticoid deficiency	*as above*
	Adrenal androgen deficiency (in females)	*as above*
	ACTH deficiency	Alabaster-like cutaneous pallor

at once present with Addisonian crisis (symptom complex due to acute adrenal deficiency).[3] The exact cause for such absence of hyperpigmentation is not clear. An intense rate of melanosome degradation in the secondary lysosomes (compound melanosomes) overwhelming the melanocyte stimulation by ACTH and α-MSH has been proposed by Kendereski et al.[8] (1999). Tarun et al.[9] (2012) found the coexistence of homozygous loss-of-function mutations in *MC1R/MC2R* in a case of familial glucocorticoid deficiency without pigmentation. Secondary adrenal insufficiency is characterized by a rather conspicuous "alabaster-like" pallor due to low ACTH levels.[7]

Box 2

Pattern of Addisonian hyperpigmentation

- Sun-exposed areas
- Pressure points (points of elbows, knees, waistline, underneath the brassiere straps)
- Darkening of the normally pigmented areas (nipples, areolae, axillae, groins, perineum and perianal regions)
- Darkening of pigmented lesions (e.g. café-au-lait spots)
- Scars
- Palmar creases
- Nails (longitudinal melanonychia)

Thyroid Diseases

Hyperthyroidism

A state of thyroid hormone excess (*thyrotoxicosis*) may be due to a hyperfunctioning thyroid gland (*hyperthyroidism*) or due to other causes. Most common cause of hyperthyroidism is Graves' disease (diffuse toxic goiter), an autoimmune disorder characterized by presence of circulating thyroid-stimulating immunoglobulins, e.g. the long-acting thyroid stimulator which bind to thyroid-stimulating hormone (TSH) receptors exerting agonistic effects. Other causes of hyperthyroidism include Plummer's disease (toxic multinodular goiter), pituitary adnoma and iatrogenic iodine excess (Jod-Basedow phenomenon). Some of the clinical manifestations **(Table 7)** are common to thyrotoxicosis due to any cause while some others like ophthalmopathy, thyroid acropachy and dermopathy are specific to Graves' disease.[3,10,11]

Pigmentary changes include facial and palmar erythema due to increased sympathetic activity, and hyperpigmentation, that is more conspicuous in dark skin, is possibly due to increased tyrosine and/or ACTH levels owing to accelerated cortisol metabolism, and hemosiderin deposition.[12-14] Hyperpigmentation of the eyelids (Jellinek's sign) has been described and vitiligo may also be seen as a coexisting autoimmune dermatosis.[3]

Table 7: Clinical manifestations of thyrotoxicosis

Symptoms	*Signs*	
	Extracutaneous	*Cutaneous*
Hyperactivity	Resting tremors	Soft, doughy and warm skin
Weight loss in spite of increased appetite	Sleeping tachycardia	Palmar and facial erythema[e,f]
Weakness	Lid lag[a]/retraction[b]	Pruritus
Heat intolerance	Ophthalmopathy (exophthalmos, conjunctival injection, periorbital edema)[c]	Hyperpigmentation
Insomnia, irritability	Thyroid acropachy[c,d]	Pretibial myxedema[c]
Amenorrhea		Thin sparse hair
Decreased libido		Plummer's nails[g]
		Alopecia areata[h], vitiligo[h]

[a]von Graefe's sign; [b]Dalrymple sign; [c]Signs specific to Graves' disease; [d]Clubbing of fingers and toes, associated with soft-tissue swelling and periosteal new bone formation in hands and feet; [e]facial suffusion may also be provoked by a substernal goiter (Pemberton sign); [f]Erythema with/without pruritus may be localized to the skin over the goiter (Maroni sign); [g]Koilonychia with onycholysis; [h]Associated autoimmune dermatoses. ***Also note:*** Pretibial myxedema, exophthalmos and acropachy are collectively known as ***Diamond's triad;*** a triad of **e**xophthalmos, pretibial **m**yxedema and hypertrophic **o**steoarthropathy is known as ***EMO syndrome***.

Hypothyroidism

Thyroid hormone deficiency, either due to decreased hormonal synthesis or resistance of the target tissue to thyroid hormones, affects women more than men. Autoimmune disorders and iatrogenic hypothyroidism are the most common among the acquired causes in nonendemic iodine-sufficient regions **(Table 8)**.[5,10]

The clinical manifestations **(Table 9)** are attributed to a hypometabolic state with reduced core body temperature, reflex cutaneous vasoconstriction, associated hyperlipidemia, and to the dermal mucin deposition (myxedema).[3,10,15]

Cutaneous pigmentary changes include a diffuse pallor **(Box 1)**, yellowish discoloration (see above), purplish lips, malar flush, melasma, and xanthomatosis secondary to hyperlipidemia.[3,5] Several cutaneous vascular phenomena like erythema ab igne,[16] cutis marmorata, purpura and punctate telangiectasia affecting the arms and finger tips are also seen producing pigmentary alterations of the skin. Persistent cutis marmorata beyond the neonatal period may be a marker of congenital hypothyroidism.[17] Purpura and ecchymoses are attributed to the loss of vasculature support secondary to dermal mucin deposition.[18] Vitiligo may coexist as an autoimmune disease.[3]

Table 8: Etiology of hypothyroidism

Primary	
Congenital	Glandular aplasia, dyshormonogenesis, TSH receptor mutation, endemic cretinism
Autoimmune	Hashimoto's thyroiditis, anti-TSH-receptor autoantibodies
Transient	De Quervain's thyroiditis, Sheehan syndrome
Iodine deficiency	Dietary deficiency in endemic areas (mountain regions)
Iatrogenic	Thyroidectomy, radiotherapy, radioiodine therapy
Infiltrative	Riedel's thyroiditis, amyloidosis, sarcoidosis
Secondary	
Pituitary	Hypopituitarism due to various causes
Hypothalamic	Tumors, infiltrations, infections
Iatrogenic	Bexarotene therapy

Abbreviation: TSH, thyroid-stimulating hormone

Diabetes Mellitus

The cutaneous manifestations of diabetes mellitus (DM) usually succeed the onset of DM, but may precede the onset of the disease as well.[19] The manifestation can be categorized into those due to the disease complications, those associated with DM, infections, and cutaneous complications of DM treatment **(Table 10)**.[19-21] In general, cutaneous infections are commonly seen in Type II DM while the cutaneous autoimmune conditions are associated with Type I DM.[22]

Cutaneous pigmentary changes can be due to the diabetic vasculopathy, associated autoimmune conditions, and as manifestations of hyperinsulinemia/insulin resistance **(Table 11)**.

Diabetic dermopathy (diabetic shin spots, pigmented pretibial papules) is the most common association with DM. It begins as multiple dull-red papules over the shins, forearms and other bony prominences that evolve into circumscribed areas of hyperpigmentation.[20] The color is due to the presence of hemosiderin-laden histiocytes.[23] Males are affected more often than females and there may be a correlation between diabetic dermopathy and internal complications of DM like nephropathy and retinopathy.[21,24] Diabetic dermopathy may also be associated with pigmented purpuric dermatosis. *Diabetic rubeosis (rubeosis faciei)* is characterized by a reddish complexion and is attributed to venous engorgement in the superficial dermal vessels as a result of decreased vascular tone or microangiopathy.[19] *Periungual telangiectasiae* occur in about 49% of cases that are attributed to loss of capillary loops with compensatory dilatation of the remaining ones. These are often accompanied by nail fold erythema, finger tip tenderness and ragged cuticles.[25] Well-demarcated *erysipelas-like erythema* may be seen over the legs which may be accompanied by underlying bony destruction due to vascular insufficiency. It is usually seen in elderly diabetics with long-standing disease.[21] Non-enzymatic glycosylation of dermal collagen and nail bed tissue has been proposed to be the cause for the *yellowish hue to skin and nails (distal end of the toe nail)* that may be seen in about 2–5% of patients.[19,25]

PIGMENTARY DERANGEMENTS IN METABOLIC DISORDERS

Porphyrias

Porphyrias are a group of inherited metabolic disorders (except for porphyria cutanea tarda), each occurring due to deficiency of a specific enzyme involved in the heme biosynthetic pathway **(Flow chart 1)**. The clinical manifestations are secondary to the accumulation of porphyrins or porphyrin precursors in the concerned tissues and based on the manifestations, porphyrias can be grouped into acute (acute intermittent porphyria) and cutaneous porphyrias [porphyria cutanea tarda (PCT), congenital erythropoietic porphyria (CEP)]. Hereditary coproporphyria and variegate porphyria present with both cutaneous features and acute neurovisceral episodes. The cutaneous manifestations of porphyria are attributed to the phototoxic properties of the porphyrins that accumulate in the skin **(Table 12)**.[21,26,27]

Table 9: Clinical manifestations of hypothyroidism

Cutaneous features	*Extracutaneous features*	*Associated diseases*
Pale, cold, xerotic skin	Weakness	***Autoimmune:*** Pernicious anemia, vitiligo, alopecia areata, autoimmune polyglandular syndromes I–III
Hypohidrosis	Cold intolerance	***Endocrinopathies:*** Diabetes mellitus, Addison's disease, acanthosis nigricans with insulin resistance
Pigmentary changes (see text)	Weight gain despite reduced appetite	***Connective tissue diseases:*** Lupus erythematosus, scleroderma, dermatomyositis, polymyositis, Sjögren's syndrome
Myxedema (puffiness of face anc extremities)	Constipation	***Others:*** Cowden syndrome, atopic dermatitis, chronic urticaria, palmoplantar pustulosis, Crow-Fukase syndrome, granuloma annulare
Thin, brittle and slow-growing nails	Menorrhagia and infertility	
Sparse, thin hair (may progress to diffuse alopecia)	Anemia and hyperlipidemia	
Macroglossia	Poor concentration and decreased libido	
Gingival swelling (in cretinism)	Carpal tunnel syndrome	

Table 10: Cutaneous manifestations of diabetes mellitus

Manifestations of diabetic vasculopathy	Diabetic wet gangrene, reactive perforating collagenosis, necrobiosis lipoidica, pigmentary changes (see text and Table 11), nail changes (Beau's lines, splinter hemorrhages, yellowish discoloration)
Manifestations of diabetic neuropathy	Bullous diabeticorum, non-healing ulcers, paresthesiae, hypohidrosis with compensatory hyperhidrosis
Infections	Staphylococcal infections (furuncle, carbuncle); streptococcal (erysipelas, cellulitis); invasive pseudomonal (malignant otitis externa); candidal (vulvovaginitis, balanoposthitis); deep fungal infections (mucormycosis)
DM associated dermatoses	Granuloma annulare, scleredema (type II), acrochordons, xanthomatosis, acanthosis nigricans
DM associated autoimmune diseases	Vitiligo, lichen planus (Grispan syndrome)
Manifestations of diabetic treatment	Sulfonylureas related (maculopapular rash, urticaria, photosensitivity, lichenoid reactions); localized reactions to insulin (lipodystrophy) and insulin hypersensitivity
Others	Hemochromatosis, xerosis, pruritus, diabetic thick skin, Huntley's papules (pebbling on or around the knuckles)

Table 11: Cutaneous pigmentary alterations in diabetes mellitus

Manifestations of diabetic vasculopathy	Diabetic shin spots, diabetic rubeosis, pigmented purpuric dermatosis, palmar erythema, periungual telangiectasia, erysipelas-like erythema
Manifestations of hyperinsulinemia	Acanthosis nigricans
Associated autoimmune disease	Vitiligo
Others	Yellowish skin and nails

Flow chart 1: The heme biosynthetic pathway, enzymes involved and their deficiency porphyrias

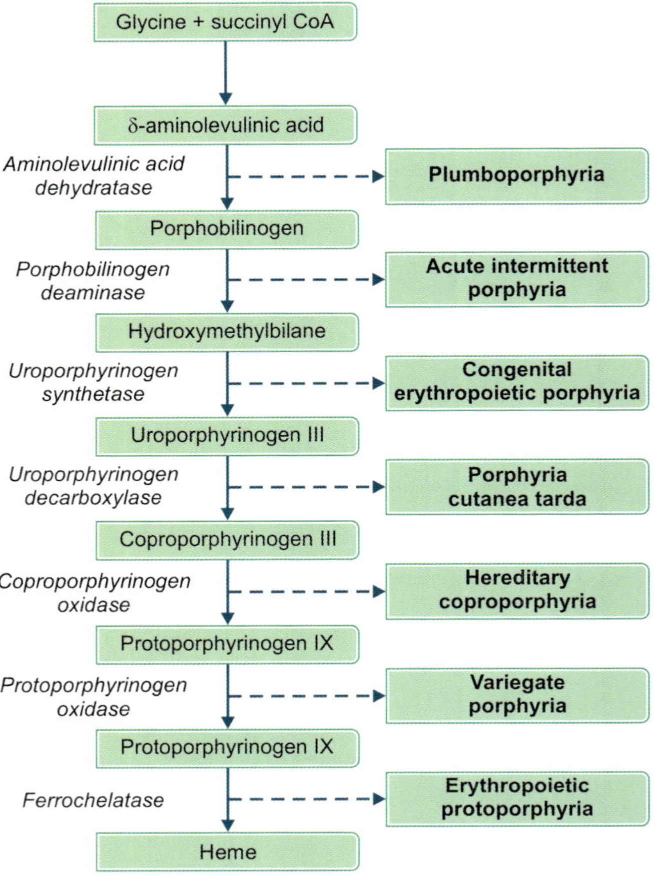

Cutaneous pigmentary alterations in PCT include hyperpigmentation, a purplish facial erythema and hair darkening. The hyperpigmentation is usually melasma-like involving the centrofacial region and may also be accompanied by hypopigmentation in a mottled pattern. A rather conspicuous purplish-red erythema involving the central part of the face particularly around the eyes may accompany the melasma-like hyperpigmentation.[28] Shafralli et al (2002) observed darkening of previously gray hair in two patients of PCT.[29]

Apart from the pathognomonic staining of the deciduous and permanent teeth (erythrodontia), a patchy hypo- and hyperpigmentation of sun-exposed body parts is the other pigmentary change observed in CEP.[28]

Amyloidosis

Amyloidosis refers to extracellular deposition of an insoluble amorphous, misfolded, fibrillar proteinaceous material (amyloid) in the tissues and organs leading to their functional impairment and morbidity. Based on the origin, type of amyloid deposit, and extent of tissue affection, amyloidosis can be classified as described in **Table 13.**[21,30-32]

Among the systemic amyloidoses, specific cutaneous pigmentary changes occur in primary systemic amyloidosis. Some of the familial amyloidoses, and rarely hemodialysis associated amyloidosis are also associated with pigmentary changes **(Table 14)**.[21]

Purpura and ecchymoses, presenting as pigmentary changes, are the most common cutaneous manifestations of primary systemic amyloidosis. Capillary fragility due to amyloid infiltration into the vessels and clotting factor X deficiency are the underlying causes of purpura and ecchymoses. Clotting factor X deficiency may be both quantitative (reduced synthesis by liver secondary to hepatic amyloidosis) and qualitative (binding of amyloid to factor X and rendering it nonfunctional).[31] Periorbital ("raccoon" eyes), flexural and the anogenital regions are frequently affected. Rupture of the fragile capillaries may be precipitated by trauma (pinch purpura), and maneuvers that increase intravascular pressure like Valsalva maneuver, rectal biopsy or proctoscopy (post-proctoscopic palpable purpura). Other pigmentary changes include pallor (due to anemia), icterus (due to hepatic involvement) and hyperpigmentation (secondary to hemorrhage and cardiac failure).[21]

Lysosomal Storage Disorders

Lysosomal storage disorders are an inherited group of disorders characterized by deficiency of lysosomal hydrolases and accumulation of the respective compounds in the lysosomes leading to progressive multisystem disease. Among the various lysosomal storage disorders, mucopolysaccharidoses (MPS), sphingolipidoses and glyco-proteinoses are of dermatological significance.

Mucopolysaccharidoses are autosomal recessive disorders (except Hunter's syndrome which is X-linked) characterized by deficiency of lysosomal enzymes that degrade the glycosaminoglycans which are the components of connective tissue protoglycans leading to their accumulation (mainly dermatan sulfate, keratin sulfate and heparan sulfate). Dermatological manifestations common to all the MPS include thick coarse skin and lips, hypertrichosis, and macroglossia. Specific cutaneous pigmentary disorders include the ivory-white reticulate pebbling of Hunter syndrome that involves the region between the posterior axillary line and angle of scapula bilaterally,[33] and the Mongolian spots of Hurler (and Hunter) syndrome that fade away more gradually than in the normal population and involving extrasacral regions like upper back, trunk and limbs.[21]

The principal dermatological manifestation of the sphingolipidoses (Fabry's disease being the prototype) and some of the glycoproteinoses is the angiokeratomas, whose onset and extent of involvement differs in different disorders. The Mongolian spots, as described above, have also been reported in some of the sphingolipidoses like GM1-gangliosidosis and Niemann-Pick disease. Other cutaneous

Table 12: The porphyrias

Porphyria	*Inheritance*	*Enzyme deficiency*	*Clinical features*	
			Systemic	*Cutaneous*
Acute intermittent porphyria (AIP)	Autosomal dominant	Porphobilinogen deaminase	Acute and relapsing neuropsychiatric symptoms like abdominal pain, constipation, vomiting, and autonomic neuropathy (tachycardia, hypertension, paralytic ileus). Respiratory failure is the most common cause of death	—
Congenital erythropoietic porphyria	Autosomal recessive	Uroporphyrinogen synthetase	—	Early onset recurrent cutaneous phototoxic reactions like erythema, blistering, skin fragility with consequent scarring, sclerodactyly, mutilation and pigmentary changes
Porphyria cutanea tarda (PCT)	Sporadic	Uroporphyrinogen decarboxylase	—	Late onset skin fragility, milia, scarring and mottled pigmentation
Hereditary coproporphyria	Autosomal dominant	Coproporphyrinogen oxidase	Systemic features are similar to AIP and seen in 10–20% of cases	Similar to PCT
Variegate porphyria	Autosomal dominant	Protoporphyrinogen oxidase	Similar to PCT	Cutaneous features are similar to PCT and seen in about 17% of cases
Erythropoietic protoporphyria	Autosomal recessive	Ferrochelatase	—	Edema on sun exposure, purpura, crusting, vesicles and chronic complications like scarring and sclerotic changes

pigmentary alterations described in sphingolipidoses include yellow-brown pigmentation, petechiae and purpura (Gaucher's disease, Niemann-Pick disease), xanthomas and café-au-lait macules (Niemann-Pick disease).[21]

Dyslipidemias

Primary dyslipidemias are a heterogeneous group of disorders of lipid and lipoprotein metabolism. Diabetes, hypothyroidism, renal failure, drugs (retinoids, protease inhibitors and hormonal contraceptives) and hepatic disease may cause disordered lipid metabolism secondarily. Most of the dyslipidemias are associated with atherosclerosis and cardiovascular complications. Dermatologically, yellowish subcutaneous lipid deposits—the xanthomata **(Table 15)**, are the principal manifestations that are morphologically specific to individual dyslipidemias and possibly have correlation with systemic affections **(Table 16)**.[21,34]

Disorders of Amino Acid Metabolism

Phenylketonuria

Phenylketonuria (PKU) is a rare inherited disorder due to deficiency of phenylalanine hydroxylase (PAH) leading to defective hydroxylation of phenylalanine to tyrosine with consequent accumulation of the former which has pathogenic effects. The principal manifestations of PKU are neurological, characterized by developmental delay, mental retardation, seizures and extrapyramidal symptoms which directly correlate the brain phelylalanine levels. Owing to the impaired melanin synthesis, most of the patients have fair skin and hair. Other dermatological manifestations include sclerodermoid changes, recurrent pyodermas and eczema. Early diagnosis and reducing dietary phenylalanine may prevent neurological damage.[21]

Alkaptonuria

Alkaptonuria is a rare autosomal recessive disease due to deficiency of homogentisic oxidase leading to the accumulation of homogentisic acid (an intermediated product of phenylalanine and tyrosine catabolism) in various tissues. The chronological sequence of clinical manifestations in this disease is: alkaptonuria (homogentisic acid in urine), ochronosis (brownish-black dyspigmentation of tissues) and ochronotic arthropathy (mainly spondyloarthropathy). Prognostically, alkaptonuria is considerd to be a benign degenerative disease that insignificantly affects normal life expectancy.

Table 13: Amyloidosis: classification and cutaneous manifestations

	Amyloid deposit	*Origin of amyloid*	*Associated disorders/ clinical features*	*Cutaneous manifestations*	
Systemic					
Primary systemic	AL	From excessively produced Ig light chains proteins	Monoclonal B-cell dyscrasias (occult or overt)	• Smooth waxy papules on face, neck and anogenital regions (amyloid deposits). • Macroglossia, nail dystrophy and alopecia • Purpura/ecchymoses and pigmentary changes (see below)	
Secondary systemic	AA	From SAA, an acute phase protein	Chronic inflammatory diseases	—	
Hemodialysis associated	Aβ2M	From β2-M, the invariant chain of class I MHC antigens	Chronic renal failure	Sacral subcutaneous or pedunculated nodules, lichenoid papules and pigmentary changes	
Familial	Familial Mediterranean fever	AA	Same as AA	Intermittent fever, serositis, renal amyloidosis Purpuric, urticarial and vasculitic lesions	
	Muckle-Wells syndrome	AA	Same as AA	Periodic fever, arthropathy, progressive nerve deafness, renal amyloidosis Urticarial lesions and pigmentary changes	
	Heredofamilial amyloid polyneuropathy	ATTR	From mutated plasma protein TTR	Progressive peripheral sensory and motor neuropathy, autonomic neuropathy (diarrhea, orthostatic hypotension), cardiomyopathy and renal amyloidosis	• Trophic ulcers, sweat disturbance • Blepharochalasis and cutis laxa
Localized					
CNS (Alzheimer's disease)		Aβ	Ig light chains produced by locally proliferating monoclonal plasma cells		—
Cutaneous		AL			Macular, lichen, biphasic and tumid amyloidoses, and other types (concha, vitiliginous and poikilodermatous)
Ocular		AL			—
Respiratory		AL			—
Urogenital		AL			—

Abbreviations: Ig, immunoglobulin: MHC, major histocompatibility complex; SAA, serum amyloid A; β2-M, β2-microglobulin; TTR, transthyretin

The hallmark cutaneous feature is the blue-black hyperpigmentation involving the pinna, medial sclera (Osler's sign), and extensor tendons of the forearms (the pigmentation being conspicuous over the knuckles). Pigmentation of the temples and malar area, buccal mucosa and larynx are also noted. The pigmentation begins about the 4th decade involving the auricular pinna initially with subsequent affection of other structures. It is attributed to the accumulation of oxidized homogentisic acid preferentially in the fibrous and cartilaginous tissues.[21]

Table 14: Cutaneous pigmentary alterations in systemic amyloidoses	
Primary systemic amyloidosis	Purpura and ecchymoses Pallor Icterus Hyperpigmentation
Familial Mediterranean fever	Erysipelas-like erythema of the extremities Purpura
Muckle-Wells syndrome	Hyperpigmented sclerodermoid changes
Heredofamilial amyloid polyneuropathy	Lichen amyloidosis

PIGMENTARY DERANGEMENTS IN NUTRITIONAL DISORDERS

Protein-energy Malnutrition

Protein-energy malnutrition (PEM) is the result of inadequate dietary intakes of protein and energy. The "inadequate intake" may reflect the actual decreased intake that is less than that required for normal growth and development, or the greater need than that required for a particular age and sex. Severe PEM present in one of the three forms—marasmus, kwashiorkor, or marasmic kwashiorkor. In marasmus (nonedematous PEM), there is a severe deficiency of both protein and calories so that the patient appears emaciated. In

Table 15: The xanthomata

Xanthomata		*Clinical characteristics*
Eruptive xanthoma		Small yellowish papules concentrated over the extensors, chiefly over the back, buttocks and limbs associated with severe hypertriglyceridemia
Tendon xanthoma		Cholesterol accumulation deep within the tendons produces subcutaneous masses mainly involving the Achilles and knuckle. The overlying skin may appear normal
Tuberous xanthoma		Large exophytic lesions over the pressure points
Planar xanthoma	Xanthelasma	Yellowish plaques involving the upper eyelids near the inner canthus
	Intertriginous	Yellowish macules, papules and plaques over the intertriginous areas
	Palmar	Yellowish plaques involving the palms

Table 16: Classification of primary dyslipidemias with associated xanthomata

*Type**	*Dyslipidemia*	*Lipid derangements*	*Xanthoma*	*Systemic affections*
I	Familial hyperchylomicronemia	↑ Tgs	Eruptive xanthoma	Increased risk of acute pancreatitis, lipemia retinalis
IIa	Familial hypercholesterolemia	↑ TC ↑ LDL-C	Tendon, tuberous and planar (xanthelasma and intertriginous) xanthomata	Coronary heart disease and other atherosclerotic vascular diseases
IIb	Familial combined hypercholesterolemia	↑ LDL-C	As in IIa, but rarely seen	Coronary heart disease and other atherosclerotic vascular diseases
III	Familial dysbetalipoproteinemia	↑ TC	Tuberous, tuberoeruptive and planar xanthomata	Coronary and peripheral arterial diseases
IV	Familial hypertriglyceridemia	↑ Tgs**	Eruptive xanthomas, but rarely seen	Lifestyle modification reduces cardiovascular morbidity
V	Mixed hyperlipidemia	↑ TC	Eruptive xanthomas	Coronary and peripheral arterial diseases, potential risk of acute pancreatitis

*Fredrickson types; **with or without reduced high density lipoprotein-cholesterol; ↑, raised.
Abbreviations: Tgs, triglycerides; TC, total cholesterol; LDL-C, low density lipoprotein-cholesterol

Kwashiorkor (edematous PEM) however protein deficiency is relatively more than that of calories and hence patients are edematous that masks underlying wasting. Marasmic kwashiorkor has the attributes of both edematous and nonedematous PEM.[35]

Cutaneous pigmentary alterations are seen in severe form of kwashiorkor characterized by initial reddish lesions that later become purplish and exfoliate giving a "flaky paint" appearance. Hair changes include alternating bands of normal and light color (flag sign) and premature graying giving the scalp a "salt and pepper" appearance. Other pigmentary changes include hypopigmentation secondary to phenylalanine deficiency and patchy postinflammatory hyperpigmentation.[21,35]

Vitamin Deficiency

Mucocutaneous pigmentary changes are predominantly seen in cyanocobalamin (vitamin B_{12}) and folic acid deficiency. Hyperpigmentation involving the knuckles and palmar creases along with an enlarged red tongue is typical of cyanocobalamin deficiency. Similar kind of pigmentation affecting the sun-exposed areas has been observed in folic acid deficiency.

Vitamin C deficiency (scurvy) is associated with perifollicular hemorrhage and later pigmentation affecting the legs. The affected follicles show cork-screw hairs. Other manifestations include bleeding gums and occasionally large ecchymoses into the skin.

Vitamin K deficiency, although primarily rare, may be associated with chronic liver diseases and can manifest as cutaneous hemorrhage (petechiae and ecchymoses).[3,21]

PIGMENTARY DERANGEMENTS IN GASTROINTESTINAL DISORDERS

Malabsorption

Malabsorption is defined as diminished gastrointestinal absorption of one or more nutrients that is, in most of the cases, associated with steatorrohea (an increase in stool fat excretion of >6% of dietary fat intake). The causes of malabsorption are myriad **(Table 17)**.[36]

Cutaneous manifestations consequent to nutritional deficiency as a result of malabsorption can be grouped into nonspecific (pruritus, ichthyosis, pigmentary changes, etc.) and the ones associated with specific nutrient deficiency (follicular keratoses, bleeding diathesis, glossitis and acrodermatitis-enteropathica like eruption secondary to vitamin A, C, B-complex and zinc deficiencies respectively). The pigmentary changes are characterized by diffuse melanosis, and/or pallor due to anemia.[21]

Table 17: Some causes of malabsorption

Gastrointestinal	Crohn's disease, celiac disease, Whipple's disease, tropical sprue, mastocytosis, scleroderma, infections
Hepatobiliary	Obstructive jaundice, liver cirrhosis
Pancreatic	Chronic pancreatitis, cystic fibrosis
Endocrine and metabolic	Diabetes, hypoparathyroidism, adrenal insufficiency, hyperthyroidism, carcinoid syndrome
Genetic disorders	Disaccharidase deficiency, agammaglobulinemia, abetalipoproteinemia, Hartnup's disease, acrodermatitis enteropathica, pernicious anemia
Drugs	Chelating agents, bile sequestrants
Surgery	Gastrectomy, ileal resection

Intestinal Polyposis Syndromes

These are a group of familial syndromes that are characterized by intestinal hamartomatous or premalignant intestinal polyps that are associated with cutaneous hamartomas and in some instances, pigmentary lesions. The genetic defect in most of these syndromes is mutation in genes involved in tumor suppression. In some of these syndromes patients are also predisposed to extracutaneous nonalimentary malignancies **(Table 18)**.[3,37]

PIGMENTARY DERANGEMENTS IN HEPATOBILIARY DISORDERS

Inherited Liver Diseases Associated with Cutaneous Pigmentary Changes

Hemochromatosis

Hemochromatosis is an inherited disorder characterized by dysregulated intestinal iron absorption with consequent deposition of the same in various tissues of the body leading to their damage and functional impairment. In most of the cases there is an autosomal recessively inherited mutation in the *HFE* gene that possibly interacts with transferrin receptors in the basolateral membrane of intestinal epithelium and regulates the amount of transferrin-mediated iron absorption. Deficiency of functional *HFE* leads to up-regulation of enterocyte iron-specific divalent metal transporters and excessive iron absorption. Cutaneous pigmentation, diabetes (bronze diabetes) and hepatic cirrhosis are the cardinal

Table 18: Intestinal polyposis syndromes associated with cutaneous pigmentary alterations

Syndromes	*Inheritance and gene affected*	*Gastrointestinal polyposis*	*Cutaneous manifestations*	*Extracutaneous manifestations*
Peutz-Jeghers syndrome	Autosomal dominant *STK11/LKB1* gene	Hamartomatous polyps predominantly involving the small intestine manifest as pain abdomen, malena or intussusception	Lentiginosis involving the perioral, periorbital regions and conspicuously over the lips and buccal mucosa. Penile/vulval lentigens may also be seen. These are often present at birth or in early infancy	Adenocarcinoma of gastrointestinal tract and breast; uterine, cervical, pancreatic and gonadal malignancies occur with greater incidence compared to general population
Turcot syndrome	Autosomal dominant Mutation in APC or one of the mismatch repair genes	Adenomatous colorectal polyps do not exceed 100 in number but are larger and malignant change occurs 1–3 decades earlier than in familial polyposis coli	Café-au-lait macules, axillary freckling have been reported in some cases	Medulloblastomas and glioblastoma multiforme
Bannayan-Riley-Ruvalcaba syndrome	Autosomal dominant *PTEN* gene	Hamartomatous gastrointestinal polyps leading to chronic anemia, diarrhea, failure to thrive or small intestinal intussusception	Penile lentiginosis, hemangiomas, vascular malformations, subcutaneous lipomas	Macrocephaly, thyroid anomalies, joint hyperextensibility, scoliosis, pectus excavatum, and down slanting palpebral fissures
Cronkhite-Canada syndrome	Sporadic Cause unknown	Polyposis may involve entire gastrointestinal tract and carry 15% risk of cancer development commonly involving the sigmoid colon and rectum	Melanotic macules over the fingers, widespread uniform hyperpigmentation, alopecia and nail dystrophy	Hypogeusia is the initial symptom followed by diarrhea (leading to protein-losing enteropathy) and ectodermal changes

manifestations. Patients are at increased risk of hepatocellular carcinoma.[38]

Although deposition of iron can be demonstrated in the skin, the hyperpigmentation, however, is the result of excess melanin. The pigmentation initially begins in the sun-exposed areas but later may become diffuse and become more pronounced on the face, genitalia and body folds. It may be associated with oral mucosal pigmentation in 15–20% of the cases. The pigmentation is accompanied by a dry ichthyotic skin.[3,39]

Wilson's Disease

Wilson's disease (hepatolenticular degeneration) is a rare autosomal recessive disease due to mutation in *ATP7B* gene that encodes a membrane-bound copper transporting ATPase. In Wilson's disease there is an impaired biliary copper excretion and its accumulation predominantly in the liver, basal ganglia, eyes, kidneys and skeleton. The predominant features of Wilson's disease are recurrent episodes of hepatitis, neurological features, renal tubular defects and osteoporosis. The hepatitis episodes begin early in life and may eventually lead to cirrhosis. The neurological features begin at about the adolescent period and are characterized by extrapyramidal symptoms.[3,38]

Kayser-Fleischer rings, characterized by greenish discoloration of the corneal margins (due to copper deposits) are an important clinical finding seen in about 60% of cases. They eventually disappear with treatment.[38]

Cutaneous Pigmentary Changes in Chronic Liver Disease

Chronic liver diseases produce a multitude of cutaneous manifestations among which the pigmentary alterations are characteristic. These include icterus chacterized yellowish discoloration that first appears over the sclera and soft palate and later becomes generalized in proportion to the hyperbilirubinemia. It may be associated with greenish gingivae as well. A muddy gray hyperpigmentation, most prominent over the sun-exposed areas is seen in chronic hepatic disease of any cause and is attributed to increased melanin production. The pigmentation may be diffuse, blotchy, or freckle-like involving the face and palmar creases. In advanced cirrhosis males develop hypogonadism and gynecomastia which may be associated with hyperpigmented areolae. Abdominal striae similar to those seen in Cushing's syndrome (see above) may develop due to impaired hepatic metabolism of glucocorticoids.[3]

Various cutaneous vascular phenomena presenting as cutaneous pigmentary changes are also seen that include palmar erythema, spider angiomas and telangiectasia. These are attributed to hyperestrogenemia (due to impaired hepatic metabolism of estrogen), altered central vasomotor control and alcohol-induced vasodilatation. Associated vitamin C and K deficiency may produce purpura and ecchymotic lesions.[40]

Pigmentary nail changes include the Terry's nails, characterized by a proximal white and distal pink color, and a red lunula. Transverse white bands (Muehrcke's lines) due to associated hypoalbuminemia may also be seen.[3]

PIGMENTARY DERANGEMENTS IN PANCREATIC DISORDERS

Acute Pancreatitis

Severe acute necrotizing pancreatitis may be associated with retroperitoneal hemorrhage and tracking of the hemorrhagic fluid into the subcutaneous space produce cutaneous discoloration at four well-recognized sites: bluish purple discoloration of the flanks (Grey Turner sign), periumbilical bluish discoloration (Cullen's sign), and bluish-black discoloration over the upper thigh (Fox's sign) and of the scrotum (Bryant's sign or blue scrotum sign). Livedo reticularis may also be seen to be associated with both acute and chronic pancreatitis (Walzel's sign).[3]

Necrolytic Migratory Erythema

Necrolytic migratory erythema (NME) is a specific cutaneous manifestation of hyperglucagonemia, usually due to a glucagonoma (pancreatic α-cell tumor). NME is characterized by an initial faint erythematous macule that extends to form large erosive erythematous patch which may be studded with vesicles and bullae. As the lesion matures, a central postinflammatory hyperpigmentation associated with crusting of the margins are seen. Most commonly the lower abdomen, groins, upper thighs and the gluteal regions are involved. Females in fifth to sixth decade are affected frequently and have associated features like weight loss, loss of appetite, hyperglycemia, angular cheilitis and a beefy-red glossitis.[3]

PIGMENTARY DERANGEMENTS IN RENAL DISORDERS

Nephrocutaneous Syndromes

Many inherited syndromes involve the kidney and skin. Dermatological manifestations in some of them are pigmentary lesions that serve as clues to the diagnosis of the syndrome. **Table 19** outlines such nephrocutaneous syndromes in which the principal dermatological features the pigmentary lesions.

Table 19: Nephrocutaneous syndromes

Syndrome	*Renal manifestations*	*Cutaneous pigmentary lesions*
Neurofibromatosis	Renovascular hypertension	Café-au-lait macules, axillary freckling, Lisch nodules (pigmented iris hamartomas)
Tuberous sclerosis complex	Angiomyolipoma, renal cysts	Ash leaf macules, pretibial confetti macules, poliosis
Von Hippel Lindau syndrome	Renal cell carcinoma	Café-au-lait macules, hemangiomas
Nail-patella syndrome	Glomerulonephritis, predisposition to develop hemolytic uremic syndrome	Triangular lunulae, heterochromia of iris, Lester iris (hyperpigmentation of the pupillary margin of the iris)
Primary systemic amyloidosis	Kidneys are involved in up to 80% of the cases. Proteinuria, hypoalbuminemia and azotemia are the complications	*See Table 13*
Familial amyloidoses		See above
Henoch–Schönlein purpura	Glomerulonephritis	Palpable purpura
Wegener's granulomatosis	Glomerulonephritis	Palpable purpura, petechiae, strawberry gingivae

Cutaneous Pigmentary Changes Seen in Chronic Renal Failure and Dialysis

Patients with chronic renal failure (CRF) and those on dialysis demonstrate a variety of cutaneous pigmentary changes. Pallor of the skin due to decreased hematopoiesis and increased hemolysis is the earliest and the most common finding. A muddy brown hyperpigmentation of the sun-exposed areas, as a result of altered renal metabolism of β-MSH, and yellowish discoloration due to carotenemia and excess urochromes in the dermis are other pigmentary changes. Hypopigmentation of the skin and hair has been described as a paradoxical phenomenon as well and has been attributed to altered phenylalanine metabolism generating tyrosinase inhibiting metabolites.[41] The uremic frosting, due to accumulation of urea in the skin is rarely seen now-a-days.

Pigmentary nail changes include the half and half nails characterized by a proximal white zone and distal (20–60%) brownish sharp demarcation seen in about 10% or the CRF cases.

A recently described, rather specific cutaneous change associated with dialysis and some CRF patients is the nephrogenic systemic fibrosis (NSF). Indurated erythematous or yellowish plaques with characteristic pseudopodal extension into adjacent skin are the typical lesions. There may be associated internal organ involvement (hence called NSF) which accounts for increased mortality.[3]

PIGMENTARY DERANGEMENTS IN CARDIAC DISORDERS

Cutaneous lesions associated with cardiac diseases may be grouped into those as the consequences of cardiac diseases itself or conditions in which both the skin and heart are involved.

Cutaneous Pigmentary Alterations as Manifestations of the Heart Diseases

Cyanosis

Cyanosis refers to the bluish discoloration of the skin and mucous membranes as a result of increased quantity of reduced hemoglobin in the blood. Cyanosis appears most prominent over the lips, nail beds, earlobes, and malar eminence and is classified into central and peripheral cyanosis. The central cyanosis is due to presence of desaturated blood in the circulation whereas peripheral cyanosis is the result of sluggish blood flow through the constricted vessels that results in excessive extraction of the oxygen by the tissues from a normally saturated blood. Cardiac causes of central cyanosis include the congenital cyanotic heart diseases (e.g. transposition of great vessels, Fallot's tetralogy, etc) and that of peripheral cyanosis is the congestive cardiac failure.[42,43]

Erythremia

Patients with long-standing congestive heart failure often develop secondary polycythemia that imparts a "ruddy" complexion to the skin. Some patients develop a rather characteristic color change termed as "erythremia" wherein a combination of cyanosis with erythema is seen. The redness is due to excess hemoglobin and the cyanosis due to impaired saturation of this excessively produced hemoglobin. Erythremia is most obvious on lips, ear lobes, finger tips, tongue and conjunctiva. Absence of digital clubbing differentiates such pigmentary manifestation of secondary polycythemia from polycythemia vera.[44]

Cardiocutaneous Syndromes

Skin and the heart are involved in a host of inherited syndromes and systemic diseases. This section briefly outlines such cardiocutaneous conditions in which pigmentary skin lesions are associated with cardiac abnormalities **(Table 20)**.

Cutaneous Pigmentary Changes Associated with Cardiac Implants

Pallor due to anemia induced by mechanical destruction of the red blood cells by metallic prosthetic aortic valves has been described. A persistent reticulate telangiectatic erythema overlying the cardiac pacemakers and cardioverter defibrillator has been reported.

PIGMENTARY DERANGEMENTS IN DISORDERS OF THE RESPIRATORY SYSTEM

Central cyanosis is commonly associated with impaired pulmonary function. It may occur in an acute manner as in extensive pneumonia and pulmonary edema, or insidiously as in chronic obstructive pulmonary diseases (chronic bronchitis and emphysema). Cyanosis in these situations is the result of pulmonary perfusion through unventilated or poorly ventilated areas of the lungs. Other causes of central cyanosis include pulmonary arteriovenous fistula and cyanotic congenital heart diseases as discussed above.[42]

Skin and respiratory system involvement is seen in various inherited syndromes and other diseases. **Table 21** highlights such conditions with pulmonary abnormalities that are associated with pigmentary skin lesions.

Table 20: Cardiocutaneous syndromes

	Syndrome	*Cardiac manifestations*	*Cutaneous pigmentary lesions*
Inherited syndromes	LEOPARD syndrome	Hypertrophic cardiomyopathy, pulmonary stenosis, heart blocks	Lentigines: present at birth and increase in number until puberty, common over the neck and upper trunk
	NAME syndrome*	Atrial myxomas	Freckles and nevi
	LAMB syndrome*	Atrial myxomas	Lentigines, blue nevi
	Danoff syndrome*	Atrial myxomas	Lentigines
	POEMS syndrome	Cardiac failure	Hyperpigmentation (diffuse or speckled), hemangiomas
	Tuberous sclerosis	Cardiac rhabdomyomas	Ash leaf and pretibial confetti macules
	Incontinentia pigmenti	Patent ductus arteriosus, tricuspid insufficiency	Linear or whorled hyperpigmentation along the Blaschko's lines follow the vesicular and verrucous stages. The hyperpigmentation may be replaced by hypomelanosis as a fourth stage in some
	Pseudoxanthoma elasticum	Mitral valve prolapsed, angina, coronary stenosis, congestive heart failure	Yellowish confluent papules over the redundant skin on the neck, axillae and other flexures giving "plucked chicken skin" appearance
	Cornelia de Lange's syndrome	Septal defects, persistent ductus arteriosus, pulmonary stenosis	Persistent cutis marmorata and periorbital and perinasal cyanosis
Chromosomal syndromes	Down syndrome	Atrioventricular septal defect due to endocardial cushion defect is considered to be pathognomonic and its incidence is 1000-folds higher in Down's syndrome compared to normal population	Cutis marmorata, livedo reticularis and acrocyanosis due to impaired peripheral circulation
Collagen vascular diseases	Systemic sclerosis	Pericarditis, myocarditis, arrhythmias and heart failure	Hypopigmented patches with perifollicular retained pigmentation giving a "salt and pepper" appearance is the most common pigmentary change. Others include Addisonian- and acanthosis nigricans-like patterns.
	Systemic lupus erythematosus (SLE)	Libman-Sachs endocarditis is a specific cardiac manifestation in SLE. Others include conduction defects, myocarditis, pericarditis and coronary artery diseases	Malar erythema and photosensitive rash
	Dermatomyositis	Myocarditis, myocardial fibrosis, conduction defects and cardiac failure occur in about one-third of cases	Lilac colored rash over the face (heliotrope rash), Violaceous papules over the knuckles (Gottron's papules), erythema over the shoulders and upper back (Shawl's sign), hyperkeratosis and hyperpigmentation over the radial side of the fingers and thumbs (mechanics' hands)

Contd...

Contd...

	Syndrome	*Cardiac manifestations*	*Cutaneous pigmentary lesions*
Metabolic disorders	Hemochromatosis	Cardiomegaly, congestive heart failure, superventricular arrhythmia, and myocardial infarction can occur in about 15% of the cases	*See above*
	Amyloidosis	Cardiac involvement is seen in primary systemic and some of the familial amyloidoses. Arrhythmias and heart blocks are common	*See Table 13*
Infectious diseases	Infective endocarditis	Vegetations over the valve leaflets leading to their incompetence	Petechiae over the conjunctiva, palate and buccal mucosa; tender red papules over the finger and toe pads (Osler's nodes); tender erythema over the thenar and hypothenar eminences (Janeway lesions); splinter hemorrhages involving the nail beds
	Rheumatic fever	Valvular disease, pericarditis, myocarditis and congestive cardiac failure	Erythema marginatum: evanescent patchy erythema over the trunk. Successive crops may occur over few weeks that tend to be more prominent in the afternoon
	Kawasaki disease	Coronary artery aneurysm, myocarditis and conduction defects	Conjunctiva injection and red tongue with prominent papillae (strawberry tongue) follow the initial febrile stage. A morbilliform exanthema follows the second stage.

*NAME, LAMB and Danoff syndromes are collectively grouped under Careny complex

Abbreviations: LEOPARD: **l**entigines **e**lectrocardiogram anomalies, **o**cular anomalies, **p**ulmonary stenosis, **a**bnormal genitalia, **r**etardation of growth and **d**eafness; NAME: **n**evi, **a**trial myxoma, **m**yxoid neurofibroma, **e**phelides; LAMB: **l**entigines, **a**trial **m**yxoma, **b**lue nevi; POEMS: **p**olyneuropathy, **o**rganomegaly, **e**ndocrinopathy, **m**onoclonal gammopathy, **s**kin manifestations

Table 21: Conditions involving respiratory system and the skin

Syndrome	*Pulmonary manifestations*	*Cutaneous pigmentary lesions*
Tuberous sclerosis	Pulmonary lymphangioleiomyomatosis	Ash leaf and pretibial confetti macules
Amyloidosis	Amyloid infiltrates in primary systemic form and secondary amyloid deposition in chronic lung diseases	*See above*
Yellow nail syndrome	Recurrent pleural effusions, chronic bronchitis and bronchiectasis	Yellowish appearing nails due to thickening of nail plate
Dyskeratosis congenita	Fine reticulate gray-brown pigmentation on the face, neck, shoulders, upper back and thigh is characteristic which may be associated with poikiloderma	Interstitial pneumonitis, fibrosis
Ataxia telangiectasia	Bronchiectasis, recurrent sinopulmonary infections	Oculocutaneous telangiectasia, café-au-lait macules, hyperpigmentations
Bloom's syndrome	Recurrent chronic bacterial infections	Poikiloderma, café-au-lait macules
Systemic sclerosis	Pulmonary fibrosis and pulmonary hypertension (in limited cutaneous systemic sclerosis)	Hypopigmented patches with perifollicular retained pigmentation giving a 'salt and pepper' appearance is the most common pigmentary change. Others include Addisonian- and acnathosis nigricans-like patterns.

REFERENCES

1. Melmed S, Jameson JL. Disorders of anterior pituitary and the hypothalamus. In: Longo DL, Fauci AS, Kasper DL, Hauser SL, Jameson JL, Loscalzo J (Eds). Harrison's Principles of Internal Medicine, 18th edn New York: The McGraw Hill Companies; 2012. pp. 2876-2902.
2. Zanini M, Oshiro R, Paschoal L, et al. Aspectos dermatológicos da acromegalia. An Bras Dermatol. 2004;79:491-4.
3. Cox NH, Coulson IH. Systemic disease and the skin. In: Burns T, Breathnach S, Cox N, Griffiths C (Eds). Rook's Textbook of Dermatology, 8th edn. Oxford: Wiley-Blackwell; 2010. pp. 62.1-62.113.
4. Torley D, Bellus GA, Munro CS. Genes, growth factors and acanthosis nigricans. Br J Dermatol. 2002;147:1096-101.
5. Strachan MW, Walker BR. Endocrine diseases. In: Colledge NR, Walker BR, Ralston SH (Eds). Davidson's Principles and Practice of Medicine, 21st edn. Edinburgh: Churchil Livingstone Elsevier; 2010. pp. 731-94.
6. Geller JL, Braunstein GD. Dermatologic manifestations of hypopituitarism. Clin Dermatol. 2006;24:266-75.
7. Arlt W. Disorders of the adrenal cortex. In: Longo DL, Fauci AS, Kasper DL, Hauser SL, Jameson JL, Loscalzo J (Eds). Harrison's Principles of Internal Medicine, 18th edn. New York: The McGraw Hill Companies; 2012. pp. 2940-61.
8. Kendereski A, Micic D, Sumarac M, et al. White Addison's disease: what is the possible cause? J Endocrinol Invest. 1999;22:395-400.
9. Turan S, Hughes C, Atay Z, et al. An atypical case of familial glucocorticoid deficiency without pigmentation caused by coexistent homozygous mutations in MC2R (T152K) and MC1R (R160W). J Clin Endocrinol Metab. 2012;97:E771-4.
10. Jameson JL, Weetman AP. Disorders of the thyroid gland. In: Longo DL, Fauci AS, Kasper DL, Hauser SL, Jameson JL, Loscalzo J (Eds). Harrison's Principles of Internal Medicine, 18th edn. New York: The McGraw Hill Companies; 2012. pp. 2911-39.
11. James WD, Berger TG, Elston DM. Endocrine diseases. In: James WD, Berger TG, Elston DM (Eds). Andrews' Diseases of the Skin Clinical Dermatology, 11th edn. Philadelphia: Elsevier Saunders; 2011. pp. 488-96.
12. Miller R, Ashkar FS, Jacobi J. Hyperpigmentation in thyrotoxicosis. JAMA. 1970;213:299.
13. Banba K, Tanaka N, Fujioka A, et al. Hyperpigmentation caused by hyperthyroidism: differences from the pigmentation of Addison's disease. Clin Exp Dermatol. 1999;24:196-8.
14. Dogra A, Dua A, Singh P. Thyroid and skin. Indian J Dermatol. 2006;51:96-9.
15. Leonhardt JM, Heymann WR. Thyroid disease and the skin. Dermatol Clin. 2002;20:473-81.
16. Kennedy CT, Burd DA, Creamer D. Mechanical and thermal injury. In: Burns T, Breathnach S, Cox N, Griffiths C (Eds). Rook's Textbook of Dermatology, 8th edn. Oxford: Wiley-Blackwell; 2010. pp. 28.1-28.94.
17. Cohen BA. Neonatal dermatology. In: Cohn BA (Ed). Pediatric dermatology, 3rd edn. Philadelphia: Elsevier Mosby; 2005. pp. 15-66.
18. Heymann WR. Cutaneous manifestations of thyroid disease. J Am Acad Dermatol. 1992;26:885-902.
19. Al-Mutairi N. Skin diseases seen in diabetes mellitus. Bull Kuwait Inst Med Spec. 2006;5:30-9.
20. Powers AC. Diabetes mellitus. In: Longo DL, Fauci AS, Kasper DL, Hauser SL, Jameson JL, Loscalzo J (Eds). Harrison's Principles of Internal Medicine, 18th edn. New York: The McGraw Hill Companies; 2012. pp. 2968-3003.
21. Sarkany RP, Breathnach SM, Morris AA, et al. Metabolic and Nutritional Disorders. In: Burns T, Breathnach S, Cox N, Griffiths C (Eds). Rook's Textbook of Dermatology, 8th edn. Oxford: Wiley-Blackwell; 2010. pp. 59.1-59.103.
22. Paron NG, Lambert PW. Cutaneous manifestations of diabetes mellitus. Prim Care. 2000;27:371-83.
23. Baur FM, Levan NE. Diabetic dermangiopathy: a spectrum including pigmented pretibial patches and necrobiosis lipoidica diabeticorum. Br J Dermatol. 1970;83:528-35.
24. Goyal A, Raina S, Kaushal SS, et al. Pattern of cutaneous manifestations in diabetes mellitus. Indian J Dermatol. 2010;55:39-41.
25. Van Hattem S, Bootsma AH, Thio HB. Skin manifestations of diabetes. Cleve Clin J Med. 2008;75:772-87.
26. Field MJ, Burnett L, Sullivan DR, et al. Clinical biochemistry and metabolism. In: Colledge NR, Walker BR, Ralston SH (Eds). Davidson's principles and practice of medicine, 21st edn. Edinburgh: Churchil Livingstone Elsevier; 2010. pp. 425-58.
27. Desnick RJ, Balwani M. The Porphyrias. In: Longo DL, Fauci AS, Kasper DL, Hauser SL, Jameson JL, Loscalzo J (Eds). Harrison's Principles of Internal Medicine, 18th edn. New York: The McGraw Hill Companies; 2012. pp. 3167-81.
28. Bickers DR, Frank J. The Porphyrias. In: Wolff K, Goldsmith LA, Katz SI, Gilchrest BA, Paller AS, Leffell DJ (Eds). Fitzpatrick's Dermatology in General Medicine. 7th edn. New York: The McGraw-Hill Companies; 2008. pp. 1228-56.
29. Shaffrali FC, McDonagh AJ, Messenger AG. Hair darkening in porphyria cutanea tarda. Br J Dermatol. 2002;146:325-9.
30. Takayama K, Satoh T, Maruyama R, Yokozeki H. Dialysis-related amyloidosis on the buttocks. Acta Derm Venereol. 2008;88:72-3.
31. James WD, Berger TG, Elston DM. Errors in metabolism. In: James WD, Berger TG, Elston DM (Eds). Andrews' Diseases of the Skin Clinical Dermatology, 11th edn. Philadelphia: Elsevier Saunders; 2011. pp. 506-37.
32. Seldin DC, Skinner M. Amyloidosis. In: Longo DL, Fauci AS, Kasper DL, Hauser SL, Jameson JL, Loscalzo J (Eds). Harrison's Principles of Internal Medicine, 18th edn. New York: The McGraw Hill Companies; 2012. pp. 945-50.

33. Gajula P, Ramalingam K, Bhadrashetty D. A rare case of mucopolysaccharidosis: Hunter syndrome. J Nat Sci Biol Med. 2012;3:97-100.
34. White LE. Xanthomatoses and lipoprotein disorders. In: Wolff K, Goldsmith LA, Katz SI, Gilchrest BA, Paller AS, Leffell DJ (Eds). Fitzpatrick's Dermatology in General Medicine. 7th edn. New York: The McGraw-Hill Companies; 2008. pp. 1272-81.
35. Alderman H, Shekar M. Nutrition, Food Security, and Health. In: Kliegman RM, Staton BF, St.Geme III JW, Schor NF, Behrman RE (Eds). Nelson Textbook of Pediatrics. 19th edn. Philadelphia: Elsevier Saunders; 2011. pp. 170-78.
36. Binder HJ. Disorders of absorption. In: Longo DL, Fauci AS, Kasper DL, Hauser SL, Jameson JL, Loscalzo J (Eds). Harrison's Principles of Internal Medicine, 18th edn. New York: The McGraw Hill Companies; 2012. pp. 2460-76.
37. Jasperson KW, Burt RW. APC-Associated Polyposis Conditions. 1998 Dec 18 [Updated 2011 Oct 27]. In: Pagon RA, Bird TD, Dolan CR, et al., (Eds). GeneReviews™ [online]. Seattle (WA): University of Washington, Seattle; 1993. Available at http://www.ncbi.nlm.nih.gov/books/NBK1345/. [Accessed on May, 2013].
38. Collier JD, Webster G. Liver and biliary tract diseases. In: Colledge NR, Walker BR, Ralston SH (Eds). Davidson's Principles and Practice of Medicine, 21st edn. Edinburgh: Churchil Livingstone Elsevier; 2010. pp. 919-84.
39. James WD, Berger TG, Elston DM. Disturbances of pigmentation. In: James WD, Berger TG, Elston DM, (Eds. Andrews' Diseases of the Skin Clinical Dermatology, 11th edn. Philadelphia: Elsevier Saunders; 2011. pp. 847-62.
40. Bacon BR. Cirrhosis and its complications. In: Longo DL, Fauci AS, Kasper DL, Hauser SL, Jameson JL, Loscalzo J (Eds). Harrison's Principles of Internal Medicine, 18th edn New York: The McGraw Hill Companies; 2012. pp. 2592-602.
41. Adya KA, Inamadar AC, Palit A. Paradoxes in dermatology. Indian Dermatol Online J. 2013;4:133-42.
42. Loscalzo J. Hypoxia and cyanosis. In: Longo DL, Fauci AS, Kasper DL, Hauser SL, Jameson JL, Loscalzo J (Eds). Harrison's principles of internal medicine, 18th edn. New York: The McGraw Hill Companies; 2012. pp. 287-90.
43. Carlo WA. Clinical Manifestations of Diseases in the Newborn Period. In: Kliegman RM, Staton BF, St.Geme III JW, Schor NF, Behrman RE (Eds). Nelson Textbook of Pediatrics, 19th edn. Philadelphia: Elsevier Saunders; 2011. pp. e92-1-92-3.
44. McDonnell JK. Cardiac disease and the skin. Dermatol Clin. 2002;20:503–11.

5

Developmental, Nevoid, Genetically Determined and Neurocutaneous Pigmentary Disorders

Nilendu Sarma

Key Features

- Developmental defects, anomalies, malformations, nevus and syndromes are closely related but specific conditions.
- Etiology of these conditions is often unknown. Multiple factors like genetic factors (e.g. mosaicism), environmental factors like infections (e.g. TORCH infections), illness, or drug abuse are implicated.
- This chapter is dedicated to in-depth discussion on many hypo- and hyperpigmented developmental, nevoid, genetically determined and neurocutaneous pigmentary disorders.

INTRODUCTION

Developmental defect (developmental abnormality, developmental anomaly or malformation) is an embryonic developmental error, clinically presenting as a structural abnormality of any type. Anomaly is defined as a structural alteration that is markedly deviated from normal.

Malformation or anomaly is generally manifested at birth and is used almost synonymous with congenital malformation. In more than 50% of cases, etiology is unknown (sporadic). About 25% of cases, there may be multiple factors. In less than one-fourth of cases, genetic factors are implicated. Genetic factors may be inherited or may result from a new mutation. About 10% of all congenital abnormalities are due to environmental factor (or teratogen) induced, like infections (e.g. TORCH infections), illness, or drug abuse by the mother during pregnancy.

Syndrome is simply defined as group of signs involving multiple systems. In many occasions, malformations are associated multisystemic involvement (malformation syndrome).

Nevus is the Latin word for birthmark of skin and/or mucosa. This is circumscribed, stable lesion and represents a clone of abnormal cells. They are benign but malignancy may develop within a nevus. Possibly all nevi are the phenotypic manifestation of a genetic mechanism called "mosaicism".

Mosaicism is defined as presence of two or more cell populations that are karyotypically or genotypically different. Unlike chimera, that develops from two different zygotes, mosaicism results from multiplication of daughter cells from a single zygote in an individual.[1] Mosaicism is a pervasive phenomenon that is seen in almost all large multicellular organisms.[2] This can lead to development of neoplasia. Now it is known that there are some definite phenotypic patterns of mosaicism. Blaschko's lines represent the most notable pattern. Other patterns are checkerboard pattern, phylloid pattern and patchy pattern without midline separation.[3] Patterns of pigmentary nevi may slightly vary from the nevi originated from keratinocytes as shown recently.[4]

The mosaicism may result from chromosomal abnormalities, single-gene mutation, or possibly from the incorporation of extrachromosomal DNA at early postzygotic stage. Rarely, it may occur even before fertilization at the half-chromatid stage. However, confirmation of mosaicism has been done only in few conditions so far.[5]

Impact of somatic mosaicism is dependent upon many factors like the type of mutation (deletion or point mutation), type of the gene affected (housekeeping, structural or regulatory), type of affected cell types, tissues and organs, loci of mutation, time of mutation, result of mutation (heterozygosity or homozygosity) and the fate of the affected cell lineage in which it arose (migration, mingling or selection).[2] Generally, mosaicism is not inherited. However, mosaicism affecting germ line will be transmitted to next generation.

Mosaicism abnormalities resulting from mosaicism. In the next sections, some important major developmental abnormalities, syndromes and nevoid disorders of skin and mucosal pigmentation have been discussed.

Hypopigmented Disorders

- Chédiak-Higashi syndrome
- Hermansky-Pudlak syndrome (HPS)
- Griscelli syndromes
- Ash leaf macules
- Piebaldism
- Waardenburg syndrome (WS)
- Nevus depigmentosus
- Nevus anemicus
- Hypomelanosis of Ito (HI)/Pigmentary mosaicism of Ito type
- Phylloid hypomelanosis
- Cutis tricolor.

Hyperpigmented Disorders

- Nevus of Ota and nevus of Ito
- Mongolian spot
- Café-au-lait (CAL) macules
- Incontinentia pigmenti (IP) of Bloch-Sulzberger
- Linear and whorled nevoid hypermelanosis (LWNH)
- Linear atrophoderma of Moulin
- Speckled lentiginous nevi (SLN)
- Phakomatosis pigmentovascularis (PPV)
- Phakomatosis pigmentokeratotica (PPK).

HYPOPIGMENTED DISORDERS

Chédiak-Higashi Syndrome

Chédiak-Higashi syndrome is a rare, autosomal recessive disorder characterized by albinoid hypopigmentation of the skin and eye, photophobia, recurrent infections, enterocolitis, prolonged bleeding time and neurologic features.[6] Affected patients often die at early age.

Pathogenesis

This occurs due to mutation in *LYST* or *CHS1* gene (1q42-43). The mutation results in abnormal intracellular protein transport and abnormally large intracellular lysosome of leukocytes and fibroblasts, dense bodies of platelets, azurophilic granules of neutrophils, and melanosomes of melanocytes. Thus there is profound neutropenia, impaired neutrophil chemotaxis and impaired bactericidal activity and defect in melanosomes.

Clinical Features

Pigmentary abnormality is the most distinctive changes that are characterized by hypopigmentation of the skin, eyes and hair. This is indistinguishable from oculocutaneous albinism.

There are three phases in this disease. In the childhood phase incidence of infection is high and may even be fatal. Second is accelerated lymphoma-like phase and third is adult phase that is characterized by progressive neurological dysfunction.

Infections most commonly involve the skin, gum, oral mucosa (severe gingivitis, oral mucosal ulceration and periodontal disease), lungs and the respiratory tract. Most common pathogens are *Staphylococcus aureus*, *Streptococcus pyogenes* and *Pneumococcus species.*

Neurological abnormality, that often manifests in children and young adults includes and is progressive include spinocerebellar degeneration and peripheral neuropathy of both axonal and demyelinating type. Clinically it manifests with movement disorders, abnormal gait, clumsiness, seizures, mental retardation, paresthesia and peripheral neuropathy.

Death may ensue in the first decade due to infection, bleeding or development of the accelerated lymphoma-like phase. Accelerated reaction is mostly precipitated by viral infections like Epstein-Barr virus. There is nonmalignant lymphohistiocytic lymphoma-like infiltration of multiple organs, severe anemia, bleeding episodes, lymphadenopathy, hepatosplenomegaly and overwhelming infections leading to death.

Diagnosis

Clinical suspicion can be confirmed by laboratory finding of giant granules in neutrophils, eosinophils, and granulocytes (in peripheral smear) and leukocyte precursor cells (in bone marrow smear). The granules are peroxidase positive and contain lysosomal enzymes. Similar granules (basically giant melanosomes) are also seen in melanocytes. Fluorescence cytometric analysis of cellular granularity and surface molecules offer useful diagnostic information.

Management

This is mostly supportive. Pigmentary and neurological abnormalities are not corrected with any treatment. Immunodeficiency may be treated with stem cell transplantation.

Hermansky-Pudlak Syndrome

Hermansky-Pudlak syndrome is a group of autosomal recessive multisystem disorders having multiple possible loci of mutations [HPS1, AP3B1 (HPS2), HPS3, HPS4, HPS5, HPS6, DTNBP1 (HPS7), and BLOC1S3 (HPS8)].[7] Clinically these are characterized by hypo- or depigmentation of skin, eye and hair. Other components of the disease are bleeding diathesis and ceroid lipofuscin deposition within multiple organs like lung, intestine and reticuloendothelial system.

Pathogenesis

There is defect in lysosome related organelles. Thus it involves melanosomes, platelet dense granules and lytic granules in the cytotoxic T lymphocytes. In melanosome, there is abnormal protein trafficking of tyrosine (TYR), tyrosinase-related protein-1 (TYRP1), DPT (dopachrome tautomerase) and platelets are devoid of dense bodies.

Clinical Features

Intensity of pigment dilution is variable and often mimics oculocutaneous albinism (tyrosinase positive). Eye changes also include nystagmus, poor vision and photophobia.

Bleeding diathesis manifests as hemorrhage in the skin, epistaxis, gingival bleeding, postpartum hemorrhage, colonic bleeding and menometrorrhagia. This can be life-threatening. This can be induced by intake of aspirin or other prostaglandin inhibitor. Extra caution should be taken during any minor or major surgery. Abnormality in the lytic granules in the cytotoxic T lymphocytes predisposes some patients with HPS2 for repeated infections.

Apart from bleeding, development of pulmonary fibrosis, granulomatous colitis, cardiomyopathy, renal failure can be life-threatening.

With time, chronic sun exposure may lead to slight pigmentation along with coarse, thickened skin (pachydermia). Development of solar keratoses skin cancers (squamous cell carcinoma and basal cell carcinoma) is also not unusual.

Diagnosis

The diagnosis of HPS is clinical. Platelet counts are normal but platelet dense bodies are found absent in electron microscopy. Bleeding time is prolonged and coagulation factor activities are normal.

Ceroid lipofuscin, a very characteristic feature of HPS can be demonstrated in urine and bone marrow. These appear as yellow, autofluorescent, amorphous lipid-protein complex. Mutation analysis can also be performed.

Management

Supportive measure, prevention of bleeding and prompt treatment of infection are important. Platelet or red blood cell transfusions may be required during surgery or in protracted bleeding. Some patients may need lung transplantation.

Sun protection, vaccination against dreaded infections like influenza and pneumococci. Moderate exercise is advocated. Premarital counseling and prenatal diagnosis have definite role.

Griscelli Syndromes

This is manifested with hypopigmentation of skin and hair. Phenotypic expression of the disease is mimicked by Chédiak-Higashi syndrome and albinism. However, unlike the two conditions, eye pigmentation is normal. Systemic associations are neurological involvement (Type 1) and immunodeficiency (Type 2). There is another type (Type 3) that is manifested without any systemic involvement.

There is presence of large clusters of unevenly distributed pigment granules in the hair shaft and abnormal accumulation of end-stage melanosomes in the melanocytes.[8] In Type 2, there is accelerated phase in which there is uncontrolled production of lymphocytes and macrophage resulting in hemophagocytosis in many organs and death.

Pathogenesis

This is an autosomal recessive disorder characterized and caused by three different mutations involving *MYOVA* gene on 15q21 (Type 1),[9] *RAB27A* gene on 15q21(Type 2) and MLPH on 2q37 (Type 3). MYO5A and RAB27A are located very closely in the same chromosome 15q21.1 region.[10]

Diagnosis

Clinical expression of the disease is highly suggestive. Microscopic examination of hair reveals clumps of pigment granules those are larger and more irregular than those seen in CHS.

Management

Bone marrow transplantation may be life-saving in Type 1.

Ash Leaf Macules and Tuberous Sclerosis

Ash leaf macules are multiple, sharply demarcated, lanceolate shaped, depigmened or hypopigmented macule present over trunk and limbs. Their size varies from 1–12 cm and total number may be few to more than 40. They are often seen at birth and are nonprogressive. There may be associated poliosis. They are considered the earliest clinical manifestation of tuberous sclerosis (TSC) and sometimes are sometimes may be the only cutaneous findings of TSC. They are detected in 50–100% of patients with TS. Any infant with ash leaf macules with infantile spasms are strongly suggestive of TSC. However, they may be found in approximately 4.7% of normal individuals. Thus if the lesion numbers are less than 3 without any neurological manifestation, extensive investigations are not justifiable. This is also found in patients with mental retardation and occasionally in basal cell nevus syndrome.

Histology

Lesions contain normal (or rarely reduced) numbers of melanocyte. Melanocytes are poorly melanized. Melanosomes are smaller, fewer and have poorly developed dendrites.

Diagnosis

Diagnosis is not difficult in appropriate clinical setting of TS. If pigment loss is subtle, Wood's lamp examination may assist in detection.

Treatment

Not required.

Piebaldism

This is a rare autosomal dominant disorder with specific form of pigmentary abnormality.

Pathogenesis

Piebaldism results from missense and frame-shift mutations of the KIT proto-oncogene (4q12)[11] or rarely *SLUG* gene (zinc finger neural crest transcriptional factor, *SNAI2* gene on chromosome 8q11.[12] These mutations result in defective melanoblast development, proliferation, migration or survival, decreased receptor TYR kinase signaling and finally decrease in melanogenesis.[13]

Clinical Features

There are congenital sharply demarcated and roughly symmetric depigmented patches that generally affect the ventral trunk like frontal scalp, forehead, ventral chest, abdomen and extremities. The hands and feet, as well as the back, remain normally pigmented. Depigmented areas or even normally pigmented areas may have smaller hyperpigmented macules. Localized white hair or poliosis of frontal scalp or eye brows is another characteristic feature. Males and females are equally affected. Additional features are CAL macules and axillary and/or inguinal freckles. Systemic abnormalities are generally not present.

Diagnosis

This is essentially clinical. But it should be differentiated from vitiligo, NF-1 and WS. Now, prenatal diagnosis can be done with DNA-based mutation analysis of KIT proto-oncogene. Histologically this is characterized by lack melanocytes in the depigmented skin.

Waardenburg Syndrome

Waardenburg syndrome is characterized by white forelock, congenital depigmented macules, pigmentary abnormality of iris (heterochromia irides), typical facial phenotype, congenital sensoryneural deafness (one or both ear) and aganglionic megacolon. There are many subtypes as discussed below and not all the features are present in each subtype.

It is considered as more severe version of neural crest development disorder than piebaldism.

Pathogenesis

Waardenburg syndrome has variable mode of inheritance. WS1 and WS2 are transmitted as autosomal dominant disorder, WS4 is inherited as autosomal recessive condition and WS3 can be transmitted as both autosomal dominant and recessive mode.

WS1 results from mutation in PAX3. WS2 can have four different mutation loci and thus may have four different genetic subtypes. It may result from mutation on *MITF* genes (WS2A), chromosome 1p (WS2B), chromosome 8p23 (WS2C), chromosome 8q11 (*SNA12* gene, WS2D).[14] Some of the WS3 patients have homozygous mutation in *PAX3* gene. WS4 may have mutation in endothelin 3, endothelin B receptor and sox 10.

Clinical Features

Four genetic types of WS have been described having distinct clinical manifestations in each type. Pigmentary dilatation is congenital but may improve with age.

Waardenburg syndrome-1 is the classical form with typical facial phenotype characterized by lateral displacement of the inner canthi of eye without any change in the interpupillary distance (dystopia canthorum), prominent nasal root and medial eyebrows (synophrys) **(Fig. 1)**. Dystopia canthorum is called when intercanthal distance divided by interpupillary distance is more than 0.6.

Waardenburg syndrome-2 has no facial features but has pigmentation and auditory abnormalities. Pigmentary abnormality is less severe than WS1. Clinical distinction many not be possible always and may require mutation analysis **(Fig. 2)**.

Waardenburg syndrome-3 has features similar to WS1 with severe musculoskeletal abnormalities, and rarely neural tube defects.

Waardenburg syndrome-4 has features like WS2 (no facial features) along with Hirschsprung disease. It has no deafness but may have more extensive hypopigmentation. WS4 may have mutation in endothelin-3, endothelin-B receptor, sox 10, a transcription factor necessary for development of

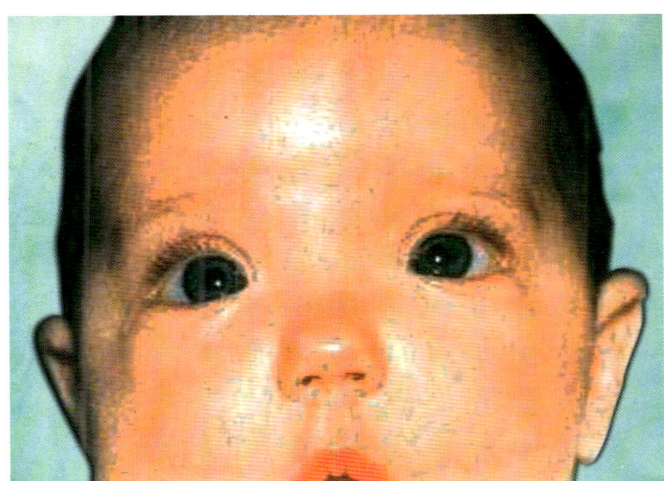

Fig. 1: One patient of Waardenburg syndrome type I (WS1) presenting with dystopia canthorum (Reproduced with permission from Read AP, Newton VE. Waardenburg Syndrome. J Med Genet. 1997;34:656-65.)

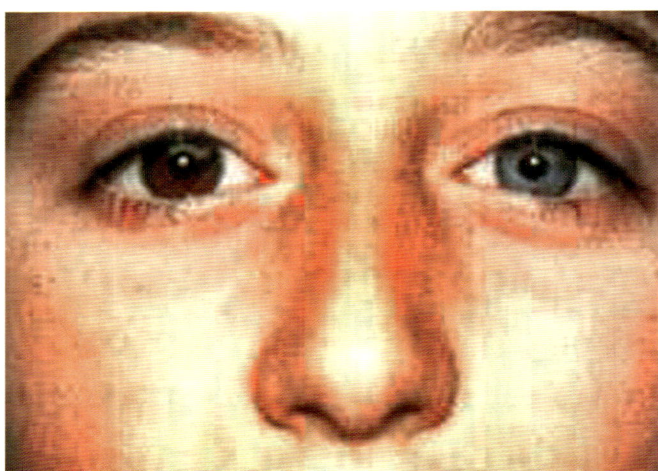

Fig. 2: A young female with type II WS caused by splice site mutation in the MITF gene presenting with blue left eye, brown right eye with sharply demarcated radial blue segment with normal facies and without any dystopica canthorum. (Reproduced with permission from Read AP, Newton VE.Waardenburg syndrome. J Med Genet. 1997;34:656-65.)

neural tube. Clinical presentation may vary according to the mutation as mentioned below:

- Peripheral demyelinating neuropathy, central demyelinating leukodystrophy, WS and Hirschsprung disease (PCWH) (*SOX10* gene mutation)
- Waardenburg-Hirschsprung disease (mutation in EDN3-receptor B gene/EDNRB)
- Albinism-Deafness syndrome/Ziprkowsky-Margolis syndrome (X-linked recessive)

Waardenburg syndrome should be differentiated from piebaldism and Tietz syndrome.

Nevus Depigmentosus

This is manifested early in life, usually before 3 years of age in 92.5% but may develop later in childhood.[15] Generally, the pigment loss is incomplete. Lesion can be single, but can also be segmental or extensive (systematized) that often shows sharp midline cutoff. They may be circumscribed, round, irregular or whorled with irregular margin. Trunk is the most common site. Associated systemic abnormality is rare but found.

Histopathology

Melanin is reduced in the lesion. Melanocyte number may be normal or reduced within the patch and there may be a functional defect in melanosome function and its transfer to keratinocytes.

Pathogenesis

This is currently unknown. Mosaicism is suggested as the etiology.

Differential Diagnosis

Vitiligo is characterized by hyperpigmented margin and late onset and progressive in nature. Segmental vitiligo is a close mimicker. This should also be differentiated from ash leaf macules, HI (in extensive disease), nevus anemicus and piebaldism. Currently there is less consensus regarding the differences between HI and systematized nevus depigmentosus

Management

Surgical management like excision, grafting especially autologous *in vitro* skin grafting may be helpful. However, pigment spread from the graft toward in between skin is poor and there is chance of depigmentation.

Nevus Anemicus

This appears as congenital hypopigmented patch, mostly on chest and in females. Although it appears hypopigmented, there is no true pigmentary abnormality. Apparent hypopigmentation is due to persistent vasoconstriction due to increased reactivity of the α-2 receptors of the lesional vasculature to catechols.

Sometimes, it may be associated with port wine stain, telangiectatic nevi (nevus vascularis mixtus)[16] and may indicate twin spotting and some genodermatoses including neurofibromatosis and PPV.[17]

Hypomelanosis of Ito/Pigmentary Mosaicism of Ito Type

This is characterized by presence of linear streaks, whorles or patches of hypopigmentation that are distributed along the lines of Blaschko.

Pathogenesis

This is considered a genetically heterogenous disease and results from chromosomal mosaicism. It is now known that numerous mutations involving different genes may result in similar phenotypic presentation of HI. It is known that mosaicism may result in many other patterns other than Blaschko's lines. However, patterns other than Blaschko's lines are not currently considered as HI. Thus a more acceptable terminology for this condition is "pigmentary mosaicism of Ito type".

Clinical Features

Hypo- or depigmented streaks that are distributed along Blaschko's line unilaterally but occasionally bilaterally. They are mostly seen at birth. In up to 70% of cases, this is detectable in infancy. Occasionally, lesions are hyperpigmented or there may be combination of hypo- and hyperpigmented patches. In fact, in many occasions, assessment of the abnormal color from the normal skin is difficult and arbitrary **(Fig. 3)**.

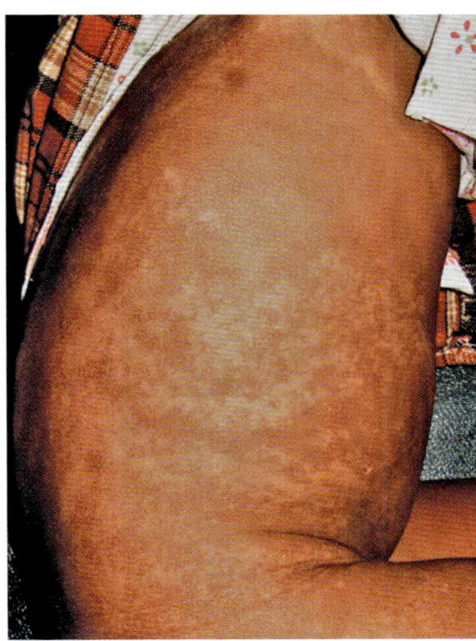

Fig. 3: A child of mosaicism of Ito type showing typical hypopigmentation along Blaschko's lines on the trunk.

Rarely this may be familial. Lesion may become more visible with time or may even fade. Disease can be localized or wide spread and intensity of pigmentation may also vary. There is no hearing defect and poliosis. Others systems like neurological, eyes, hair, teeth or musculoskeletal system may be affected. Psychomotor retardation and cognitive deficit are the most significant anomalies of the central nervous system (CNS). Other abnormalities are autism, epilepsy, language disorders, malformations like neural migration disorders, cerebral hypoplasia, cortical atrophy and agenesis of the corpus callosum.[18] Other defects are hemihypertrophy, kyphoscoliosis, genital anomalies, inguinal hernia and congenital heart defects.

Diagnosis

Diagnosis is clinical and is generally not difficult. This should be differentiated from LWNH, nevus depigmentosus and IP, piebaldism and WS.

Mosaicism can be detected with appropriate selection of affected cells. Fibroblast, lymphocytes or keratinocytes from the affected skin may be used for genetic analysis.

HI has some similarity with IP of Bloch-Sulzberger that commonly shows hyperpigmentation (3rd stage) but HI is mainly composed of hypopigmentation. Unlike IP, there is no preceding vesicular or verrucous stages.

Systematized nevus depigmentosus is another condition that may be indistinguishable from HI clinically. However, chromosomal mosaicism has not been detected in nevus depigmentosus.

Phylloid Hypomelanosis

This is a very rare condition. This may be seen at birth or develop in first year of life. Trunk is the most common site but limbs are also affected. This is caused by trisomy 13 or translocation trisomy 13.

There are round or oval hypopigmented patch distributed like floral ornament or art nouveau painting (Greek phyllon = leaf, eidos = form) or the asymmetrical leaves of a begonia. A single case of phylloid hypermelanosis that was caused by tetrasomy of chromosome 5p has been reported.[19] Usually other abnormalities like mental retardation, absence of corpus callosum, conductive hearing defect, and many craniofacial abnormalities like patchydactyly, clinodactyly and camptodactyly and severe dysmorphea are associated.

There is a hyperpigmented counterpart of this disorder called phylloid hypermelanosis. This is extremely rare and might represent a heterogeneous phenotype for different disorder.[20]

Cutis Tricolor

This condition, coined by Happle et al. in 1997 is defined as presence of both hypo- and hyperpigmentation either on same area or in close proximity to each other.[21] Cutis tricolor is a very rare condition. This is seen at birth or very early in life. Intensity of pigmentary alteration may increase for some time. This is an acquired condition except on report where two sisters were affected.

This can be a pure cutaneous trait without any other abnormality. It may be a part of a complex malformation syndrome when it is called cutis tricolor syndrome or Ruggieri-Happle syndrome. It may also be seen in association with other (e.g. vascular) skin disturbances.

In cutis tricolor syndrome, associated abnormalities include coarse facial features, dolichocephaly, urinary and fecal incontinence, hypotonia, hypoplasia of corpus callosum, mental retardation, seizure disorders and various skeletal abnormalities.

Cutis tricolorparvimaculata is a distinct type of cutis tricolor characterized by small, paired hypochromic and hyperchromic macules on a background of normal intermediate-pigmented skin. It has been described two patients with ring chromosome 15 syndrome.[22]

Pathogenesis

Possibly this reflects a genetic mechanism called twin spotting. Twin-spotting has been studied in plants, as well as in Drosophila melanogaster. The concept of twin spotting is yet to be proved in human. It is proposed that an early postzygotic mutational event results in two different autosomal recessive mutations located on the homologous chromosome making the embryo double heterozygous.

Histologically, pigmented areas demonstrate increased basal pigmentation and hyopigmented areas show less pigmentation in basal layer. No incontinence or dermal melanocytes are seen.

HYPERPIGMENTED DISORDERS

Nevus of Ota

This is blue-gray pigmented macule or patches on the upper half of face, first described by Taninoin in 1939. It develops from migration arrest of melanoblast that arises from neural crest. Pathogenesis is same in nevus of Ota, blue nevus, and Mongolian spot. Generally they develop unilaterally but bilateral involvement is also seen.

It is often present at birth. However, this may appear later. Nevus of Ota when develop later and is not associated with any eye or extracutaneous involvement is called nevus of Hori or acquired bilateral nevus of Ota like macule. Females are more commonly affected. Distribution corresponds to ophthalmic and maxillary division of trigeminal nerve. Involvement of lower part of face is rare. Pigmentation is generally diffuse and homogeneous but can also be blotchy and formed by coalescence of many smaller macules. Presence of palpable component is rare but reported. Associated pigmentation in sclera is found in about two-thirds of all cases. Pigmentation may also be present in iris (heterochromia irides), cornea and even optic nerve, meninges, periosteum, Eustachian tube, tympanic membrane, nasal mucosa, palate and in pharynx. Melanoma may develop in nevus of Ota. Malignant transformation of meninges is also repeated reported.[23] Glaucoma is a rare complication.[24]

This may be associated with nevus of Ito and other disorders like PPV, port-wine stain, Sturge-Weber syndrome, Takayasu disease, Klippel-Trenaunay syndrome and neurofibromatosis.[25,26]

Histopathology

There is presence of bipolar melanocytes that can synthesize melanin is found in the upper third of reticular dermis.

Treatment

Q-switched Nd:YAG or Q-switched ruby laser can be used.

Nevus of Ito

This is a clinically similar except the location. It is present over supraclavicular, scapular or deltoid area.

Mongolian Spot

Pathogenesis

Mongolian spots develop due to the failure of migration of the melanocytes from the neural crest to the basal layer of the epidermis. Thus, elongated dendritic dermal melanocytes are found widely scattered among normal collagen bundles.[27]

Clinical Features

This is a very common condition among children of oriental origin and is characterized by grayish-blue to grayish-black patch over the sacrococcygeal area or occasionally other areas like legs, chest or scalp. Extensive patches are called generalized dermal melanocytosis or dermal melanocytic hamartomas **(Fig. 4)**. This occurs due to the presence of functional melanocytes in the dermis. This is often present since birth or may develop shortly thereafter. Intensity of pigmentation generally increases for the first 2 years and then it regresses to become indistinguishable completely by 6–7 years of age. Only rarely it may become persistent especially over the extrasacral ones.

Generally, they have no clinical significance in most of the cases. However, they may be a feature of PPV Types II, IV and V, and have been described in the setting of Sjögren-Larsson syndrome. Extensive Mongolian spots are reported to be associated with GM1 gangliosidosis type 1[28] and with trisomy 20 mosaicism.

Treatment

Generally unnecessary. In persistent cases, Q switched Nd:YAG laser is quite effective.

Café-Au-Lait Macule

These are homogeneously brown colored macules with distinct margin that may be smooth or finely irregular. In McCune Albright syndrome, margin is prominently irregular (coast of Maine appearance) and in NF, it is more smooth (coast of California).

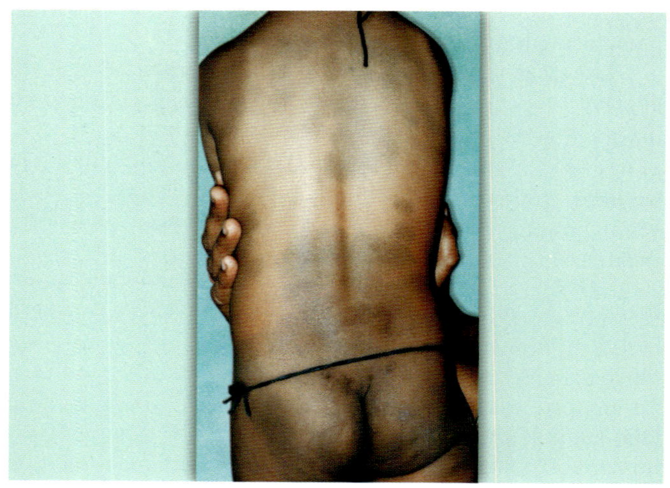

Fig. 4: Extensive Mongolian spots in a child

They are commonly distributed over trunk and buttock. Generally, head and neck area are spared.

They may be present at birth or develop during early year. However the size and number of the lesions may also increase with time. Intensity of pigmentation may increase or decrease gradually. Size is variable and often depends on the associated disease. Commonly, it is less than 1.5 cm but lesions may appear as freckles or may be very large (even up to 30 cm).

Isolated CAL is not uncommon and has no significance. Multiple CALM generally indicates presence of multisystemic involvement and some syndromes like neurofibromatosis, TSC, McCune Albright syndrome, Watson syndrome, Bloom syndrome, ring chromosome syndrome, LEOPARD syndrome, some metabolic disease like Gaucher syndrome and also rarely in nevoid basal cell carcinoma syndrome.[29] A number of 6 or more is highly indicative of NF1. **Table 1** depicts possible list of disease that may feature CAL.

Management

Q-switched Nd:YAG and Q-switched ruby laser can be attempted.

Incontinentia Pigmenti of Bloch-Sulzberger

Incontinentia pigmenti is a syndrome characterized by polydysplasia of ectodermal tissue manifesting as abnormalities of skin, teeth, hair and eyes.

This is rare and is inherited as X-linked dominant disease. Mutation in *NEMO* gene (also known as γ-subunit of the inhibitor κB kinase/IKKγ) causes the disease. This was mapped to Xp11 (IP1)[30] and more recently to Xq28 (IP2).[31]

Disease in male is generally lethal. Thus most cases are in female. It can involve, apart from skin organs like CNS (up to 50% of cases), eyes and teeth. Also noted are breast, hair (alopecia) and nail abnormality.

This has four stages:

The first stage is called vesiculobullous, or inflammatory stage with eosinophilia. This is seen in approximately 90% of all cases. Cases that have an observable stage 1, usually manifest within first 2 weeks of life and resolution occurs by 4 months of age 32. Erythema and vesicle, and rarely pustules develop in a linear fashion over limbs and trunk and sometimes on scalp sparing the face. Rarely, lesions may relapse much later for shorter period and with less severity. Lesions on limbs may progress to verrucous lesions of second stage or become atrophic of fourth stage. Trunk lesions generally heal without atrophy.

In the second stage, that generally starts at 2–6 weeks age, pustular, verrucous, lichenoid lesions develop mostly over limbs and also over eye lids and scalp.

The most characteristic of IP is the third stage that shows development of brown, slate-gray pigmented colored whorls, or stellate macules streaks arranged along Blaschko's lines. This is seen mostly around 12–26 weeks of postnatal life but may be noted at birth. This is seen in almost 98% of all cases of IP after the resolution of vesicobullous and verrucous stage. Pigmented macules are noted mostly in the torso and it is now known that they do not correspond to the previous vesicular or verrucous lesions. Thus they do not reflect postinflammatory hyperpigmentation. Even in some cases, second and third stage lesions may coexist. This stage may improve by second to third decade. Diagnostic criteria has been proposed for this condition **(Table 2)**.[32,33]

Fourth stage of the disease is hypopigmented streaks along Blaschko's lines and this develops as the sequel of the previous stage. Thus, this appears usually in the second decade. Hypopigmentation persists throughout life and mimicks HI in an adult. This stage is not seen in all and in many, only very localized involvement is noted that is detected only after careful examination.

Hair and nail are generally affected. Patchy alopecia is common.

Among the extracutaneous features dental abnormality is the most common presenting as abnormal tooth eruption and malformed crowns involving both deciduous and permanent teeth. Teeth involvement is permanent unlike skin involvement that may improve.

Eye involvement is one of the dreaded complications and it may lead to blindness due to retinal dysplasia.[33] Retinal involvement is due to vaso-occlusive changes. Some nonretinal involvement may lead to strabismus. Retinal involvement occurs early, usually within 1 year of life necessitating early intervention.

Neurological involvement is common and characteristic. There is seizure disorder that starts early in life. Other manifestations are spastic paralysis, encephalomyelitis,[34] mental and motor retardation, microcephalus, cerebellar ataxia, congenital hearing loss and muscle paresis.[33]

Management

Supportive therapy is required. For neonatal seizures, opinion of pediatric neurologist should be sought. Retinal abnormality like proliferative retinopathy may be treated with laser photocoagulation or cryotherapy. Retinal detachment is an emergency.

Linear and Whorled Nevoid Hypomelanosis

First described by Kalter in 1988,[35] this is characterized by swirls and whorls of hyperpigmented macules along Blaschko's lines that generally develop within a few weeks of birth but pigmentation may progress for the next few years. In some cases, pigmentary alteration may be reticulated. Male and females are equally affected.

Pattern of pigmentary alteration mimicks HI and systematized nevus depigmentosus but both these disorders are hypomelanotic. This is also known as zebra-

Table 1: Café-au-lait and associated diseases and syndrome[29]			
Syndrome	*Gene or locus*	*Cutaneous clinical features*	*Systemic clinical features*
NF1	NF1	Multiple café-au-lait (>6), skin-fold freckling, cutaneous and plexiform neurofibromas	Macrocephaly, optic pathway glioma, skeletal dysplasia
NF2	NF2	Café-au-lait macules seen but not a criterion for diagnosis, neurofibromas	Acoustic neuromas, schwannomas, meningiomas, juvenile posterior subcapsular lenticular opacity
Multiple familial Café-au-lait	Unknown	Multiple café-au-lait	Without other stigmata of NF1
Legius (NF-1 like) syndrome	SPREADI	Multiple café-au-lait, skin-fold freckling	Without other stigmata of NF1
McCune Albright syndrome	GNAS1	Segmental café-au-lait	Precocious puberty, other endocrinopathies polyostotic fibrous dysplasia
Constitutional MMR deficiency syndrome	MLH1, MSH2, MSH6, PMS2	Multiple café-au-lait	Adenomatour colonic polyps, multiple malignancies (medulloblastoma, lymphoma, glioblastoma)
Ring chromosome syndrome	Chromosomes[7,11,12,15,17]	Multiple café-au-lait	Microcephaly, mental retardation, short stature
Leopard/multiple lentigines syndrome	PTPN11	Café-au-lait, Café-noir, lentigines	Cardiac conduction defects, ocular hypertelorism, pulmonary stenosis, growth retardation, hearing loss
Cowden syndrome	PTEN	Café-au-lait spots, facial trichilemmomas, soft tissue tumors (lipomas, neuromas)	Cobblestoning of the oral mucosa, gastrointestinal polyps, breast carcinoma, thyroid adenoma and cancer
Banayan-Riley-Ruvalcaba syndrome	PTEN	Pigmented genital macules, facial trichilemmomas	Oral papillomas, gastrointestinal polyps. Macrocephal vascular anomalies
Weak Association			
NAME (naevi, atrial mixoma, ephelides) syndrome	Unknown	Nevi, ephelides	Atrial mixoma
Ataxia telangiectasia	ATM	Cutaneous and ocular telangiectasias	Cerebellar ataxia, immunodeficiency hypogonadism, lymphoreticular malignancy
Epidermal nevus syndrome	Unknown	Linear epidermal nevus	Mental retardation, seizures, movement disorders
Turner syndrome	X-chromosomal anomalies (XO karyotype or Xp deletion)	Cutaneous lymphatic malformations	Short stature, broad chest, low hairline, low-set ears and webbed necks, swelling, gonadal dysfunction, congenital heart disease, hypothyroidism.
Silver-Russell syndrome	Unknown	Multiple café-au-lait macules	Short stature, craniofacial and body asymmetry, microcephaly, congenital cardiac defects
Fanconi anemia	FANCA, FANCB/C/D locus on chromosome 3, FANCE/F/G/H	Hyper- and hypopigmentation of the skin, mucocutaneous squamous cell carcinomas	Bone marrow failure multiple congenital anomalies, mental retatrdation, microcephaly
Westerhof syndrome	Unknown	Hypopigmented and hyperpigmented macules	Retarded growth and mental deficiency

Contd...

Contd...

Syndrome	*Gene or locus*	*Cutaneous clinical features*	*Systemic clinical features*
MEN1/Men 2B	RET	Multiple malignancies	
Bloom syndrome	RECQL3	Hypo- and hyperpigmented spots; telangiectasias	Mental retardation, short stature
Gaucher disease	Chromosome 1	Yellowish-brown skin pigmentation	Astenia, diarrhea, ataxia, splenomegalia hemorrhages, muscular atrophia
Hunter disease	X-linked	Skin eruptions	Macrocephaly, mental retardation, valvular dysfunction
Watson syndrome	NF1	Axillary/inguinal freckling	Mental retardation, short stature, pulmonary valvular stenosis, Lisch nodules

Source: With prior permission from Ponti G, Tomasi A, Pastorino L, et al. Diagnostic and pathogenetic role of café-au-lait macules in nevoid basal cell carcinoma syndrome. Hereditary Cancer in Clinical Practice. 2012;10:15

Table 2: Diagnostic criteria of incontinentia pigmenti

Family history	*Major criteria*	*Minor criteria*
No evidence of IP in a first-degree female relative*	Typical neonatal rash: Erythema and vesicles with eosinophilia Typical hyperpigmentation mainly on trunk, following lines of Blaschko, fading in adolescence Linear, atrophic, hairless lesions	Dental anomalies Alopecia Abnormal nails Retinal disease
Evidence of IP in a first-degree female relative†	Suggestive history or evidence of typical rash, hyperpigmentation, atrophic hairless lesions Vertex alopecia Dental anomalies Retinal disease Multiple male miscarriages	

*At least one major criterion is necessary for diagnosis in cases with no apparent family history. Minor criteria support and diagnosis; complete lack thereof should induce a degree of uncertainty.

†Presence of any one or more of the major criteria strongly suggests a diagnosis of incontinentia pigmenti in cases with definitive family history.

Source: With prior permission from Berlin AL, Paller AS, Chan LS. Incontinentia pigmenti: A review and update on the molecular basis of pathophysiology. J Am Acad Dermatol. 2002;47:169-87.

like hyperpigmentation. In some occasions, both hypo- and hypermelanosis is simultaneously present. Whether this indicates simultaneous presence of HI and LWNH is unknown. Classically, pigmentary alterations are generalized and usually detected within few weeks of life. A localized unilateral form exists that is known as progressive cribriform and zosteriform hyperpigmentation and it usually starts in 2nd decade. Extracutaneous systemic involvement is generally not found but reported occasionally.[36] Reported associations are neurological (seizure, psychomotor delay, cerebral palsy) and cardiac involvement (dextrocardia, atrial septal defects), deafness, skeletal and ocular abnormalities.

Pathogenesis

This is caused by chromosomal mosaicism or chimerism.

Histopathology

Hyperpigmented areas show epidermal alterations like presence of increased basal layer pigmentation, melanocytic vacuolation without any pigmentary incontinence.

Linear Atrophoderma of Moulin

Linear atrophoderma of Moulin is a rare disorder described by Moulin in 1992.[37] The current term "linear atrophoderma of Moulin" was coined by Baumann et al.[38] This is clinically characterized by unilateral atrophic and variably hyperpigmented plaques forming a band and distributed along Blaschko's line without any preceding inflammation or sclerotic appearance. This generally appears in childhood or adolescence and is nonprogressive. There is no induration, no preceding inflammation and erythema. In histology, there is increased basal pigmentation. Characteristically, there is absence of any other abnormality including abnormality in dermal collagen and subcutaneous tissue. There are some atypical presentations also. In occasional cases, it may develop postadolescent age and may be bilateral.[39]

This should be differentiated from LWNH, IP of Bloch-Sulzberger, idiopathic atrophoderma of Pasini and Pierini (IAPP) and linear scleroderma. The latter two show typical histological changes of collagen and atrophy. After the original cases described by Moulin et al. many subsequent cases have been described. Some of these cases had histological signs of atrophy thus making it more difficult to differentiate from IAPP and scleroderma. IAPP shows pigmentation and atrophy and no induration and are not distributed along Blaschko's lines. Linear morphea, in contrast shows induration initially before developing atrophy and are also not distributed along Blaschko's lines. It shows inflammation and lilac color initially. Thus they can be differentiated.

Distribution of the lesions indicates that this is caused by mosaicism but the involved gene is not identified so far. Apart from cutaneous pigmentary changes, no other abnormalities have been described so far. Anecdotal reports mentioned partial improvement with intravenous penicillin along with topical PUVA therapy, oral potassium para-aminobenzoate, vitamin E (400 IU/day), topical clobetasol propionate and topical calcipotriol.[40]

There is no well accepted successful treatment for this condition so far.

Speckled Lentiginous Nevi

Speckled lentiginous nevus is possibly a subtype of congenital melanocytic nevus. This is generally present at birth but may appear after birth. For this reason, many consider this as acquired nevi and not a subtype of CMN. Even when seen at birth, the initial presentation is that of a CAL macule and pigmented superimposed macules/papules develop later.

Clinical Features

Speckled lentiginous nevus is characterized by a background diffuse light tan to dark brown pigmentation that develops earlier, even at birth. This may represent a CAL macule. Pigmentation may darken with sun exposure. The size varies from 3–6 cm and shape may be variable like oval, block-like, zosteriform or linea and may be distributed along the lines of Blaschko. Occasionally, it may involve both upper and lower eyelid.

The second component is the darker smaller spots distributed on the background patch. They may be composed of either macules or papules. Color may vary from blue, brown or black. Histology of the speckles may be variable and show characters of lentigines, junctional, compound or dermal nevi, blue nevi or even Spitz nevi.

Speckled lentiginous nevus is sometimes a component of other syndromes. SLN (macular) may be associated in PPV Type III along with nevus flammeus with or without nevus anemicus. It may be seen (papular type) in PPK along with an organoid nevus with sebaceous differentiation. The proposed mechanism for this association of SLN in PPV and PPK is "twin spotting".

In addition, SLN syndrome was described by Happle in 2002[41] as a separate entity that is characterized by presence of SLN along with many other cutaneous or systemic disorders like ipsilateral sensory and/or motor neuropathy, spinal muscular atrophy or hypertrophy, hyperhidrosis over the SLN area. The close spatial relation hints at their inherent association. This occurs as sporadic trait. But several members of a family may be affected by the genetic mechanism called paradominant inheritance.[42]

Differential Diagnosis

It should be differentiated from agminated lentiginosis, agminated spitz nevi. This should be differentiated from partial unilateral lentiginosis with segmental neurofibromatosis.[43]

Histopathology

There is simple lentiginous pigmentation of the basal layer and rarely few nevus cells in the background pigmentation. Darker speckles (macules) demonstrate melanocytic nests at the dermoepidermal junction at the tips of the papillae and the papules show dermal or compound melanocytic nevi.

Treatment

Q-switched ruby, Nd:YAG or alexandrite laser can be attempted.

Phakomatosis Pigmentovascularis

This is characterized by presence of nevus flammeus along with different types of pigmentary nevi like nevus of Ota, nevus spilus, and Mongolian spots. This was described by Ota in 1939.[44]

Phakomatosis pigmentovascularis has been classified into four types based on various combinations as mentioned below:

Type I: Combination of nevus flammeus, nevus depigmentosus and verrucous epidermal nevus.

Type II: Combination of nevus flammeus, dermal melanocytosis (nevus of Ota/nevus of Ito/aberrant Mongolian spots) with or without nevus anemicus. This is the most common form and nevus of Ota is a part of this.

Type III: Combination of nevus flammeus and nevus spilus with or without nevus anemicus.

Type IV: Combination of nevus flammeus, dermal melanocytosis, nevus spilus with or without nevus anemicus.

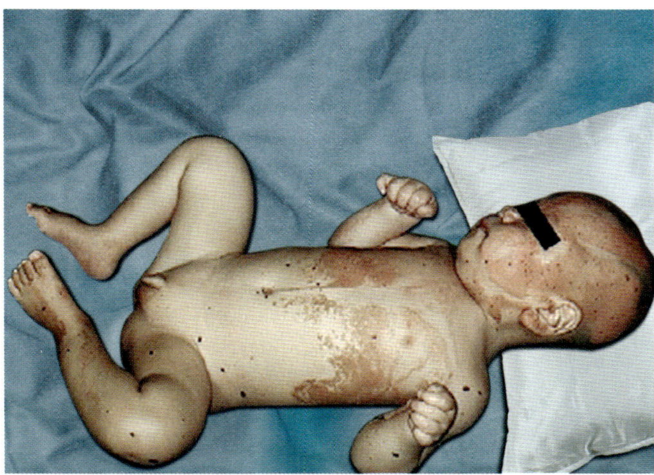

Fig. 5: A 4-month-old boy with phakomatosis pigmentokeratotica showing epidermal nevus of sebaceous differentiation along with nevus spilus papulosus. (Reproduced with permission from Happle R. The group of epidermal nevus syndromes Part I. Well defined phenotypes. J Am Acad Dermatol. 2010;63:1-22)

A fifth type has been recently proposed. It consisted of cutis marmorata telangiectatica congenita, dermal melanocytosis. Association of PPV Type V with nevus spilus has also been reported.

Subtype "a" indicates only cutaneous manifestation and "b" indicates systemic involvement.

Pathogenesis

This possibly reflects a specific genetic mutation called twin spotting affecting caused by developmental aberration in the neural crest-derived vasomotor nerves and melanocytes.

Differential Diagnosis

This should be differentiated from Sturge-Weber syndrome, Klippel-Trenaunay syndrome.

Phakomatosis Pigmentokeratotica

Phakomatosis pigmentokeratotica is a rare type of nevus syndrome that is characterized by combination of two different types of nevi, organoid nevus with sebaceous differentiation and SLN. The first one is distributed along Blaschko's lines and the second one shows a checkerboard pattern **(Fig. 5)**. Based on the presence of absence of extracutaneous involvement, this has been divided into two subtypes. It can involve neurological, ophthalmological and musculoskeletal systems. Neurological involvement may manifest with hemiatrophy, weakness, dysesthesia. Ophthalmologic changes include internal strabismus, ptosis but unlike Schimmelpenning syndrome, there is no coloboma and epibulbar lipodermoid.[45] There may be localized hyperhidrosis over SLN.

This occurs because of a genetic mechanism twin spotting theory where there are two simultaneous homozygous recessive mutations. Underlying gene mutations are yet unknown. Heterozygous mutations have been identified involving HRAS c.37G > C (p.Gly13Arg) HRAS c.182A>G (p.Gln61Arg).[46]

It should be differentiated from Schimmelpenning syndrome that lacks lentiginous nevi and has major neurological changes and features specific eye abnormalities like conjunctival lipodermoid, and/or coloboma.[47]

REFERENCES

1. Happle R. What is a nevus? A proposed definition of a common medical term. Dermatology. 1995;191:1-5.
2. Hall JG. Review and hypotheses: somatic mosaicism: observations related to clinical genetics. Am J Hum Genet. 1988;43:355-63.
3. Happle R. Mosaicism in human skin-Understanding the patterns and mechanisms. Arch Dermatol. 1993;129:1460-70.
4. Sarma N. Pigmentary nevi on face have unique patterns and implications: the concept of Blaschko's lines for pigmentary nevi. Indian J Dermatol. 2012;57(1):30-4.
5. Happle R. Dohi Memorial Lecture: new aspects of cutaneous mosaicism. J Dermatol. 2002;29:681-92.
6. Introne W, Boisset RE, Gahl WA. Clinical,molecular and cell biological aspects of Chédiak-Higashi syndrome. Mol Gen Metab. 1999;68:283-303.
7. Huizing M, Helip-Wooley A, Westbroek W, et al. Disorders of lysosome-related organelle biogenesis: clinical and molecular genetics. Annu Rev Genomics Hum Genet. 2008; 9:359-86.
8. Ménasché G, Ho CH, Sanal O, et al. Griscelli syndrome restricted to hypopigmentation results from a melanophilin defect (GS3) or a MYO5A F-exon deletion (GS1). J Clin Invest. 2003;112:450-6.
9. Pastural E, Barrat FJ, Dufourcq-Lagelouse R, et al. Griscelli disease maps to chromosome 15q21 and is associated with mutations in the myosin-Va gene. Nat Genet. 1997;16: 289-92.
10. Pastural E, Ersoy F, Yalman N, et al. Two genes are responsible for Griscelli syndrome at the same 15q21 locus. Genomics. 2000;63:299-306.
11. Giebel LB, Spritz RA. Mutation of the KIT (mast/stem cell growth factor receptor) protooncogene in human piebaldism. ProcNatlAcadSci USA. 1991;88:8696-9.
12. Spritz RA. Molecular basis of human piebaldism. J Invest Dermatol. 1994;103(Suppl):137S-140S.
13. Spritz RA. Genetic hypomelanoses: disorders characterized by congenital white spotting — piebaldism, Waardenburg syndrome, and related genetic disorders of melanocyte development — Clinical aspects, 2nd edn. In: Nordlund JJ, Boissy RE, Hearing VJ, King RA, Oetting WS, Ortonne J-P (Eds). The Pigmentary System. Blackwell, Malden, MA. 2006. pp. 541-50.

14. Pingault V, Ente D, Dastot-Le Moal F, et al. Review and update of mutations causing Waardenburg syndrome. Hum Mutat. 2010;31:391-406.
15. Lee HS, Chun YS, Hann SK. Nevus depigmentosus: clinical features and histopathologic characteristics in 67 patients. J Am Acad Dermatol. 1999;40:21-6.
16 Ruggieri M, Milone P, Pavone P, et al. Nevus vascularis mixtus (cutaneous vascular twin nevi) associated with intracranial vascular malformation of the Dyke-Davidoff-Masson type in two patients. Am J Med Genet A. 2012;158A:2870-80.
17. Ahkami RN, Schwartz RA. Nevus anemicus. Dermatology. 1999;198(4):327-9.
18. Parisi L, Di Filippo T, Roccella M. Hypomelanosis of Ito: neurological and psychiatric pictures in developmental age. Minerva Pediatr. 2012;64(1):65-70.
19. Hansen LK, Brandrup F, Rasmussen K. pigmentary mosaicism with mosaic chromosome 5p tetrasome. Br J Dermatol. 2003;149:414-6.
20. Happle R, Franco-Guío MF, Santacoloma-Osorio G. Phylloid Hypermelanosis: A Cutaneous Marker of Several Different Disorders? Pediatr Dermatol. 2012. doi: 10.1111/pde.12053. (Epub ahead of print).
21. Baba M, Seckin D, Akcali C, et al. Familial cutis tricolor: a possible example of paradominant inheritance. Eur J Dermatol. 2003;13:343-5.
22. Boente Mdel C, Bazan C, Montanari D. Pediatr Dermatol. Cutis tricolor parvimaculata in two patients with ring chromosome 15 syndrome. 2011;28(6):670-3.
23. Rahimi-Movaghar V, Karimi M. "Meningeal melanocytoma of the brain and oculodermal melanocytosis (nevus of Ota): case report and literature review," Surgical Neurology. 2003;59(3):200-10.
24. Magarasevic L, Abazi Z. Unilateral open-angle glaucoma associated with the ipsilateral nevus of Ota. Case Rep Ophthalmol Med. 2013;2013:924-37
25. Alvarez-Cuesta CC, Raya-Aguado C, Vázquez-López F, et al. "Nevus of Ota associated with ipsilateral deafness," J Am Acad Dermatol. 2002;47:S257-9.
26. Sharma G, Nagpal A. Nevus of Ota with rare palatal involvement: a case report with emphasis on differential diagnosis. Case Rep Dent. 2011;2011:670-9.
27. Okawa Y, Yokota R, Yamauchi A. On the extracellular sheath of dermal melanocyte in nevus fuscoceruleus acromio-deltoideus (Ito) and Mongolian spot. J Invest Dermatol. 1979;73:224-30.
28. Beattie RM, Harvey D. Extensive and unusual Mongolian blue spots in a child with GM1 gangliosidosis type one. J R Soc Med. 1992;85(9):574-5.
29. Ponti G, Tomasi A, Pastorino L, et al. Diagnostic and pathogenetic role of café-au-lait macules in nevoid basal cell carcinoma syndrome. Hered Cancer Clin Pract. 2012;10:15.
30. Cannizzaro LA, Hecht F. Gene for incontinentia pigmenti maps to band Xp11 with an (X;10)(p11;q22) translocation. Clin Genet. 1987;32:66-9.
31. Sefiani A, Abel L, Heuertz S, et al. The gene for incontinentia pigmenti is assigned to Xq28. Genomics. 1989;4:427-9.
32. Landy SJ, Donnai D. Incontinentia pigmenti (Bloch-Sulzberger syndrome). J Med Genet. 1993;30:53-9.
33. Alexander L, Paller AS, Chan LS. Incontinentia pigmenti: A review and update on the molecular basis of pathophysiology. J Am Acad Dermatol. 2002;47:169-87.
34. Brunquell PJ. Recurrent encephalomyelitis associated with incontinentia pigmenti. Pediatr Neurol. 1987;3:174-7.
35. Kalter DC, Griffiths WA, Atherton DJ. Linear and whorled nevoid hypermelanosis. J Am Acad Dermatol. 1988;19:1037-44.
36. Nehal KS, PeBenito R, Orlow SJ. Analysis of 54 Cases of Hypopigmentation and Hyperpigmentation Along the Lines of Blaschko. Arch Dermatol. 1996;132:1167-70.
37. Moulin G, Hill MP, Guillaud V, et al. Bandes pigmente´es atrophiques acquises suivant les lignes de Blaschko. Ann Dermatol Venereol. 1992;119:729-36.
38. Baumann L, Happle R, Plewig G, et al. Atrophodermia linearis Moulin: Ein neues Krankheitsbild, das den Blaschko- Linien folgt. Hautarzt. 1994;45:231-6.
39. Patsatsi A, Kyriakou A, Chaidemenos G, et al. Linear atrophoderma of Moulin: a case report and review of the literature. Dermatol Pract Concept. 2013; 3(1):7-11.
40. Wongkietkachorn K, Intarasupht J, Srisuttiyakorn C, et al. Linear atrophoderma of Moulin: a case report and review of the literature. Case Rep Dermatol. 2013;5:11-4.
41. Happle R. Speckled lentiginous nevus syndrome: delineation of a new distinct neurocutaneous phenotype. Eur J Dermatol. 2002:12;133-5.
42. Happle R. Paradominant inheritance: a possible explanation for Becker's pigmented hairy nevus. Eu J Dermatol. 1992:2;39-40.
43. Wong SS. Bilateral segmental neurofibromatosis with partial unilateral lentiginosis. Br J Dermatol. 1997;136:380-3.
44. Ota M. Nevus fusco-caeruleus ophthalmo-maxillaris. Jpn J Dermatol. 1939;46:369-74.
45. Happle R. The group of epidermal nevus syndromes Part I. Well defined phenotypes. J Am Acad Dermatol. 2010;63: 1-22.
46. Groesser L, Herschberger E, Sagrera A, et al. Phacomatosis Pigmentokeratotica Is Caused by a Postzygotic HRAS Mutation in a Multipotent Progenitor Cell. J Invest Dermatol. 2013;133(8):1998-2003.
47. Oh GN, Kim JY, Choi JE, et al. Phacomatosis pigmento-keratotica without extracutaneous abnormalities: a case study involving a preterm baby. J Korean Med Sci. 2012;27: 1444-6.
48. Read AP, Newton VE, Waardenburg syndrome. J Med Genet. 1997;34:656-65.

6

Metabolic Disorders of Pigmentation

Imran Majid

Key Features

Though many metabolic diseases have some symptoms related to skin pigmentation, only a few diseases have specific diagnostic features by way of pigmentary morphology.

- Often, pigmentary changes in a given clinical setting with other associated features give valuable clues to a diagnosis.
- In the individual patient the approach, and the extent to which investigations should be carried out, depend on the disease suspected.
- An overall knowledge of metabolic diseases as well as their common and rare external features is invaluable to the dermatologist.
- Further advances in genomics and proteomics in the future may unravel the mysteries and linkage of some of the genetic disorders with pigmentary changes and multi-system involvement.

INTRODUCTION

Metabolic disorders are a group of disorders characterized or caused by an abnormal metabolic process or step in the human body. Metabolic disorders can be congenital, due to an inherited enzyme abnormality or a defective gene, or can be acquired, secondary to some disorder of an endocrine organ. Both these types of metabolic disorders can be associated with some pigmentary changes in the skin and/or mucosal surfaces. These pigmentary changes can be broadly classified into hypomelanosis, hypermelanosis and non-melanin pigmentation of skin or mucosae. This chapter will try to give a broad outline of these metabolic disorders and their effect on skin and mucosal pigmentation. The main aim would be to aid the clinician in arriving at a possible diagnosis by looking at the pattern of skin or mucosal dyspigmentation. For the purpose of simplicity we would describe the disorders under two headings:

I. Disorders causing hypopigmentation
II. Disorders causing hyperpigmentation

HYPOPIGMENTATION

Hypopigmentation caused by metabolic disorders can be generalized or localized. The most important of these disorders are described in **Box 1**.

Box 1

Metabolic disorders associated with hypopigmentation of skin

1. Phenylketonuria
2. Homocystinuria
3. Histidinemia
4. Cystinosis
5. Infantile sialic acid storage disease
6. Selenium deficiency
7. Copper deficiency

Phenylketonuria

Phenylketonuria is the most common genetic disorder of amino acid metabolism.[1] It is inherited as an autosomal recessive trait and is thus more common in children born from consanguineous marriages. The basic defect is a deficiency of the enzyme "phenylalanine hydroxylase" (PAH) which is involved in the conversion of phenylalanine to tyrosine **(Fig. 1)**. Due to this non-conversion, there is a progressive accumulation of phenylalanine in the body fluids.[2,3] In fact, classic phenylketonuria is defined by plasma phenylalanine levels exceeding 1,000 μmol/L (normal < 120 μmol/L). The incidence of phenylketonuria is about 5 in 100,000 births.[3,4]

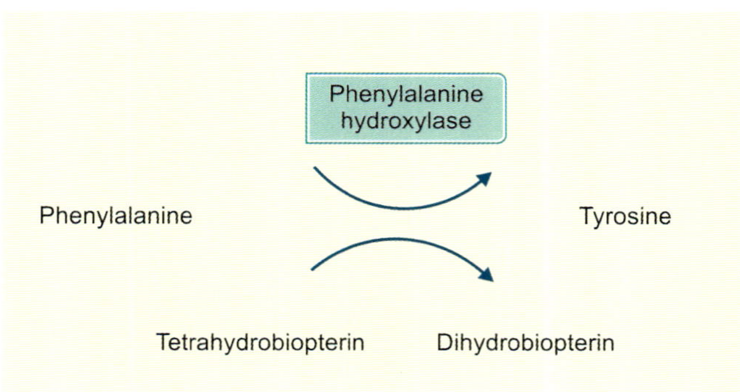

Fig. 1: Phenylalanine metabolism pathway

Two forms of phenylketonuria are described **(Box 2)**; while the more common one is due to inherited deficiency of PAH enzyme, the other rarer variant is due to a defect in tetrahydrobiopterin synthesis, which is an important co-enzyme in the process of conversion of phenylalanine to tyrosine **(Fig. 1)**.

Box 2

Phenylketonuria

- Phenylketnonuria is caused by deficiency of Phenylalanine hydroxylase enzyme.
- Progressive pigment dilution of the skin is the classical cutaneous manifestation
- Central nervous system manifestations are the major cause of morbidity
- Prognosis is good if the diagnosis is made and treatment started early in life

Clinical Presentation

A child born with phenylketonuria is usually normal at birth but with age there is a progressive developmental delay and mental retardation. If the diagnosis is delayed there is significant intellectual disability and this is the most common mode of presentation to a physician.[5] Additionally, the patient may also suffer from seizures (50%) and extrapyramidal symptoms like Parkinsonism. Moreover, there is a classical "musty" or "mousy" odor that aggravates after the patient takes a diet rich in phenylalanine.

Skin and Mucosal Manifestations

The most common presentation in skin and mucosa is a progressive dilution in melanin pigmentation which results in fair skin and blonde hair.[4,5] The child is usually fairer and more blond than his/her parents as well as brothers/sisters. This dilution in skin and hair pigmentation is more striking in black or colored races. Caucasian children with this disease almost invariably have blond hair, blue eyes, fair skin, and photosensitivity. However, the ability of these children to tan is normal. Additional cutaneous features include scleroderma like plaques, hair loss, keratosis pilaris, decreased number of pigmented nevi and eczema mimicking atopic dermatitis.[6]

Mechanism of Pigment Dilution

The mechanism for the pigment dilution in skin and hair is thought to be a competitive inhibition of the binding of tyrosine to tyrosinase by excess phenylalanine or a decreased amount of tyrosine.

Diagnosis

Diagnosis of phenylketonuria is done on the basis of the clinical features with the characteristic musty odor and demonstration of high levels of phenylalanine in the patient's blood. A screening test is now available for the diagnosis of phenylketonuria in newborns and this test is routinely done in many developed nations as a part of normal newborn screening. The test is known as "Guthrie inhibition assay" test. Prenatal diagnosis is also possible by performing amniocentesis or chorionic villus sampling.

Prognosis and Treatment

With a low-phenylalanine diet, the abnormality in skin color, photosensitivity, odor, and eczema are reversible. However, if the diagnosis is delayed there is irreversible damage to the central nervous system and deleterious effects on the patient's intellect.[7,8]

Implementing a diet low in phenylalanine early in infancy can dramatically reduce the chances of mental retardation. Tyrosine treatment causes darkening toward normal color within 1–2 months.[7,8]

Homocystinuria

Homocystinuria is a disorder of methionine metabolism, leading to an abnormal accumulation of homocysteine and its metabolites in blood and urine. It is inherited as an autosomal recessive trait and is basically due to a defect in transfer of the sulfur from methionine to homocysteine.[9] Three forms of homocystinuria are known and they are called as homocystinuria I, II and III depending upon the specific genetic defect.

The clinical presentation of homocystinuria is varied and the disease can present as mental retardation, psychiatric disturbances, developmental delay, seizures and skeletal or ophthalmological abnormalities.[10] Skin manifestations include a generalized hypopigmentation, livedo reticularis of the legs, tissue paper scars on hands and fine, brittle hair.

Hypopigmentation in homocystinuria results from the inhibition of tyrosinase by homocysteine and is usually reversible on treatment.[11,12]

Histidinemia

Histidinemia is a rare autosomal recessive metabolic disorder caused by a deficiency of the enzyme "histidase" which is needed for the metabolism of histidine.

Histidinemia is characterized by increased levels of histidine in blood, urine and CSF and decreased levels of the metabolite urocanic acid in blood, urine, and skin cells.[13]

Usually asymptomatic, some children may present with neurological dysfunction and generalized hypopigmentation.[14,15] The cause of this hypopigmentation is not known with certainty but it is postulated to be due to deficient levels of adrenocorticotropic hormone (ACTH) and melanocyte-stimulating hormones (MSH). The hypopigmentation is most apparent on the skin of the nipple, areola and genitalia and in contrast with anemia, the mucous membranes retain their normal color. There is an increased tendency of sunburns and lack of tanning of the skin.

In addition to the dilution of skin pigment other dermatological features include loss of terminal hair due to decreased gonadotropin secretion. This is observed in almost all patients, first in the axillae and later, in the pubic area as well. There is also fine wrinkling and dryness of the skin simulating advanced age.

Cystinosis

Cystinosis is a lysosomal storage disorder caused by defective transport of the amino acid cysteine out of lysosomes. The disease is inherited as an autosomal recessive trait and affects multiple organ systems of the body. Cysteine that accumulates is poorly soluble and crystallizes within the lysosomes of many cell types leading to cell damage and consequently a widespread tissue and organ damage ensues.[16,17]

Patients usually present during the first year of life with polyuria, polydipsia, dehydration, metabolic acidosis, hypophosphatemic rickets and failure to thrive. If untreated, renal failure develops by age 7–10 years.

Patients with infantile cystinosis have hypopigmentation with blond hair, blue eyes and a clear skin. However some patients, in particular African Americans have no such hypopigmentation. Additionally, there is no correlation between cutaneous phenotype and the severity of renal disease in cystinosis. The cause of hypopigmentation in cystinosis has not been so far elucidated.

Infantile Sialic Acid Storage Disease

Infantile sialic acid storage disease (ISSD) is a rare, autosomal recessive inborn error of metabolism characterized by early onset developmental delay, skin hypopigmentation, coarse facial features, hepatosplenomagaly, seizures and failure to thrive.[18]

Deficiency Disorders Causing Hypopigmentation

In addition to the metabolic disorders described above, there are many deficiency diseases that are associated with hypopigmentation. These include selenium deficiency that causes loss of hair and hypopigmentation and copper deficiency which is also associated with hypopigmentation of the skin and hair. Copper deficiency is related to hypopigmentation because tyrosinase is a copper-dependent enzyme. However, as multiple nutritional deficiencies tend to co-exist, it is often difficult to pinpoint a single nutrient deficiency as a cause of skin dyspigmentation.

HYPERPIGMENTATION

Increased pigmentation is a feature of many metabolic disorders but in most of these, the mechanism of hyperpigmentation is obscure. In some of these disorders, however, elevated level of β-MSH-like immunoreactivity is seen.

Hypermelanosis in metabolic disorders may be diffuse or localized. It may be confined to the epidermis, when the skin appears brown in color, or else it may involve the dermis, when the skin is a slate-gray or blue in color. Additionally, pigments other than melanin may also be present.

Metabolic disorders causing hyperpigmentation are listed in **Table 1**.

Porphyria Cutanea Tarda (Box 3)

Porphyria cutanea tarda (PCT) is a metabolic disorder which occurs due to deficient activity of enzyme uroporphyrin decarboxylase (UROD), an important enzyme in heme synthesis pathway.[19] Deficiency of this enzyme leads to accumulation of uroporphyrin and other carboxylated porphyrins in the blood and tissues. Three main forms of PCT

Table 1: Metabolic causes of hyperpigmentation

Localized hyperpigmentation	*Generalized hyperpigmentation*
Pellagra	Alkaptonuria (ochronosis)
Porphyria cutanea tarda (PCT)	Hemochromatosis
	Addison's disease
	Gaucher's disease
	Niemann-Pick disease
	Vitamin A deficiency
	Wilson's disease
	Chronic renal disease

are known as Type 1 or sporadic form which occurs secondary to an acquired deficiency of UROD in hepatocytes; Type 2 or familial type in which the enzyme deficiency is inherited and is present in all body tissues and lastly Type 3 which is a rare type characterized by hereditary deficiency of UROD limited to hepatocytes.[19,20] Sporadic form of PCT is the most common type accounting for about three-fourths of all cases of PCT and it can be associated with hepatotrophic viral infections like HCV. While the sporadic type of PCT commonly presents in middle age the familial type can occur at a very young age.

Clinical Presentation

Clinically, the patients present with increased skin fragility on photo-exposed parts of the body and bullous eruptions which resolve spontaneously over weeks to leave atrophic scars and milia formation. Other features that are sometimes seen include hypertrichosis on the face especially on the forehead and ears, scarring alopecia, morphea like plaques, onycholysis and even scarring alopecia on the scalp.

In addition, a variety of changes are seen as far as the sin and mucosal pigmentation is concerned. A diffuse hyperpigmentation can occur that is accentuated on the sun exposed parts of the body or else one can see a reticulate macular hyperpigmentation on the photo-exposed parts of the body.[21] Additionally, a melasma like pigmentation can occur on the cheeks and the periorbital region especially in females.[22]

Box 3

Porphyria cutanea tarda

- Three forms are known—Type 1 or Sporadic form; Type 2 or Familial form and Type 3.
- Increased skin fragility and blister formation on photo-exposed parts of the body are the classical clinical features.
- Hyperpigmentation of the skin may be seen which is more pronounced on sun-exposed parts.
- Low-dose chloroquine and venesections are the main treatment options.

Diagnosis

Diagnosis is confirmed by the presence of uroporphyrins in urine, plasma spectrofluorometry and stool analysis especially in cases with renal failure. In addition to this screening, the patient needs to be investigated for the presence and the severity of liver disease especially HCV infection, hemochromatosis, alcohol abuse, etc.

Treatment

Treatment of PCT involves the treatment of the underlying cause in addition to the treatment of porphyria. For the primary condition two main treatment options are favored; chloroquine or its derivatives and repeated venesections. Chloroquine is considered to be the drug of first choice in PCT and it is given in a lower dose (125–250 mg twice weekly) than that used in malaria.[23,24] The drug is given over about 6–18 months and then discontinued slowly. Usually the disease goes into remission and remains so for months together (up to 2 years) after chloroquine therapy.[24,25]

Venesection is preferred over chloroquine in patients who have significant hepatitis C virus (HCV) hepatitis as they require iron depletion to prevent further liver damage and also in patients who do not show a good response to chloroquine.[26] Venesection, when indicated, is usually performed every week or fortnightly and about 500 mL of blood is removed at every session. The treatment is continued till transferring saturation reaches 15% and plasma ferritin levels reach below 25 µg/L.[27]

Alkaptonuria (Box 4)

Alkaptonuria is a rare metabolic disorder which occurs due to deficiency of the enzyme homogentisic acid oxidase.[28] The cardinal features of the disorder include urine that turns dark on standing, pigmentation of skin, cartilage and connective tissues and arthritis predominantly involving the axial skelton.[28]

Epidemiology and Genetics

Alkaptonuria is a rare disorder with an incidence of 1 in 200,000 births and the disease has been reported from multiple regions of the world. The disease is inherited as an autosomal recessive trait and the gene responsible for the disorder has been localized to chromosome 3q (3q21-23). [28]

Pathogenesis

Hemogentisic acid is an intermediate in the metabolism of phenylalanine and tyrosine and secondary to the enzyme deficiency of homogentisic acid oxidase, homogentisic acid cannot be metabolized further leading to its accumulation in body fluids and tissues. This leads to the deposition of oxidized homogentisic acid pigment throughout the body, particularly in fibrous and cartilaginous tissues. This pathological deposition is known as "ochronosis" which literally means "ochre like" (pale yellow) referring to the color of connective tissue when viewed through microscope. As a result of this deposition, the cartilages including the larynx, articular cartilage as well as the intervertebral discs and trachea attain a black color.[29,30] In addition the urine as well as the sweat becomes discolored especially after exposure to air. Changes in the articular cartilage are responsible for the characteristic arthropathy that develops in later life in these patients.[31]

Clinical Presentation

Alkaptonuria is usually a silent disease until adult life and the only manifestations in childhood are discoloration of the urine and "spotting or staining" of the napkins or clothing. Cutaneous changes of the disorder are rarely seen prior to 12–15 years of age and usually become apparent in the fourth decade of life. The earliest sign is thickening of the ear cartilage, associated with blue-black or gray-blue discoloration. In the skin, earliest signs of pigmentation are usually seen in the axillae which can attain a blue or brown color. Later the whole face may show a brown, mottled pigmentation and this pigmentation can extend on to the neck and even trunk.[29,30] In some cases, the ochronotic pigmentation on the face is limited to the butterfly area only. In addition to the skin and ears, one of the earliest signs of the disease is bluish discoloration of the sclera and conjunctiva. In later stages of the disease, pigmentation may even be seen on the palmar and plantar skin.

Box 4

Alkaptonuria

- It is a rare metabolic disease due to deficiency of enzyme 'homogentisic acid oxidase'?
- Characterized by the deposition of pigment in body tissues known as 'ochronosis'
- Clinically silent till adulthood when it presents with sclera, auricular or skin pigmentation.
- Arthropathy and renal failure are late complications.
- Vitamin C in high doses can be given as treatment.

Extracutaneous manifestations of the disorder include an arthropathy that first involves the axial skeleton and presents with chronic back pain and stiffness usually in the fourth decade of life.[31,32] Radiography at this stage shows flattened and calcified intervertebral discs. In later stages, arthropathy can extend to involve the large peripheral joints to cause a rheumatoid like joint involvement. The disease is known to resemble rheumatoid arthritis clinically but osteoarthritis radiographically because of the degenerative changes in joints. Renal complications can ensue in later life with an increased incidence of renal calculi and there may be cardiovascular complications as well with valvular involvement and aortic and mitral valve calcification and even atherosclerosis. Involvement of the ossicles and ear drum with ochronosis can lead to deafness in the involved patients.

Diagnosis

Diagnosis of alkaptonuria is made on the basis of clinical presentation especially on the basis of achronotic deposition in skin and ears/eyes. The diagnosis is confirmed by urine analysis and enzyme assays. In addition the patient may also need a skin biopsy to demonstrate the classical histopathological changes of ochronosis.

Treatment

There is no specific treatment for alkaptonuria and the commonest treatment that is offered in these patients is Vitamin C (ascorbic acid) in a dose of 1–1.5 g per day.[33] The drug is supposed to inhibit the oxidation of homogentisic acid and also gives some protection against the degenerative effect of ochronotic pigment deposition in tissues. Physiotherapy for joints, analgesics, Vitamin B_{12} and Nitisinone (an inhibitor of homogentisic acid production) have also been described as treatment options in this disorder.

Hemochromatosis

Hemochomatosis is a disorder characterized by the pathological deposition of iron in body tissues. Literally "hemochromatosis" means "pigmentation derived from blood" and this term was first coined by von Recklinghausen in 1899.[34]

The disease basically occurs due to increased absorption of iron with secondary deposition in different organs of the body. Clinical manifestations occur because of the deposition of iron in the liver, pancreas, heart and endocrine organs. As a consequence the patient may present with cirrhosis of liver, cardiac failure or diabetes.[34,35]

Two main forms of hemochromatosis are known as the hereditary or idiopathic type and acquired type which occurs due to alcohol abuse or hemosiderosis. The hereditary form of the disease is most commonly seen in males above 40 years of age. Skin involvement is seen as diffuse pigmentation that either involves or is the most prominent on the exposed areas of the body first but becomes generalized later on.[35] Due to the classical pigmentation that occurs in the skin, the disease is also known as "bronze diabetes". Pigmentation that occurs in skin has a typical gray hue and is basically due to dermal melanosis rather than hemosiderin pigment deposition. Blackish stasis dermatitis and black keratin cysts have also been described in hemochromatosis.[36,37]

Wilson's Disease

Wilson's disease is a rare autosomal recessive disorder of copper metabolism in which there is an excessive absorption of copper from small intestines and excretion by liver. This leads to deposition of copper in liver, brain and other tissues of the body. The disease most commonly presents as unexplained chronic liver disease with neuropsychiatric symptoms.[38]

Skin involvement is seen in the form of a reticulate brownish pigmentation usually involving the legs.[38] In addition there is a bluish discoloration at the base of finger nails (azure lunula) and premature graying of hair. Eye examination reveals yellowish discoloration (jaundice) and greenish-gold to brown pigmentation of the cornea (Kayser Fleischer ring). Other signs of liver disease like spider angiomas and palmar erythema can also be seen. Copper chelating agents and oral zinc are used as treatment options.[39]

Gaucher's Disease

Gaucher's disease is a lysosomal storage disease that occurs secondary to deficiency of the enzyme "glucocerebrosidase". Deficiency of this enzyme leads to accumulation of glycosphingolipids, principally glucocerebrosides in the body tissues especially in spleen, liver, bone marrow, alveolar spaces and brain tissue.[40] Clinically, the disease presents as anemia, thrombocytopenia, bone demineralization, jaundice with hepatosplenomegaly and neurologic effects like ataxia and seizures.

In the skin and mucosae, the disease causes a diffuse light-brown pigmentation or brownish macular lesions.[41] Rapid tanning of the skin has also been reported. [41]

Niemann-Pick Disease

Niemann-Pick disease is an inherited metabolic disease caused by the deficiency of sphingomyelinase. The disorder is transmitted as an autosomal recessive trait and many of these affected patients especially those with a severe variant of the disease usually die in early childhood only. Deficiency of the enzyme sphingomyelinase leads to accumulation of sphingomyelin in histiocytes in multiple organ systems of the human body with resultant organ dysfunction. In the skin patients may show patches of waxy induration and yellowish-brown pigmentation. In addition, popular, papulonodular and even suppurative lesions, cafe-au-lait macules, Mongolian spots and xanthomas and xanthogranulomas have also been described.[42,43]

Chronic Renal Disease

Chronic renal disease is frequently accompanied by increased pigmentation of the skin. This hypermelanosis is diffuse and brown in color. It is most intense on the hands and face. Hyperpigmented macules are also common on the palms and soles.[44]

Elevated levels of β-MSH are found in the plasma due to slow clearance by the kidney rather than increased production by the pituitary. Lipochromes and carotenoids deposited in the skin may also play a part.[45]

Deficiency Disorders

Deficiency disorders associated with hyperpigmentation include Pellagra and vitamin A deficiency.

Pallegra is the classic clinical manifestation of niacin deficiency. The condition is characterized by photosensitivity with erythema and hyperpigmentation of sun-exposed sites. The affected skin becomes hard, dry and cracked and in extreme cases is black in color.

The sites of involvement are the sun-exposed skin of the face, neck, dorsa of hands and feet, and sometimes the forearms. Mucosal sites are also affected.[46,47]

Hyperpigmentation is also seen in Vitamin A deficiency in addition to the typical eye changes. The classical cutaneous manifestation of vitamin A deficiency is xerosis of skin along with hyperpigmentation of the face and limbs.[48] Keratosis pilaris, desquamation of the skin, conjunctival pigmentation is also seen in these patients.[49]

REFERENCES

1. Williams RA, Mamotte CDS, Brunett JR. Phenylketonuria: An Inborn Error of Phenylalanine Metabolism. Clin Biochem Rev. 2008;29:31-41.
2. Kaufman S. A model of human phenylalanine metabolism in normal subjects and in phenylketonuric patients. Proc Natl Acad Sci USA. 1999;96:3160-4.
3. Kaufman S, Holtzman NA, Milstien S, et al. Phenylketonuria due to a deficiency of dihydrobiopterin reductase. N Engl J Med. 1975;293:785-90.
4. Yu JS. Phenylketonuria: a review. Postgrad Med J. 1970;46: 430-46.
5. Pitt DB, Danks DM. The natural history of untreated phenylketonuria. J Paediatr Child Health. 1991;27:189-90.
6. Jablonska S, Stachow A, Suffczynska M. Skin and muscle indurations in phenylketonuria. Arch Dermatol. 1967;95: 443-50.
7. Smith I. Recommendations on dietary management of phenylalanine. Report of MRC Working Party on phenylketonuria. Arch Dis Child. 1993;68:426-7.
8. Kang ES, Sollee ND, Gerald PS. Results of treatment and termination of the diet in phenylketonuria (PKU). Paediatrics. 1970;46:881-90.
9. Carson NAJ, Cusworth DC, Dent CE, et al. Homocystinuria. Arch Dis Child. 1963;38:425-36.
10. Schoonderwaldt HC, Boers GHJ, Cruysberg JRM, et al. Neurologic manifestations of homocystinuria. Clin Neurol Neurosurg. 1981;83:153-62.
11. Reish O, Townsend D, Berry SA, et al. Tyrosinase inhibition due to interaction of homocysteine with copper: The mechanism for reversible hypopigmentation in homocystinuria due to cystathione β-synthase deficiency. Am J Hum Genet. 1995;57:127-32.
12. Mudd SH, Edwards WA, Loeb PM, et al. Homocystinuria due to cystathionine synthase deficiency: the effect of pyridoxine. J Clin Invest. 1970;49:1762-73.
13. Woody NC, Snyder CH, Harris JA. Histidinemia. Amer J Dis Child. 1965;110:606.
14. Gatfield PD, Knights RM, Devereux M, et al. Histidinemia: report of four new cases in one family and the effect of low histidine diets. Can Med Assoc J. 1969;101:71-5.
15. Holton JB, Lewis FJW, Moore GR. Biochemical Investigation of Histidinaemia. J Clin Path. 1964;17:671.
16. Newbold PC. The skin in genetically controlled metabolic disorders. J Med Genet. 1973;10:101-11.

17. Wilmer MJ, Schoeber JP, van den Heuvel LP, et al. Cystinosis: practical tools for diagnosis and treatment. Pediatr Nephrol. 2011;26:205-15.
18. Varki A. Sialic acids in human health and disease. Trends Mol Med. 2008;14:351-60.
19. Elder GH. Porphyria cutanea tarda. Semin Liver Dis. 1998;18:67-75.
20. Kauppinen R. Porphyrias. Lancet. 2005;365:241-52.
21. Mascaro JM, Herrero C, Lecha M, et al. Uroporphyrinogen-decarboxylase deficiencies: porphyria cutanea tarda and related conditions. Semin Dermatol. 1986;5:115-24.
22. Doyle JA, Friedman SJ. Porphyria and scleroderma. A clinical and laboratory review of 12 patients. Australas J Dermatol. 1983;24:109-14.
23. Shaffrali FC, McDonagh AJ, Messenger AG. Hair darkening in porphyria cutanea tarda. Br J Dermatol. 2002;146:325-9.
24. Ashton RE, Hawk JLM, Magnus IA. Low-dose oral chloroquine in the treatment of porphyria cutanea tarda. Br J Dermatol. 1984;111:609-13.
25. Scholnick PL, Epstein J, Marver HS. The molecular basis of the action of chloroquine in porphyria cutanea tarda. J Invest Dermatol.1973;61:226-32.
26. Wennersten G, Ros AM. Chloroquine in treatment of porphyria cutanea tarda. Long-term efficacy of combined phlebotomy and high-dose chloroquine therapy. Acta Derm Venereol Suppl (Stockh). 1982;100:119-23.
27. Ratnaike S, Blake D, Campbell D, et al. Plasma ferritin levels as a guide to the treatment of porphyria cutanea tarda by venesection. Australas J Dermatol. 1988;29:3-7.
28. Fernandez-Canon JM, Granadino B, Beltron-Valero de Bernabe D, et al. The molecular basis of alkaptonuria. Nat Genet. 1996;14:19-24.
29. Lee PJ, Brenton DP. Inborn errors of amino acid and organic acid metabolism. In: Warrell DA, Cox TM, Firth JD (Eds). Oxford Textbook of Medicine, 4th edn. Oxford: Oxford University Press; 2003. pp. 9-31.
30. Quyoom S, Jehangir M, Hassan I, et al. Ochronosis. Indian J Dermatol Venereol Leprol. 2003;69:76-7.
31. O'Brien WM, La Du BN, Bunim JJ. Biochemical, pathologic and clinical aspects of alkaptonuria, ochronosis and ochronotic arthropathy. Review of world literature. Am J Med. 1963;34:813-38.
32. Capkin E, Karkucak M, Yayli S, et al. Ochronosis in differential diagnosis of patients with chronic backache: a review of the literature. Rheumatol Int. 2007;28:61-4.
33. Wolff JA, Barshop B, Nyhan WL, et al. Effects of ascorbic acid in alkaptonuria: alterations in benzaquinone acetic acid and ontogenic effect in infance. Pediatr Res. 1989;26: 140-4.
34. Bacon BR. Hemochromatosis: diagnosis and management. Gastroenterology. 2001;120:718-25.
35. Tavill AS, Sharma BK, Bacon BR. Iron and the liver: genetic hemochromatosis and other hepatic iron overload disorders. Prog Liver Dis. 1990;9:281-305.
36. Leyden JJ, Lockshin NA, Krebel S. The black keratinous cyst: a sign of hemochromatosis. Arch Dermatol. 1972;106: 379-81.
37. Soderberg KI, Sharp M, Carrington PR. Brown and black scaly patches on the lower leg. Arch Dermatol. 2007;143: 1441-6.
38. Danks DM. Steely hair, mottled mice and copper metabolism. N Engl J Med. 1975;293:1147-8.
39. Hoogenraad TU, van der Hamer CJA, Hattum JV. Effective treatment of Wilson's disease with oral zinc sulphate: two case reports. BMJ. 1984;289:273-6.
40. Rooney PJ. Hyperlipidemias, lipid storage disorders, metal storage disorders, and ochronosis. Curr Opin Rheumatol. 1991;3:166-71.
41. Goldblatt J, Beighton P. Cutaneous manifestations of Gaucher disease. Br J Dermatol. 1984;111: 331-4.
42. Sibulkin D, Olichney JJ. Juvenile xanthogranuloma in a patient with Niemann-Pick disease. Arch Dermatol. 1973;108:829-34.
43. Boustany RMN, Kaye E, Alroy J. Ultrastructural findings in skin from patients with Niemann-Pick disease, type C. Pediatric Neurology. 1990;6:177-83.
44. Gilchrest BA, Stern RS, Steinman TI, et al. Clinical features of pruritus among patients undergoing maintenance haemodialysis. Arch Dermatol. 1982;118:154-60.
45. Thomas EA, Thomas PA. A prospective study of cutaneous abnormalities in patients with chronic kidney disease. Indian J Nephrol. 2012;22:116-20.
46. Bean WR, Spies TD, Vilter RW. Asymmetric cutaneous lesions in pellagra. Arch Dermatol Syphilol. 1944;49:335-45.
47. Wan p, Moat S, Anstey A. Pellagra: a review with emphasis on photosensitivity. Br J Dermatol. 2011;164:1188-200
48. Frazier CN, Hu CK. Cutaneous lesions associated with a deficiency in vitamin A. Arch Intern Med. 1931;48:507-9.
49. Miller S. Nutritional deficiency of the skin. J Am Acad Dermatol. 1989;21:1-30.

7

Endocrinal Pigmentary Disorders

Raghunatha Reddy R, Shashikumar BM

Key Features

- Endocrine-related pigmentary disorders are not so uncommon; most of them may have near similar manifestations except for a few. It could be an early predictor for an endocrine disorder and its early diagnosis and management could be of great help to the patient.
- A thorough knowledge of the other clinical and dermatological manifestations of the endocrine disorder is very essential to arrive at a clinical diagnosis of endocrine-related pigmentation.
- It is important to have a proper knowledge and nearest differential diagnosis to evaluate specifically and to order for relevant diagnostic tests.

INTRODUCTION

Physiology and pathophysiology of pigmentation is a complex process regulated by endocrine, paracrine and autocrine factors apart from environmental effect. The endocrine system consists of hormone producing glands which includes pituitary, thyroid, parathyroid, pancreas, adrenal gland, testes and ovaries. Pituitary hormones like melanocortins (α-melanotropins, β-melanotropins, γ-mela-notropins, β-lip otropins), adrenocorticotropic hormone (ACTH) and estrogens (α-estradiol, β-estradiol and estradiol) have direct stimulatory action on melanogenesis. Malfunction of these glands may present as abnormal pigmentation.

ROLE OF MELANOCORTINS, ACTH, AND MELANOCORTIN RECEPTORS IN MELANOGENESIS

Proopiomelanocortin (POMC) peptides like melanocortins (melanocyte-stimulating hormone, MSH) and adrenocorticotropins have regulatory role in melanogenesis. Structurally, MSH peptides (that include α-MSH, β-MSH, and γ-MSH peptides) and ACTH have common amino acid sequence "His-Phe-Arg-Trp" which is critical for melanotropic activity.[1,2] In animals, α-MSH and β-MSH induces darkening of the skin. MSH peptides stimulate both melanogenesis and the switching of the pheo- to the eumelanogenic pathway. Also, α-MSH is shown to specifically stimulate follicular melanogenesis and tyrosinase activity at the transcriptional, translational, or post-translational level, depending on genotype and hair cycle in hamsters.[1-3] In humans, the systemic administration of α-MSH, β-MSH or ACTH stimulates skin pigmentation, predominantly in sun-exposed areas.[4,5] Clinical observations have shown that the pathologically increased levels of plasma ACTH in Addison's disease, or the excessive ACTH production by tumors (Nelson syndrome), are accompanied by hyperpigmentation and skin atrophy. In most patients with excess ACTH/α-MSH, even though the hyperpigmentation is generalized, it is most prominent in sun-exposed areas. In contrast, patients with pituitary POMC gene mutations leading to defective production of the POMC protein have red hair pigmentation.

Table 1: Etiology of Addison's diseases[10]

• *Adrenal dysgenesis:* Congenital adrenal hypoplasia (CAH) mutations of steroidogenic factor, adrenocorticotropic hormone (ACTH) unresponsiveness.
• *Adrenal destruction:* Autoimmune polyglandular syndrome (APS), adrenoleukodystrophy (ALD), adrenal hemorrhage, adrenal metastases, infections, and amyloidoses.
• *Impaired steroidogenesis:* Congenital adrenal hyperplasia (CAH), mitochondrial disorders, Smith-Lemli-Opitz syndrome (SLOS)

Melanocortin (MC) receptors (MC1 to MC5) are 45 kDa seven transmembrane G protein-coupled receptors. MC receptors are coupled to adenyl cyclase. MC receptors have different pharmacological profiles of activation by MSH and ACTH peptides; MC1R has the highest affinity for α-MSH and ACTH and is the most important in the regulation of melanogenic activity.[6] MC2R has specific affinity for ACTH, and its messenger ribonucleic acid (mRNA) is predominantly expressed in the cortex of adrenal gland. Expression and activity of MSH receptors in mammalian pigment cells are also regulated by intrinsic and extrinsic factors of which the most important is UV radiation.

The phenotypic effects of MSH and ACTH peptides in melanocytes are mediated via interactions with cell surface receptors containing seven transmembrane domains linked to the G_S protein and cyclic adenosine monophosphate (cAMP)-dependent pathways through activation of protein kinase A (PKA) and phosphorylation/dephosphorylation reactions.[1,7] Increased intracellular cAMP leads to increased tyrosinase activity and melanin production, stimulation of dendrite formation, and inhibition or stimulation of cell proliferation.

Endocrine disorders may result from an excess or deficiency of particular hormone or a lack of responsiveness to the hormone in the target organ. Since hormones are involved in a wide range of metabolic and regulatory process, abnormalities in hormone levels tend to have profound consequences, affecting many different organ systems. In this section, we restrict our discussion to endocrine disorders leading to dyspigmentation alone.

ADDISON'S DISEASE

Addison's disease (*Synonyms: chronic adrenal insufficiency, Primary adrenal insufficiency, hypocortisolism, hypoadrenalism*) is a chronic, rare disorder due to insufficient secretion or supply of adrenocortical hormones.

Etiology

The prevalence of Addison's disease is 2 in 10,000 in the general population. Approximately one half of these cases are acquired, most common cause being autoimmune destruction of the adrenal glands; the other one half are genetic, most commonly caused by distinct enzymatic blocks in adrenal steroidogenesis affecting glucocorticoid synthesis (i.e. congenital adrenal hyperplasia).[8] But in India and other developing countries tuberculosis is still the leading cause of Addison's disease.[9] Other infectious causes include human immunodeficiency virus (HIV), *Cytomegalovirus (CMV), Cryptococcus* and histoplasmosis **(Table 1)**.

Clinical Features

Addison's diseases commonly manifests with relatively nonspecific signs and symptoms **(Table 2)** such as fatigue and loss of energy, often resulting in delayed or missed diagnoses (e.g. as depression or anorexia).

A distinguishing feature of primary adrenal insufficiency is hyperpigmentation, which is caused by excess ACTH stimulation of melanocytes. Hyperpigmentation is gradual in onset and generalized but more pronounced in skin areas

Table 2: Clinical features of Addison's disease[10,11]

Symptoms	*Signs*	*Biochemical abnormalities*
• Fatigue • Muscular weakness • Abdominal pain • Nausea, vomiting • Diarrhea • Salt craving • Behavior changes • Headache • Sweating • Depression • Muscle and joint pain • Cessation of menses	• Postural hypotension • Weight loss • Sparse axillary hair • Generalized pigmentation, • Associated vitiligo and/or goiter	• *CBC:* Eosinophilia • Lymphocytosis, anemia • *Serum chemistry:* Hyponatremia, hyperkalemia, hypoglycemia, hypercalcemia • High (supine) plasma renin and/or increased night time adrenocorticotropic hormone (ACTH) levels • Low plasma cortisol levels • Low ACTH stimulated cortisol responses

Table 3: Pattern of Addisonian pigmentation

- *Sun-exposed areas:* Face and extensor aspects of upper extremities
- *Frictional areas:* Elbow, knee, waistline, under bra straps
- Pressure areas
- *Accentuation of normally high pigmented areas:* Genital, perineum, axillae, areolae, umbilicus.
- *Creases:* Palmar and plantar
- Scars
- Darkening of existing pigmented lesions like nevi
- Eruptive lentigines
- *Mucous membrane:* Spotty pigmentation mainly on tongue and buccal mucous
- *Hairs and nails:* Longitudinal melanonychia

exposed to increased friction or shear stress and is increased by sunlight **(Table 3)**. Adjective "Addisonian pigmentation" is used to describe classical pattern of pigmentation of the condition. This characteristic pattern of pigmentation is seen in 95–100% of cases of Addison's disease.[12,13] Few reports of Addison's disease without pigmentation[14] and localized melasma-like pigmentation[15] have been described.

Mucosal involvement is seen in most of the cases with brown patches on gingiva, vermillion border of the lips, buccal mucosa, palate and tongue.[16] Oral involvement may represent the first signs of Addison's disease in few cases.[17]

Nails show diffuse brown discoloration and longitudinal melanonychia. Darkening of hairs can be seen in few cases.

Similarly, Addisonian pigmentation is noted in Nelson's syndrome and tumors which secrete ectopic ACTH, whereas, in secondary adrenal insufficiency, the skin has paleness due to lack of ACTH secretion.

Diagnosis

The diagnosis of adrenal insufficiency is established by the short cosyntropin test but random serum cortisol measurements are of limited value. Once confirmed, adrenal CT, adrenal autoantibodies and chest X-ray are useful to detect etiology. Skin biopsy is nonspecific and not diagnostic. The histopathology of pigmented area shows increased amounts of melanin in basal and spinous layers. Melanocytes counts are normal but melanophages may be seen in papillary dermis.

Treatment

Treatment includes glucocorticoid and mineralocorticoid replacement therapy. Hyperpigmentation of skin regresses slowly over months to years but mucosal pigmentation and pigmentation over scars may persist. Decrease in intensity of pigmentation during replacement therapy is one of the most sensitive indices for changing the maintenance dose of corticosteroids.

ACROMEGALY

Acromegaly is a syndrome resulting from an excess of growth hormone (GH) or somatotropin in adults. More than 99% of cases result from a pituitary adenoma.

Clinical Features (Table 4)

Skin involvement was described in 1899 by Steinberg.[18] Skin changes have been considered a classic finding in acromegaly.

Table 4: Clinical and lab features in acromegaly

Cutaneous	*Others*	*Lab*
• Gigantism • *Facies:* Prognathism, frontal bossing, widely spaced teeth • *Lips:* Large, thickened and protruded • *Eyelid:* Thickened • *Tongue:* Large and furrowed • *Ears:* Large, triangular • Elongated fingers • Skin tags • Oily skin • Hypertrichosis • Acne • Cutis verticis gyrata • Seborrheic keratoses • Addisonian hyperpigmentation • Acanthosis nigricans	• Headache • Visual field loss • Arthropathy • Carpal tunnel syndrome • Proximal myopathy • *Cardiovascular system (CVS):* Hypertension, cardiomyopathy, Sleep apnea, Hyperlipidemia	• Insulin-like growth factor↑ • Serum GH↑ (Not suppressed by oral glucose) • Prolactin↑ • Blood glucose↑ • *MRI brain:* Adenoma is greater than 90% • *X-ray fingers:* Tufting

One of the earliest signs is an edematous and doughy feeling, most noticeable in face, palms and soles.

Hyperpigmentation is noted in around 50% of patients and it is mainly of Addisonian pattern.[19]

Treatment

Treatment consists of surgery to resect the tumor.

HYPERTHYROIDISM

Hyperthyroidism is due to increased thyroid hormone due to various causes. Autoimmune thyroiditis (Graves' disease) is one of the most common causes. Other causes include adenoma, multinodular goiter or exogenous production of thyroid hormone.

Hyperthyroidism is associated with a wide variety of skin manifestations. Hyperpigmentation has been reported in 2% of hyperthyroidism patients[20] with an even higher incidence reported in Japanese patients.[21] Various degrees of pigmentation ranging from generalized to localized pigmentation on the face have been described. But Addisonian pattern of pigmentation is well recognized. This pigmentation differs from Addison's disease pigmentation in that the involvement of the mucous membranes is uncommon and pigmentation of nipples and genital skin is less striking.[22,23] Pituitary ACTH released as compensation for accelerated cortisol degradation is incriminated as the reason for hyperpigmentation in thyrotoxicosis. Also, vitiligo has been reported to be more commonly associated with autoimmune Graves' diseases.

PHEOCHROMOCYTOMA

Pheochromocytomas are rare neuroendocrine tumors. They have a highly variable clinical presentation, most common presentation being episodes of headaches, sweating, palpitations, and hypertension. Nearly 80–85% of pheochromocytomas arise from the adrenal medulla, whereas about 15–20% are from extra-adrenal chromaffin tissue.[24,25] Addisonian pattern of pigmentation was described in malignant pheochromocytomas. In a report, slate-grey macular pigmentation on the forehead, cheeks, nose, lips, helices of the ears, and dorsum of the hands, with prominence over the knuckles and the skin over the interphalangeal joints, elbows, and knees were noted. Also the scars of acne and previous injuries over the legs and mucosa were pigmented.[26] Pigmentation is due to ectopic ACTH and MSH production by the tumor which fades gradually after resection of tumor.

DIABETES MELLITUS

Diabetes mellitus is the most common endocrine disease and India is having the largest number of diabetics in the world. Mainly there are two types of diabetes mellitus, type I diabetes mellitus [insulin-dependent diabetes mellitus (IDDM) or "juvenile diabetes"] is due to autoimmune destruction of beta islet cells leading to insulin deficiency and type II diabetes mellitus [non-insulin-dependent diabetes mellitus (NIDDM) or "adult-onset diabetes"] is due to insulin resistance. The skin is one of the major organ systems involved in diabetes. Almost all diabetic patients eventually develop skin complications from the long-term effects of diabetes mellitus.[27]

Cutaneous manifestations of diabetes mellitus generally appear subsequent to the development of the disease, but they may be the first presenting signs and in some cases they may precede the primary disease manifestation by many years.[28] Prevalence of cutaneous disorders associated with diabetes ranges between 30 and 71%.[29-31] Multiple factors play a role in the manifestations of cutaneous signs of diabetes mellitus. Abnormalities in the metabolism of carbohydrates, alteration of metabolic pathways, vascular involvement in the form of atherosclerosis, microangiopathy and neuronal involvement in the form of sensory, motor and autonomic neuropathies and impaired host mechanisms, all play a role.

Vitiligo has been associated with both type 1 and type 2 diabetes mellitus and there is an increased association of vitiligo with a proven or presumed autoimmune disease.[32] Yellowish discoloration of skin is due to carotenemia which is seen in 10% of diabetics. This abnormal deposition of yellow pigment is due to diabetic diet, impaired conversion of carotene to vitamin A in the diabetic liver; or hyperlipidemia accompanying diabetes.[33,34] One of the most common cutaneous manifestations of diabetes is diabetic dermopathy or diabetic shin spots, which arise due to a trivial trauma seen most commonly over the shin and will remain as thin atrophic hyperpigmented scars.

CARCINOID SYNDROME

Carcinoids are slow-growing tumors arising from the enterochromaffin or Kulchitsky cells and, in most cases, originate in the gastrointestinal (GI) tract or the lungs. Carcinoid syndrome is the term used to describe a constellation of symptoms caused by the secreted bioactive substances and is present in less than 10% of patients with carcinoid tumors. Episodic cutaneous flushing is the hallmark of the carcinoid syndrome and is seen in 85% of patients.[35] Diffuse pigmentation is seen in gastric and thymic carcinoid secondary to MSH-production. Also, pellagra like rash with associated pigmentation is noted. Most of the pigmentary changes are due to niacin deficiency associated with this condition.

PIGMENTARY CHANGES IN PREGNANCY

Hyperpigmentation is one of the most common cutaneous changes that occur during pregnancy, occurring in up to 90% of women. Mild to moderate, localized, and generalized hyperpigmentation, with accentuation of normally hyperpigmented regions, such as the areolae of the breasts, axillae, and genitalia are common. Pigmentation of linea alba and scars is also observed in pregnancy. Pigmentation of the neck is also noted but less often.[36,37] Melasma or chloasma was observed in 50–75% of pregnant women.[37-39] Darkening and enlargement of nevi is also noted.[40,41] Also, Type b pigmentary demarcation lines are known to appear for the first time during pregnancy.[42] Most pregnancy-related skin hyperpigmentation is benign and is usually resolves within a year after delivery.

REFERENCES

1. Eberle A (Ed). The Melanotropins: Chemistry, Physiology and Mechanism of Action. Karger Publishing, Basel; 1988. pp. 73-8.
2. Hadley ME. Hormonal control of calcium homeostasis. In: Hadley ME (Ed). Endocrinology. Prentice-Hall, Englewood Cliffs, New Jersey; 1984. pp. 182-207.
3. Cone RD, Lu D, Koppula S, et al. The melanocortin receptors: agonists, antagonists, and the hormonal control of pigmentation. Recent Prog Horm Res. 1996;51:287-318.
4. Lerner AB, McGuire J. Effect of alpha- and beta-melanocyte stimulating hormones on the skin color of mean. Nature. 1961;189:176-9.
5. Levine N, Sheftel SN, Eytan T, et al. Induction of skin tanning by subcutaneous administration of a potent synthetic melanotropin. JAMA. 1991;266:2730-6.
6. Gantz I, Konda Y, Tashiro T, et al. Molecular cloning of a novel melanocortin receptor. J Biol Chem. 1993;268:8246-50.
7. Cone RD, Mountjoy KG, Robbins LS, et al. Cloning and functional characterization of a family of receptors for the melanotropic peptides. Ann NY Acad Sci. 1993;680:342-63.
8. Williams GF, Dluhy RG. Disorders of adrenal cortex. In: Fauci AS, Braunwald E, Kasper DL (Eds). Harrison's Principles of Internal Medicine, 17th edn. New York: The McGraw-Hill Companies, Inc; 2008. pp. 2247-69.
9. Bhatia E, Jain SK, Gupta RK, et al. Tuberculous Addison's disease: Lack of normalization of adrenocortical function after anti-tuberculous chemotherapy. Clin Endocrinol. 1998;48:355-9.
10. Ten S, New M, Maclaren N. Clinical review 130: Addison's disease 2001. J Clin Endocrinol Metab. 2001;86:2909-22.
11. Levin NA, Greer KE. Cutaneous manifestations of endocrine disorders. Dermatol Nurs. 2001;13:185-96.
12. Dunlop D. Eighty-six cases of Addison's disease. Br Med J. 1963;12:887-9.
13. Mattingly D. In: Recent Advances in Medicine, 15th edn. London: JA Churchill; p. 146.
14. Goodwin TJ, Kind PR, Bogomoletz VW. Addison's disease without pigmentation. Postgrad Med J. 1973;49:305-8.
15. Bari AU, Mahmood T. Addison's disease may present to a dermatologist as melasma. JPAD. 2006;16:56-9.
16. Lanza A, Heulfe H, Perillo L, et al. Oral pigmentation as a sign of Addison's disease: a brief reappraisal. The Open Dermatology Journal. 2009;3:3-6.
17. Nieman LK, Chanco Turner ML. Addison's disease. Clin Dermatol. 2006;24:276-80.
18. Centurion S, Schwartz R. Cutaneous signs of acromegaly. Int J Dermatol. 2002;41:631-4.
19. Cox NH, Coulson IH. Systemic disease and the skin. In: Burns T, Breathnach S, Cox N (Eds). Rook's Textbook of Dermatology, 8th edn. UK: Wiley-Blackwell; 2010. pp. 62.1-112.
20. Locke W. Unusual manifestations of Graves's disease. Med Clin North Am. 1967;51:915-24.
21. Arakawa T, Wada Y, Tada K, et al. Hyperpigmentation of the skin with DOPA-uria of a newborn. Tohoku J Exp Med. 1963;80:329-37.
22. Freedberg IM, Vogel LN. The skin in thyrotoxicosis. In: Braverman LE, Utiger RD (Eds). The Thyroid, 6th edn. Philadelphia: JB Lippincott Co; 1991. pp. 731-3.
23. Youmans JB. Changes in the skin in thyrotoxicosis. J Med Sci. 1931;181:681-92.
24. Whalen RK, Althausen AF, Daniels GH. Extra-adrenal pheochromocytoma. J Urol. 1992; 147:1-10.
25. Pacak K, Linehan WM, Eisenhofer G, et al. Recent advances in genetics, diagnosis, localization, and treatment of pheochromocytoma. Ann Intern Med. 2001;134:315-29.
26. Zawar VP, Walvekar R. A pheochromocytoma presenting as generalized pigmentation. Int J Dermatol. 2004;43: 140-2.
27. Hussain F, Arif M, Ahmad M. Skin Care Knowledge, Attitude and Practices among Pakistani Diabetic Patients. Egyptian Dermatology Online Journal. 2010;6(1):5.
28. Pavloviae MD, Milenkoviae T, Diniae M, et al. The prevalence of cutaneous manifestations in young patients with type 1 diabetes. Diabetes Care. 2007;30:1964-7.
29. Giligor RS, Lazarus GS. Skin manifestations of diabetes mellitus. In: Rifkin H, Raskin P (Eds). Diabetes Mellitus. Louana: Brady Co; 1981. pp. 313-21.
30. Sehgal VN, Sanker P. Some aspects of skin diseases and diabetes mellitus. Indian J Dermatol Venereol. 1965;31: 264-9.

31. Romano G, Morretti G, Dibenedetto A. Skin lesions in diabetes mellitus: Prevalence and clinical correlations. Diabetes Res Clin Pract. 1998;39:101-6.
32. Owen VJ. Diabetes mellitus. Br J Dermatol. 1969;81:9-13.
33. Sibbald RG, Schachter RK. The skin and diabetes mellitus. Int J Dermatol. 1984;23:567-84.
34. Patterson JW. Skin changes in diabetes mellitus: a review. Mil Med. 1983;148:135-40.
35. Jabbour SA, Davidovici BB, Wolf R. Rare syndromes. Clin Dermatol. 2006;24:299-316.
36. Martin AG, Leal-Khouri S. Physiologic skin changes associated with pregnancy. Int J Dermatol. 1992;31:375-8.
37. Wong RC, Ellis CN. Physiologic skin changes in pregnancy. J Am Acad Dermatol. 1989;8:7-11.
38. Winton GB, Lewis CW. Dermatoses of pregnancy. J Am Acad Dermatol. 1982;6:977-98.
39. Black MM, Wilkinson JD. Skin diseases in pregnancy. In: Kaminetzky HA (Ed). Principles and Practice of Obstetrics and Perinatology. Philadelphia: John Wiley; 1987. pp. 1361-79.
40. Foucar E, Bentley TJ, Laube DW, et al. A histopathologic evaluation of nevocellular nevi in pregnancy. Arch Dermatol. 1985;121:350-4.
41. Ellis DL, Wheeland RG. Increased nevus estrogen and progesterone ligand binding related to oral contraceptives and pregnancy. J Am Acad Dermatol. 1986;14:25-31.
42. Ruiz-Villaverde R, Blasco Melguizo J, et al. Pigmentary demarcation lines in a pregnant Caucasian woman. Int J Dermatol. 2004;43:911-2.

8

Chemical, Occupational and Drug-induced Pigmentary Disorders

Sanjay Ghosh, Saurav Kundu

Key Features

- Chemical leukoderma, an underdiagnosed condition, should always be excluded before stamping a case as "idiopathic" vitiligo.
- Householders consumer products rather than industrial chemicals especially in developing countries could induce this ailment commonly.
- Chemical leukoderma can spread beyond the site of contact to remote place.
- Occupational hyperpigmentation may be induced by pigmented contact dermatitis, metal deposition in skin, tattoos, chemical exposure.
- Pigmented contact dermatitis occurs mostly from sensitizing fragrances and chemicals in cosmetics predominantly in dark complexion individuals.
- Drug may cause mucocutaneous dyspigmentation which, although of limited degree of morbidity, is very much cosmetically disturbing to the patient.

CHEMICAL INDUCED HYPOPIGMENTATION

Introduction

Chemical leukoderma denotes an acquired vitiligo-like depigmentation due to repeated exposure to specific chemical compounds.[1,2]

This chemical effect remains independent of their sensitizing potential and is distinctly separate from post-inflammatory depigmentation and Koebner in vitiligo.[3]

Chemical leukoderma has been reported from many countries of the world, developing as well as developed, induced probably by "globalization processes".[4]

Chemical leukoderma remains an under-diagnosed common condition often inducing clinical dilemma with idiopathic vitiligo in dermatological practice. This ailment has been increasing rapidly in incidence in recent decades in developing countries like India.[4]

History

Oliver et al. in 1939[5] first identified chemical leukoderma in a leather manufacturing company in workers who used "acid-cured" rubber gloves. Monobenzylether of hydroquinone (MBH), an antioxidant used in the rubber industry, was the culprit agent. In later decades, several reports of occupational leukoderma caused by phenolic compounds were published from various countries.[6]

Para-tertiary butylphenol (PTBP) and para-tertiary octylphenol (PTOP) were reported offending chemicals from Japan,[7] whereas from Russia PTBP and para-tertiary butylphenol formaldehyde (PTBPF) resins were reported.[8] Occupational depigmentation in tappet assembly workers exposed to para-tertiary butyl catechol (PTBC) was mentioned by Gellin et al.[9] Depigmentation from certain phenolic detergent germicides such as PTBP and para-tertiary amyl phenol (PTAP) was reported by Kahn.[10] Vitiligo caused by PTBP and homologues has been reported by Malten et al.[11]

Chemical leukoderma from semi-permanent and permanent hair colors and rinses was first published in 1993 by Taylor et al.[12] Offending chemicals were paraphenylene diamine (PPD) and benzyl alcohol.

From India, chemical leukoderma was first reported by Pandhi and Kumar [13] induced by adhesive "*bindi*" (decorative color used on the forehead by Asian females) and footwear.[13] Bajaj et al. were the first to report chemical leukoderma from free PTBP contained in *bindi* adhesive,[14] from MBH in synthetic wallets causing depigmentation of the breast from the habit of keeping wallets inside blouses,[15] from MBH causing footwear depigmentation,[16] from PPD in hair dye,[17] from azo dye in "*alta*" (a decorative color used by Asian females on their feet)[18] and from solvent yellow 3, an azo dye, used in "*alta*" and other domestic objects such as watch straps, spectacles, and hearing aids.[19]

Etiopathogenesis

Predisposing factors for the development of chemical leukoderma predominantly constitutes genetic factors which render the melanocytes more fragile. Precipitating factors, which in comparison to idiopathic vitiligo are evident in chemical leukoderma, initiate programmed cell death, or apoptosis of melanocytes **(Flow chart 1)**.[20]

Tyrosinase-related protein-1 (TYRP1), by catalytic conversion of chemicals, produces radical oxygen species. This oxidative stress triggers activation of cellular free radical scavenging pathway to prevent cell death. Genetic inability of melanocytes to tolerate and/or respond to oxidative stress may underlie etiology of chemical leukoderma.[21]

Elevated tumor necrosis factor related apoptosis-inducing ligand (TRAIL) death receptor expression and heat shock protein (HSP) play important role in onset of chemical leukoderma and later its generalization by systemic autoimmunity.

Melanocyte exposed to 4-tertiary butyl phenol (TBP) induces elevated TRAIL expression. TRAIL expression is strongly positive even in peri-leukoderma skin.

Dendritic cells (DC) effector functions also take pivotal role in spreading of leukoderma. Stressed melanocytes mediate DC inactivation by releasing heat shock protein (HSP70). DC function is partially inhibited by antibody to TRAIL **(Flow chart 2)**.[22]

Melanocyte-stimulating hormones (MSH)-induced microphthalmia-associated transcription factor (MITF) up-regulates expression of TYRP1 and increases sensitivity to 4-TBP. Normal melanocytes respond to 4-TBP by reducing expression of MITF and TYRP1. Thus Manga et al. hypothesized that melanocytes in vitiligo demonstrate reduced ability to withstand oxidative stress due, partly, to a disruption in MITF regulation of TYRP1.[23]

Flow chart 1: Precipitating factors: Chemical leukoderma and vitiligo compared

Predisposing factors = Genetic factors render the melanocyte fragile
Precipitating factors = Initiates programmed cell death or apoptosis

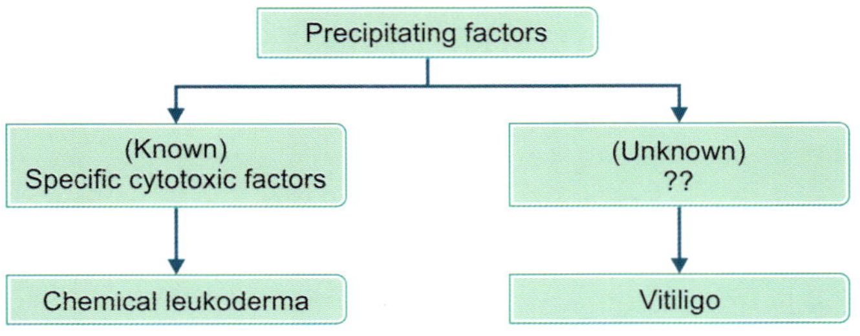

Flow chart 2: Pathogenesis of chemical leukoderma: Elevated TRAIL and HSP[22]

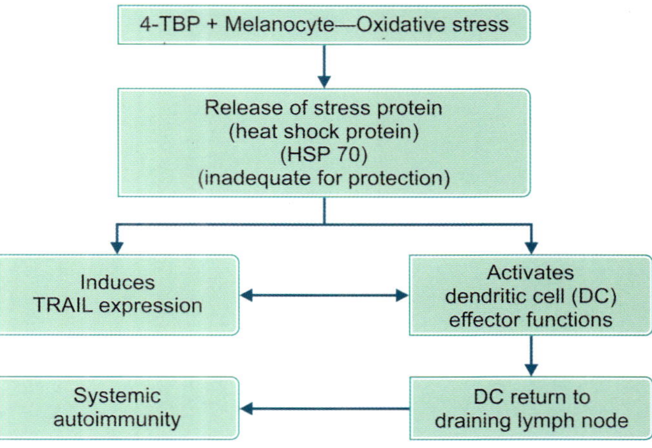

Many drugs act as potential exogenous sources of reactive oxygen species (ROS), especially when metabolized by cytochrome P450 (CYP) enzymes, as they produce reactive quinones and semiquinones.[24] Proton pump inhibitors (PPI) have recently been shown to reactivate vitiligo by producing free radicals[25] or pH changes.[26]

Contributory Agents

Common chemical contributory agents responsible for chemical leukoderma have been shown in **Table 1**. Common substances causing chemical leukoderma have been depicted in **Table 2**. Non-industrial household objects reported to induce chemical leukoderma have also been listed in **Table 3**.

In a recent Indian publication etiological agents for chemical leukoderma identified were hair dye 27.4% (21% self-use; 6.4% not self-use) **(Fig. 1)**, deodorant and spray perfume 21.6% **(Fig. 2)**, detergent and cleansers 15.4%, adhesive *bindi* 12%, rubber *chappal* 9.4% **(Fig. 3)**, black socks and shoes 9.1% **(Fig. 4)**, eyeliner 8.2%, lipliner 4.8%, rubber condoms 3.5%, lipstick 3.3% **(Fig. 5)**, fur toys 3.1%, toothpaste 1.9%, insecticides 1.7%, "*alta*" 1.2%, and amulet string color 0.9% **(Fig. 6)**.[4]

In contrast to the western literature, in the above study, household chemical exposure was a much more common inducing agent than occupational chemical exposure. Non-technical or non-industrial occupations had more involvement than those in technical or industrial occupations. The probable reasons for these discrepancies of data between developed and developing countries could be:

- Lack of quality control in consumer products in developing countries (cheaper ingredients to compete in market even by multinational companies)

Table 1: Chemical leukoderma: Contributory chemicals	
Most potent phenol/catechol derivatives • Monobenzyl ether of hydroquinone (MBH) • Hydroquinone *p-tert*-Butylcatechol (PTBC) *p-tert*-Butylphenol (PTBP) *p-tert*-Amylphenol (PTAP)	
Additional phenol/catechol derivatives • Monomethyl ether of hydroquinone (MMH) • Monoethyl ether of hydroquinone (MEH) • *p*-Phenylphenol • *p*-Octylphenol • *p*-Cresol	
Sulfhydryls • Cysteamine • Sulfanilic acid • Cystamine dihydrochloride	
Miscellaneous • Mercurials • Arsenic • Cinnamic aldehyde • Paraphenylenediamine (PPD) • Corticosteroids • Chloroquine • Soymilk and derived protein (Inhibits PAR2)	• Tretinoin • Benzoyl peroxide • Ammoniated mercury • Azelaic acid • Fluorouracil • Brilliant lake red R • Thiotepa
Ortonne[1] and Miyamoto and Taylor [21]	

Table 2: Chemical leukoderma: Common sources[20]	
Germicidal detergents	Rubber antioxidants
Varnish and lacquer resins	Motor oil additives
Synthetic oils	Deodorants
Duplicate paper	Formaldehyde resins
Soap antioxidants	Latex gloves
De-emulsifiers (oil-field)	Plasticizers
Insecticides	Printing inks
Disinfectants	Paints
Photographic chemicals	Adhesives

- Lack of reporting from industrial set-up:
  - *From owner's view:* Fear of compensation
  - *From worker's view:* Fear of losing job
  - *From doctor's view:* Lack of awareness
- Lack of industrialization.

Table 3: Chemical leukoderma: Contributory non-industrial household objects
• Hair dye [Paraphenylenediamine (PPD)]
• Toothpaste (cinnamic)
• Tattoo [(Paraphenylenediamine (PPD)]
• Nickel
• Artificial nails (Methacrylate)
• Swim goggles (Neoprene rubber)
• Rubber (***Hawaii***) Sandal (Mercapto and Thiuram)
• Perfume
• *Bindi* [Para-tertiary butylphenol (PTB)]
• Wallet (synthetic leather: MBH) (breast)
• Footwear
• *Alta* (feet decorative cosmetic) (Azo dye)
• Amulet string color (Azo dye)
• Stethoscope earpieces
• Oxygen nasal cannula

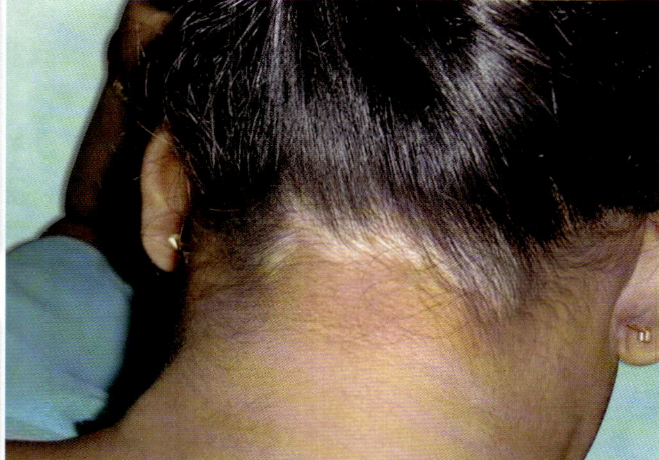

Fig. 1: Chemical leukoderma: Hair dye [Paraphenylenediamine (PPD)]

Clinical Features

Chemical leukoderma should be considered in the differential diagnosis of every case of idiopathic vitiligo or leukomelanoderma. Chemical leukoderma develops not only at the site of chemical contact, but also remotely.[27]

The mechanism responsible for this distant spread of the disease could be: (i) sensitization,[28] (ii) autotransfer or heterotransfer of the chemical from patients themselves and people close to them.

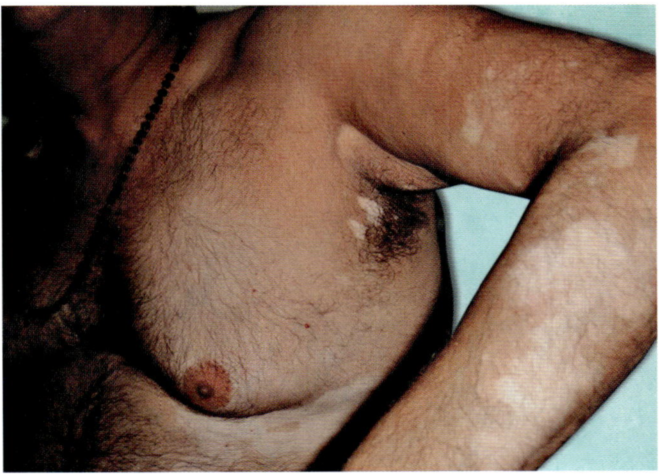

Fig. 2: Chemical leukoderma: Deodorants

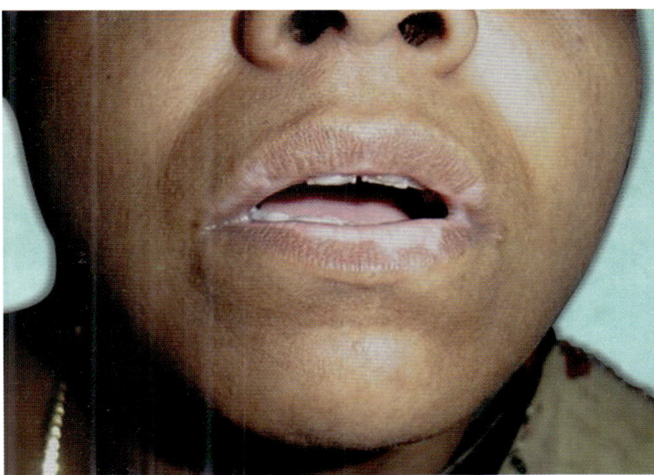

Fig. 5: Chemical leukoderma: Lipstick

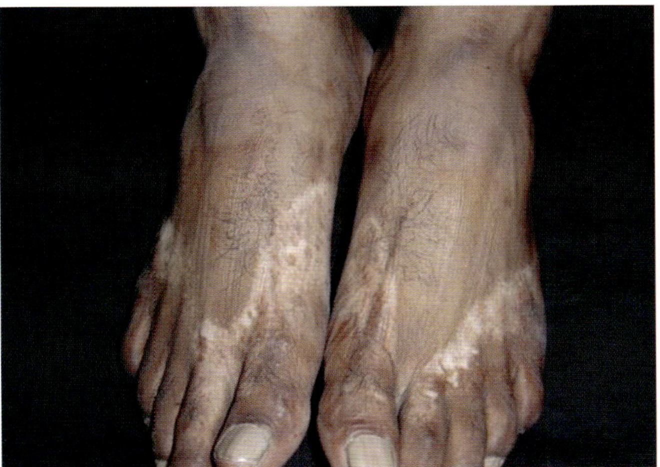

Fig. 3: Chemical leukoderma: Rubber sandals

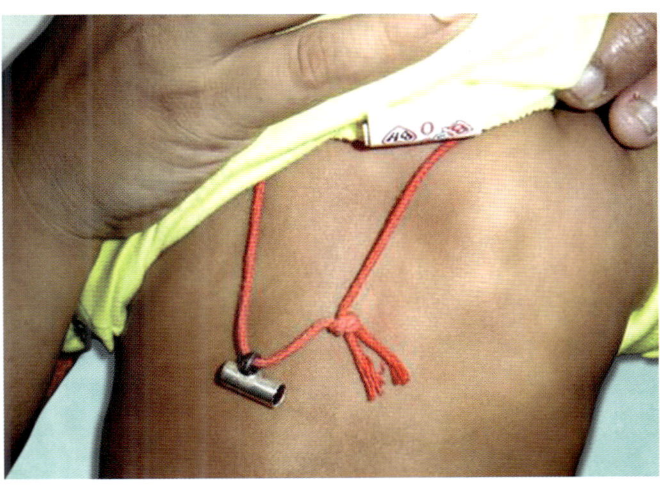

Fig. 6: Chemical leukoderma—from Amulet String Color (in two and half month old child)

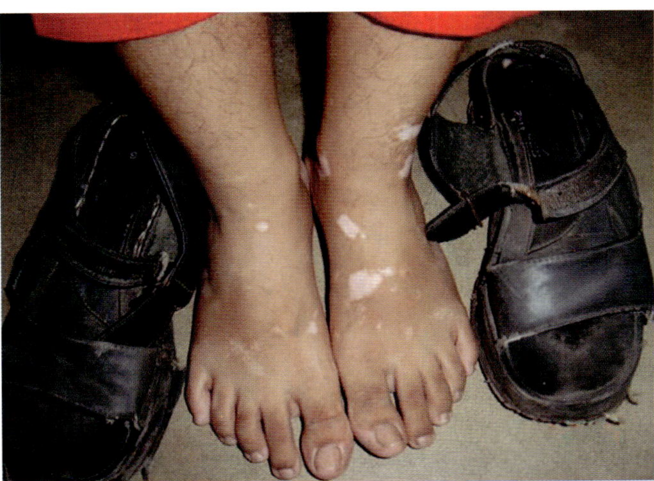

Fig. 4: Chemical leukoderma: Black shoes [Paraphenylenediamine (PPD)]

Chemical leukoderma patches may be symmetrical or asymmetrical. Occasionally, surrounding hyperpigmentation (leukomelanoderma) may be present.

Differential diagnosis of chemical leukoderma includes: (a) vitiligo (b) Koebnerization in vitiligo (c) post-inflammatory leukoderma (d) condition with Confetti macules.

Clinicohistopathologically, no absolute criteria can differentiate chemical leukoderma from vitiligo. However, chemical leukoderma can be diagnosed clinically by a history of repeated exposure to a known or suspected depigmenting agent at the primary site, distribution of macules corresponding to chemical exposure, and the presence of numerous acquired confetti or pea-sized macules **(Fig. 7) (Table 4)**.[28]

Chemical leukoderma can be compared with "Koebner in vitiligo" by the following features in the latter: (1) history of single chemical exposure or trauma, (2) usually linear, and (3) pre-existing vitiligo.[28]

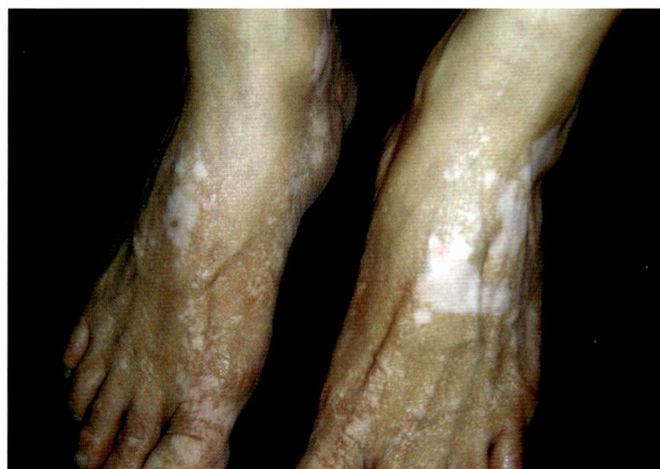

Fig. 7: Chemical leukoderma: Confetti macules

Table 4: Chemical leukoderma: Clinical comparison with vitiligo

	Chemical leukoderma	*Vitiligo*
Trichome	--	+
Leukotrichia	--	+
Koebner	--	+
Confetti macules	+	--
Ocular changes	--	+

(*Source:* Mosher[28] and Ortonne[1])

Chemical leukoderma can be differentiated from post-inflammatory leukoderma by the clinical features of the latter: (1) primary rash always limited to the original area and (2) no Confetti or remote macules.[28]

The presence of numerous acquired confetti or pea-sized macules is characteristic, although not diagnostic, of chemical leukoderma. In an Indian study,[4] a considerable number of patients (88.4%) showed confetti macules, which thus represents an important diagnostic clue for chemical leukoderma.

Contact dermatitis is not a prerequisite for the development of chemical leukoderma.[28] However, in some cases of concurrent contact dermatitis and chemical leukoderma the same offending chemical may cause contact dermatitis as well as chemical leukoderma in some patients but by a different pathomechanism.

Chemical Leukoderma or Contact Leukoderma or Occupational Leukoderma?

There prevails some confusion regarding the varying terminology of chemical leukoderma or occupational leukoderma. The term "contact leukoderma" may be confusing as the adjective "contact" may indicate that leukoderma is confined only to the site of contact, which is baseless as shown in the various studies.[4,28] The term "contact" may also signify that regarding pathogenesis this is similar to contact dermatitis, which again is not true. The term "occupational leukoderma" may be misleading as the majority of cases in the large study[4] were induced by non-occupational household objects. Thus, "chemical leukoderma" remains as more rational and justified term to describe the disease.

Chemical Vitiligo

Some patients who, despite the omission of all contributory toxic chemicals for more than 1 year, still develop vitiliginous patches in different parts of their body. These cases can be termed as "chemical vitiligo" to represent the vitiliginous process, which was switched on initially by the chemicals and continued even after stopping use of the chemicals.[4]

Chemical Leukoderma Syndrome

A syndromic classification of chemical leukoderma similar to allergic contact dermatitis syndrome[29] has been described,[4] which can explain all the clinical features and pathomechanisms adequately, which is termed as "chemical leukoderma syndrome (CLS)." The detail of this proposal is outlined in **Table 5**. Boissy[30] has commented that this staging system seems very appropriate for occupational/contact leukoderma.

Chemical Leukoderma: Clinical Diagnostic Criteria

Chemical leukoderma has to be excluded with certainty from every case of idiopathic vitiligo.[28] However, the differentiating

Table 5: Chemical leukoderma syndrome[4]

- *Stage I:* Chemical leukoderma only at site of contact **(Fig. 8)**
- *Stage II:* Local spread of chemical leukoderma through lymphatics beyond site of contact **(Fig. 9)**
- *Stage IIIA:* Distant spread of chemical leukoderma through hematogenous spread beyond site of contact **(Figs 10A and B)**
- *Stage IIIB:* Distant spread of chemical leukoderma through hematogenous spread beyond the site of contact along with systemic organ involvement
- *Stage IIIC[a]:* Systemic introduction (injection, inhalation or ingestion) other than skin contact causing chemical leukoderma with or without systemic organ involvement (Systemic chemical leukoderma)
- *Stage IV:* Distant spread of vitiligo-like patches even after 1 year of strictly withholding exposure to offending chemicals (Chemical vitiligo)

[a]This stage is a hypothesis or probability, not yet proved

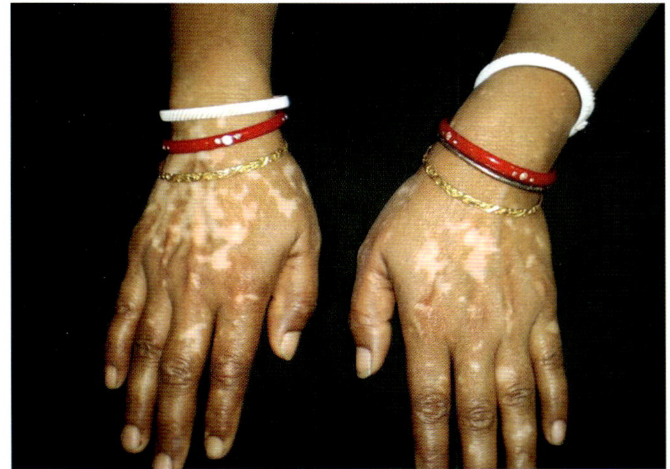

Fig. 8: Stage I: Chemical leukoderma

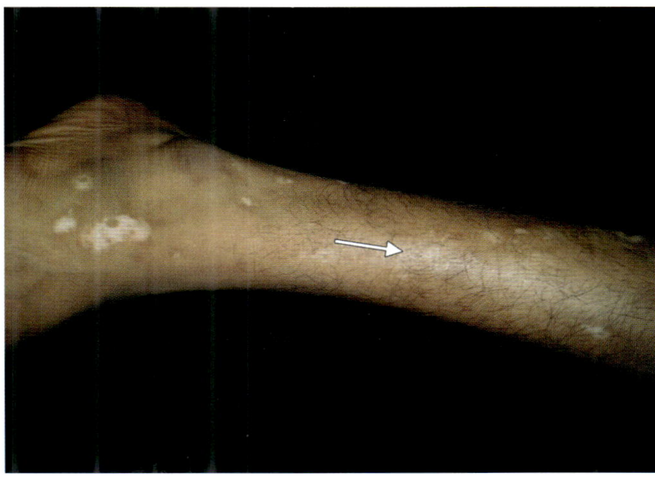

Fig. 9: Stage II: Chemical leukoderma

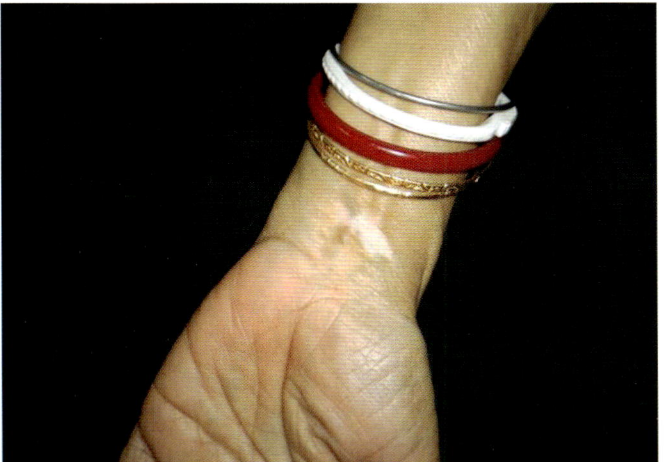

Fig. 10A: Stage IIIA: Chemical leukoderma

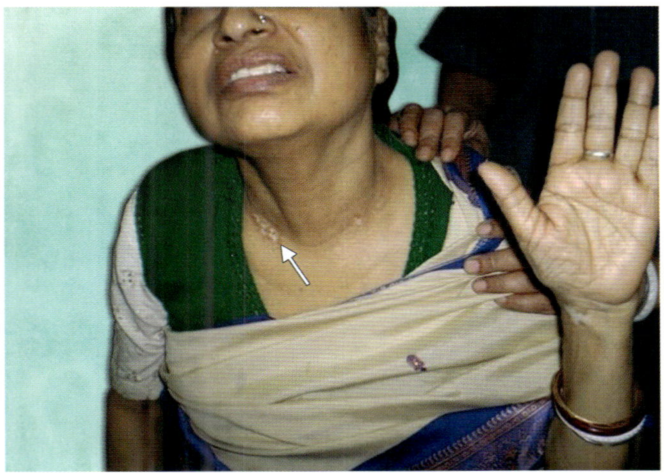

Fig. 10B: Stage IIIA: Chemical leukoderma (Remote vitiligo macule)

factors between chemical leukoderma and vitiligo often remain clinically obscure, which often leads to misdiagnosis of chemical leukoderma syndrome (CLS) as vitiligo. The clinical criteria of diagnosis of chemical leukoderma have not yet been specifically outlined. The proposed clinical diagnostic criteria of chemical leukoderma have been outlined in **Table 6**.

Management

Management of chemical leukoderma includes: (a) counseling of the patients emphasizing the non-idiopathic nature of the diseases and thus differentiating from idiopathic vitiligo, (b) getting detail history of the patients about the exposure of both occupational as well as household objects to detect the causes, (c) strict and permanent removal of causes.

Table 6: Clinical diagnostic criteria of chemical leukoderma syndrome[4]

1. Acquired vitiligo-like depigmented lesion(s)
2. History of repeated exposure to specific chemical compound(s)
3. Patterned vitiligo-like macule(s) conforming to site of exposure
4. Confetti Macules
Any three of the above four criteria should be present to diagnose a case of chemical leukoderma.

Therapeutic management may be phototherapy either psoralen and UVA light therapy [(PUVA) (Topical or systemic)] or ultraviolet B narrowband (UVB NB). Low-dose steroid pulse therapy has been attempted by some authors.[31]

Prognosis of early cases remains good, if etiological factors are completely withdrawn. After repigmentation recurrence is rare until inducing factors are restricted.[1,28]

Chemical Leukoderma versus Idiopathic Vitiligo

The relationship between chemical leukoderma and idiopathic vitiligo seems quite intriguing. Gellin[9] commented that some persons with "idiopathic vitiligo" may actually have an environmentally or occupationally induced leukoderma. Some cases of idiopathic vitiligo may be due to unsuspected inhalation or ingestion of chemicals that produce contact leukoderma as observed by Fisher.[32] Some forms of vitiligo vulgaris are in fact chemical leukoderma caused by unidentified melanocytotoxic chemicals in the environment.[33]

Depigmentation in both cases occurs from loss of melanocytes in the epidermis. Depigmentation in chemical leukoderma spreads to remote sites not exposed to the offending chemicals in the same way as generalized idiopathic vitiligo.[34]

Understanding the mechanisms by which 4-TBP causes melanocyte death may elucidate the pathology underlying contact vitiligo in specific and idiopathic vitiligo in general as predicted by Manga et al.[23]

Glassman[34] has shown some similarities between idiopathic vitiligo and chemical leukoderma. Exogenous oxidants have been incriminated in pathogenesis of chemical leukoderma and shared mechanisms might elucidate trigger factors and reasons for progression and chronic nature in idiopathic vitiligo.

Conclusion

As in developing countries like India the patent loads of chemical leukoderma have been increasing in recent years and this skin ailment resembles vitiligo very closely causing psychosocial reaction, the clinicoetiological diagnosis of this skin disorder is very much warranted.[27]

OCCUPATIONAL HYPERPIGMENTATION

Occupational hyperpigmentation can be classified into four groups:

1. Pigmented contact dermatitis.
2. Metal deposition in skin.
3. Tattoos.
4. Chemical exposure.

Pigmented Contact Dermatitis

The term was coined by Osmundsen in 1970 when he described an epidemic of intense bizarre hyperpigmentation caused by contact allergy with an optical whitener, Tinopal CH 3566 used in washing powders and was later validated with positive patch test results.

Pigmented contact dermatitis occurs mostly from sensitizing fragrances and chemicals in cosmetics. It is usually seen in dark complexion individuals. In fair skinned individuals eczematous changes predominate.[35] Pigmented contact dermatitis also occurred in textile mill workers from azo dye coupling agent Naphthol AS[36,37] and insoluble cutting oils have been reported to cause occupational melanoderma. The histology is consistent with melanodermatitis toxica caused by tar and industrial oils.

Paraphenylenediamine, a rubber antioxidant was described as a cause of reticular brownish black pigmentation in Japanese ferry boat captain contacting a rubber peephole of a radarscope.[38]

A case report of ashy dermatosis associated with cobalt alloys in a plumber should be taken as example of pigmented contact dermatitis.[39] The clinical features and histology was compatible with ashy dermatosis. Patch testing was positive to cobalt chloride.

A case of prurigo pigmentosa caused by contact allergy to chromium component of acupuncture needle has been reported.[40] Erythema and subsequent pigmentation was induced by patch testing with potassium dichromate and resumption of acupuncture caused flare up both at the previous patch test site and initial dermatitis over back.

List of chemicals causing pigmented contact dermatitis has been shown in **Table 7**.

Metal Deposition in Skin

Occupational deposits metals in skin that cause pigmentary changes are rare.[41] The discoloration may result from either the metal deposition in the skin or stimulation of melanin synthesis.[42,43]

Silver: Argyria results from deposition of silver in skin causing blue to slate gray discoloration especially of face and hands

Table 7: Chemicals causing pigmented contact dermatitis
• Optical whitener
• Naphthol AS
• Azo dyes: Sudan I
• Vacanceine red
• Insoluble cutting oils
• Tars
• Paraphenylenediamine
• Cobalt chloride
• Chromium

with relative sparing of skin folds. Pigmentation may occur in the gingiva, oral mucosa, conjunctiva, sclera and nails.[44] Onset ranges from several months to several years.[45] Several cases of occupational argyria reported in past during handling of silver by silversmith or from oral suctioning of silver nitrate solution in silver polishers.[46]

Localized argyria may result from exposure to topical silver salts as in silversmiths[47] and in photographic developers.[48]

Mercury: Mercury causes gray brown pigmentation which is equally prominent in light exposed and light protected areas and increased in skin folds. Generally, pigmentation is more pronounced in eyelids, nasolabial folds and folds of neck.[49] This pigmentation results from mercury containing topical preparation and also from industrial exposure.[50] Systemic administration of mercury compounds can result in diffuse blue gray or black gingival pigmentation similar to that produced by lead and bismuth.[51]

Gold: Chrysiasis results from the deposition of gold in skin resulting from excessive use of therapeutic gold injection. The pigmentation is slate like, bluish gray or may show a purplish hue. Sun exposure is essential for the development of gold pigmentation. Oral mucosa is not affected.[52] Clinically, the pigmentation of chrysiasis differs from that of argyria in that gold-induced pigment is more prominent around eyes and is limited to sun-exposed areas.[43]

Bismuth: It is reported to cause a generalized gray pigmentation of the skin and also the conjunctiva and oral mucosa.[43] A distinctive blue gingival line produced by bismuth similar to lead line but differentiated by occupational history and associated symptoms. Occupationally bismuth is employed in preparation of metal alloys. Bismuth was once used parenterally in the treatment of venereal disease and to promote healing of peptic ulcer. In 1993, Zala et al. reported generalized metal gray pigmentation of skin and mucosa without signs of chronic bismuth poisoning following long-term bismuth injection for pneumocytosis cystoides intestinalis.[53]

Chromates: The skin and nails of electroplaters, leather tanners, lithographers who contact bichromates develop a pale "ochre" yellow tint.[46]

Copper: Copper dust causes a greenish black discoloration of hair, skin and teeth of copper smelters.[54]

Cadmium: Cadmium solution coming in contact with skin may turn skin black.[54]

Tellurium: Occupational absorption of tellurium was reported by Blackadder and Nanderson (1975) in two research workers who shared signs of tellurium intoxication, the characteristic smell of garlic in breath and excreta. Other findings include bluish black discoloration of finger webs and streaks on face and neck.[55]

Tattoos

Pigmented foreign particles may accidentally be introduced as contaminants of wounds or may, at high velocity, with explosive or abrasive forces penetrate previously intact skin. Carbon is the most common material leaving black or blue blemishes, depending on depth of deposit. Another common example of accidental tattooing is seen in abrasion in road accidents with embedding of asphalt.[56]

"Collier stripes" are distinctive occupational marks found in coal miners. They are seen as blue-black, bluish-gray irregularly shaped linear or angular scars seen at the sites of abrasion or small scratches as a result of tattooing coal dust into the skin.[57]

"Pigmented scars" are also observed in iron, stone, silver and flour mill employees. Hare (1951) reported red brown punctuate perifollicular pigmentation from deposition granules on the forearm of a metal worker employed in "pickling" of metal in hydrochloric acid which contained iron salts in acid medium.[58]

Chemical Exposure

Exposure to certain chemicals produces hyperpigmentation. Examples include arsenic and certain halogenated aromatic hydrocarbons. Occupational arsenic exposure may be seen following certain types of works, which have been tabulated in **Table 8**.[59]

Although respiratory tract is the most common portal of entry, skin and gastrointestinal routes are also possibilities. The pigmentary changes in the skin are seen as "bronze" colored hyperpigmented patches with characteristic 1–2 mm hypopigmented rain-drop like macules. The pigmentation tend to affect nipples, axillae, groin, pressure point and areas around scars but oral mucosa is spared which helps to differentiate from Addison's disease.[60] Pigmentation results from deposit of melanin formed from arsenic altered cell metabolism in skin.

Hyperpigmentation from halogenated aromatic hydrocarbon has been reported with exposure to dioxin (TCDD) and polychlorinated biphenyl (PCB). They are found in products such as hydraulic fluids, lubricants, plasticizers,

Table 8: Occupational causes of arsenic exposure
• Agriculture (as a cotton desiccant)
• Animal husbandry (as a sheep dip and growth promotion of swine and poultry)
• Rodenticide, Fungicide
• Copper and lead smelters
• Glass, ceramic and leather workers
• Painters

adhesives, sealants, herbicides, etc.[61] The exact mechanism of hyperpigmentation is not known. Color may vary from brown to gray with face, neck and dorsum of hand most obviously involved. Similar pigmentation of the nails and conjunctiva has been found in 2–3% of industrial PCB poisoning.[59,62]

COSMETIC INDUCED HYPERPIGMENTATION

History

During World War I, in the spring of 1917, Riehl identified approximately 17 patients who had striking dark-brown to grayish-brown facial pigmentation that was most pronounced on the lateral aspects of the face and neck and primarily concentrated on the forehead, ears, temple, and zygomatic regions.[63,64]

Later, Hoffmann and Habermann described a condition referred to as melanodermatitis toxica that was hypothesized to be a form of contact dermatitis associated with the use of certain oils and hydrocarbons. Minami and Noma described a pigmented dermatitis in Asian women unrelated to the war and named the condition melanosis faciei femineae.[65] In 1970, Osmundsen subsequently reported seven patients who had a similar bizarre hyperpigmentation that occurred as a result of contact dermatitis to an optical whitener, Tinopal CH 3566, in washing powder and called the condition pigmented contact dermatitis (PCD).[66] Subsequently in 1973, Nakayama introduced the term pigmented cosmetic contact dermatitis for cases that were ascribed to the use of certain cosmetics.

Although the majority of the literature suggests that Riehl melanosis is synonymous with pigmented contact dermatitis, this is an erroneous assumption because the cases reported by Riehl appear to be a distinct entity related to nutritional alterations that occurred in World War I, with no further case reports noted after the war ended. Pigmented contact dermatitis, on the other hand, is caused by an allergic contact dermatitis to a variety of topical and airborne allergens.[64-67]

Pathophysiology

The cosmetic-induced hyperpigmentation is postulated to be caused by frequent and repeated contact with small amounts of sensitizing allergens primarily in cosmetics. Nakayama hypothesized that allergens used in commercial products were too low in concentration to produce typical eczematous dermatitis, but rather accumulation of these allergens resulted allergic contact dermatitis, a type IV cytolytic reaction.[68,69] This later reaction is characterized by vacuolar degeneration of the basal layer of the epidermis associated with pigment incontinence in the superficial dermis. The melanin pigment is slowly engulfed by macrophages; therefore, resolution of the hyperpigmentation is a prolonged process. Because most cases occur in patients with a darker complexion, one hypothesis is that various pigment-genetic interactions contribute to the development of this condition.[66] Furthermore, Imokawa and Kawai have provided clinical evidence that various allergens implicated in allergic contact dermatitis can stimulate melanogenesis.[70]

Clinical Features

Many cases are preceded by mild erythema, edema, and pruritus,[64] followed by a diffuse-to-reticulated pattern of hyperpigmentation. The pigmentation varies dependent upon the causal agent and can be brown, slate-gray, gray-brown, red-brown, or blue-brown.[64,66,71]

The site of pigmented contact dermatitis also depends on the allergen responsible. Pigmented cosmetic dermatitis more commonly involves the face. Additionally, hyperpigmentation is most pronounced in individuals with darker complexions.

Ultraviolet (UV) exposure may contribute to the hyperpigmentation in select cases, which is supported by the fact that some of the chemicals implicated are known photosensitizers, and, in these cases, the pigmentation appears to be most pronounced in sun-exposed areas.[64,66]

Causes

A variety of contact allergens have been implicated in pigmented cosmetic dermatitis, as described in **Tables 9 to 11**.[66] Although the majority of cases occur because of direct contact with these allergens, a few cases secondary to contact with airborne allergens have been described.[66,71,72]

Cases of pigmented contact dermatitis have been reported in the Indian literature, and the most common allergen to be implicated is kumkum, a colored cosmetic used by Hindu women that is applied most often to the central forehead and along the hair line.[66,78] Only commercially available red kumkum can sensitize and cause pigmented contact dermatitis. Components of kumkum include azo dyes, coal tar dyes, toluidine red, erythrosine, lethal red calcium salt, fragrances, tumeric powder, groundnut oil, tragacanth gum, Cananga oil, and parabens.[66]

Laboratory Studies

- *Patch test:* Closed patch testing is performed with the standard series, cosmetic series, fragrance series, and patient's personal products.
- *Photo-patch test:* Done when photo aggravation is suspected.
- *Provocative use test or repeated open application test (ROAT):* This test is performed when closed patch testing results are equivocal or negative. The concentration of the allergen (e.g. preservatives, fragrances) may be too low in the cosmetic series to produce a positive reaction on the back.[66]

Table 9: List of cosmetic allergens[73]
• *D&C Red 31:* Pigment
• *Brilliant Lake Red R:* Pigment in lipsticks and rouges[74,75]
• *D&C Yellow No. 11 and 10:* Pigment
• *PAN (phenyl-azo-2-naphthol):* Impurity in azo pigments
• *Chromium hydroxide:* Pigment
• *Carbanilides (trichlorocarbanilide and Irgasan CF3):* Bactericidal
• *Aniline dyes:* Pigment
• Hair dyes
• *Ricinoleic acid (castor oil acid):* Bactericide (deodorants, lipstick, military camouflage)[76]
• *Kumkum (red):* Cosmetic powder and liquid (Hindu women)[77]
• Fragrances

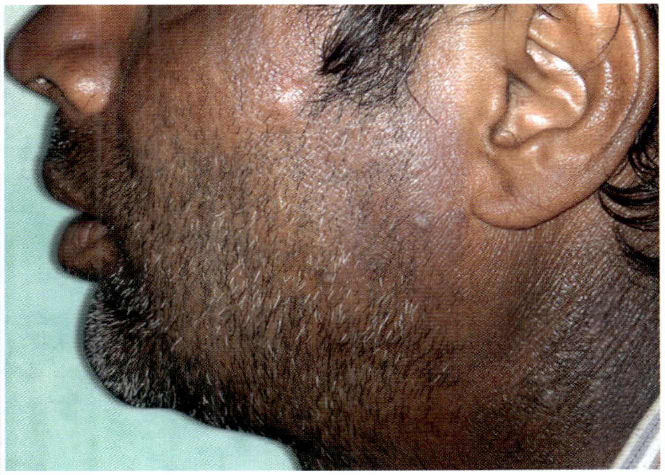

Fig. 11: Musk ambrette-induced pigmentation

Table 10: List of fragrance allergens
• Jasmine absolute
• Benzyl salicylate
• Hydroxycitronellal
• Ylang-ylang oil
• Cinnamic alcohol
• Musk ambrette[72,78] **(Fig. 11)**
• Cananga oil
• Sandalwood oil
• Synthetic sandalwood (containing bornyl methoxy cyclohexanol)
• Geraniol oil
• Eugenol
• Isoeugenol
• Balsam of Peru
• Lavender oil
• Lemon oil[79,80]
• Methoxycitronellal
• Benzyl alcohol
• Cinnamic derivatives

Table 11: List of miscellaneous allergens
• *Chromate (K dichromate):* Leather, soaps
• *Nickel/nickel sulfate:* Component metal products and jewelry
• Paratertiary Butyl-Phenol Formaldehyde Resin (PTBPFR) (Neoprene adhesive in leather products[81]
• *Minoxidil 5%:* Topical vasodilator for hair loss treatment.[82,83]

Management

The suspected allergens are to be avoided strictly, and removal of these agents often leads to gradual improvement. Use of allergen-free apparel, soaps, and cosmetics are warranted.

In some situations, topical creams containing 2–5% hydroquinone combined with tretinoin may hasten the resolution of the hyperpigmentation. Glycolic acid has also been reported as helpful.[84]

DRUG-INDUCED HYPERPIGMENTATION

Adverse cutaneous reactions to medications are a common reason for consultation with dermatologist. Drug may cause abnormal pigmentation of the skin and mucosa. Although pigmentary changes caused by drugs usually result in a limited degree of morbidity, these changes can be very much cosmetically disturbing to the patient.

Pathophysiology

Multiple pathologic mechanisms are responsible for drug-induced pigmentation disorders. Most cases of pharmacologic pigmentation are not immunologically mediated.

The pathogenesis of drug-induced pigmentation can be categorized into three mechanisms: (1) Drug or drug metabolite deposition in the dermis or epidermis (2) Enhanced melanin production with or without an increase in the number of active melanocytes (3) Drug-induced post-inflammatory changes in the skin.

Epidemiology: Drug-induced skin pigmentation is estimated to account for 10–20% of all cases of acquired pigmentation. Drug-induced pigmentation is not generally associated with mortality or morbidity, although it may result in considerable psychological and social impairment. Drug-induced pigmentation can occur in persons of any race, but people with darker skin often exhibit more intense hyperpigmentation than individuals with fair skin. No difference was found in the prevalence among males and females. Drug-induced pigmentation is seen in persons of all age.[85]

History Taking

A thorough history is essential to determine the cause of a pigmentary disorder. A patient should be questioned about: (a) temporal relationship of medications and the development of pigmentation. Drug-induced pigmentation is an acquired disease that tend to spread insidiously over time as the patient has further exposure to the drug (b) associated symptoms and comorbid illnesses, as lichenoid or bullous eruptions often accompany drug-induced dyschromias (c) any medications taken in the 6 months preceding the dyspigmentation should be documented, including herbal drugs and over the counter (OTC) medications (d) any prior history of adverse drug reactions and about resolution of symptoms after with-drawal of therapy as the pigmentary changes should fade with time (e) recent exposure to excess sunlight or artificial UV light which can aggravate cutaneous pigmentation.

Physical Examination

Specific clues in the physical examination of a dyschromic patient may indicate drug specific etiology. Most importantly, drug-related pigmentation usually has a characteristic topographic distribution (e.g. confined to pretibial areas or scars) and may cause prominent discoloration in sun-distributed areas, mucous membrane, sclera, cartilage and/or nails.

Patchy dyspigmentation limited to the sun exposed areas is caused by amiodarone, daunorubicin, gold, methotrexate, psoralens, 5-fluorouracil. Generalized dyspigmentation, similar to that seen in Addison's disease is seen with minocycline use. Pigmentation mainly affecting the palm and soles, mucous membrane or teeth is seen with iron, silver or topical hydroquinone or in previous scars as seen with hydroxyurea. Flagellate pigmentation is usually caused by bleomycin.

Color of the lesion can also give us a clue regarding the offending drug: (a) amiodarone: slate gray (b) minocycline: blue black (c) quinacrine: yellow (d) clofazimine: red.

Acanthosis nigricans can sometimes be mistaken for hyperpigmentation because it appears as dark velvety patches and plaques in the axillae, inguinal creases, neck and upper back. Certain drugs such as somatotrophin, testosterone, nicotinic acid, oral contraceptives have been associated with development of acanthosis nigricans.

Clinical Features

A large number of drugs are well known for their tendency to induce mucocutaneous dyspigmentation. These medications tend to be associated with distinct clinical and histological patterns largely dependent on their underlying pathogenesis. Antimalarials, chemotherapeutic agents, heavy metals, psychotropic drugs and miscellaneous medications (e.g. amiodarone, zidovudine, minocycline, clofazimine, psoralens) and are among the most commonly implicated medications in acquired dyschromia.

Antimalarials

Hyperpigmentation is considered one of the most notorious and frequent adverse cutaneous effect of this group. These drugs are frequently used in dermatology practice to treat autoimmune disorders such as lupus erythematosus and rheumatoid arthritis. This group includes chloroquine, hydroxychloroquine, amodiaquin and quinacrine.

About 25% of patients receiving these drugs for at least 4 months will develop bluish-gray or purple pigmentation. Pigmentation appears most frequently in the pretibial areas but can also involve the nail bed, nose, cheeks, forehead, ears and oral mucosa especially the hard palate. Initial lesions are discrete oval macules which eventually coalesce into large patches. Pigmentation is usually reversible within several months of stopping the inciting agent. Histology reveals increased epidermal melanin and hemosiderin deposition in the dermis.

Patients ingesting quinacrine develop a characteristic yellow discoloration that extends to the conjunctiva and oral mucosa. It is commonly mistaken for jaundice and serum bilirubin estimation may help in differentiating the conditions. It usually resolves 1–4 months of drug discontinuation.[86]

Chemotherapeutics

Cancer chemotherapeutic agents can cause various adverse cutaneous effects, including photosensitivity and diffuse and localized hyperpigmentation of skin nails and mucous membrane.

Pathogenesis is not clearly known. Proposed mechanism include direct stimulation of melanin production and post-inflammatory hyperpigmentation after drug-induced toxicity to the keratinocytes

Agents known to cause skin dyspigmentation include bleomycin, busulfan, doxorubicin, daunorubicin, 5-Fluorouracil (FU), cyclophosphamide, carmustine and docetaxel.[87]

Bleomycin: A cytotoxic antibiotic used to treat malignancies such as testicular carcinoma and Hodgkin's disease. Hyperpigmentation occurs in up to 20% of patients. Hyperpigmentation usually occurs within 1 to 9 weeks of drug administration and can be accompanied by pruritus. Skin discoloration varies from generalized hypermelanosis to focal pigmentation over pressure points or linear flagellated bands on trunk. These flagellated bands are a distinct feature associated with this drug and are thought to be associated with minor trauma caused by scratching; however some patients deny having pruritus.[88] Histologic examination demonstrates increased epidermal melanin without an increase in epidermal melanocytes and little dermal pigment incontinence.

5-Fluorouracil: An antimetabolite chemotherapy used for treatment of breast and gastrointestinal (GI) cancer. When used systemically up to 5% individuals develop a photosensitivity reaction in sun exposed areas, followed by hyperpigmentation in those areas. Additionally, hyperpigmentation may also develop in skin near infusion or portal irradiation sites or on the dorsal aspects of hands, palm, soles and trunk.[89] This has been termed "serpentine supravenous hyperpigmentation" and may also be associated with alkylating agents, antibiotics, protease inhibitors and antimitotic.

Adriamycin: It may cause pigmented patches in the oral mucosa, particularly the lateral aspect of tongue.

Hydroxyurea: They may cause nail bed and/or lunula hyperpigmentation and tongue pigmentation.

Pemetrexed: It has been reported to cause hyperpigmentation of palm and soles.[90]

Epidermal Growth Factor Receptor Inhibitor

It has been associated with telangiectasias, which on resolution have been associated with hyperpigmentation.

Heavy Metals

The heavy metals gold, silver, bismuth and mercury are well known for their ability to cause pigmentary disturbance. Their prevalence is gradually decreasing as their use is limited nowadays.

Silver sulphadiazine commonly used in burns can result in slate-gray pigmentation due to systemic absorption, if used for large surface areas. Pigmentation is accentuated in sun exposed areas with sparing of skin folds. Nails, sclera and mucosa may also be involved.[7] Histologically, silver granules are found deposited in the basement membrane, on the lamina propria of the eccrine glands as well as in the elastic fibers; the granules are thought to stimulate melanin synthesis in adjacent melanocytes.[91]

Gold is rarely used nowadays as an alternative therapy for patients with pemphigus vulgaris or rheumatoid arthritis. It can lead to blue gray hyperpigmentation of sun exposed areas on prolonged use. Pigmentation is most prominent around eyes but does not affect the nail or mucosa. Biopsies demonstrate gold particles within dermal macrophage lysosomes and surrounding blood vessels.

Injection of iron salts into the dermis can cause focal blue gray discoloration. It can occur after administration of ferric subsulfate (Monsel's solution) as a hemostatic agent. Biopsies show deposition of iron particles into the macrophages or along collagen fibers in dermis.

Tetracyclines

Pigmentary disturbances are disconcerting adverse events associated with the tetracycline drug group, particularly with minocycline ingestion.[92,93] Tetracyclines, including minocycline, have been associated with brown discoloration of the teeth in children. Use of these medications in children younger than 9 years is discouraged.

Minocycline

It is a lipid-soluble antibiotic with anti-inflammatory properties that is frequently used in the treatment of acne or other inflammatory conditions; adverse cutaneous effects from its use are common, with hyperpigmentation **(Fig. 12)** occurring in roughly 3–5% of all patients using it long-term.

In addition to a prolonged period of ingestion, other risk factors such as higher cumulative dose, excessive sun exposure, and prior inflammatory skin changes have been shown to increase the risk of minocycline-related hyperpigmentation.[92]

Minocycline has three classic and distinct patterns of dyspigmentation:

I. Type I is blue-black discoloration localized to scars and post-inflammatory sites; this discoloration is proposed to be the result of hemosiderin and/or iron chelate deposition in dermis.

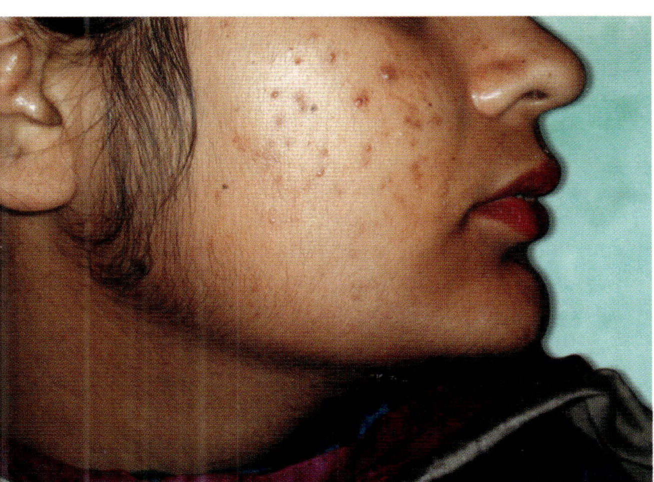

Fig. 12: Minocycline-induced pigmentation

II. Type 2 is blue-gray pigmentation of normal skin on the extremities, especially the anterior shins (which may mimic antimalarial pigmentation). These changes are derived from deposition of melanin and iron-containing granules in the dermis and subcutis.
III. Type 3 is generalized "muddy" brown hyperpigmentation seen most prominently in sun-exposed skin, thought to result from increased basal layer melanin (without evidence of iron deposition).

In addition to these clinical patterns, other tissues such as the sclera, oral mucosa, thyroid, breast, aorta, bones, and lymph nodes may exhibit dyspigmentation.[93]

Histopathologic findings are largely dependent on the clinical type of discoloration.

Cessation of minocycline therapy typically results in a gradual fading of dyspigmentation, although in some cases symptoms never completely resolve.

In recent years, Q-switched lasers such as the Q-switched ruby, alexandrite, and Nd:YAG have had success in reducing or clearing minocycline induced dyspigmentation.[94]

Amiodarone

Amiodarone, a coronary vasodilator used in the treatment of cardiac arrhythmias, can induce blue-gray or violaceous pigmentation of sun-exposed skin and yellow-brown stippling of the cornea. Pigmentary changes usually develop after long-term therapy (≥6 month); the risk of such adverse cutaneous effects increases with a longer duration of use and at doses greater than 400 mg/d. Many times dyspigmentation is preceded by a photoallergic reaction.

Histopathologic examination reveals focal deposition of yellow-brown granules and lipofuscin within dermal macrophages; electron microscopy further demonstrates the granules contained within intralysosomal laminated inclusion bodies.

Pigmentation has been shown to slowly resolve months to years after withdrawal of therapy, although the dyspigmentation can be permanent.[95]

Antiretrovirals

Azidothymidine, otherwise known as AZT or zidovudine, is commonly used in highly active antiretroviral therapy (HAART) for patients with HIV disease. It causes a reversible dyspigmentation of the nails and occasionally brown mucocutaneous hyperpigmentation. Reported nail changes associated with this drug include diffuse blue pigmentation and longitudinal or transverse banding that begins in the proximal nailbed.

Histologically, pigmented skin lesions demonstrate increased melanin deposition along the epidermal basal layer and within dermal histiocytes.

Skin and nail discoloration have been shown to gradually resolve with drug discontinuation.

Emtricitabine (FTC) is known to cause skin pigmentation in African Americans at an incidence of 8% and in Asians at an incidence of 4%. The pigmentation was asymptomatic and often located on the distal extremities.[96]

Clofazimine

Clofazimine is a phenazine dye used to treat discoid lupus, leprosy, and other mycobacterial infections; it regularly induces a diffuse, reddish cutaneous and conjunctival discoloration within the first few weeks of use.

With prolonged ingestion, affected patients typically develop violet-brown or bluish cutaneous pigmentation most apparent in lesional skin **(Fig. 13)**.

Histological findings that correlate with these progressive skin changes include initial drug deposition within macrophages and subcutaneous and visceral fat; enhanced epidermal melanin deposition with ceroid lipofuscinosis is seen with continued medication use.

Gradual fading of pigmentary changes is seen with withdrawal of the drug usually within 2 years.[97]

Psychotropic Drugs

Antipsychotic medications produce adverse cutaneous effects in approximately 5% of patients; patients taking phenothiazines, imipramine, or desipramine most frequently develop a progressive slate or blue-gray pigmentation in sun-exposed areas of the skin.

Among the phenothiazines, the low-potency antipsychotic chlorpromazine is the most commonly implicated drug. It is known to induce a purple discoloration of the face and extremities, with marked sparing of the facial wrinkles. Pigmentation may involve the nail beds and exposed portions of the eye. Dyspigmentation tends to develop after a prolonged course of high doses of the drug and has been

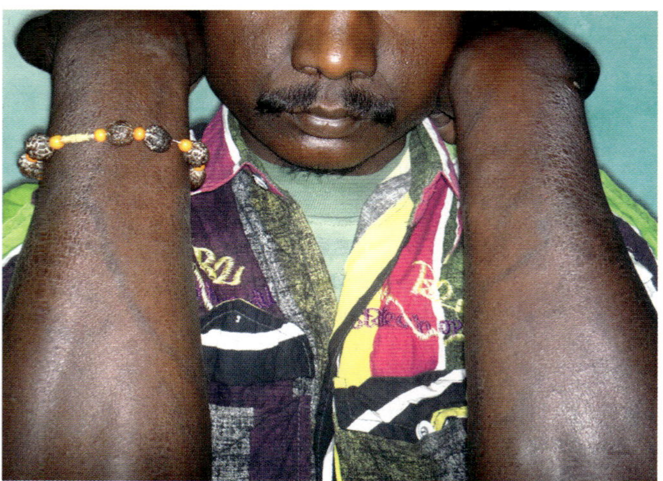

Fig. 13: Clofazimine-induced pigmentation

shown to slowly resolve if switched to another neuroleptic, such as levomepromazine.

Histologically, pigmented granules are visible in dermal macrophages around the superficial capillaries, and ultrastructural analysis has found that the electron-dense granules are composed of melanin and complexes of melanin and drug metabolite.[98]

Tricyclic Antidepressants

Tricyclic antidepressants particularly imipramine and desipramine, may also induce blue or slate-gray pigmentation in sun-exposed skin. Histopathology reveal brown granules composed of drug-melanin complexes free in the dermis (along the basement membrane) and deposited within dermal macrophages. Replacement of the inciting drugs with alternative antidepressants has been successful in resolving the patient's skin discoloration.[99] Additionally, the Q-switched alexandrite laser has shown promising results in treating pigmentation caused by prior imipramine use.

Miscellaneous Drugs

Other drugs associated with mucocutaneous dyspigmentation include oral contraceptives,[100] psoralens, and topical hydroquinone. Approximately 30% of all women using oral estrogen therapy report the development of melasma like facial pigmentation. Discontinuation of the hormonal therapy in conjunction with strict sun avoidance promotes resolution of the hyperpigmentation.

One case of diffuse facial hyperpigmentation was noted after the administration of adalimumab.[101]

Psoralens

These are plant extracts currently used in the treatment of psoriasis and vitiligo. When used with UV light, these chemicals cause a predictable pigmentation of the skin via proliferation of follicular melanocytes and increased production and transfer of melanin.

Hydroquinone

It is a hydroxyphenolic bleaching chemical normally used in the treatment of skin hyperpigmentation. Blue-black pigmentation similar to that seen in inherited ochronosis has been shown to develop with topical application in darker-skinned individuals.[102]

Topical Ophthalmic Medications (Latanoprost and Bimatoprost)

These topical preparation used to treat glaucoma have been reported to cause periocular and diffuse facial hyperpigmentation as well as darkening of the iris.[103]

Imatinib (Gleevec)

This drug, a tyrosine kinase inhibitor, has been reported on several occasions to cause mucosal pigmentation that stains positively with both Fontana-Masson and Prussian blue stains, similar to minocycline.[104] It has also been associated with both hypopigmentation and hyperpigmentation, and it has been suggested that cases of hyperpigmentation may be due to imatinib mediated increases in c-Kit signaling resulting in melanogenesis.[105]

Histologic Findings

The histologic findings of several forms of drug-induced pigmentation have been reported. The patterns of histologic abnormalities are often drug specific and have been described as hyperpigmentation of the basal cell layer, pigment incontinence within the dermis, and accumulation of pigment-laden macrophages around blood vessels and eccrine glands. The pigment within macrophages may be positive for the Fontana-Masson stain, indicating the presence of melanin, or may be positive for Perls Prussian blue stain, indicating the presence of iron; on occasion, both results may be positive with both stains.

Minocycline type I reactions demonstrate pigment-laden macrophages within the dermis or scar that are only positive with Perls' staining. Minocycline type II reactions demonstrate pigment-laden macrophages around blood vessels and eccrine glands that stain with both Fontana-Masson and Perls stains, indicating the presence of both melanin and iron. Minocycline type III reactions have been characterized by the presence of increased epidermal basal cell layer melanin pigmentation.

Amiodarone pigmentation is a result of a form of photodistributed lipofuscinosis with accumulation of lysosomal laminated bodies within macrophages. These granules within macrophages stain positively with periodic acid-Schiff stain.

Phenothiazine pigmentation results from the accumulation of pigment-laden macrophages around superficial blood vessels. These macrophages stain with Fontana-Masson stain, but not Perls' stain.

Chemotherapeutic agent–induced pigmentation may result from interface dermatitis, resulting in incontinence of pigment.

Antimalarial pigmentation demonstrates pigment granules extracellularly and within dermal macrophages that stain for hemosiderin, melanin, or both.

Management

The most important factor in the management of drug-induced dyspigmentation involves the identification and discontinuation of the offending drug. Most mucocutaneous pigmentation is reversible and spontaneously resolves with avoidance of the inciting drug.

In a scenario in which several drugs may be implicated as the cause of dyspigmentation, a decision must be made between the physician and patient to stop all non-essential medications. Decreasing the dose of any essential, life-saving treatment is often sufficient to diminish drug-related dyschromia. Additionally, merely explaining the benign nature of the cutaneous reaction may alleviate patient anxiety and allow time to determine the offending medication.

In addition, exposure to sun or UV light may increase pigmentation, especially after sensitization with a photosensitizing medication. Sunscreen use and vigilant avoidance of the sun are helpful to prevent progression or recurrence of pigmentary changes.

Finally, topical depigmenting agents and laser treatments (e.g. Q-switched alexandrite laser, Q-switched ruby laser) have been reported to improve cases of permanent dyspigmentation. The use of these therapies is controversial because they have shown inconsistent results; further evaluation is needed.

REFERENCES

1. Ortonne JP, Bahadoran P, Fitzpatrick TB, et al. Hypomelanosis and hypermelanosis. In: Freddberg IM, Eisen AZ, Wolft K, Austen KF, Goldsmith LA, Katz SI (Eds). Fitzpatricks' Dermatology in General Medicine. New York: McGraw Hill; 2003. pp. 836-81.
2. Jimbow K, Jimbow M. Chemical and pharmacologic agents. In: Norlund JJ, Boissy RE, Hearing VJ (Eds). The Pigmentary System: Physiology and Pathophysiology. New York: Oxford University Press; 1998. pp. 618-24.
3. Beck MH, Wilkinson SM. Contact dermatitis: allergic. In: Burns T, Breathnack S, Cox N, Griffiths C (Eds). Rook's Textbook of Dermatology. Oxford: Blackwell; 2004. pp. 20.1–20.124.
4. Ghosh S, Mukhopadhyay S. Chemical leucoderma: A clinic aetiological study of 864 cases in the perspective of a developing country. Br J Dermatol. 2009;160:40-7.
5. Oliver EA, Schwartz L, Warren LH. Occupation leukoderma. J Am Med Assoc. 1939;113:927-8.
6. Bajaj AK. Chemical leukoderma. In: Valia RG, Valia A (Eds). What's New in Dermatology, STDs and Leprosy? Mumbai: Fulford; 2004. pp. 3-5.
7. Okmura Y, Shirai T. Vitiliginous lesions occurring among workers in a phenol derivative factory. Jpn J Dermatol. 1962;7:617-9.
8. Chumakov NN, Babanov GP, Simarov AG. Vitiliginoid dermatoses in workers of phenol formaldehyde resin workers. In: Chumakov NN, Babanov GP, Simarov AG (Eds). Bulletin of Dermatology. Moscow: State Publishing Firm of Medical Literature; 1962. p. 14.3.
9. Gellin GA, Possick PA, Davis IH. Occupational depigmentation due to 4-tertiarybutyl catechol (TBC). J Occup Med. 1970;12:386-9.
10. Kahn G. Depigmentation caused by phenolic detergent germicides. Arch Dermatol. 1970;102:177-87.
11. Malten KE, Seutter E, Hara I, et al. Occupational vitiligo due to paratertiary butylphenol and homologues. Trans St Johns Hosp Dermatol Soc. 1971;57:115-34.
12. Taylor JS, Maibach HJ, Fisher AA, et al. Contact leukoderma associated with the use of hair colors. Cutis. 1993;52:273-80.
13. Pandhi RK, Kumar AS. Contact leukoderma due to '*bindi*' and footwear. Dermatologica. 1985;170:260-2.
14. Bajaj AK, Gupta SC, Chatterjee AK. Contact depigmentation from free para-tertiary-butylphenol in *bindi* adhesive. Contact Dermatitis. 1990;22:99-102.
15. Bajaj AK, Gupta SC, Chatterjee AK. Contact depigmentation of the breast. Contact Dermatitis. 1991;24:58.
16. Bajaj AK, Gupta SC, Chatterjee AK. Footwear depigmentation. Contact Dermatitis. 1996;35:17-8.
17. Bajaj AK, Gupta SC, Chatterjee AK, et al. Hair dye depigmentation. Contact Dermatitis. 1996;35:56-7.
18. Bajaj AK, Pandey RK, Misra K, et al. Contact depigmentation caused by an azo dye in alta. Contact Dermatitis. 1998;38: 189-93.
19. Bajaj AK, Misra A, Misra K, et al. The azo dye solvent yellow 3 produces depigmentation. Contact Dermatitis. 2000;42:237-8.
20. Boissy RE, Manga P. On the etiology of contact occupational vitiligo. Pigment Cell Res. 2004;17:208-14.
21. Miyamoto L, Taylor JS. Chemical leukoderma. In: Hann SK, Nordlund JJ (Eds). Vitiligo: A Comprehensive Monograph on Basic and Clinical Science. London: Blackwell Science; 2000. pp. 269-80.
22. Kroll TM, Bommiasamy H, Boissy RE, et al. 4-Tertiary butyl phenol exposure sensitizes human melanocytes to dendritic cell-mediated killing: relevance to vitiligo. J Invest Dermatol. 2005;124:798-806.
23. Manga P, Sheyn D, Yang F, et al. A role for tyrosinase-related protein 1 in 4-tert-butylphenol-induced toxicity in melanocytes. Am J Pathol. 2006;169:1652-62.
24. Namazi MR. Cytochrome-P450 enzymes and autoimmunity: expansion of the relationship and introduction of free radicals as the link. J Autoimmun Dis. 2009;6:4.
25. Namazi MR. Proton pump inhibitors may trigger vitiligo by rendering melanocytes prone to apoptosis. Br J Dermatol. 2008;158:844-5.
26. Schallreuter KU, Rokos H. From the bench to the bedside: proton pump inhibitors can worsen vitiligo. Br J Dermatol. 2007;156:1371-3.
27. Ghosh S. Chemical leukoderma: what's new on etiopathological and clinical aspects? Indian J Dermatol. 2010:55:255-8.
28. Mosher DB, Fitizpatrick TB. Chemical leukoderma. In: Sober AJ, Fitzpatrick TB (Eds). Yearbook of Dermatology. Boston: Mosby; 1994. pp. 3-13.
29. Lachapelle JM. The spectrum of diseases for which patch testing is recommended. In: Lachapelle JM, Maibach HI (Eds). Patch Testing, Prick Testing: A Practical Guide. Berlin: Springer; 2003. pp. 7-26.

30. Boissy RE. Occupatinal vitiligo. In: Picardo M, Taieb A (Eds). Vitiligo; 2009. pp. 175-80.
31. Jung JY, Yeom KB, Eun HC. Chemical Leukoderma Improved by Low-dose Steroid Pulse Therapy. Ann Dermatol. 2010;22:241-4.
32. Fisher AA. Differential diagnosis of idiopathic vitiligo: Part III: Occupational leukoderma. Cutis. 1994;53:278-80.
33. Cummings MP, Nordlund JJ. Chemical leukoderma: fact or fancy. Am J Contact Derm. 1995;6:122.
34. Glassman SJ. Vitiligo, reactive oxygen species and T-cells. Clinical Science. 2011;120:99-120.
35. Pinol-Aguade J. Dermatitis por blanquedoresn opticos. Med Cutan. 1971;5:249-68.
36. Ancona-Alayon A, Escobar-Marques R, Gonzalez-Mendoza A, et al. Occupational pigmented contact dermatitis from Naphthol AS. Contact Dermatitis. 1976;2:129-34.
37. Fujimoto K, Hashimoto S, Kozuka T, et al. Occupational pigment contact dermatitis from azo dyes. Contact Dermatitis.1985;12:15-7.
38. Hamada T, Horiguchi S. Chronic melanodermatitis due to rubber peephole of a ship radaroscope. Contact Dermatits.1978;4:245-6.
39. Zenorola P, Bisceglia M, Lomuto M. Ashy dermatosis associated with cobalt allergy. Contact Dermatitis. 1994; 31:53-5.
40. Tanni T, Kono T, Katoh J, et al. Acase of prurigo pigmentosa considered to be contact allergy to chromium in acupuncture needle. Acta Derm Venereol.1991;71:66-7.
41. Schwartz L. Occupational pigmentary changes in the skin. Arch Dermatol Syphilol. 1947;56:592-600.
42. Wahlberg JE. Metals and skin. In: Maibach HI (Ed). Occupational and industrial dermatology, 2nd edn. Chicago; 1987. pp. 348-50.
43. Bleehen SS, Gould DJ, Harrington CI, et al. Occupational argyria: Light and electron microscopic studies and X-ray microanalysis. Br J Dermatol. 1981;104:19-26.
44. Granstein RD, Sober AJ. Drug and heavy metal induced hyperpigmentation. J Am Acad Dermatol.1981;5:1-18
45. Grawkrodger DJ. Pigmentary changes related to occupation. In: English JSC (Ed). A colour handbook of occupational dermatology. London: Manson; 1998. pp. 147-58.
46. White RP. Silver, arsenic, chromates. In: The Dermatergoses. London: HK Lewis and Co; 1934. pp. 140-54.
47. Lewin G. Localised argyria oin workers in silver plate. Ann Dermatol Venereol. 1987;6:363-8.
48. Buckley WR. Localised argyria. Arch Dermatol. 1963;88: 531-9.
49. Lamar LM, Bliss BR. Localised pigmentation of skin due to topical mercury. Arch Dermatol. 1966;93:450-3.
50. Kennedy C, Molland EA, Henderson WJ, et al. Mercury pigmentation from industrial exposure. Br J Dermatol. 1997;96:367-74.
51. Everett MA. Metal discolouration. In: Dermis DJ (Ed). Clinical Dermatology. Hagerstown: Harper and Row Inc. 1979;4:124-8.
52. Burrows D, Adams RM. Metals. In: Adams RM (Ed). Occupational Skin Disease, 2nd edn. Philadelphia: Saunders; 1990. pp. 349-86.
53. Zala L, Hunziker T, Broather LR. Pigmentation following long term bismuth therapy for pneumatosis cystoides intestinalis. Dermatology.1993;184:288-9
54. Browning E. Toxicity of industrial metals, 2nd edn. London: Butterworth; 1969. p. 149
55. Blackadder ES, Nanderson WG. Occupational absorption of tellurium: Report of 2 cases. Br J Indust Med. 1975;39: 59-61.
56. Agris J. Adventitious tattooing. J Dermatol Surg. 1976;2:72-4.
57. Bettlen FR. Collier's stripes-the coal miner's dermatosis. Br J Dermatol Syphilis.1940;52:129-30.
58. Hare PJ. A case of occupational iron pigmentation of the skin. Br J Dermatol. 1951;63:63-6.
59. Ruxin TA, Taylor JS. Other occupational dermatosis: acne, pigmentary disorders, skin cancer, infection, reaction to temperature and humidity, scleroderma and nail changes. In: Hogan DJ (Ed). Occupational skin disorder. New York: Igaku-Shoin; 1994. pp. 89-103.
60. Adams RM. Occupational dermatosis and disorders due to chemical agents. In: Fitzpatrik TB, Eisen AZ ,Wolff K, et al. (Eds). Dermatology in General Medicine, 4th edn. New York: McGraw Hill; 1993. pp. 903-5.
61. Brodkin RH, Schwartz RA. Cutaneous signs of dioxin exposure. Cutis. 1984;30:189-94.
62. Gladen BC, Taylor JS, Wu YC, et al. Dermatological finding in children exposed transplacentally to heat degraded polychlorinated biphenyl in Taiwan. Br J Dermatol. 1990;122: 799-808.
63. Riehl G. Uber eine eigenartige melanose. Wien Klin Wochensschr. 1917;30:280-1.
64. Rorsman H. Riehl's melanosis. Int J Dermatol. Mar 1982;21:75-8.
65. Nakayama H. Pigmented Contact Dermatitis and Chemical Depigmentation. In: Rycroft R, Menne T, Frosch P, Lepoittevin J (Eds). Textbook of Contact Dermatitis, 3rd edn. New York: Springer; 2001. pp. 319-33.
66. Shenoi SD, Rao R. Pigmented contact dermatitis. Indian J Dermatol Venereol Leprol. 2007;73:285-7.
67. Osmundsen PE. Pigmented contact dermatitis. Br J Dermatol. 1970;83:296-301.
68. Nakayama H, Harada R, Toda M. Pigmented cosmetic dermatitis. Int J Dermatol. 1976;15:673-5.
69. Nakayama H, Matsuo S, Hayakawa K, et al. Pigmented cosmetic dermatitis. Int J Dermatol. 1984;23:299-305.
70. Imokawa G, Kawai M. Differential hypermelanosis induced by allergic contact dermatitis. J Invest Dermatol. 1987;89:540-6.
71. Ebihara T, Nakayama H. Pigmented contact dermatitis. Clin Dermatol. 1997;15:593-9.
72. Hayakawa R, Matsunaga K, Arima Y. Airborne pigmented contact dermatitis due to musk ambrette in incense. Contact Dermatitis. 1987;16:96-8.

73. el Sayed F, Manzur F, Bazex J. Pigmented contact dermatitis from cosmetics. Contact Dermatitis. 1995;32:111-3.
74. Kozuka T, Tashiro M, Sano S, et al. Brilliant Lake Red R as a cause of pigmented contact dermatitis. Contact Dermatitis. 1979;5:297-304.
75. Sugai T, Takahashi Y, Takagi T. Pigmented cosmetic dermatitis and coal tar dyes. Contact Dermatitis. 1977;3:249-56.
76. Leow YH, Tan SH, Ng SK. Pigmented contact cheilitis from ricinoleic acid in lipsticks. Contact Dermatitis. 2003;49: 48-9.
77. Nath AK, Thappa DM. Kumkum-induced dermatitis: an analysis of 46 cases. Clin Exp Dermatol. 2007;32:385-7.
78. Parodi G, Guarrera M, Rebora A. Lichenoid photocontact dermatitis to musk ambrette. Contact Dermatitis. 1987;16: 136-8.
79. Naganuma M, Hirose S, Nakayama Y, et al. A study of the phototoxicity of lemon oil. Arch Dermatol Res. 1985;278: 31-6.
80. Serrano G, Pujol C, Cuadra J, et al. Riehl's melanosis: pigmented contact dermatitis caused by fragrances. J Am Acad Dermatol. 1989;21:1057-60.
81. Ozkaya-Bayazit E, Buyukbabani N. Non-eczematous pigmented interface dermatitis from para-tertiary-butyl-phenol-formaldehyde resin in a watchstrap adhesive. Contact Dermatitis. 2001;44:45-6.
82. Trattner A, David M. Pigmented contact dermatitis from topical minoxidil 5%. Contact Dermatitis. 2002;46:24-7.
83. Perez-Bernal A, Munoz-Perez MA, Camacho F. Management of facial hyperpigmentation. Am J Clin Dermatol. 2000;1: 261-8.
84. Kobori T, Araki, Toda K. Photoleukomelanodermatitis (Kobori) caused by benzothiazidiazine derivatives. Jap J Dermatol. 1966;76:665-7.
85. Halder RM, Nandeker MA, Neal KW. Pigmentary disorders in ethnic skin. Dermatol Clin. 2003;21:617-28.
86. Koranda FC. Antimalarials. J Am Acad Dermatol. 1981;4: 650-5.
87. Bronner AK, Hood AF. Cutaneous complications of chemotherapeutic agents. J Am Acad Dermatol. 1983;9:645-63.
88. Fernandez-Obregon AC, Hogan KP, Bibro MK. Flagellate pigmentation from intrapleural bleomycin. A light microscopic and electron microscopic study. J Am Acad Dermatol. 1985;13:464-8.
89. Hrushesky WJ. Unusual pigmentary changes associated with 5-fluorouracil therapy. Cutis. 1980;26:181-2.
90. Schallier D, Decoster L, de Greve J. Pemetrexed induced hyperpigmentation of the skin. Anticancer Res. 2011;31: 1753-5.
91. Tanita Y, Kato T, Hanada K, et al. Blue macules of localized argyria caused by implanted acupuncture needles. Electron microscopy and roentgenographic microanalysis of deposited metal. Arch Dermatol. 1985;121:1550-2.
92. McGrae JD, Zelickson AS. Skin pigmentation secondary to minocycline therapy. Arch Dermatol. 1980;116:1262-5.
93. Pepine M, Flowers FP, Ramos-Caro FA. Extensive cutaneous hyperpigmentation caused by minocycline. J Am Acad Dermatol.1993;28:292-5.
94. Green D, Friedman KJ. Treatment of minocycline induced cutaneous pigmentation with the Q-switched Alexandrite laser and a review of the literature. J Am Acad Dermatol. 2001;44:342-7.
95. Trimble JW, Mendelson DS, Fetter BF, et al. Cutaneous pigmentation secondary to amiodarone therapy. Arch Dermatol.1983;119:914-8.
96. Ward HA, Russo CG, Shrum J. Cutaneous manifestation of antiretroviral therapy. J Am Acad Dermatol. 2002;46:284-93.
97. Job CK, Yoder L, Jacobson RR, et al. Skin pigmentation from clofazimine therapy in leprosy patients: a reappraisal. J Am Acad Dermatol.1990;23:236-41.
98. Wolf ME, Richer S, Berk MA, et al. Cutaneous and ocular changes associated with use of chlorpromazine. Int J Clin Pharmacol Ther Toxicol. 1993;31:365-7.
99. Ming ME, Bhawan J, Stefanato CM, et al. Imipramine induced hyperpigmentation: four cases and a review of literature. J Am Acad Dermatol. 1999;40:159-66.
100. Baker H. Adverse cutaneous reaction to oral contraceptives. Br J Dermatol. 1969;81:946-9.
101. Blomberg M, Zachariae CO, Gronhaj F. Hyperpigmentation of face following adalimumab treatment. Acta Derm Venereol. 2009;89:546-7.
102. Kramer KE, Lopez A, Stefanato CM, et al. Exogenous ochronosis. J Am Acad Dermatol. 2000;42:869-71.
103. Chien KH, Lu DW, Chen JT. Extensive facial skin pigmentation after latanoprost treatment. Cutan Ocul Toxicol. 2009;28:185-7.
104. Li CC, Malik SM, Blaeser BF, et al. Mucosal pigmentation caused by imatinib: Report of three cases. Head Neck Pathol. 2011;6:231-7.
105. Dereure O. Drug induced skin pigmentation. Epidemiology, Diagnosis and Treatment. Am J Clin Dermatol. 2001;2:253-62.

9

Infective and Post-inflammatory Pigmentary Disorders

Sunil Dogra, Rahul Mahajan

Key Features

- Pigmentary alterations in various infectious diseases like superficial dermatomycoses, leprosy, post-kala-azar dermal leishmaniasis (PKDL), treponematoses, and onchocerciasis offer important diagnostic clues, the recognition of which helps in making an early diagnosis and initiating appropriate treatment.
- The pathogenesis of pigmentary changes varies from neurological in leprosy, oxidative damage in PKDL, direct inhibition of melanocytes by *Malassezia* and its pigments, to post-inflammatory in treponematoses and onchocerciasis.
- However, despite adequate treatment of the infections, some of these pigmentary changes are long lasting and even may become permanent.
- Post-inflammatory hyper- and hypopigmentation secondary to various inflammatory dermatoses are an important subset of dyschromias, the incidence of which is on the rise probably due to the proliferating use of dermatological procedures like lasers.
- Their occurrence depends on an individual's chromic tendency as well as the type of dermatosis; deeper the inflammation, more intense will be the pigmentary change.
- Management of post-inflammatory hyperpigmentation involves use of sunscreen, pre- and postprocedure application of demelanizing agents and using lasers with appropriate fluencies.

INTRODUCTION

The color of skin is important to an individual for both social and cultural reasons. It is determined primarily by presence of melanin; and by few other pigments like oxyhemoglobin, reduced hemoglobin and carotenoids. Dermatoses which involve changes in the melanin content of the skin present as either hypermelanosis (excess melanin) or hypomelanosis (deficient melanin). Among the various causes of altered pigmentation, infections form a significant group especially in tropical countries like India. The typical discoloration produced helps not only in the diagnosis of the condition but also an early and effective intervention is an important step in preventing cosmetic disfigurement due to pigmentary changes. Similarly post-inflammatory pigmentary changes are frequently encountered secondary to various dermatoses and therapeutic interventions. The present chapter focuses on the infectious dermatoses leading to pigmentary alterations and the post-inflammatory pigmentary changes, their pathomechanisms and management.

INFECTIVE

Among the infectious dermatoses manifesting with pigmentary anomalies, common ones include fungal infections like pityriasis versicolor and tinea nigra; bacterial infections like leprosy, syphilis and pinta; protozoal infections like post-kala-azar dermal leishmaniasis; and parasitic infestations like onchocerciasis.

PITYRIASIS VERSICOLOR

Pityriasis versicolor is a common superficial dermatomycosis caused by the genus *Malassezia* that is characterized by presence of typical discolored macules on the skin covered with branny scales. In the tropical regions, the disease is seen throughout the year where as in the temperate areas, it is more common in warmer seasons. In India, the maximum incidence is seen in the months between June and August.[1]

The genus *Malassezia* consists of 13 species which are differentiated from each other on the basis of morphologic, cellular, biochemical and genetic characteristics, *M. furfur, M. globosa, M. obtusa, M. restricta, M. slooffiae, M. sympodialis, M. pachydermatis, M. dermatis, M. yamatoensis, M. japonica, M. nana, M. caprae and M. equina.*[2-7] *M. globosa* has been found to be the most common isolated species in various studies. The fungus exists in both yeast as well as mycelia forms.

Various factors have been implicated in predisposing a person towards development of pityriasis versicolor. These include increased amounts of corticosteroids, either endogenous or exogenously administered,[8] a genetic predisposition, poor nutritional state, chronic infections, greasy skin and excessive sweating, pregnancy and immunodeficiency. Park et al. evaluated the differences of skin characteristics between pityriasis versicolor patients and normal healthy subjects using noninvasive bioengineering methods and concluded that transepidermal water loss (TEWL) and sebum excretion rate differ significantly between pityriasis versicolor lesions (both hypo/hyperpigmented) and normal skin.[9]

Although all ages may be affected, it is more common in young and middle aged adults. The disease may manifest in various clinical forms, hypopigmented, hyperpigmented, leukoderma like erythematous or dark brown with different colors occasionally, seen in the same patient. The common sites of involvement are chest, abdomen and trunk although face, axillae, dorsa of hands, penis, perineal region and groins may be involved uncommonly.[10] Face is the most common site in children in up to 40% cases.[11] Skin lesions are characterized by asymptomatic or mildly itchy, yellow-brown or dark brown scaly macules which coalesce to form large sheets with geographic margins and few discrete lesions present at the periphery. The disease has to be differentiated from pityriasis rosea **(Figs 1 and 2)**, pityriasis alba, vitiligo, post-kala-azar dermal leishmaniasis (PKDL) and other common causes of hypopigmentation.

Depigmentation can occur during or after healing of lesions of the hyperpigmented and hypopigmented form of pityriasis versicolor (pityriasis versicolor alba).[12] In most cases, it tends to be long lasting (3 weeks–6 months).[13-15] It can also occur without any hyperpigmented pre-stage. Seventy-two percent of children exhibit the hypopigmented or depigmented pattern. In contrast to vitiligo, depigmented lesions in pityriasis versicolor alba are less sensitive to ultraviolet (UV) light, do not develop erythema during UV irradiation and are resistant to repigmentation even after addition of a photosensitizing agent.[16] Atrophying pityriasis versicolor, another atypical clinical form of pityriasis versicolor is characterized by lesions of pityriasis versicolor with overlying skin atrophy. It may occur due to injudicious topical steroid use or it may represent a delayed-type hypersensitivity reaction to antigens derived from the *Malassezia* species and the atrophy is induced by elastases secreted by histiocytes at the site of inflammation.[17]

Mechanism of Pigmentary Changes

The species of *Malassezia* yeasts does not determine the color of the lesions; instead it is the interactions between the organism and the skin barrier materials, which leads to hypopigmentation or hyperpigmentation. Initially depigmentation was thought to result from the light filtering effect by the scales and the fungal layer. Later, many authors believed that hypopigmented lesions seen in pityriasis versicolor are due to the production of dicarboxylic acids, especially azelaic acid.[18] However, many studies have observed that concentrations of azelaic acid *in vivo* are too low for inhibition of tyrosinase and or damage to melanocytes.[19] De Luca[20] proposed the effects of lipid

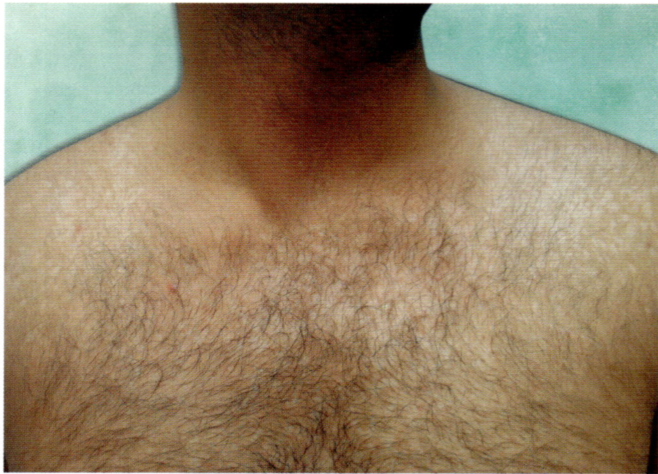

Fig. 1: Hypopigmented pityriasis versicolor; presenting with typical macules over the seborrheic areas coalescing at places and satellite lesions at the periphery

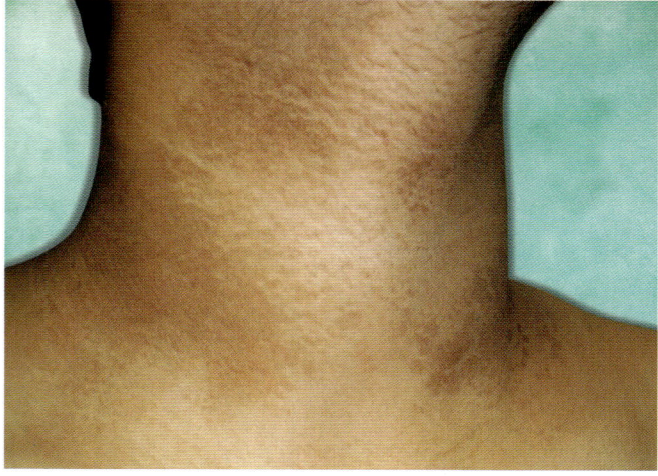

Fig. 2: Hyperpigmented pityriasis versicolor; resembling the atopic dirty neck

peroxides and byproducts causing damage to melanocytes. An interesting observation has been the newly discovered tryptophan-dependent secondary metabolites of *M. furfur*, pityriacritine and pityrialactone, which possess potent broad-spectrum ultraviolet effect. This might explain why patients with pityriasis versicolor alba do not get sunburn in the depigmented areas. Under UV light, this pigment exhibits yellowish-green fluorescence which explains the slightly yellowish depigmentation in pityriasis versicolor.[21] On chromatographic separation of the pigment, a variety of differently colored bands as well as fluorochromes are revealed. This again corresponds to the multitude of colors visible in lesions of pityriasis versicolor. Moreover, these pigments have been shown to inhibit tyrosinase activity *in vitro*. During further thin-layer chromatographic separation enzyme inhibition was reproducibly assigned to a particular band (R_f = 0.39–0.43 in fraction 6) and finally to a single peak on high-performance liquid chromatography separation of this thin-layer band.[22] Malassezin, a pigment produced by *M. furfur* has been shown to damage melanocyte.[23]

In fair skinned as well as in darker skinned population, the lesions are hyperpigmented macules. The exact reason for this is not fully understood but numerous theories have been put forward. It has been suggested that hyperpigmentation occurs due to the increased thickness of stratum corneum.[24] Alternatively, the inflammatory cell infiltrate may lead to stimulation of melanocytes. *Malassezia* yeasts hydrolyze triglycerides into free fatty acids which are then converted back into medium and long chain fatty acids. These in turn release arachidonic acid, the precursor of inflammatory cytokines like prostaglandins and leukotrines. Electron microscopic studies have revealed larger than normal melanosomes in hyperpigmented lesions and smaller ones in hypopigmented lesions.[25] Concluding, pigment production might elucidate some phenomena of the disease like fluorescence, hyperpigmentation, depigmentation and their coexistence, and hypopigmentation as a transitional state between pigment synthesis by the yeasts and suppression of melanogenesis.

The diagnosis of pityriasis versicolor is essentially clinical which can be confirmed by Wood's lamp examination and direct microscopy. Florescence on Wood's lamp examination is seen in only 33% of cases; where the causative agent is *M. furfur*. Direct microscopy with 10% potassium hydroxide (KOH) reveals the characteristic "banana and grapes" or "spaghetti and meat balls" appearance. The various topical medications used in the treatment of pityriasis versicolor are 25% sodium thiosulphate (hyposulfite), 2.5% selenium sulfide shampoo, Whitfield's ointment, 1–2% imidazole creams and 2% terbinafine cream.[26] These agents need to be applied once or twice daily for at least 2 weeks for clinical and mycological cure. The appearance of normal pigmentation may take months to occur and the patient should be counseled regarding this fact. Oral antifungals are routinely used in treating *Malassezia* infections since topical creams need to be applied over large body surface area and is cumbersome. Oral fluconazole and itraconazole are most commonly employed. Fluconazole in a dose of 400 mg daily for 1–3 days has been recommended. Alternatively, itraconazole in a dose of 200 mg daily for 5–7 days can be tried. Depigmentation in pityriasis versicolor alba is difficult to treat. Jung and Bohnert described repigmentation during UV therapy within 3 weeks.[15] Another study evaluating 79 patients of pityriasis versicolor showed no effect of an additional UV therapy or an additional combination of UV therapy and photosensitizing agent (meladinine) versus antifungal treatment alone.[14] It is therefore recommended that patients with pityriasis versicolor should receive therapy as soon as possible in order to minimize the effect of the disease on skin pigmentation. If considered, UV therapy should be given only after complete eradication of the fungus.

TINEA NIGRA

Tinea nigra is another superficial dermatomycosis that is caused by two dematiaceous fungi, *Hortaea werneckii* and *Stenella araguata*.[27] The former has been successfully cultured from soil, sewage, and wood and decaying vegetation but not the latter.[28] The incubation period varies from 2–7 weeks. Human infection by *H. werneckii* is thought to result from direct inoculation after minor skin trauma. Individuals with hyperhidrosis are at increased risk and may be the reason for the palmoplantar localization of lesions.[29] The disease is more common in children and young adults with a female predilection. It presents as an asymptomatic, unilateral or less commonly bilateral circumscribed solitary, mottled, brown to black macule 1–5 mm in diameter beginning on the palms and rarely on other body sites such as neck, chest and dorsa of hands and phalanges. The macule may enlarge with peripheral extension with little scaling and inflammation although the advancing borders acquire a relatively darker pigmentation than trailing parts. This benign condition needs to be differentiated from acral lentiginous melanoma which is more indurated, post-inflammatory hyperpigmentation, syphilis, pinta, and skin staining from dyes and pigments.[30]

Direct microscopy reveals olive brown, septate, branching hyphae, and moderate numbers of elongated budding cells. A few intercalary chlamydoconidia may also be seen. The fungus is grown in SDA at 25–30°C as it does not grow at 37°C. Whitfield's ointment and other preparations containing salicylic acid effectively clear the disease. Other options include topical 10% thiabendazole, clotrimazole, miconazole, or oxiconazole.[31]

LEPROSY

Leprosy is a chronic infectious disease caused by *Mycobacterium leprae* which can express itself in different clinicopathologic forms. The invading *M. leprae* has three main targets, the peripheral neural tissues, endothelial cells and macrophage-monocyte system. The diagnosis of leprosy is made clinically by presence of any one of the following three cardinal features—definite loss of sensation in a hypopigmented or reddish skin patch, thickened or enlarged peripheral nerve, with loss of sensation and/or weakness of the muscles supplied by that nerve and the presence of acid-fast bacilli in a slit skin smear.[32]

The Indian classification of leprosy includes six clinico-pathologic variants, indeterminate leprosy, tuberculoid leprosy, maculo-anesthetic leprosy, borderline leprosy, lepromatous leprosy and pure neuritic leprosy. Indeterminate leprosy is seen mostly in children and presents as slightly hypopigmented or erythematous macules 1–3 in number with variable size from 1–5 cm in diameter or even larger. The lesions are widely distributed over body, often symmetrically and characteristically over trunk and outer sides of the extremities, have an ill-defined margins and smooth surface. Lesions are typically flat, when thickening present, the macule has passed into one of the determinate forms. Sensory impairment is slight, in only few of the patches. It represents unstable disease, may disappear spontaneously or may evolve into any of the determinate forms of leprosy. Hypopigmented macules and patches are a consistent feature of almost all clinical types of leprosy although lesional morphology with respect to the degree of infiltration and anesthesia varies in different forms. The cause of hypopigmentation in leprosy is relatively less well studied **(Fig. 3)**. It was earlier hypothesized that the local inflammatory infiltrate may interfere with pigment formation. Alternatively, *M. leprae* may divert dihydroxyphenylalanine (DOPA) from melanin synthesis pathway for its own metabolic needs although this was refuted by many authors.[33] Singh et al. observed that degree of hypopigmentation was proportional neither to the degree of infiltrate nor to the vascular involvement by the infiltrate. They concluded that the most plausible hypothesis was that the hypopigmentation was related to neural involvement.[34] Another interesting observation is the relatively high prevalence of vitiligo in leprosy (approximately 10% in multibacillary leprosy).[35] Both leprosy and vitiligo may induce pigment loss, via different mechanisms. The loss of nervous control of melanogenesis could be one of the mechanisms due to nervous damage in leprosy. Autoimmune disorders may occur in both diseases, as circulating autoantibodies have been described in vitiligo and leprosy. The treatment of leprosy has been simplified with the introduction of highly effective World Health Organization-multi drug treatment (WHO-MDT) regimen. For up to five skin lesions, paucibacillary regimen (PBR) is given for 6 months and for more than five skin lesions, multibacillary regimen (MBR) is administered for 12 months.

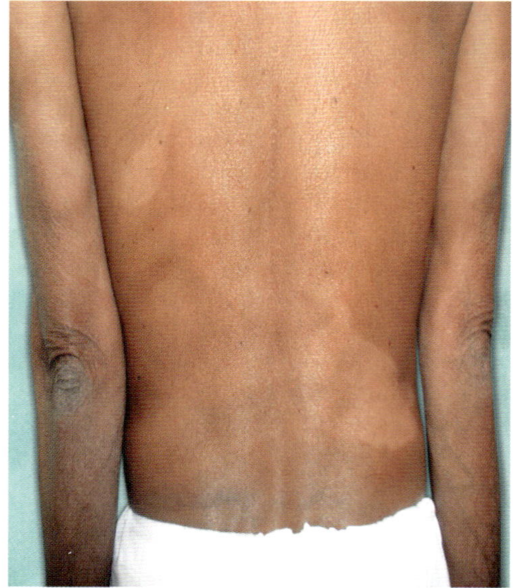

Fig. 3: Hypopigmented lesion of borderline tuberculoid Hansen with lesional anesthesia and dry rough surface

POST-KALA-AZAR DERMAL LEISHMANIASIS

Post-kala-azar dermal leishmaniasis is a complication of visceral leishmaniasis (VL) and is seen in patients who have recovered from VL but are otherwise well. It is seen mainly in Sudan and India, where it follows VL in 50% and 5–10% of cases respectively. The causative organism is *Leishmania donovani*. It plays an important role in inter-epidemic periods of VL, acting as reservoir of infection. The disease appears to be immunologically mediated as high concentrations of serum IL-10 in VL patients predict development of PKDL. Further, production of IFN-γ by peripheral blood mononuclear cells (PBMC) after treatment of VL coincides with appearance of PKDL lesions.[36]

The clinical presentation is typical. In Sudan, most common morphologic presentation is a papular or nodular rash (51%). Other presentations include maculopapular (23%), micropapular/measles like (17%) and macular (9%) rash. In India, the most common presentation is persistent erythema and induration on butterfly area of face which shows photosensitivity, multiple symmetric hypopigmented macules over face and trunk which may coalesce **(Fig. 4)**, and a combination of papules, nodules and plaques. Uncommon morphologic types include annular, warty, papillomatous, fibroid or xanthomatous types. Ulceration is not a feature of PKDL.[36,37] In less than 10% of patients, PKDL may present with depigmented macules as the sole manifestation which may be localized, generalized or extensive in distribution.[38] Even after adequate treatment of PKDL, these macules take a long time to repigment. The degree of pigment loss can be considerable and may simulate vitiligo.

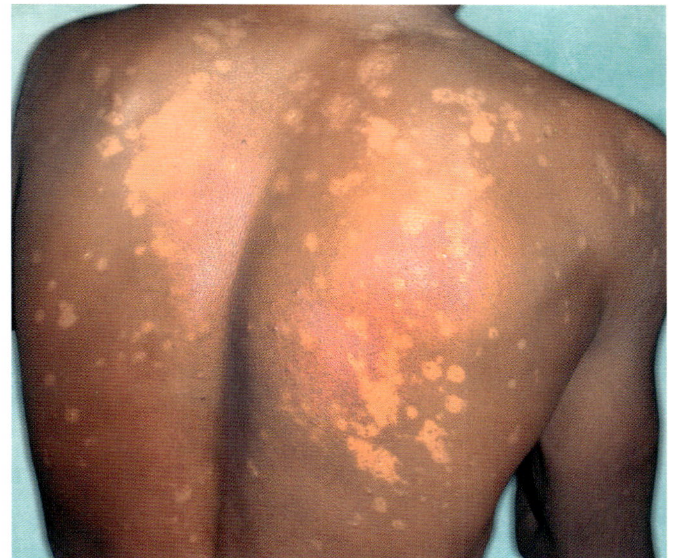

Fig. 4: Hypopigmented macules of post-kala-azar dermal leishmaniasis with irregular margins

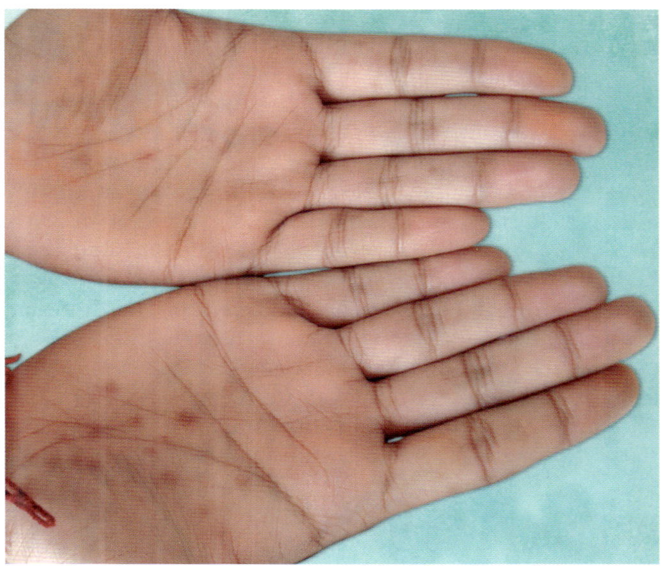

Fig. 5: Macular syphilid over palms

The cause of hypopigmentation in PKDL has been less well studied.[38] Although the pigment loss correlates with the density of the dermal infiltrate on histopathology, this is not manifested clinically as nodules show minimal or no hypopigmentation. In addition, functional abnormalities of melanosomes are also seen.[37] It is hypothesized that oxidative burst mechanism of host macrophages in order to kill the parasite generates many superoxide radicals that may be toxic to melanocytes.[39] Increased protease secretion in *L. donovani* isolates from PKDL patients[40] has been shown to degrade the extracellular matrix components fibronectin and collagen type IV, which can lead to poor melanocyte adhesion and damage to dendrites, affecting melanosomal transfer. The diagnosis is based on the demonstration of the organism either in tissue smears or in culture. Leishmanin skin test is negative in Indian PKDL and positive in Sudanese PKDL. Histopathology shows decreased number of pigmented granules from the hypopigmented lesions. Dermis reveals the presence of well-organized epithelioid cell granuloma and significant perivascular fibrous reaction. Leishman-Donovan (LD) bodies may or may not be visible in specimen from the hypopigmented macules but are usually seen in more infiltrated lesions. The most sensitive and specific tests are polymerase chain reaction (PCR) on lesional skin and enzyme-linked immunosorbent assay (ELISA) on serum samples, using rk39, a *Leishmania*-specific recombinant antigen. The treatment of choice is intravenous administration of sodium stibugluconate in a dose of 20 mg/kg/day for 4 months. Recently oral miltefosine has also been tried.[36]

TREPONEMATOSES: SYPHILIS AND PINTA

Syphilis is caused by *Treponema pallidum* and is acquired most commonly through unprotected sexual contact with an infected partner. Although the incidence of syphilis has considerably decreased in the last century, it still continues to be a significant health problem. In untreated individuals, treponemes proliferate at the site of entry in the chancre to produce primary chancre. This is followed by spirochetemia and their dissemination throughout the body which leads to appearance of secondary lesions. This rash in secondary syphilis may appear as reddish brown macules on the palms and soles **(Fig. 5)**. In such cases, it may be confused with tinea nigra. Pigmentary cutaneous lesions are not uncommonly seen in secondary syphilis in the form of leukoderma syphiliticum.[41] It occurs as sequel of macular syphilide or roseolar rash, the most common morphologic manifestation of secondary syphilis. The lesions of macular syphilis are symmetrical, coppery red and asymptomatic and when they resolve, they leave behind a characteristic pattern of depigmentation on a background of hyperpigmentation, called as leukoderma syphiliticum. Over the sides of neck, such depigmentation was earlier termed as "necklace of Venus." Primary and secondary syphilis can be successfully treated with a single intramuscular injection of 2.4 mega units of benzathine penicillin.

The etiologic organism of pinta is *T. pallidum carateum*. The disease is endemic in only a few parts of the world

(Central and South America).[42] Like syphilis, pinta has an early (primary and secondary) infectious stage. The primary stage is characterized by erythematous papules or plaques develop. This is followed by the secondary stage after several months or years which manifests as hyperpigmented lesions of varying colors (brown, blue, black or gray), and infiltration. Late in the course of the disease, atrophy may be seen in the lesions with irregular areas of confetti like depigmentation (tertiary stage). Pinta needs to be differentiated from erythema dyschromicum perstans, pityriasis alba, vitiligo, and tuberculoid leprosy. The World Health Organization recommends that patients and contacts over 10 years of age are given a single intramuscular injection of 1,200,000 IU of benzathine penicillin, and those under 10 years should receive 600,000 IU. In individuals allergic to penicillin, tetracyclines and erythromycin are alternatives.[43]

ONCHOCERCIASIS

Onchocerciasis is a filarial disease caused by *Onchocerca volvulus*. The disease is endemic in Africa and certain parts of Central and South America.[44] The vectors of the disease are black flies of the Simuliidae family. The most common symptoms and signs are pruritus, onchocercal dermatitis, nodules and, in areas of high endemicity blindness.[45] The disease may be detectable as early as 6 months of age, and presents with pruritus, often confined to a limb or other circumscribed body site, and a non-specific papular rash worsened by scratching. The skin changes have been classified as acute papular onchodermatitis (APOD), chronic papular onchodermatitis (CPOD), lichenified onchodermatitis (LOD), atrophy and hypopigmentation.[46] Early in the course of the disease, the skin appears infiltrated over the shoulders and around the pelvis; and less commonly as acute swelling on the face and cheeks with erythema and itching. Over the next few months and years, localized areas of scarring with hyperpigmentation, CPOD and lichenified onchodermatitis are seen. Depigmentation is a common feature of late-stage onchodermatitis commonly seen bilaterally over the pretibial region, but may affect the inguinal regions, bony prominences and the shoulders.[47] The patches of hypopigmentation are spotty, with islands of normal appearing skin, but large coalescent sheets of depigmentation are present in late-stage disease.[48] The name leopard skin is used to describe this change. In Central America, an inflammatory rash accompanied by hyperpigmentation known as "mal morado" is observed.

Clinically, the diagnosis is usually evident. Histological examination of nodules may be examined for adult worms and microfilariae. The filarial ELISA is positive in 60–90% of cases. Ivermectin is the drug of choice, given orally in a single dose of 100–200 μg/kg. Patients may be retreated after 6–12 months. The alternative drug regimen, now rarely used, involves the use of diethylcarbamazine (DEC), which may cause severe exacerbation of skin and eye disease, even blindness.

POST-INFLAMMATORY

Post-inflammatory pigmentary changes refer to a reactive state of transient/permanent hypermelanosis or hypomelanosis that occurs as sequel of a variety of inflammatory skin conditions. This occurs due to an altered production of melanin into the epidermis or dermis by labile melanocytes. The darker Indian skin (with Fitzpatrick skin types III–V) has a propensity to develop these pigmentary alterations following a variety of dermatologic disorders.[49] The sizes and the shapes of the pigmented lesions tend to correspond to the shapes of

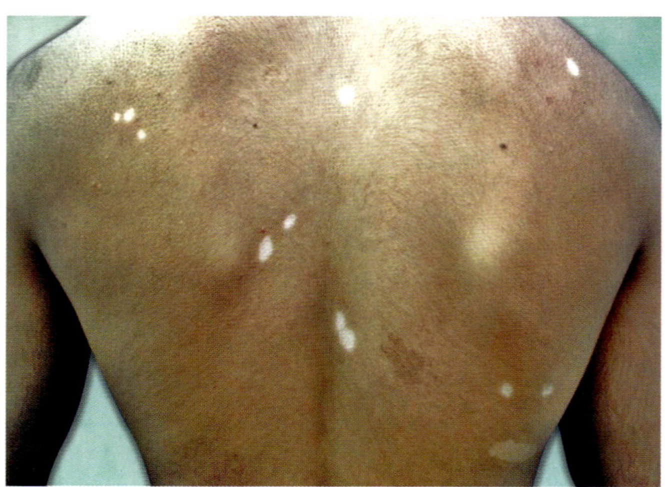

Fig. 6: Post-inflammatory depigmentation resembling vitiligo following psoriasis

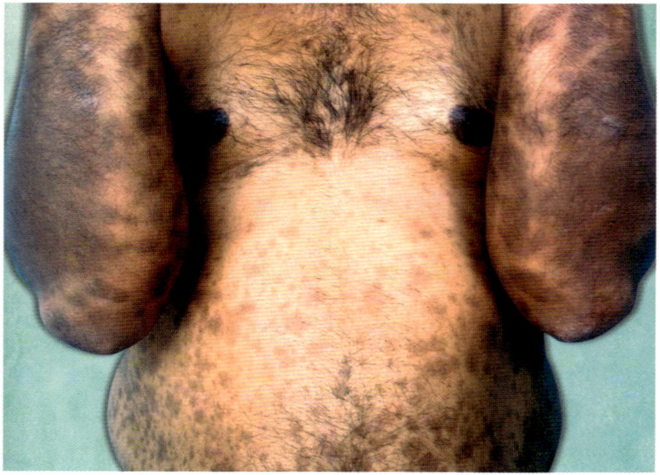

Fig. 7: Post-inflammatory hyperpigmentation in a patient with severe psoriasis vulgaris

the original lesions and thus in some cases; it may be possible to speculate on the original disease responsible for the post-inflammatory sequel. The intensity of post-inflammatory pigmentation is not necessarily related to the degree of previous inflammation.[50] However, it may be worsened by certain environmental factors like exposure to sunlight, and photosensitizing medication and chemicals. In diseases like scabies, contact dermatitis, psoriasis and atopic dermatitis, post-inflammatory pigmentary changes **(Figs 6 and 7)** tend to be less intense, transient and generally disappear without any treatment. In contrast, in few dermatoses like lichen planus and fixed drug eruption, the hyperpigmentation produced tends to be darker, persistent and somewhat resistant to treatment.[51,52] Even after the active disease has been controlled, these dyschromias serve as a frequent source of impaired quality of life of the patients, particularly with ethnic skin.[53]

Mechanism of Post-inflammatory Pigmentary Changes

The mechanisms which stimulate excess production or conversely inhibit adequate synthesis of melanin after inflammation are not well elucidated. The most accepted hypothesis is the effect of inflammatory cytokines like prostaglandins (PGE1, PGE2 and PGD2) and other arachidonic acid-derived leukotrienes (LTs) and thromboxanes (TXs), on the regulation of melanin synthesis.[54] Exposure to these cytokines leads to increase in the size of melanocytes as well as more number of dendritic processes. In addition, other cytokines such as interleukin (IL)-1, IL-6, tumor necrosis factor alpha (TNF-α), epidermal growth factor and nitric oxide can stimulate synthesis of melanosomes by melanocytes.

Individual Chromatic Tendency

Ruiz-Maldonado and Orozco-Covarrubias proposed that whether a patient develops hypopigmentation or the more common hyperpigmentation or shows no pigment alteration post an inflammatory process depends on individual chromatic tendency.[55] According to them, melanocytes in an individual can be strong or weak; and thus the post-inflammatory response can be normochromic, hypo/hyperchromic. Individuals with weak or labile melanocytes have a tendency towards hypopigmentation as their melanocytes get easily damaged after trauma or inflammation. Conversely, patients with strong melanocytes respond with hyperpigmentation. An individual's chromatic tendency shows no consistent relationship with one's inherent color, that is, a dark complexioned individual may have labile melanocytes and a light skinned individual may be strong melanocytes.

POST-INFLAMMATORY HYPERPIGMENTATION

It is an acquired excess of pigment in the skin after an inflammatory process. Various factors that determine the character of pigmentation include the depth at which pigment excess occurs—epidermal or dermal, degree of inflammation and the causative inflammatory disease.[55] The color of pigmentation depends on the location of melanin, brown in case of epidermal location and bluish-gray in case of dermal deposition. Secondly, severe inflammation leading to melanocyte destruction leads to hypopigmentation whereas less severe inflammation may result in hyperpigmentation. Finally dermatoses like lupus erythematosus and lichen planus which are associated with disruption of basal cell layer usually **(Figs 8 and 9)** lead to significant dyspigmentation.

Post-inflammatory hyperpigmentation commonly occurs in Fitzpatrick skin phototypes (SPT) III to VI and can have a considerable impact on quality of life. Although the majority of cases improve spontaneously, this may take several months or even years to resolve and in some cases, the pigmentation becomes permanent. The lesions may be symmetric or asymmetric with hazy margins. Dermatoses which heal with post-inflammatory hyperpigmentation include infections like impetigo, syphilis, pinta, pityriasis versicolor, onchocerciasis, herpes zoster, inflammatory diseases like atopic dermatitis, psoriasis, immunobullous diseases, phototoxic drug eruptions, Steven-Johnson syndrome, physical or chemical injuries and others like acne, lichen planus **(Fig. 9)** and

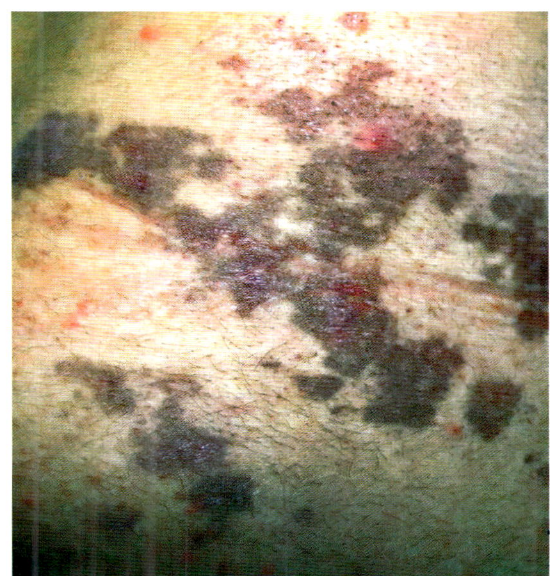

Fig. 8: Lichen planus healing with surrounding post-inflammatory hyperpigmentation

hyperpigmentation, it might be reduced and the total number of treatment sessions increased in order to maintain efficacy and safety.

POST-INFLAMMATORY HYPOPIGMENTATION

It refers to an acquired partial or total loss of melanocytes secondary to cutaneous inflammation. The dermatoses mentioned earlier which lead to post-inflammatory hyperpigmentation can also result in hypopigmentation and both can be seen in the same patient at the same time. As mentioned earlier, although intrinsic chromatic tendency is important, individual dermastosis also plays its part in development of hypopigmentation.[53] Screening of ultraviolet rays by the hyperkeratosis and parakeratosis in pityriasis alba contributes towards development of hypopigmentation. As with post-inflammatory hyperpigmentation, the localized or generalized patches of post-inflammatory hypopigmentation tend to be symmetric, asymptomatic and corresponding to the original dermatosis.

Post-inflammatory hypopigmentation is more apparent in dark skinned individuals and hence a source of embarrassment. In view of the social stigma attached with vitiligo, post-inflammatory hypopigmentation needs to be differentiated from it. In contrast to the scalloped margins seen in vitiligo, lesions of post-inflammatory hypopigmentation have feathery margins and are less depigmented. Others diseases which need to be excluded include hypopigmented mycosis fungoides and sarcoidosis. Histological evaluation can aid the diagnosis in such cases. Treatment of post-inflammatory hypopigmentation is challenging. Although many areas with slight hypopigmentation resolve on their own within a few weeks, more extensive and severely hypopigmented lesions are slow to resolve and may become permanent. If functional melanocytes are still present narrow-band UVB phototherapy or topical psoralen and UVA light therapy (PUVA) may be a useful option.

REFERENCES

1. Dutta S, Bajaj AK, Basu S, et al. Pityriasis versicolor: socioeconomic and clinicomycologic study in India. Int J Dermatol. 2002;41:823-4.
2. Guého E, Midgley G, Guillot J. The genus *Malassezia* with description of four new species. Antonie van Leeuwenhoek. 1996;69:337-55.
3. Guillot J, Gueho E. The diversity of *Malassezia* yeasts confirmed by rRNA sequence and nuclear DNA comparisons. Antonie van Leeuwenhoek. 1995;67:297-314.
4. Hirai A, Kano R, Makimura K, et al. *Malassezia nana* sp. nov., a novel lipid-dependent yeast species isolated from animals. Int J Syst Evol Microbiol. 2004;54:623-7.
5. Sugita T, Tajima M, Takashima M, et al. A new yeast, *Malassezia yamatoensis*, isolated from a patient with seborrheic dermatitis, and its distribution in patients and healthy subjects. Microbiol Immunol. 2004;48:579-83.
6. Sugita T, Takashima M, Kodama M, et al. Description of a new yeast species, *Malassezia japonica*, and its detection in patients with a topic dermatitis and healthy subjects. J Clin Microbiol. 2003;41:4695-9.
7. Sugita T, Takashima M, Shinoda T, et al. New yeast species, *Malassezia dermatis*, isolated from patients with atopic dermatitis. J Clin Microbiol. 2002;40:1363-7.
8. Gupta AK, Batra R, Bluhm R, et al. Skin diseases associated with *Malassezia* species. J Am Acad Dermatol. 2004;51:785-98.
9. Park HJ, Lee YW, Choe YB, et al. Skin characteristics in patients with pityriasisversicolor using non-invasive method, MPA5. Ann Dermatol. 2012;24:444-52 .
10. Khaddar RK, Cherif F, Ben Hadid R, et al. Penile shaft involvement in pityriasis versicolor. Acta Dermatoven APA. 2008;17:86-8.
11. Terragni L, Lasagni A, Oriani A, et al. Pityriasis versicolor in the pediatric age. Pediatr Dermatol. 1991;8:9-12.
12. Thoma W, Krämer HJ, Mayser P. Pityriasis versicolor alba. J Eur Acad Dermatol Venereol. 2005;19:147-52.
13 Adamson HG. Pityriasis versicolor with subsequent leukodermic patches. Br J Dermatol. 1949;61:322.
14. El-Gothamy Z, Abdel-Fattah AF. Tinea versicolor hypopigmentation: histochemical and therapeutic studies. Int J Dermatol. 1975;14:510-5.
15. Jung EG, Bohnert E. Mechanism of depigmentation on pityriasis versicolor alba. Arch Dermatol Res. 1976;256:333-4.
16. Bouassida S, Boudaya S, Ghorbel R. Pityriasis versicolor in children: a retrospective study of 164 cases. Ann Dermatol Venereol. 1998;125:581-4.
17. Yang YS, Shin MK, Haw CR. Atrophying Pityriasis Versicolor: Is this a new variant of pityriasis versicolor? Ann Dermatol. 2010; 22:456-9.
18. Bojanowsky A, Bohnert E, Jung EG. Pityrosporumorbiculare: ErregerverschiedenerklinischerBilder und Modell einer Depigmentierungsart. Act Dermatol. 1979;5:19-25.
19. Robins EJ, Breathnach AS, Bennet D. Ultrastructural observations on the effect of azelaic acid on normal human melanocytes and human melanoma cell line in tissue culture. Br J Dermatol. 1987;113:687-97.
20. De Luca C, Picardo M, Breathnach A, et al. Lipoperoxidase activity of *Pityrosporum*: characterisation of by-products and possible role in pityriasis versicolor. Exp Dermatol. 1996;5:49-56.
21. Keddie FM. Tinea versicolor. A historical survey based on selections from the writings of the nineteenth century. In: Robinson (Ed). The Diagnosis and Treatment of Fungal Infections. Illinois: CC Thomas; 1974. pp. 169-84.
22. Thoma W, Trinkaus M, Mayser P. Tyrosinase inhibition durch Stoffwechselprodukte von *M. furfur*. Haut- und Geschlechtskrankheiten 2000;75:473.

23. Podobinska M, Krämer HJ, Bartsch A. A cytotoxic metabolite from *Malassezia furfur*. Isolation and chemical identification as malassezin. Arch Dermatol Res. 2003; 294:512.
24. Galadari I, El Komy M, Mousa A, et al. Tineaversicolor: histologic and ultrastructural investigation of pigmentary changes. Int J Dermatol. 1992;31:253-6.
25. Aljabre SH, Alzayir AA, Abdulghani M, et al. Pigmentary changes of tinea versicolor in dark-skinned patients. Int J Dermatol. 2001;40:273-5.
26. Gupta AK, Kogan N, Batra R. Pityriasis versicolor: a review of pharmacological treatment options. Expert Opin Pharmacother. 2005;6:165-78.
27. Superficial infections. In: Rippon JW (Ed). Medical mycology. The pathogenic fungi and pathogenic actinomycetes, 2nd edn. London: WB Saunders Company; 1982. pp. 145-53.
28. Keddie F. Cladosporiumwernickii: Infection and *in vivo* culture. Arch Dermatol. 1964; 89:432-5.
29. Velsor HV, Singletary H. Tinea nigra palmaris: a report of 15 cases from coastal North Carolina. Arch Dermatol. 1964;90:59-61.
30. Vaffee AS. Tinea nigra palmaris resembling malignant melanoma. N Engl J Med. 1970;283:1112.
31. Carr JF, Lewis CW. Tinea nigra palmaris. Arch Dermatol. 1975;111:904-5.
32. Ramesh V, Kumar J. Systemic manifestations. In: Kar HK, Kumar B (Eds). IAL Textbook of leprosy, 1st edn. New Delhi: Jaypee Brothers. 2010; pp. 293-304.
33. Prabhakaran K. Hypopigmentation of skin lesions in leprosy—a hypothesis. Lepr India. 1977;49:462-3.
34. Singh K, Iyenger B, Singh R. Hypopigmentation in leprosy. Lepr India. 1983;55:675-9.
35. Boisseau-Garsaud AM, Vezon G, Helenon R, et al. High prevalence of vitiligo in lepromatous leprosy. Int J Dermatol. 2000;39:837-9.
36. Singh S, Sharma U, Mishra J. Post-kala-azar dermal leishmaniasis: recent developments. Int J Dermatol. 2011;50: 1099-108.
37. Ganguly S, Das NK, Barbhuiya JN, et al. Post-kala-azar dermal leishmaniasis—an overview. Int J Dermatol. 2010; 49:921-31.
38. Ramesh V, Ramam M, Singh R, et al. Hypopigmented post-kala-azar dermal leishmaniasis. Int J Dermatol. 2008;47:414-6.
39. Schallreuter KU, Wood JM, Pitelkow MR. Regulation of melanin biosynthesis in human epidermis by tetrahydrobipterin. Science. 1994; 263:1444-6.
40. Salotra P, Duncan RC, Singh R. Upregulation of surface proteins in *Leishmania donovani* isolated from patients of post-kala-azar dermal leishmaniasis. Microbes Infect. 2006;8:637-44.
41. Kent ME, Romanelli F. Reexamining syphilis: an update on epidemiology, clinical manifestations, and management. Ann Pharmacother. 2008;42:226-36.
42. Koff AB, Rosen T. Nonvenereal treponematoses: yaws, endemic syphilis, and pinta. J Am Acad Dermatol. 1993;29: 519-35.
43. Antal GM, Lukehart SA, Meheus AZ. The endemic treponematoses. Microbes Infect. 2002;4:83-94.
44. Benton B. Economic impact of onchocerciasis control through the African Programme for Onchocerciasis Control: an overview. *Ann Trop Med Parasit.* 1998;92:S33-9.
45. Coffeng LE, Fobi G, Ozoh G, et al. Concurrence of dermatological and ophthalmological morbidity in onchocerciasis. Trans R Soc Trop Med Hyg. 2012;106:243-51.
46. Murdoch ME, Asuzu MC, Hagan M, et al. Onchocerciasis: the clinical and epidemiological burden of skin disease in Africa. Ann Trop Med Parasitol. 2002;96:283-96.
47. Okello DO, Ovuga EB, Ogwal-Okeng JW. Dermatological problems of onchocerciasis in Nebbi District, Uganda. East Afr Med J. 1995;72:295-8.
48. Carme B, Ntsoumou-Madzou V, Samba Y, et al. Prevalence of depigmentation of the shins: a simple and cheap way to screen for severe endemic onchocerciasis in Africa. Bull World Health Organ. 1993;71:755-8.
49. Bleehen SS, Ebling FJG, Champion RH. Disorders of the Skin Colour. In: Champion RH, Burton JL, Ebling FJG (Eds). Textbook of Dermatology. London: Blackwell Scientific Publications; 1992. pp. 1561-1622
50. Takiwaki H, Shirai S, Kohnn H, et al. The degrees of UVA-induced erythema and pigmentation correlate linearly and are reduced in a parallel manner by topical anti-inflammatory agents. J Invest Dermatol. 1994;103:42-6.
51. Levine N. Pigmentary abnormalities. In: Schachner L, Hansen R (Eds). Pediatric Dermatology, 4th edn. New York: Churchill Livingstone; 2011. pp. 539-82.
52. Eimpunth S, Wanitphadeedecha R, Manuskiatti W. A focused review on acne-induced and aesthetic procedure-related postinflammatory hyperpigmentation in Asians. J Eur Acad Dermatol Venereol. 2013;27:S7-18.
53. Grimes E. Management of hyperpigmentation in darker racial ethnic groups. Semin Cutan Med Surg. 2009;28: 77-85.
54. Tomita Y, Maeda K, Tagami HT. Leukotrienes and thromboxane A2 stimulate normal human melanocytes *in vitro*: possible inducers of post-inflammatory hyperpigmentation. Tohoku J Exp Med. 1988;156:303-4.
55. Ruiz-Maldonado R, de la Luz Orozco-Covarrubias M. Post-inflammatory hypopigmentation and hyperpigmentation. Sem Cut Med Surg. 1997;16:36-43.
56. Wong CK, Guerrier CJ, MacMillan DC. An electron microscopical study of Bloch-Sulzberger syndrome (incontinentiapigmenti). Acta Derm Venereol. 1971;51:161-8.
57. Masu S, Seigi M. Pigmentary incontinence in fixed drug eruptions. J Am Acad Dermatol. 1983;8:525-32.
58. Lacz NL, Vafaie J, Kihiczak NI. Postinflammatory hyperpigmentation: a common but troubling condition. Int J Dermatol. 2004;43:362-5.
59. Ho SG, Yeung CK, Chan NP. A retrospective analysis of the management of acne post-inflammatory hyperpigmentation using topical treatment, laser treatment, or combination

topical and laser treatments in oriental patients. Lasers Surg Med. 2011;43:1-7.

60. Halder RM, Nootheti PK. Ethnic skin disorders overview. J Am Acad Dermatol. 2003;48:S143-8.
61. Taylor SC. Utilizing combination therapy for ethnic skin. Cutis. 2007;80:15-20.
62. Rossi AB, Leyden JJ, Pappert AS. A pilot methodology study for the photographic assessment of post-inflammatory hyperpigmentation in patients treated with tretinoin. J Eur Acad Dermatol Venereol. 2011;25:398-402.
63. Manuskiatti W, Triwongwaranat D, Varothai S. Efficacy and safety of a carbon-dioxide ablative fractional resurfacing device for treatment of atrophic acne scars in Asians. J Am Acad Dermatol. 2010;63:274-83.
64. Chapas AM, Brightman L, Sukal S. Successful treatment of acneiform scarring with CO_2 ablative fractional resurfacing. Lasers Surg Med. 2008;40:381-6.
65. Kaiser MR, Davis SC, Mertz BA. Effect of ultraviolet radiation-induced inflammation on epidermal wound healing. Wound Repair Regen. 1995;3:311-5.
66. Nordback I, Kulmala R, Jarvinen M. Effect of ultraviolet therapy on rat skin wound healing. J Surg Res. 1990;48:68-71.
67. Hasan AT, Eaglstein W, Pardo RJ. Solar-induced post-inflammatory hyperpigmentation after laser hair removal. Dermatol Surg. 1999;25:113-5.
68. West TB, Alster TS. Effect of pretreatment on the incidence of hyperpigmentation following cutaneous CO_2 laser resurfacing. Dermatol Surg. 1999;25:15-7.
69. Negishi K, Akita H, Tanaka S. Comparative study of treatment efficacy and the incidence of post-inflammatory hyperpigmentation with different degrees of irradiation using two different quality-switched lasers for removing solar lentigines on Asian skin. J Eur Acad Dermatol Venereol; 2011.
70. Maeda K, Naganuma M. Topical trans-4-aminomethyl cyclohexanecarboxylic acid prevents ultraviolet radiation-induced pigmentation. J Photochem Photobiol B. 1998;47:136-41.
71. Papa CM, Kligman AM. The behavior of melanocytes in inflammation. J Invest Dermatol. 1965;45:465-73.
72. Manuskiatti W, Eimpunth S, Wanitphakdeedecha R. Effect of cold air cooling on the incidence of postinflammatory hyperpigmentation after Q-switched Nd:YAG laser treatment of acquired bilateral nevus of Ota like macules. Arch Dermatol. 2007;143:1139-43.
73. Callender VD, Surin-Lord S, Davis EC, et al. Postinflammatory hyperpigmentation: etiologic and therapeutic considerations. Am J Clin Dermatol. 2011;12:87-99.
74. Chandra M, Levitt J, Pensabene CA. Hydroquinone therapy for post-inflammatory hyperpigmentation secondary to acne: not just prescribable by dermatologists. Acta Derm Venereol. 2012;92:232-5.
75. Bulengo-Ransby SM, Griffiths CE, Kimbrough-Green CK. Topical tretinoin (retinoic acid) therapy for hyperpigmented lesions caused by inflammation of the skin in black patients. N Engl J Med. 1993;328:1438-43.
76. Grimes P, Callender V. Tazarotene cream for postinflammatory hyperpigmentation and acne vulgaris in darker skin: a double-blind, randomized vehicle-controlled study. Cutis. 2006;77:45-50.
77. Katsambas AD. RALGA (Diacneal), a retinaldehyde and gly colic acid association and postinflammatory hyperpigmentation in acne—a review. Dermatology. 2005;210:S39-45.
78 Spann CT. Ten tips for treating acne vulgaris in Fitzpatrick skin types IV–VI. J Drugs Dermatol. 2011;10:654-7.
79. Grimes PE. The safety and efficacy of salicylic acid chemical peels in darker racial-ethnic groups. Dermatol Surg. 1999; 25:18-22.
80. Garg VK, Sinha S, Sarkar R. Glycolic acid peels versus salicylic-mandelic acid peels in active acne vulgaris and post-acne scarring and hyperpigmentation: a comparative study. Dermatol Surg. 2009;35:59-65.
81. Battle EF, Soden CE. The use of lasers in darker skin types. Semin Cutan Med Surg. 2009;28:130-40.
82. Kim S, Cho KH. Treatment of facial post-inflammatory hyperpigmentation with facial acne in Asian patients using a Q-switched neodymium-doped yttrium aluminum garnet laser. Dermatol Surg. 2010;36:1374-80.
83. Cho SB, Park SJ, Kim JS. Treatment of post-inflammatory hyperpigmentation using 1064-nm Q-switched Nd:YAG laser with low fluence-report of three cases. J Eur Acad Dermatol Venereol. 2009;23:1206-7.
84. Taylor CR, Anderson RR. Ineffective treatment of refractory melasma and post-inflammatory hyperpigmentation by Q-switched ruby laser. J Dermatol Surg Oncol. 1994;20:592-7.
85. Katz TM, Goldberg LH, Firoz BF. Fractional photothermolysis for the treatment of post-inflammatory hyperpigmentation. Dermatol Surg. 2009;35:1844-8.
86. Kroon MW, Wind BS, Meesters AA, et al. Nonablative 1550 nm fractional laser therapy not effective for erythema dyschromicum perstans and post-inflammatory hyperpigmentation: a pilot study. J Dermatolog Treat. 2012; 23: 339-44.
87. Rokhsar H, Ciocon DH. Fractional photothermolysis for the treatment of post-inflammatory hyperpigmentation after carbon dioxide laser resurfacing. Dermatol Surg. 2009; 35:535-7.
88. Park JM, Tsao H, Tsao S. Combined use of intense pulsed light and Q-switched ruby laser for complex dyspigmentation among Asian patients. Lasers Surg Med. 2008; 40:128-33.
89. Kono T, Chan HH, Groff WF. Prospective direct comparison study of fractional resurfacing using different fluences and densities for skin rejuvenation in Asians. Lasers Surg Med. 2007;39:311-4.
90. Hantash BM, Bedi VP, Sudireddy V. Laser-induced transepidermal elimination of dermal content by fractional photothermolysis. J Biomed Opt. 2006;11:041115.

10

Neoplasms with Pigmentary Changes or Discoloration

Prasad Kumarasinghe, Daniel Hewitt

Key Features

- Many neoplasms of skin show changes in level of pigmentation, many are hyperchromic, a smaller number are hypochromic.
- Change of color of the lesions may be due to melanin or other pigment.
- Malignant melanoma is the most dreaded pigmented skin tumor.
- Among fair skinned Caucasians most melanomas occur on the trunk, head and neck or proximal limbs, whereas the most common melanoma in dark skinned races is acral lentiginous melanoma on soles or the palms.
- The main goals in management of melanoma are prevention, early detection, optimal initial surgical treatment and subsequent adjuvant treatment.
- Hypopigmented mycosis fungoides is more common among dark skinned races.

INTRODUCTION

Many dermatological conditions, including neoplasias have pigmentary changes. Some cutaneous neoplasms are hyperchromic (increased pigmentation), some are hypochromic (decreased color) and the others have no increase or decrease in color.

Dyspigmentation is more pronounced in pigmented races (skin of color). Melanoma is the most significant neoplastic condition with pigmentary changes. Advanced melanoma carries a poor prognosis. Some pigmentary changes are not characteristic but are significant associated features, e.g. leukoderma associated with malignant melanoma. Many color changes in neoplasms are due to an increase or a decrease of melanin pigment, but some others are due to other reasons, e.g. xanthomas having a yellowish color due to fatty material in the cells, subcutaneous vascular tumors giving a bluish gray appearance and superficial vascular tumors giving a reddish discoloration due to hemoglobin.

Some pigmentary neoplastic conditions are more common among dark skinned races, e.g. hypopigmented mycosis fungoides. Some conditions are more commonly seen in dark skinned races but do occur in all races in the same frequency, e.g. acral lentiginous melanoma. Acral lentiginous melanoma is the most common type of melanoma in dark skinned races.

Where there are changes of hypopigmentation or lightening of skin due to lesions, they become more obvious in dark skinned races. Likewise darkly pigmented lesions are more visible in light skinned individuals, e.g. malignant melanoma.

Some neoplastic conditions can have both hypopigmented/depigmented areas as well as hyperpigmented areas, e.g. malignant melanoma, pigmented squamous cell carcinoma, mammary and extramammary Paget's disease.

In this chapter more emphasis will be given to malignant melanoma as it is the most dangerous skin malignancy.

HYPERCHROMIC NEOPLASTIC CONDITIONS

Many hyperchromic conditions are due to increased melanin, but some are due to hemoglobin or hemosiderin. Some lesions give a pigmented appearance due to an optical illusion, e.g. subcutaneous cysts. The following is a list of hyperchromic neoplastic lesions (in alphabetical order):

- Angiokeratomas
- Basal cell carcinoma-pigmented
- Bowenoid papulosis
- Chloroma/cutaneous myeloid sarcoma

- Dermatofibromas
- Glomus tumor
- Hemangiomas, subcutaneous
- Kaposi's sarcoma
- Lymphomatoid papulosis
- Malignant melanoma, lentigo maligna, melanosis secondary to advanced melanoma
- Mastocytomas
- Melanoacanthoma
- Melanocytic nevi
- Merkel cell carcinoma, although not a true melanocytic tumor it can appear purplish or reddish in color
- Mycosis fungoides; hyperpigmented
- Neurofibromas
- Paget's disease with hyperpigmentation
- Pilomatricomas
- Squamous cell carcinoma *in situ*, pigmented
- Seborrheic keratoses and its variant dermatosis papulosis nigra
- Skin tags (acrochordons)
- Syringomas, in dark skinned persons
- Tumors with rapid growth with hemorrhage inside.

HYPOCHROMIC NEOPLASTIC CONDITIONS

Some hypochromic conditions are due to reduced melanin, whereas some are due to other material (e.g. xanthoma). The following is a list of hypochromatic lesions:

- Arsenical keratoses and associated neoplasms with rain drop depigmentation
- Halo nevi
- Lymphangioma circumscriptum
- Melanoma with regression and associated leukoderma
- Mycosis fungoides; hypopigmented
- Porokeratosis
- Stucco keratosis
- White fibrous papulosis
- White sponge nevus of oral mucosa
- Sebaceoma
- Xanthomas.

MIMICS OF NEOPLASTIC DYSCHROMIC LESIONS

- Epidermoid cysts; optical illusion giving a blue-black color, or an open punctum showing oxidized blackish sebaceous material
- Fibromatosis including knuckle pads
- Lichen planus, hypertrophic, pigmented
- Keloids-pigmented, minocycline induced pigmentation of keloids
- Longitudinal melanonychia
- Porokeratoses
- Prurigo nodularis
- Solar lentigo
- Subungual hematoma
- Viral warts-pigmented
- Xanthogranuloma.

DIAGNOSIS AND MANAGEMENT

Management of each condition depends on correct diagnosis. Most of the conditions are fairly straightforward at clinical examination for an astute clinician, e.g. seborrheic keratoses, pigmented basal cell carcinoma. Some conditions require urgent action such as excision of the tumor as in the case of a malignant melanoma. Some conditions need biopsy for a definitive diagnosis. Dermoscopy is helpful in some other conditions (e.g. malignant melanoma). Minimally pigmented melanomas and lentigo maligna melanoma lesions can be diagnosed more easily with confocal microscopy, although the equipment is rather expensive for routine use.

Management of all the different conditions is not dealt here in detail. However, management of malignant melanoma is discussed as it is the most significant tumor of the melanocyte. It is well known that advanced melanoma has a very poor prognosis. Melanoma incidence has been increasing in the Western Countries in the last few decades. Acral lentiginous melanoma is the type that occurs most commonly in the pigmented races. As the awareness of this is inadequate, late presentation of ALM is not uncommon in countries with predominantly dark skinned people.

The following segment of the chapter will discuss some potentially fatal neoplastic conditions and some common conditions with pigmentary changes.

MALIGNANT MELANOMA[1-37]

Malignant melanoma is the most dangerous of the common skin malignancies.[1-7] It is most common in Caucasian populations. Australia has the world's highest incidence, although the incidence has been steady in high incidence countries for the last decade.[7]

In Western countries, earlier detection has led to an improvement in survival but prevention and early diagnosis remain a challenge.

Mortality is related to metastatic spread, which can occur at a variable time from onset of initial disease. Ideally this is prevented, but treatments for metastatic disease are improving. The goals in management of melanoma are prevention, early detection, optimal initial surgical treatment and subsequent adjuvant treatment.

Melanomas are divided into four main and several less common clinical and histological subtypes. The individual subtype is not independently related to prognosis, but these subtypes show the various presentations of malignant melanoma.

Melanoma Subtypes[1,7]

Major Subtypes (Figs 1 to 5)

- Lentigo maligna melanoma
- Superficial spreading melanoma
- Nodular melanoma
- Acral lentiginous melanoma

Other Subtypes

- Amelanotic melanoma
- Mucosal melanoma
- Subungual melanoma
- Desmoplastic melanoma
- Melanoma arising from blue nevi
- Melanoma arising from congenital melanocytic nevi
- Nevoid melanoma
- Metastatic melanoma of unknown primary
- Melanoma of other sites (e.g. eyes, gastrointestinal tract, genitourinary tract, leptomeninges)

Prevention

A key to prevention is to understand risk factors. Behavioral risk factors are amenable to modification by public awareness campaigns. The most important behavioral risk factor in the fair skinned persons is the number of blistering sunburns that have occurred. Recently, regular sunscreen use has been related to a decreased incidence of melanoma compared to discretionary use.[2] Intermittent sun exposure, high total cumulative exposure, childhood ambient ultraviolet exposure and use of tanning booths also confer an increased risk, although individually these seem to confer a lower relative risk than the factors above.

Melanoma Risk Factors

Melanoma Constitutional Risk Factors

- Personal history of melanoma
- Personal history of solar keratosis or nonmelanoma skin cancer
- Immunosuppression (especially transplant patients)
- Inherited gene mutations (CDKN2A, p16INK4A, p14ARF, MC1R, BRAF, MITF, BRCA2)
- Atypical nevus syndrome (>5 atypical nevi)
- Numerous nevi
- Family history of melanoma (first degree relative)
- Light skin color (Fitzpatrick Type I)
- Red or blonde hair compared to brown or black hair
- Blue or green eyes compared to brown eyes
- Numerous freckles
- Male sex
- Age over 50.

Melanoma Behavioral Risk Factors; in Lighter Skinned Persons

- Number of blistering sunburns
- Intermittent sun exposure
- Total cumulative sun exposure
- Tanning bed use
- Lack of regular sunscreen use.

Screening

Education of primary care physicians and of members of the public is likely to improve mortality. Most melanomas, when diagnosed early, are curable. It is sensible to be more vigilant

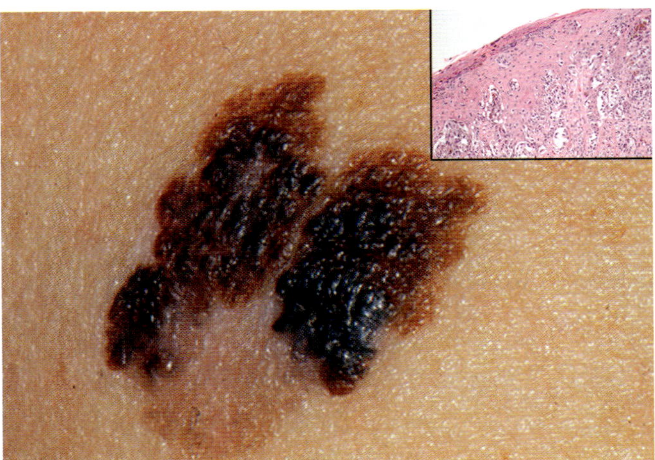

Fig. 1: Superficial spreading malignant melanoma. (*Photomicrograph Source:* Dr Minh Lam, Dermatopathologist, Perth, Australia)

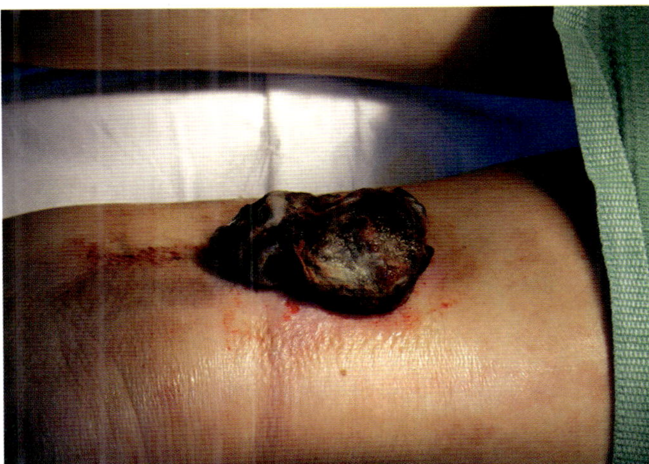

Fig. 2: Nodular malignant melanoma

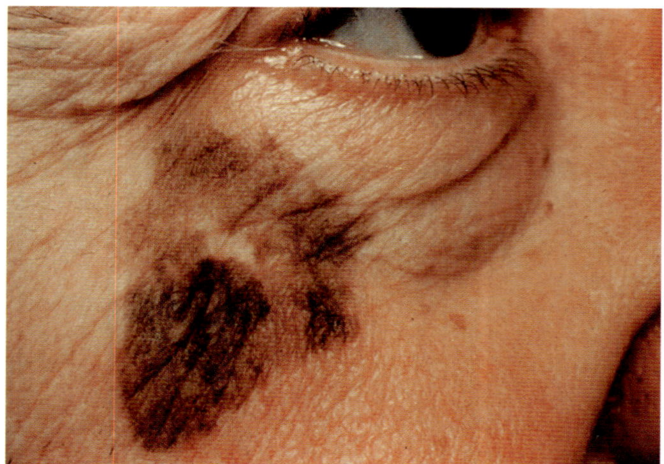

Fig. 3: Lentigo maligna

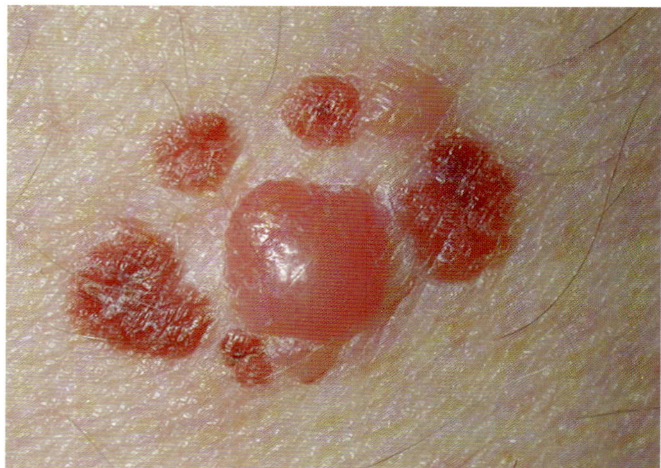

Fig. 4: Cutaneous secondary deposits from a melanoma. Note that some secondaries appear non-pigmented

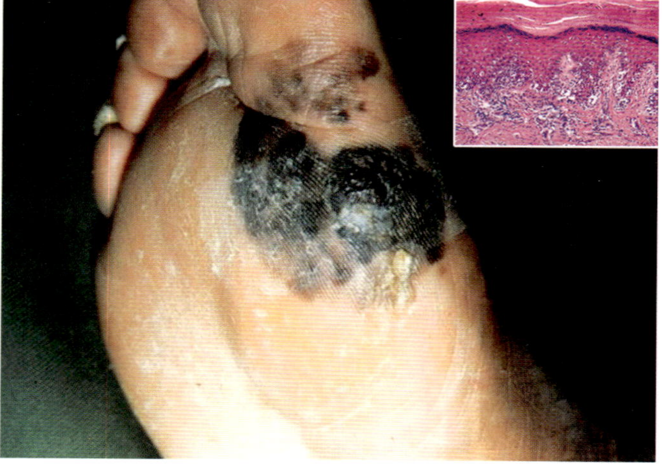

Fig. 5: Acral lentiginous melanoma. (*Histopathology photomicrograph Source:* Dr Joyce Lee, National Skin Centre, Singapore)

in those who have known risk factors. Melanomas detected on screening examinations by physicians are generally thinner than those detected in other ways. Therefore, encouragement to have regular professional skin examinations is important particularly in Fitzpatrick Type I and Type II skin.

Diagnosis

Early clinical diagnosis relies on clinical acumen. Formal diagnosis relies on histological examination. A routine skin examination involves examination of the entire skin surface. Bright natural light or white light is essential. Magnification and dermoscopy increase diagnostic accuracy in experienced hands.

Table 1: Melanoma diagnosis: The ABCD criteria

A - Asymmetry	One-half unlike the other half
B - Border	Irregular, scalloped or poorly defined border
C - Color	Varied from one area to another; shades of tan, brown, and black; sometimes white, red, or blue
D - Diameter	Melanomas are usually greater than 6 mm when diagnosed

Most melanomas present with an early macular phase. Their features have been summarized with the ABCD rule **(Table 1)**.

Approximately half of all melanomas are first noticed by the patient.[4] The presenting history in these cases is almost always of a changing lesion.

Approximately 15% of melanomas present as an enlarging lesion that does not display any of the 'ABCD' criteria. These melanomas contribute disproportionately to melanoma mortality[5] due to their rapid progression in a vertical growth phase and higher potential for metastasis. It is very important to recognize them. Their features elevated, firm and growing (EFG) are summarized with the acronym EFG.[6]

Initial Treatment

Local surgical clearance is the most important first step in treatment.[7] Once a lesion has been identified as suspicious for melanoma, the first imperative is to excise it. Most guidelines recommend this be done with a two millimeter clinical margin. The entire lesion should be excised if at all possible to minimize any possible sampling error. Punch biopsies are

Table 2: Recommended melanoma clinical excision margins based on Breslow thickness

Melanoma *in situ*	0.5 cm
Melanoma <1.0 mm	1.0 cm
Melanoma 1.0–4.0 mm	1.0–2.0 cm
Melanoma >4.0 mm	2.0 cm

Table 3: Melanoma staging and prognosis[7,8]

Stage	
0 or Melanoma *in situ*	Melanoma confined to the epidermis
I	Melanoma confined to the skin up to 1.0 mm in Breslow thickness
II	Melanoma confined to the skin greater than 1.0 mm in Breslow thickness
III	Regional disease, melanoma has spread to local lymph nodes
IV	Distant disease, melanoma has spread beyond local lymph nodes, to internal organs or to skin far from the original tumor

generally inappropriate. If complete excision is not feasible, generous incisional biopsy must include the most atypical part of the lesion and as much of the lesion as possible.

For large macular lesions, such as lentigo maligna melanoma, complete excision may be difficult. A large shave biopsy may be preferable as it enables a much larger sample to be obtained than an incisional biopsy. It is essential that a large sample of the dermoepidermal junction is taken. The wound generally heals well given there is still dermis at its base. Generally, if a melanocytic proliferation is seen histologically, formal excision of the entire lesion should be undertaken. If there happens to be dermal involvement, a shave biopsy will possibly not give an accurate reading of the Breslow thickness, but invasion to mid or deep dermis is uncommon with lentigo maligna melanoma

A full histopathological report with synoptic summary should be produced. The most important aspect of this is the Breslow thickness, the measurement in millimeters from the granular layer of the epidermis to the lowest apparent melanoma cell. The remaining lesion or scar is then re-excised with margins determined by the Breslow thickness **(Table 2)**. These margins are measured clinically. Histologically, margins often measure approximately 30% smaller.

Prognosis can be determined based on the stage of melanoma. For level I melanomas, the Breslow thickness is the most important prognostic indicator **(Table 3)**. Tumor, lymph nodes and metastases (TNM) classification is used for staging melanoma as well.[7,9] For example, T1a N0 M0 is a melanoma without superficial ulceration or mitoses which is less than 1 mm in thickness, without any palpable lymph nodes or metastases, T4b, N 2b M 1c is a melanoma greater than 4 mm thick, with ulceration, 2–3 palpable lymph nodes, with metastases in other visceral sites or distant metastases to any site combined with an elevated serum lactate dehydrogenase (LDH) level.

Investigations

After a diagnosis of primary cutaneous melanoma there is no evidence to support the use of any particular investigation routinely. The whole skin must be thoroughly examined and all major lymph node beds and the liver and spleen should be palpated.

Ultrasound is more accurate than palpation for detecting lymph node metastases greater than 4.5 mm in diameter but its low yield does not justify its cost. Blood tests, such as lactate dehydrogenase, full blood count, serum electrolytes and liver function tests are not helpful. Chest X-ray, CT scanning and positron emission tomography (PET) scanning only rarely identify occult stage IV disease. All of these investigations can often give equivocal or false positive results and are therefore not routinely recommended.

Sentinel lymph node biopsy is the most accurate method to identify occult regional lymph node metastasis. Some authors now recommend it in patients with melanomas greater than 1.0 mm in Breslow thickness.[10] Routine use of sentinel lymph node biopsy cannot be justified with our current evidence and understanding. At present, no survival benefit has been shown with this procedure, although it does provide prognostic information. Generally, it has been recommended that those with positive sentinel lymph node biopsy go on to have complete lymph node dissection. This does have associated morbidity, depending on the site, and there is no proven survival benefit in this group compared to those that did not have sentinel lymph node biopsy.

The benefit of sentinel lymph node biopsy depends on a melanoma metastasizing via a sentinel node, or the first node of lymphatic drainage from the primary melanoma. The proportion of melanomas that actually do this is not precisely known, but it may be only 50%. It is known that some melanomas metastasize hematogenously and contiguously. Circulating tumor cells have been detected in melanoma patients even after removal of the primary melanoma. Panels of melanoma cellular markers are being evaluated, e.g. MLANA, ABCB 5 correlate with disease recurrence and progression.[11]

Metastatic melanoma does occur in the brain, an organ without lymphatics. Furthermore, lymphatic drainage from some locations, such as the head and neck, can be very variable over time. In this sense, a negative sentinel lymph node biopsy should not provide absolute reassurance of excluding metastatic disease.

Lymph nodes are a natural focus of immunity. It is possible for melanoma cells to be detected here and prevented from further metastasis. Conversely, nevus cells have been identified in lymph nodes. In this sense sentinel lymph node status is not as important a prognostic indicator as distant metastatic disease.

Clinically or ultrasonographically suspected lymph node metastasis needs fine needle aspiration biopsy to accurately stage the patient. If locoregional disease is identified, a detailed history and examination are required as imaging investigations are indicated for any symptoms that may suggest metastatic disease.

Positron emission tomography scanning is generally superior to CT scanning in the detection of metastatic disease, although there is a false positive rate of approximately 10%. CT scanning does seem superior in the detection of small lung metastases and provides more accurate anatomical information. MRI scanning provides more accurate imaging of metastases in the brain than CT scanning. Combining CT and PET scanning may offer the best imaging technique, when both are available.

In stage IV disease imaging and other investigations need to be individualized. Generally they should be seen as a tool to help determine changes in management.

Adjuvant Therapy

Patients with stage IIB, IIC, and IIIC should be considered for adjuvant therapy due to their high risk of recurrence and mortality. Adjuvant interferon-alpha therapy has known activity in the systemic treatment of melanoma. It improves relapse free survival by 10% at 5 years but does have considerable toxicity. This toxicity, although reversible, needs to be weighed against the modest benefits of therapy.

Treatment for Stage III Disease

For lymph node disease, complete lymph node dissection is recommended. Locoregional disease (between the primary site and the lymph node basin) should also be surgically cleared when possible. For the cleared lymph node basin, postoperative adjuvant radiotherapy may confer additional benefit when more than three lymph nodes are involved or there are other adverse pathological findings.

Locoregionally recurrent melanoma that is melanoma occurring again at the excision site, between the excision site and a regional lymph node site or at the lymph node site should be surgically excised whenever possible. For involved limbs where regional control is not possible, isolated limb perfusion using melphalan under hyperthermic conditions has produced response rates of almost 90%.

Treatment for Stage IV Disease[14-18]

The median survival of stage IV melanoma is 6–9 months. Dacarbazine has been the standard chemotherapy until the last few years. Response rates were reported up to 20%, but only 5% showed complete response and it was of short duration. Interferon-alpha, interleukin-2, fotemustine and temozoloamide have also been used, alone and in combination but have been generally disappointing.[7]

Radiotherapy can be useful in palliation of metastases of bone, brain, skin, lymph nodes, liver and the adrenal gland. This may be indicated where there are localized symptoms from these metastases.

Vemurafenib works via the *BRAF* pathway and decreases production of a protein in this pathway responsible for melanoma growth. BRAF mutations present in up to half of melanoma patients. So far it shows a 63% improvement in mortality at three months compared to chemotherapy. Significant side effects, such as skin irritation and joint pain, occur in less than 10%.

Ipilimumab is a monoclonal human antibody. It inhibits cytotoxic T-lymphocyte associated antigen and thereby it increases T-cell activation and interleukin-2 secretion; thus stimulating the body's immune response to melanoma. Early studies show an average four months improvement in survival.

Follow-up

It is important to follow-up all melanoma patients. They are at risk of recurrence, secondary spread and further primary melanoma. A new primary occurs in 2–8% of those with previous melanoma. 80% of recurrences of melanoma occur in the first three years. Patients with stage I disease should be followed up 6 monthly for 5 years and yearly thereafter. For higher stages, they should be followed up 4 monthly for 5 years and yearly thereafter.

Melanoma in Skin of Color[19-37]

Acral lentiginous melanoma (ALM) is the most common type of malignant melanoma in dark skinned races. Etiologically it has no relationship with sun exposure. It occurs in equal proportions in all races, but other types of melanomas are uncommon in dark skinned races. These have a characteristic appearance histologically. In the radial growth phase, lesions are characterized by acanthosis, expanded stratum corneum, elongation of rete ridges and lentiginous proliferation of atypical melanocytes along basal layer of epidermis at the borders of the tumor. Intraepidermally large atypical melanocytes with large nuclei and nucleoli and cytoplasm filled with melanin granules can be seen.[1]

Clinically, ALM occurs on the palms of hands, soles of the feet or subungually. As the awareness of malignant melanoma is relatively lacking among the countries with dark skinned people, often these patients present late in the course of disease leading to a poorer prognosis.[20] In contrast, in fair skinned communities as the melanoma awareness is much better, melanomas are diagnosed and treated early, leading to a better prognosis.

Management of ALM is similar to management of other types of melanoma. However, when a finger or a toe is involved, to achieve safe excision margins amputation of a part of a digit may be required. More conservative surgery, avoiding digital amputation is also advocated by some. Margins of ALM on palms and soles can be rather indistinct, similar to Hutchinson's melanocytic freckles (lentigo maligna melanoma). Confocal laser microscopy may be useful in ascertaining the borders in such cases. Multiple mapping biopsies may be required in large lesions of ALM, before deciding on the margins of excision.

In certain genetically determined skin diseases, such as xeroderma pigmentosum, the incidence of melanoma is very high even in dark skinned patients.

It is an exciting time of melanoma research. After decades of efforts with vaccines, chemotherapeutics and biologic agents that showed little or no survival benefit, we are now entering an era where newer agents are showing clear survival benefit. Precise selection of patients and further understanding of the specific treatment or combination of treatments likely to help them will further improve mortality and quality of life of patients with metastatic melanoma. More awareness will hopefully lead to early detection and appropriate treatment of melanoma in light skinned individuals as well as dark skinned individuals.

PIGMENTED BASAL CELL CARCINOMA[38-44]

Pigmented basal cell carcinoma (PBCC) is the most common type of BCC found among the dark skinned races.[38,39] They can occur in sun exposed areas as well as sun protected areas **(Fig. 6)**. The pigmentation is not due to any excess of melanocytes but is due to increased melanin production by the melanocytes and dispersion of this melanin in the epidermal keratinocytes, melanophages and interstitium. It is not clear how the melanization is upregulated in pigmented BCC. These BCC can become ulcerated and nodular as they advance over months or years. Generally these BCC are not deeply infiltrative. Pigmented BCC may be mistaken as pigmented seborrheic keratosis particularly in the head and neck region. Distant metastases have not been reported in PBCC, but extremely rarely other types of BCC metastasise. Treatment of PBCC is just like for any other type of BCC. Surgical excision is the first line of treatment. Radiotherapy, serial curettage and cautery, cryotherapy, and imiquimod are other options of treatment.

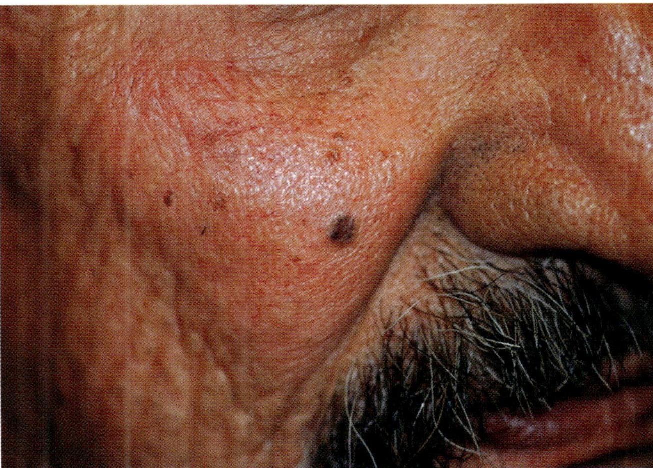

Fig. 6: Pigmented basal cell carcinoma

MYCOSIS FUNGOIDES[45-68]

Mycosis fungoides (MF) is the most common primary cutaneous T-cell lymphoma. Generally it has an indolent clinical course. Most cases occur in adults; however it can occur in children as well. In dark skinned races MF lesions are often hypopigmented. Many reports from Asian countries indicate that hypopigmented MF is the most common presentation in these countries.[45-55] It can mimic other hypopigmented skin conditions such as progressive macular hypomelanosis, post-inflammatory hypopigmentation and leprosy. Mycosis fungoides usually presents as ill defined erythematous, hypopigmented or even hyperpigmented ill defined patches or plaques **(Fig. 7)**. As the disease progresses some patients develop nodular lesions. Some patients progress to have systemic involvement which may lead to a fatal outcome. Multiple skin biopsies are often required for accurate diagnosis. On many occasions initial biopsies (early disease) may not be conclusive of MF histopathologically, but months or years later as the disease evolves repeat biopsy histopathology may show sufficient features to diagnose mycosis fungoides. T-cell gene rearrangement studies are also useful, if facilities are available.

A small proportion of cases of lymphomatoid papulosis may progress into mycosis fungoides or Sezary syndrome. The lymphomatoid papulosis lesions may initially heal (wax and wane) with hyperpigmented or hypopigmented scars over many years before some of them evolving into T-cell lymphomas.

The first line of treatment after diagnosis is topical steroids and ultraviolet light therapy. Most centers administer narrowband ultraviolet (UV) treatment rather than UVA. Although this controls the lesions from visual point of view, the natural history of disease progression is not altered by topical steroids or UV treatment. For advanced disease chemotherapy with newer agents have been attempted with variable success, e.g. vorinostat, a histone deacetylase inhibitor has shown some promising results.[68] Electron beam

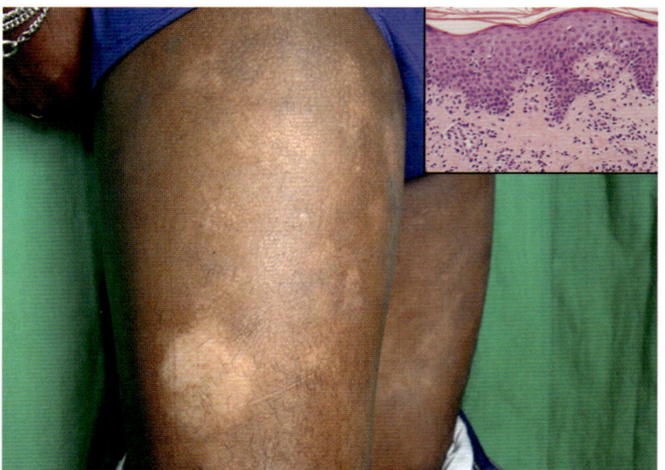

Fig. 7: Hypopigmented mycosis fungoides. (*Clinical photograph Source:* Dr Ranthilaka Ranawaka, Sri Lanka *Histopathology photomicrograph Source*: Dr Joyce Lee, National Skin Centre, Singapore)

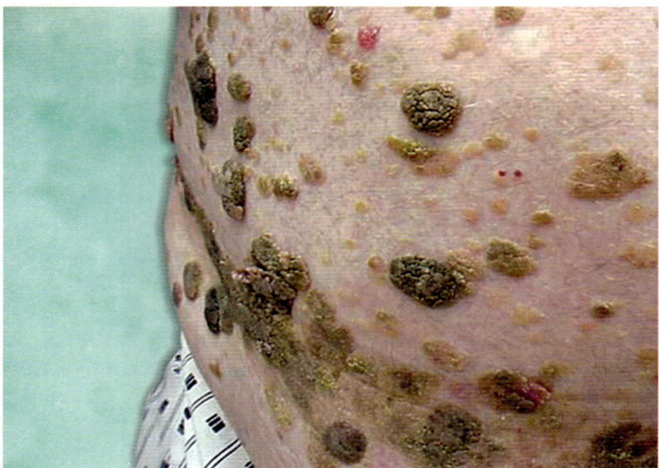

Fig. 8: Pigmented seborrheic keratoses

therapy is also useful to contain disease if the cutaneous lesions are extensive.

SOME COMMON BENIGN NEOPLASTIC CONDITIONS WITH PIGMENTARY CHANGES[69-78]

- Seborrheic keratosis and variants including dermatosis papulosis nigra (DPN)
- Skin tags
- Dermatofibromas.

Seborrheic Keratoses[69-78]

These are common benign tumors. They are very common in the elderly. In the pigmented races the pigmentation can be intense, mimicking a primary melanocytic tumor. Histopathologically several types are recognized; acanthotic, hyperkeratotic, reticulated, clonal, irritated and melanoacanthoma. Hyperkeratosis, acanthosis and papillomatosis are common features. There can be an eruption of seborrheic keratoses as a non-metastatic manifestation of internal malignancies. This is termed Leser Trélat sign. However, some authors believe that this association may be due to chance occurrence in the elderly.

Most commonly seborrheic keratoses occur on the head and neck region and upper trunk. However they can occur practically anywhere on the body except on the palms and the soles **(Fig. 8)**.

Seborrheic keratoses do not need to be treated, other than for cosmetic reasons. However, some may become inflamed due to friction with clothing, scratching, etc. If treatment is required cryotherapy, electrocautery under topical anesthesia (if very superficial) or local anesthesia, laser treatment, or shave excision under local anesthesia may be done according to the situation.

Occasionally, there can be collision tumors such as basal cell carcinoma or squamous cell carcinoma in the same site.[76-78] Therefore, careful examination is warranted, particularly if there is a history of bleeding, pain, itching or asymmetric enlargement. Dermatoscopy can be useful in ruling out other associated malignancies. If in doubt a deep shave biopsy or a punch biopsy is indicated to confirm the diagnosis.

Stucco keratoses are a variant of seborrheic keratoses more commonly seen on the lower extremities. Sometimes they are seen on the upper limbs as well. They appear as firm keratinous flat ashy or brownish multiple lesions. They are more resistant to destructive methods of treatment such as cryotherapy. It is best to explain the condition to the patient and leave them alone, as more destructive methods are likely to cause more unsightly scars and dyspigmentation.

Dermatosis papulosis nigra is another clinical variant of seborrheic keratosis. They are more commonly seen in dark skinned races. DPN is characterized by numerous small 0.5–3 mm small papules in the head and neck region and upper chest **(Fig. 9)**. They are most common on the face and neck of Negroid races. However, they do occur in Indian, oriental and fair skinned people as well, in descending order. They can be electrocauterized under EMLA topical anesthesia. Larger lesions can also be treated with cryotherapy. However one has to be careful about cryotherapy in dark skinned patients as it can lead to depigmentation or hypopigmentation. Strong trichloroacetic acid (e.g 80% TCA) can also be used, (using fine end of tooth picks) to treat small DPN lesions, however the operator has to be careful not to allow the acid to spread to the normal skin.

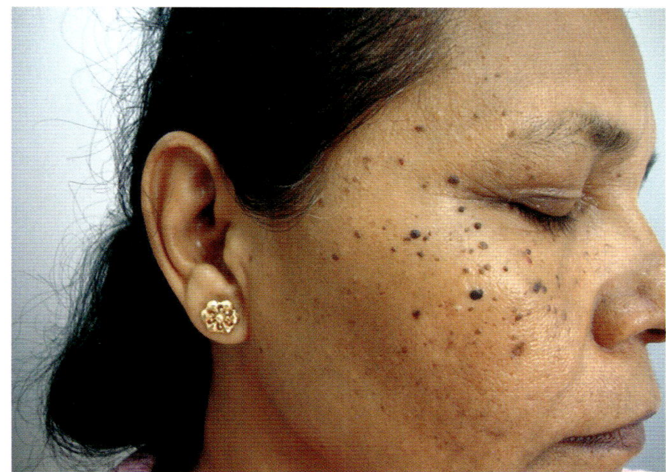

Fig. 9: Dermatosis papulosis nigra
(*Source:* Dr Ranthilaka Ranawaka, Sri Lanka)

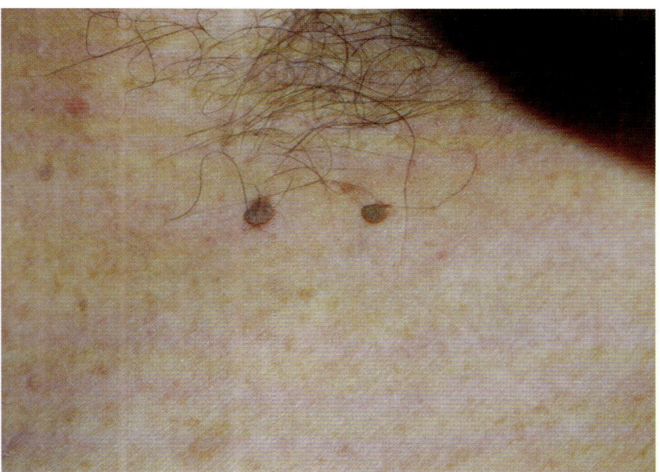

Fig. 10: Acrochordons (skin tags)

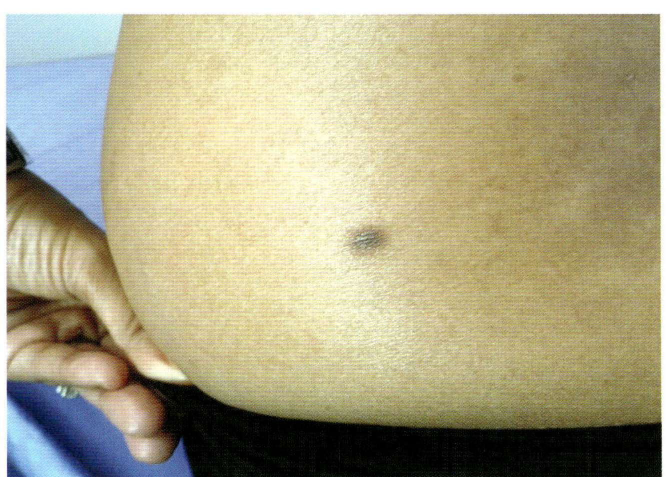

Fig. 11: Dermatofibroma with hyperpigmentation

Skin Tags (Acrochordons)

These benign, pedunculated or stalked "outpouchings" of the skin are common in all races.[79-83] Histopathologically, the epidermis shows papillomatosis and acanthosis. Larger lesions may show dermal fat in the deeper layers. Multiple lesions are often associated with obesity and insulin resistance. In pigmented races they can appear hyperpigmented. Most commonly skin tags occur on the neck, axillae and submammary regions **(Fig. 10)**. However, they can occur almost anywhere on the body. They may be removed for cosmetic reasons. Otherwise they can be left alone as they are benign. Simple snip excision under local anesthesia and electrocautery of the base is probably the best way to treat them. If they are small, electrocautery under EMLA topical anesthesia or cryotherapy may also be used. In pigmented skin, excessive deep cryotherapy can leave depigmented scars.

Dermatofibromas[84-86]

These are firm skin colored or hyperpigmented benign papules or nodules that occur commonly on the limbs **(Fig. 11)**. They can occur on the trunk as well. These lesions can be extremely pruritic in some cases. Typically when the adjacent skin on the two opposing sides of the lesion is gently pushed towards the lesion dermatofibromas dimple or pucker. In dark skinned patients dermatofibromas can appear deeply pigmented, mimicking a melanocytic tumor. Dermatoscopy is useful to differentiate in difficult cases. Sometimes a desmoplastic malignant melanoma can mimic a dermatofibroma.

Histopathologically, epidermis is usually acanthotic and the dermis may show a fibrous infiltrate, a cellular infiltrate, or a vascular pattern. These lesions are best left alone as scars from excisions are often more unsightly. However, if a patient is keen to get a lesion removed, a simple excision may be performed. A rapidly growing ill defined larger lesion should raise the possibility of a dermatofibrosarcoma protuberans (DFSP) which is a highly malignant tumor. If this is suspected the lesion should be excised and the specimen sent for histopathological examination. If confirmed as a DFSP wider excision would be required.

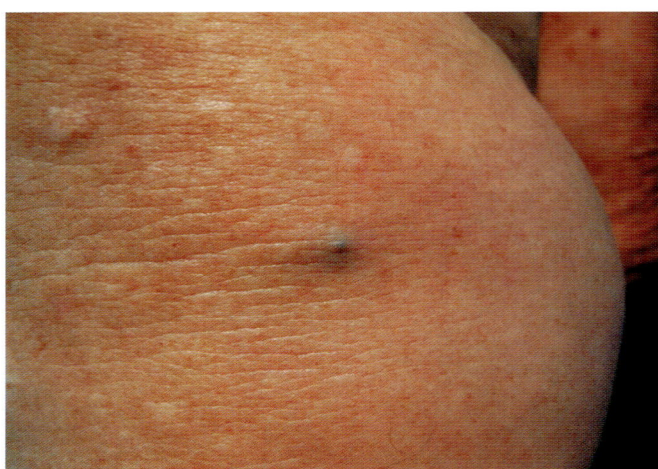

Fig. 12: An epidermoid cyst mimicking the appearance of a pigmented lesion

Some non-neoplastic lesions such as cysts can also mimic pigmented tumor **(Fig. 12)**.

CONCLUSION

Many neoplastic conditions have increased localized pigmentation. Some have associated hypopigmentation. Clinically melanoma is the most important malignant tumor arising in the skin. It can have a fatal outcome if not diagnosed and treated early. Prevention of melanoma is very important in fair skinned persons as it may account for about 75% of skin cancer deaths among the fair skinned persons. Early detection and appropriate treatment of melanoma are important in all cases of melanoma in all skin types. Of the hypopigmented skin malignancies, hypopigmented mycosis fungoides is the most important condition clinically. A good knowledge of the conditions that cause secondary pigmentary change is also very important for accurate diagnosis and to avoid unnecessary surgery.

REFERENCES

1. Le Boit PE, Burg G, Weedon D, et al. WHO Classification of Tumours: Pathology and Genetics Skin Tumours. Lyon: IARC Press; 2006. pp. 73-5.
2. Green AC, Williams GM, Logan V, et al. Journal reduced melanoma after regular sunscreen use: randomized trial follow-up. J Clin Oncol. 2011;29(3):257-63.
3. Friedman RJ, Rigel DS, Kopf AW. Early detection of malignant melanoma: the role of physician examination and self-examination of the skin. CA Cancer J Clin. 1985;35(3):130-51.
4. McPherson M, Elwood M, English DR, et al. Presentation and detection of invasive melanoma in a high-risk population. J Am Acad Dermatol. 2006;54(5):783-92.
5. Chamberlain AJ, Fritchi L Giles GG, et al. Nodular type and older age as the most significant associations of thick melanoma in Victoria, Australia. Arch Dermatol. 2002;138(5):609-14.
6. Kelly JW, Chamberlain AJ, Staples MP, et al. Nodular melanoma. No longer as simple as ABC. Aust Fam Physician. 2003;32(9):706-9.
7. Australian Cancer Network Melanoma Guidelines Revision Working Party. Clinical Practice Guidelines for the Management of Melanoma in Australia and New Zealand. Cancer Council Australia and Australian Cancer Network, Sydney and New Zealand Guidelines Group, Wellington (2008).
8. Lens MB, Dawes M, Newton-Bidhop JA, et al. Tumour thickness is a predictor of occult lymph node metastases in patients with stage I and II melanoma undergoing sentinel lymph node biopsy. Br J Surg. 2002;89(10):1223-7.
9. AJCC. American Joint Committee Cancer Staging Manual, 6th edn. New York: Springer-Verlag; 2002.
10. Morton DL. Overview and update of the phase III Multicenter Selective Lymphadenectomy Trials (MSLT-I and MSLT-II) in melanoma. Clin Exp Metastasis. 2012;29(7): 699-706.
11. Reid AL, Millward M, Pearce R, et al. Markers of circulating tumour cells in the peripheral blood of patients with melanoma. BJD. 2013;168:85-92.
12. Cornett WR, McCall LM, Petersen RP, et al. Randomized multicentre trial of hyperthermic isolated limb perfusion with melphalan alone compared with melphalan plus tumor necrosis factor: American College of Surgeons Oncology Group Trial Z00200. J Clin Oncol. 2006;24(25):4196-201.
13. Balch CM, Soong SJ, Gershenwald JE, et al. Prognostic factors analysis of 17,600 melanoma patients: validation of the American Joint Committee on Cancer melanoma staging system. J Clin Oncol. 2001;19(16):3622-34.
14. Chapman PB, Hauschild A, Robert C, et al. Improved survival with vemurafenib in melanoma with BRAF V600E mutation. N Eng J Med. 2011;364(26):2507-16
15. Robert C, Thomas L, Bondarenko I, et al. Ipilimumab plus dacarbazine for previously untreated metastatic melanoma. N Eng J Med. 2011;364(26):2517-26.
16. Francken AB, Bastiaannet E, Hoekstra HJ. Follow-up in patients with localised primary cutaneous melanoma. Lancet Oncol. 2005;6(8):608-21.
17. Ferrone CR, Ben Porat L, Panageas KS, et al. Clinicopathological features of and risk factors for multiple primary melanomas. JAMA. 2005;294(13):1647-54.
18. Puzanov I, Flaherty KT. Targeted molecular therapy in melanoma. Semin Cutan Med Surg. 2010;29(3):196-201.
19. Soon SL, Washington CV. Melanoma of skin of color. In: Kelly AP, Taylor SC (Eds). Dermatology for skin of color. New York: McGraw-Hill; 2009. pp. 283-90.
20. Wu XC, Eide MJ, King J, et al. Racial and ethnic variations in incidence and survival of cutaneous melanoma in the United states 1999-2006. J Am Acad Dermatol. 2011; 65: S26-37.

21. Lee HY, Chay WY, Tang MB, et al. Melanoma: differences between Asian and Caucasian patients. Ann Acad Med Singapore. 2012;41(1):17-20.
22. Pailoor J, Mun KS, Leow M. Cutaneous malignant melanoma: clinical and histopathological review of cases in a Malaysian tertiary referral centre. Malays J Pathol. 2012;34(2): 97-101.
23. Puig-Butillé JA, Badenas C, Ogbah Z, et al. Genetic alterations in RAS-regulated pathway in acral lentiginous melanoma. Exp Dermatol. 2013;22(2):148-50.
24. Egger ME, McMasters KM, Callender GG, et al. Unique prognostic factors in acral lentiginous melanoma. Am J Surg. 2012;204(6):874-9.
25. Sureda N, Phan A, Poulalhon N, et al. Conservative surgical management of subungual (matrix derived) melanoma: report of seven cases and literature review. Br J Dermatol. 2011;165(4):852-8.
26. Loosemore MP, Morales-Burgos A, Goldberg LH. Acral lentiginous melanoma of the toe treated using Mohs surgery with sparing of the digit and subsequent reconstruction using split-thickness skin graft. Dermatol Surg. 2013;39(1 Pt 1):136-8.
27. Chow WT, Bhat W, Magdub S, et al. *In situ* subungual melanoma: digit salvaging clearance. J Plast Reconstr Aesthet Surg. 2013;66(2):274-6.
28. Chiba FB, Schettini AP, Delfino AC, et al. Clinical and epidemiological profile of cutaneous malignant melanomas in two referral institutions in the city of Manaus, Brazil. An Bras Dermatol. 2011;86(6):1239-41
29. Durbec F, Martin L, Derancourt C, et al. Melanoma of the hand and foot: epidemiological, prognostic and genetic features. A systematic review. Br J Dermatol. 2012;166(4): 727-39.
30. Bradford PT, Goldstein AM, McMaster ML, Tucker MA. Acral lentiginous melanoma: incidence and survival patterns in the United States, 1986-2005. Arch Dermatol. 2009;145(4):427-34.
31. Oh TS, Bae EJ, Ro KW, et al. Acral Lentiginous Melanoma Developing during Long-standing Atypical Melanosis: Usefulness of Dermoscopy for Detection of Early Acral Melanoma. Ann Dermatol. 2011;23(3):400-4.
32. Yamaguchi M, Harada K, Ando N, et al. Marked response to imatinib mesylate in metastatic acral lentiginous melanoma on the thumb. Clin Exp Dermatol. 2011;36(2):174-7.
33. Nishi H, Inoue Y, Kageshita T, et al. The expression of human high molecular weight melanoma-associated antigen in acral lentiginous melanoma. Biosci Trends. 2010;4(2):86-9.
34. Kundu RV, Kamaria M, Ortiz S, et al. Effectiveness of a knowledge-based intervention for melanoma among those with ethnic skin. J Am Acad Dermatol. 2010;62(5):777-84.
35. Albreski D, Sloan SB. Melanoma of the feet: misdiagnosed and misunderstood. Clin Dermatol. 2009;27(6):556-63.
36. Phan A, Dalle S, Touzet S, et al. Dermoscopic features of acral lentiginous melanoma in a large series of 110 cases in a white population. Br J Dermatol. 2010;162(4):765-71.
37. Sneyd MJ, Cox B. Melanoma in Maori, Asian, and Pacific peoples in New Zealand. Cancer Epidemiol Biomarkers Prev. 2009 18(6):1706-13.
38. Forman SB, Garrett AB. Basal Cell Carcinoma. In: Kelly AP, Taylor SC (Eds). Dermatology for Skin of Color. New York: McGrawHill; 2009. pp. 296-9.
39. Tan WP, Tan AW, Ee HL, et al. Melanization in basal cell carcinomas: microscopic characterization of clinically pigmented and non-pigmented tumours. Australas J Dermatol. 2008;49(4):202-6.
40. Dourmishev LA, Rusinova D, Botev I. Clinical variants, stages, and management of basal cell carcinoma. Indian Dermatol Online J. 2013;4(1):12-7.
41. Lyseng-Williamson KA, Keating GM. Vismodegib: a guide to its use in locally advanced or metastatic basal cell carcinoma Am J Clin Dermatol. 2013;14(1):61-4.
42. Jain M, Madan NK, Agarwal S, et al. Pigmented basal cell carcinoma: Cytological diagnosis and differential diagnoses. J Cytol. 2012;29(4):273-5.
43. Chang JM, Gao XM. Clinical and histopathological characteristics of basal cell carcinoma in Chinese patients. Chin Med J (Engl). 2013;126(2):211-4.
44. Kikuchi A, Shimizu H, Nishikawa T. Clinical histopathological characteristics of basal cell carcinoma in Japanese patients. Arch Dermatol. 1996;132(3):320-4.
45. McDonald HC, Pandya AG. Cutaneous T cell lymphoma. In: Kelly AP, Taylor SC (Eds). Dermatology for skin of color. New York: McGraw-Hill; 2009. pp. 300-305.
46. Patel AB, Kubba R, Kubba A. Clinicopathological correlation of acquired hypopigmentary disorders. Indian J Dermatol Venereol Leprol. 2013:79(3) 376-82.
47. Koorse S, Tirumalae R, Yeliur IK, et al. Clinicopathologic profile of hypopigmented mycosis fungoides in India. Am J Dermatopathol. 2012;34(2):161-4.
48. Willemze R, Jaffe ES, Burg G, et al. WHO-EORTC classification for cutaneous lymphomas. Blood. 2005;105(10):3768-85.
49. Tan ES, Tang MB, Tan SH. Retrospective 5-year review of 131 patients with mycosis fungoides and Sézary syndrome seen at the National Skin Centre, Singapore. Australas J Dermatol. 2006; 47(4):248-52.
50. Tan E, Tay YK, Giam YC. Profile and outcome of childhood mycosis fungoides in Singapore. Pediatr Dermatol. 2000; 17(5):352-6.
51. Tang M, Tan SH, Lim LC. Leukoderma associated with Sézary syndrome: a rare presentation. J Am Acad Dermatol. 2003;49(5 Suppl):S247-9.
52. Tan SH, Tham SN, Goh CL. Skin cancers at Tertiary Referral Skin Hospital in Singapore. Int J Dermatol. 1995;34(11):770-6.
53. Willemze R. Thirty years of progress in cutaneous lymphoma research. G Ital Dermatol Venereol. 2012;147(6): 515-21.
54. Benner MF, Jansen PM, Vermeer MH, et al. Prognostic factors in transformed mycosis fungoides: a retrospective analysis of 100 cases. Blood. 2012;119(7):1643-9.

55. Olsen EA, Whittaker S, Kim YH, et al. Clinical end points and response criteria in mycosis fungoides and Sézary syndrome: a consensus statement of the International Society for Cutaneous Lymphomas, the United States Cutaneous Lymphoma Consortium, and the Cutaneous Lymphoma Task Force of the European Organisation for Research and Treatment of Cancer. J Clin Oncol. 2011;29(18):2598-607.
56. Benner MF, Willemze R. Applicability and prognostic value of the new TNM classification system in 135 patients with primary cutaneous anaplastic large cell lymphoma. Arch Dermatol. 2009;145(12):1399-404.
57. Ladizinski B, Olsen EA. Mycosis fungoides. Mayo Clin Proc. 2013;88(3):e27.
58. Kim YH, Liu HL, Mraz-Gernhard S, et al. Long-term outcome of 525 patients with mycosis fungoides and Sezary syndrome: clinical prognostic factors and risk for disease progression. Arch Dermatol. 2003;139(7):857-66.
59. AlGhamdi KM, Arafah MM, Al-Mubarak LA, et al. Profile of mycosis fungoides in 43 Saudi patients. Ann Saudi Med. 2012;32(3):283-7.
60. Wongpraparut C, Setabutra P. Phototherapy for hypopigmented mycosis fungoides in Asians. Photodermatol Photoimmunol Photomed. 2012;28(4):181-6.
61. Ranawaka RR, Abeygunasekara PH, de Silva MV. Hypopigmented mycosis fungoides in Type V skin: a report of 5 cases. Case Rep Dermatol Med. 2011;2011:190572.
62. Stone ML, Styles AR, Cockerell CJ, et al. Hypopigmented mycosis fungoides: a report of 7 cases and review of the literature. Cutis. 2001;67(2):133-8.
63. Neuhaus IM, Ramos-Caro FA, Hassanein AM. Hypopigmented mycosis fungoides in childhood and adolescence. Pediatr Dermatol. 2000;17(5):403-6.
64. McCarty MJ, Vukelja SJ, Sausville EA, et al. Lymphomatoid papulosis associated with Ki-1-positive anaplastic large cell lymphoma. A report of two cases and a review of the literature. Cancer. 1994;74(11):3051-8.
65. Cardoso J, Duhra P, Thway Y, et al. Lymphomatoid papulosis type D: a newly described variant easily confused with cutaneous aggressive CD8-positive cytotoxic T-cell lymphoma. Am J Dermatopathol. 2012;34(7):762-5.
66. Gan EY, Tang MB, Tan SH. Lymphomatoid papulosis: is a second lymphoma commoner among East Asians? Clin Exp Dermatol. 2012;37(2):118-21.
67. Kempf W, Pfaltz K, Vermeer MH, et al. EORTC, ISCL, and USCLC consensus recommendations for the treatment of primary cutaneous CD30-positive lymphoproliferative disorders: lymphomatoid papulosis and primary cutaneous anaplastic large-cell lymphoma. Blood. 2011;118(15):4024-35.
68. Steinhoff M. Beyer M, Roewert-Huber J, et al. Complete clinical remission of tumor stage mycosis fungoides after extensive skin necroses, granulomatous reaction, and fever under treatment with bexarotene, vorinostat and high dose fenofibrate. J Am Acad Dermatol. 2008;58:S88-91.
69. Schaffer JV, Bolognia JL. Common benign neoplasms of melanocytes. In: Nordlund JJ, Boissy RE, Hearing VJ, King RA, Oetting WS, Ortonne JP (Eds.) The Pigmentary System, 2nd edition. Oxford: Blackwell; 2006. pp. 1093-163.
70. Luba MC, Bangs SA, Mohler AM, et al. Common benign skin tumors. Am Fam Physician. 2003;67(4):729-38.
71. Rajesh G, Thappa DM, Jaisankar TJ, et al. Spectrum of seborrheic keratoses in South Indians: a clinical and dermoscopic study. Indian J Dermatol Venereol Leprol. 2011;77(4):483-8.
72. Saraiya A, Al-Shoha A, Brodell RT. Hyperinsulinemia Associated with Acanthosis Nigricans, Finger Pebbles, Acrochordons, and the Sign of Leser-Trelat. Endocr Pract. 2013;20:1-15. [Epub ahead of print]
73. Ahlgrimm-Siess V, Cao T, Oliviero, et al. Seborrheic keratosis: Reflectance confocal microscopy features and correlation with dermoscopy. J Am Acad Dermatol. 2013. pii: S0190-9622(12)02379-1.
74. Wood LD, Stucki JK, Hollenbeak CS, et al. Effectiveness of cryosurgery vs curettage in the treatment of seborrheic keratoses. JAMA Dermatol. 2013;149(1):108-9.
75. Abakka S, Elhalouat H, Khoummane N, et al. Uterine leiomyosarcoma and Leser-Trélat sign. Lancet. 2013;381(9860):88.
76. Rajabi P, Adibi N, Nematollahi P, et al. Bowenoid transformation in seborrheic keratosis: A retrospective analysis of 429 patients. J Res Med Sci. 2012;17(3):217-21.
77. Terada T, Kamo M, Baba Y, et al. Microinvasive squamous cell carcinoma arising within seborrheic keratosis. Cutis. 2012;90(4):176-8.
78. Yap WM, Tan PH, Ong BH. Malignancy arising in seborrheic keratosis: a report of two cases. Ann Acad Med Singapore. 1997;26(2):235-7.
79. Senel E, Salmanoğlu M, Solmazgül E, et al. Acrochordons as a cutaneous sign of impaired carbohydrate metabolism, hyperlipidemia, liver enzyme abnormalities and hypertension: a case-control study. J Eur Acad Dermatol Venereol; 2011.
80. Boza JC, Trindade EN, Peruzzo J, et al. Skin manifestations of obesity: a comparative study. J Eur Acad Dermatol Venereol. 2012;26(10):1220-3.
81. Kurek KC, Howard E, Tennant LB, et al. PTEN hamartoma of soft tissue: a distinctive lesion in PTEN syndromes. Am J Surg Pathol. 2012;36(5):671-87.
82. Hildenbrand C, Burgdorf WH, Lautenschlager S. Cowden syndrome diagnostic skin signs. Dermatology. 2001;202(4):362-6.
83. Romano C, Schepis C. PTEN gene: a model for genetic diseases in dermatology. Scientific World Journal. 2012; 2012:252457.
84. Hsi ED, Nickoloff BJ. Dermatofibroma and dermato-fibrosarcoma; an immunohistochemical study reveals distinctive antigenic profiles. J Dermatol Sci. 1996;11(1):1-9.
85. Ferrari A, Argenziano G, Buccini P, et al. Typical and atypical dermoscopic presentations of dermatofibroma. J Eur Acad Dermatol Venereol; 2012.
86. Han TY, Chang HS, Lee JH et al. A clinical and histopathological study of 122 cases of dermatofibroma (benign fibrous histiocytoma). Ann Dermatol. 2011;23(2):185-92.

11

Nutritional Pigmentary Disorders

Vineet Relhan, Khushboo Goel Mahajan

Key Features

Nutritional deficiencies may lead to numerous cutaneous manifestations with pigmentary changes being one of them:

- Knowledge of these pigmentary changes may save the patient from numerous investigations to rule out other systemic disorders and help him with treatment by supplementation of the causative nutritional substance.
- Nutritional pigmentary changes, though specific for a particular vitamin, may show overlapping features with other vitamin deficiency and sometimes supplementation should include a combination of vitamins.
- Most common nutritional disorders associated with pigmentary changes are vitamin B_{12} and nicotinic acid deficiency and protein energy malnutrition.
- There are no specific tests to diagnose nutritional pigmentary disorders, but causal association can be drawn through therapeutic challenge.
- Vitiligo, an autoimmune disorder, has also shown an association with various nutritional factors and these may be used as adjuvants with the therapy.

INTRODUCTION

Nutritional deficiencies may be associated with various cutaneous findings. Nutritional deficiencies usually lead to secondary deficiency of vitamins which are necessary organic molecules for human life and growth. The deficiency of vitamins may lead to various cutaneous manifestations including the pigmentary ones which may be specific for a vitamin or show overlapping features. The pigmentary changes seen in the skin due to malnutrition may result in hyperpigmentation, or hypopigmentation. These pigmentary changes may be secondary to amino acid imbalance in malabsorption or through photosensitization or thickening of the horny layer in ichthyosiform reaction.[1] Discoloration may also be a result of loss of nutrients through sweat glands, sebaceous glands, and hair follicles and through epidermal desquamation. This chapter discusses the pigmentary changes in relation to specific nutritional deficiencies and also brings about the recent developments in the role of nutrition in pigmentary disorders like vitiligo.

VITAMIN DEFICIENCIES ASSOCIATED WITH PIGMENTARY CHANGES

Vitamin B_{12}

There are several causes of vitamin B_{12} deficiency including fatty stool, malabsorption syndromes and decreased levels of vitamin B_{12} in maternal milk or malnutrition in infancy. There have also been reports of pigmentation due to a vitamin B_{12} deficiency caused by postgastrectomy malabsorption.[2] Vitamin B_{12} deficiency may also be caused by malabsorption secondary to pernicious anemia, in which intrinsic factor is deficient. Megaloblastic anemia is the most important disease resulting from vitamin B_{12} deficiency. Vitamin B_{12} deficiency may affect bone marrow, gastrointestinal tract and nervous system leading to systemic manifestations such as anemia, neutrophil hypersegmentation, mouth ulcers, altered bowel habit, anorexia, weight loss, glove and stocking sensory loss and corticospinal or posterior column impairment. Dermatological conditions, such as vitiligo and poliosis, are also associated with pernicious anemia.

Skin manifestations of vitamin B_{12} deficiency were first described by Baker et al.[3] in 1963 where found in 21 patients from India. Pigmentation due to vitamin B_{12} deficiency may be seen anywhere on the body, but is most prominent on the acral regions, i.e. the dorsal aspect of hands and feet especially affecting the fingers and toes. Pigmentation is specially accentuated over the digit joints. There may also be the involvement of face, neck, axilla, abdomen or buccal mucosa. The pigmentation may be patchy or diffuse, and the shade may vary from deep brown to brownish-black depending on skin color of the patient. The nail and the nail bed are usually spared, however they have been shown to be involved in few cases. In blacks suffering from pernicious anemia, hyperpigmentation is best seen on the palms and soles.[4]

The exact mechanism of increased pigmentation in vitamin B_{12} deficiency is unknown. It has been suggested that vitamin B_{12} deficiency causes a decrease in intracellular reduced glutathione (GSH) levels, which normally inhibits tyrosinase activity in melanogenesis. Lack of this inhibitor permits an increase in melanogenesis.[5] Another possibility could be a defect in melanin transport and its incorporation into keratinocytes with subsequent pigment incontinence.[6] The change in location and distribution of melanin from the epidermis to the dermis might lead to clinically evident hyperpigmentation.

Histological examination reveals epidermal thinning, vacuolar change of keratinocytes and enlargement of the nuclei of many keratinocytes. There is large amount of pigment within upper dermal melanophages and relatively little epidermal melanin.[6]

The hyperpigmentation often resembles with Addison's disease, however, no correlation has been found with hypoadrenalism[7] or betamelanocyte stimulating hormone levels. In fact, pigmentation clears after few months of therapy with vitamin B_{12}, thus establishing a causal association.

Folic Acid

Folic acid (FA) acts as a coenzyme in the catabolism of numerous amino acids and is necessary for deoxyribonucleic acid (DNA) synthesis. Deficiency of FA may be physiological as in pregnancy or in infants on exclusive goat milk; pathological as seen in those on dialysis; or pharmacological due to intake of drugs like methotrexate which inhibits its metabolism. Also, patients with vitamin B_{12} deficiency manifest concurrent FA deficiency by causing decreased absorption of FA, eventually resulting in the development of megaloblastic anemia.

Since the deficiencies are concurrent, skin manifestations are similar to those seen in vitamin B_{12} deficiency.[1] The pathogenesis of hyperpigmentation in FA deficiency has been explained by Griepp,[8] according to whom deficiency of FA results in elevated levels of biopterin which is an important substrate for hydroxylation of phenylalanine. The resulting increased levels of hydroxylated phenylalanine leads to an increase in melanin synthesis which manifests clinically as hyperpigmentation.

Nicotinic Acid

Nicotinic acid (niacin) is a water-soluble vitamin, also known as vitamin B_3. Two substances, nicotinic acid and nicotinamide, are called pellagra-preventing factors. One third of the nicotinamide comes from food, and two thirds comes from tryptophan by endogenous synthesis that requires vitamin cofactors (B_1, B_2, B_6).[9] Niacin is required for glycolysis, protein and amino acid metabolism. As cellular functions in multiple organs and tissues are affected by niacin deficiency, the clinical expression of pellagra is diverse.[10]

Pellagra can be primary or secondary depending on whether the deficiency of niacin is due to inadequate dietary intake or inadequate absorption respectively.

Inadequate dietary niacin or its precursor, tryptophan is seen in alcoholics and vegetarians whose diet is low on animal proteins and in people on strict maize diet, as maize is tryptophan-poor and contains nicotinic acid in a bound form.

Absorption or processing of niacin may be altered in certain disease conditions like prolonged diarrhea, anorexia nervosa, chronic alcoholism, chronic colitis, severe ulcerative colitis, regional ileitis, hepatic cirrhosis, carcinoid tumor, Hartnup's syndrome, and tuberculosis of the gastro-intestinal tract.[11] Drugs including isoniazid, sulfonamides, anticonvulsive drugs, antidepressants, 6-mercaptopurine and 5-fluorouracil may also cause pellagra by interfering with the tryptophan-niacin pathway.[11-13] The phototoxic reaction seen commonly in pellagra may be induced by a deficiency of urocanic acid and/or cutaneous accumulation of kynurenic acid.[14]

The classic triad of pellagra consists of 3D's: dermatitis, diarrhea and dementia. Skin changes are present in 75% of the patients[15] and usually begin on exposed areas. There may be bilateral symmetric brown-red colored "butterfly" eruption on the face, or an exudative eruption on the dorsa of the hands or lower legs. A characteristic finding is "Casal's necklace" which is a well-marginated symmetric hyperpigmented scaly eruption on the front of the neck and sternal area forming a collar.[1] The dermatitis typically begins as painful erythema which changes to an exudative eruption with pruritus and burning. Initial bright red well-demarcated erythema changes to cinnamon-brown in color. Besides hyperpigmentation on the hands, neck and feet, there may be diffuse hyperpigmentation on sun-protected areas of the body as seen in Addison's disease.[15] In the later stages, the skin may become hard, rough, cracked and brittle look, like that of "goose skin" and give a yellowish-brown hue.[10] The lips, tongue and mouth are inflamed and covered with small vesicles and ulcers. The lesions become worse in summer, often disappear in winter, and recur in spring.

Histopathological examination from older lesions in "pellagra" shows basket weave hyperkeratosis, patchy parakeratosis, acanthosis and a split in the lucidal corneal zone and an increased melanisation of basal layer. Eventually, there may be epidermal atrophy overlying dermal fibrosis, sebaceous gland atrophy and a chronic lymphohistiocytic perivascular infiltrate.[10] The pigmentation seen in pellagra is usually the summation of melanin pigment together with oxidized lipid.[16] The collagen was found to be edematous and the elastin fragmented.[16]

Though there are no chemical tests to definitively diagnose pellagra, diagnosis can be strongly suggested by examining levels of serum niacin, tryptophan, nicotinamide adenine dinucleotide and nicotinamide adenine dinucleotide phosphate. A combined excretion of *N*-methylnicotinamide and pyridone of less than 1.5 mg in 24 hours indicates severe niacin deficiency.

Treatment consists of exogenous administration of niacin (nicotinic acid) or nicotinamide in a dose of 100 mg orally every 6 hours till resolution of major acute symptoms, followed by the oral administration of 50 mg every 8–12 hours until all skin lesions heal. For children, a dose of 10–50 mg orally every 6 hours is sufficient until resolution of the symptoms and signs of pellagra. Therapy should also include other B vitamins, zinc and magnesium as well as a diet rich in calories.

Vitamin B_2 (Riboflavin)

Riboflavin is a water-soluble vitamin which acts in the Krebs cycle and is a cofactor in fatty acid and amino acid metabolism. Its deficiency can be physiological caused by an increased intake of carbohydrates and lipids with relative protein deficiency as seen in chronic alcoholism[9] or pathological like in liver cirrhosis. Riboflavin deficiency typically leads to "oculoorogenital syndrome" which manifests as cheilitis, angular stomatitis; dry, atrophic "magenta tongue", seborrheic dermatitis like eruption in the nasolabial folds, and eczematous changes followed by hyperpigmentation of the scrotum or vulva as seen in zinc deficiency.[17] Pellagra-like hyperpigmentation could be produced in rats receiving riboflavin free diet.[15]

Vitamin B_6 (Pyridoxine)

The active metabolite of vitamin B_6 is pyridoxal 5-phosphate, which acts as a cofactor in tryptophan metabolism, resulting in production of nicotinic acid. Pyridoxal is a coenzyme for numerous enzymes important for cellular metabolism like alanine aminotransferase, cocarboxylases, deaminases, etc. Isoniazid has a chemical structure similar to vitamin B_6, but induces a vitamin deficiency resembling a nicotinic acid deficiency.[18] Canned protein rich food also induces a relative B6 and nicotinic acid deficiency. The cutaneous manifestations of vitamin B_6 deficiency resembles with zinc and vitamin B_2 deficiency and leads to pellagra-like dermatitis, periorificial seborrheic dermatitis, angular stomatitis, cheilitis, glossitis and oral erosions. Topically applied nicotinamide can be used for treatment of dermatitis.[19] A therapeutic trial with 1 gm of vitamin B_6 by intravenous or oral daily administration helps confirm the diagnosis further.[9]

Vitamin C

Vitamin C or ascorbic acid is an important cofactor for proline hydroxylation and thus essential in collagen formation. It also plays an important role in iron metabolism, tyrosine synthesis and cytochrome metabolism of exogenous substances.[20] Ascorbic acid keeps tetrahydrofolic acid in its reduced form, and its deficiency aggravates anemia because of folate deficiency.[17] Vitamin C deficiency may be due to malnutrition, chronic alcoholism, or dietary abnormalities.

Skin manifestations of scurvy manifests as follicular hyperkeratosis, hemorrhages, gingivitis, cheilitis and may show melasma-like hyperpigmentation.[21]

Being a strong reducing agent, vitamin C inhibits the various oxidative reactions in the synthesis of melanin and also converts black melanin to its brown reduced form. It has been shown to be decreased in vitiliginous skin[22] and also reduces the degree of hyperpigmentation in Addison's disease.[1]

Vitamin D

The main action of vitamin D is in regulating calcium and phosphorus metabolism. The skin plays an important role in the synthesis, storage, and release of vitamin D.[23] Administration of more than 1,00,000 IU daily over prolonged period leads to hypervitaminosis D which manifests as vomiting, diarrhea, headache, bone changes, and diffuse hyperpigmentation, the exact pathogenesis of which is not clear.[15] The role of vitamin D in vitiligo has been discussed later.

TRACE ELEMENTS AND SKIN PIGMENTATION

Trace elements may have a role in skin pigmentation as suggested by high zinc levels found in melanized structures of the body such as choroid of the eye, pigmented moles and melanosomes.[24] These are essential for normal function of various metalloenzymes and deficiency, though relatively rare, may be secondary to malabsorption, marked proteinemia or severe burns. Copper, another trace element also plays a role in skin pigmentation as it interferes with production of enzyme tyrosinase (which converts tyrosine to melanin) when deficient. Zinc has also been shown to catalyze few steps of melanin synthesis and it may act as a link between melanin and the protein component.

Hyperpigmented skin lesions have been reported in patients with abnormalities of trace element metabolism, such as in Wilson's disease[25] and hemochromatosis. Some of the hyperpigmentary conditions, like xeroderma pigmentosa and melanosis secondary to pregnancy or oral contraceptives have been shown to be associated with high copper levels, but not all conditions with hypercupremia show pigmentary changes. Lightening in hair color seen in kwashiorkor showed no significant difference in quantitative values of copper or zinc values in depigmented hair pre- and postrecovery.[26] Association of depigmentation of hair with whitish skin also has been observed in neonatal copper deficiency syndromes.[27]

Chronic selenium (Se) deficiency as seen with total parenteral nutrition may lead to whitening of the fingernail beds, which resolves with Se supplementation.

Arsenic (As) intake either as Fowler's solution given for treatment of psoriasis in former times or as a contamination of wines from grapes treated with as containing pesticides may lead to a typical, dirty looking discoloration and spotty hyperpigmentation of skin.

PIGMENTARY CHANGES SECONDARY TO PROTEIN ENERGY MALNUTRITION

Protein energy malnutrition encompasses two major terms: marasmus which is secondary to caloric malnutrition, and kwashiorkor which is secondary to protein deficiency with a relative excess of carbohydrate. Kwashiorkor is defined as a total body weight of 60–80% that expected for age and height with either edema and/or hypoalbuminemia. Though mainly a problem of developing countries it remains a devastating problem globally. Affected children show delayed development and growth associated with anorexia, diarrhea, nausea and increased susceptibility to infections. Classic cutaneous finding is a "flaky paint dermatoses" or crazy pavement dermatoses which presents as diffuse fine reddish-brown scaling over the body especially over pressure areas.[28] Other features include, fluid filled lesions and erosions in areas of friction, variable areas of hyper- and hypopigmentation and "flag sign" in hair comprising of alternating lighter and darker areas of hair pigmentation, reflecting inconsistent states of nutritional intake.[29] In white-skinned children there is erythema in the beginning succeeded by small purple patches, which later darken and have a waxy feel, sharp raised edges giving the features of enamel paint areas. Within a few days these spots change from their original florid color to dark brown, reddish-brown or black. In pellagra the skin changes are found in exposed areas, whereas in crazy pavement dermatosis the lesions are found over pressure areas.[28] In the pigmented areas melanin is found in the stratum lucidum. Ultrastructural studies of depigmented skin in kwashiorkor have shown the thickness of the malpighian layer to be less than that of controls, probably due to changes in the kinetics of cell migration in kwashiorkor.[30] Diffuse dyspigmentation may be seen in African and Indian children and this may be sometimes difficult to distinguish from genetic hypopigmentation.

VITILIGO AND NUTRIENTS

Vitamin B_{12} and Folic Acid

It is thought that patients with vitiligo are more likely to have pernicious anemia and vitamin B_{12} deficiency. A nutritional deficiency in either of these two vitamins results in hyperhomocysteinemia.[31] Homocysteine interferes with melanogenesis and thus has a role in pathogenesis of vitiligo by two mechanisms: it inhibits the histidase and tyrosinase activity of the skin and also leads to accumulation of melanocytotoxic compounds by generation of reactive oxygen species by homocysteine oxidation.[32] However, there are conflicting reports about homocysteine, vitamin B_{12} and FA levels in vitiligo. Kim et al.[33] reported that serum B_{12} and FA levels were not different in their vitiligo group compared with controls. However, Karadag et al.[34] found that serum B_{12} levels were significantly lower and serum homocysteine levels were significantly higher in the vitiligo group, but FA levels were not different between the control and vitiligo groups. Balci et al. found no significant difference in the levels of homocysteine between 48 patients with vitiligo and the control group.[35]

Antioxidants

Antioxidants may be used as an adjuvant in treatment of vitiligo as the pathogenesis of melanocyte degeneration in vitiligo involves an imbalance in the antioxidant system and free radical-mediated damage. Phototherapy, commonly used to treat vitiligo has been shown to further increase this oxidative damage as firstly, photosensitizing agents are known to generate reactive oxygen species, secondly, it is seen that *in vivo* ultraviolet exposure of human epidermis causes increased levels of oxidative stress by causing changes in the enzymatic antioxidant defence system[36] and thirdly, psoralen ultraviolet A (PUVA) therapy causes depletion of GSH levels in the skin which is associated with decreases in tyrosine hydroxylase activity and melanin production in the skin.[37] Therefore, some studies have advocated the use of antioxidants as adjuvant to phototherapy to achieve repigmentation and prevent oxidative distress resulting from PUVA therapy.

The epidermal levels of ubiquinol, vitamin E, reduced GSH, and catalase (CAT) activity have been found to be reduced in vitiligo patients, however the blood levels of these, other vitamins like A, C and E and polyunsaturated fatty acids of phospholipids involved in antioxidant defence mechanism have been found to be similar to healthy age matched controls. Thus, it may be postulated that an imbalance of the intracellular redox status and a depletion of antioxidants are predominantly localized to epidermis of vitiligo patients. Jalel et al. supplemented the vitiliginous mice with antioxidants and found that the oxidative stress caused by the photochemical reaction in these vitiliginous mice was inhibited by vitamin A, C and E as an antioxidant in addition to polyphenol, zinc and selenium which are enzymes cofactors for GSH peroxidise and CAT which are melanocyte antioxidant defence keys.[38] Therefore, antioxidants may be kept in mind as an adjuvant in the treatment of vitiligo patients.

Vitamin D

It is a well-known fact that autoimmunity plays an important role in the pathogenesis of vitiligo and many studies have found the existence of other autoimmune disorders in patients with vitiligo.[39,40] Meanwhile, many autoimmune diseases have been found to be associated with reduced vitamin D levels.[41] These findings have led to the hypothesis that vitamin D levels may be associated with vitiligo. A study by Silverberg et al.[42] found that patients with vitiligo who had additional autoimmune diseases, had lowered levels of 25(OH)D, suggesting that vitamin D deficiency may be a risk factor for the development of vitiligo. In a further study by Li et al.[43] significantly decreased levels of 25(OH)D were observed in the patients with vitiligo as compared to controls. However, there have not been additional studies that have investigated the association between vitiligo and 25(OH)D levels. These findings suggest that a deficiency in 25(OH) D may contribute to the development of vitiligo. Vitamin D analogues are now also used in the topical therapy of vitiligo and appear to be effective. Studies have revealed two underlying mechanisms for this. Firstly, vitamin D analogs can control the activation, proliferation and migration of melanocytes. Secondly, vitamin D analogs can modulate T-cell activation, resulting in reduced autoimmune damage of melanocytes.[43-45] However, further studies are required to evaluate the exact relationship of serum vitamin D levels and vitiligo, as well as to elucidate the effects of vitamin D in treatment of vitiligo.

PIGMENTATION DISORDERS DUE TO NUTRITION EXCESS

Pigmentary changes are commonly seen with increased amounts of carotene in the diet or of lycopene which is a structural isomer of beta-carotene. Dietary sources of carotene includes carrots, spinach, corn, apples, butter, eggs, yellow beans, kale, pumpkins, yellow turnips, sweet potatoes and papaya and that of lycopene includes, tomatoes and other reddish foods. Pigmentary changes are mainly seen in children and presents as diffuse yellow discoloration over body sparing the sclera and oral cavities (cf. Jaundice).[1,46] Carotene is a yellowish lipochrome that is normally present in keratin and subcutaneous fat and in hypercarotinemia, yellow pigmentation is seen on the tip of the nose, palms, soles, nasolabial folds and forehead due to the high lipid content of corneum and its affinity to carotene, which is lacking in the mucosa. If the offending foods are reduced or eliminated, the skin color will return to normal in 2–6 weeks.[47]

WORK-UP OF A PATIENT WITH NUTRITIONAL PIGMENTARY DISORDER

A basic work-up of a patient presenting with pigmentary disorder suspected to be due to nutritional disorder would include, hemoglobin, RBC indices, peripheral smear, total leukocyte count, platelet count, serum vitamin B_{12} of less than 50 pg/mL (normal range, 180–900 pg/mL), serum folate, iron, total iron binding capacity, ferritin, cortisol, adrencorticotropic hormone, routine chemistries and glucose-6-phosphate dehydrogenase levels.

The differential diagnosis for skin hyperpigmentation includes endocrine disorders, like Addison's disease, myxedema, Grave's disease; liver diseases, like cirrhosis, hemochromatosis, Wilson's disease; metabolic disorders like porphyrias; exogenous chemical exposure and occult malignancy, and these causes should be actively excluded.

REFERENCES

1. Burg G, Bergner T. Pigmentary disorders associated with nutritional deficiency states. Clin Dermatol. 1989;7(2):36-43.
2. Mori K, Ando I, Kukita A. Generalized hyperpigmentation of the skin due to Vitamin B_{12} deficiency. J Dermatol. 2001;28(5): 282-5.
3. Baker SJ, Johnson S, Ignatius M, et al. Hyperpigmentation of skin: A sign of vitamin B_{12} deficiency. Br Med J. 1963;1(5347):1713-5.
4. Ogbuawa O, Trowel J, Williams JT, et al. Hyperpigmentation of pernicious anemia in blacks. Arch Intern Med. 1978;138(3):388-9.
5. Niiyama S, Mukai H. Reversible cutaneous hyper-pigmentation and nails with white hair due to vitamin B_{12} deficiency. Eur J Dermatol. 2007;17(6):551-2
6. Marks VJ, Briggaman RA, Wheeler CE. Hyperpigmentation in megaloblastic anemia. J Am Acad Dermatol. 1985;12(5 Pt 2):914-7.
7. Baker SJ, Mathar VI, Abe K. Beta-melanocyte stimulating hormone levels in subjects with hyperpigmentation associated with megaloblastic anemia. Blood. 1970;35(1):83-5.
8. Griepp PR. Hyperpigmentation syndromes (diffuse hypermelanosis). Arch Intern Med. 1978;138(3):356-7.
9. Bousquet E, Larregue M, Barthelemy JP, et al. Pellagroid syndrome with vitamin B_6 deficiency. Biological and clinical study of a case. Ann Biol Clin (Paris). 1972;30(6):585-92.
10. Hegyi J, Schwartz RA, Hegyi V. Pellagra: Dermatitis, dementia, and diarrhea. Int J Dermatol. 2004;43(1):1-5.
11. Castiello RJ. Lynch PJ. Pellagra and the carcinoid syndrome. Arch Dermatol. 1972; 105(4):574-7.
12. Darvay A, Basarab T, McGregor JM, et al. Isoniazid induced pellagra despite pyridoxine supplementation. Clin Exp Dermatol. 1999;24(3):167-9.
13. Stevens HP, Ostlere LS, Begent RH, et al. Pellagra secondary to 5-fluorouracil. Br J Dermatol. 1993;128(5):578-80.

14. Dogliotti M, Liebowitz M, Downing DT, et al. Nutritional influences of pellagra on sebum composition. Br J Dermatol. 1977;97(1):25-8.
15. Schaaf F. Uber die Bedeutung der Vitamine in der Dermatologie. Zentralbl Hautkr. 1933;46:657-784.
16. Zawahry MEL, Zawahry BEL. Pellagra: A clinicopathological study of an advanced case. In: Wilkinson DS, Mascaro JM, Orfanos CE (Eds). Clinical Dermatology Berlin CMD Case Collection. Stuttgart: Schattauer; 1987. pp. 382-3.
17. Barthelemy H, Chouvet B, Cambazard F. Skin and mucosal manifestations in vitamin deficiency. J Am Acad Dermatol. 1986;15(6):1263-74.
18. Marche J. Drug-induced pellagra. Prophylaxis and treatment. Therapie. 1968;3(1):9-27.
19. Comaish JS, Felix RH, McGrath H. Topically applied nicotinamidein isoniazid-induced pellagra. Arch Dermatol. 1976;112(1):70-2.
20. Leboulanger I. Les vitamines. Neuilly, France, Laboratoires Roche. 1976.
21. Hruszek H. Zur Ursache des Chloasma gravidarum oder uterinum, seiner Verhiitung und Bekiimpfung. Miinch Med Wochenschr. 1937;84:1336-7.
22. Ratnam AV, Saatry PB, Satyanarayana BV. Ascorbic acid and melanogenesis. Br J Dermatol. 1977;97(2):201-4.
23. Pavlovitch JH, Delescluse C. Vitamin D and the metabolism of epidermis. Int J Dermatol. 1983;22(2):98-100.
24. Molokhia MM, Portnoy B. Trace elements and skin pigmentation. Br J Dermatol. 1973;89(2):207-9.
25. Leu ML, Strickland T, Wang CC, et al. Skin pigmentation in Wilson's disease. JAMA. 1970;211(9):1542-3.
26. Bradfield RB, Soo Hoo T, Baertl JM. Effect of hypo-chromotrichia on hair copper and zinc during kwashiorkor. Am J Clin Nutr. 1980;33(6):1315-7.
27. Ashkenazy A, Levin St, Djaldetti M, et al. The syndrome of neonatal copper deficiency. Pediatrics. 1973;52(4):525-33.
28. Henington VM, Caroe E, Derbes V, et al. Kwashiorkor; report of four cases from Louisiana. AMA Arch Derm. 1958; 78(2):157-70.
29. Heath ML, Sidbury R. Cutaneous manifestations of nutritional deficiency. Curr Opin Pediatr. 2006;18(4):417-22.
30. Sims RT. The ultrastructure of depigmented skin in kwashiorkor. Br J Dermatol. 1968;80(12):822-32.
31. Montes LF, Diaz ML, Lajous J, et al. Folic acid and vitamin B_{12} in vitiligo: a nutritional approach. Cutis. 1992;50(1):39-42.
32. Ortonne JP. Vitiligo and other disorders of hypopigmentation. In: Bolognia JL, Jorizzo JL, Rapini RP (Eds). Dermatology, 1st edn. New York: Mosby; 2003. pp. 947–73.
33. Kim SM, Kim YK, Hann SK. Serum levels of folic acid and vitamin B_{12} in Korean patients with vitiligo. Yonsei Med J. 1999;40(3):195-8.
34. Karadag AS, Tutal E, Ertugrul DT, et al. Serum holotrans-cobalamine, vitamin B_{12}, folic acid and homocysteine levels in patients with vitiligo. Clin Exp Dermatol. 2012;37(1):62-4.
35. Balci DD, Yonden Z, Yenin JZ, et al. Serum homocysteine, folic acid and vitamin B_{12} levels in vitiligo. Eur J Dermatol. 2009;19(4):382-3.
36. Punnonen K, Autio P, Kiistala U, et al. *In vivo* effects of solar-stimulated ultraviolet irradiation on antioxidant enzymes and lipid peroxidation in human epidermis. Br J Dermatol. 1991;125(1):18-20.
37. Benathan M, Virador V, Furumura M, et al. Co-regulation of melanin precursors and tyrosinase in human pigment cells: Roles of cysteine and glutathione. Cell Mol Biol (Noisy-le-grand). 1999;45(7):981-90.
38. Jalel A, Soumaya GS, Hamdaoui MH. Vitiligo treatment with vitamins, minerals and polyphenol supplementation. Indian J Dermatol. 2009;54(4):357-60.
39. Le Poole IC, Wankowicz-Kalinska A, van den Wijngaard RM, et al. Autoimmune aspects of depigmentation in vitiligo. J Investig Dermatol Symp Proc. 2004;9(1):68-72.
40. Weiss GR, Fehrenkamp SH, Tokaz LK, et al. Vitiligo and Graves' disease following treatment of malignant melanoma with recombinant human interleukin 4. Dermatology. 1996;192(3):283-5.
41. Adorini L, Penna G. Control of autoimmune diseases by the vitamin D endocrine system. Nat Clin Pract Rheumatol. 2008;4(8):404-12.
42. Silverberg JI, Silverberg AI, Malka E, et al. A pilot study assessing the role of 25 hydroxy vitamin D levels in patients with vitiligo vulgaris. J Am Acad Dermatol. 2010;62(6):937-41.
43. Li K, Shi Q, Yang L, et al. The association of vitamin D receptor gene polymorphisms and serum 25-hydroxyvitamin D levels with generalized vitiligo. Br J Dermatol. 2012;167(4):815-21.
44. Amano H, Abe M, Ishikawa O. First case report of topical tacalcitol for vitiligo repigmentation. Pediatr Dermatol. 2008;25(2):262-4.
45. Parsad D, Kanwar AJ. Topical vitamin D analogues in the treatment of vitiligo. Pigment Cell Melanoma Res. 2009;22(4):487-8.
46. Congdon PJ, Kelleher J, Edwards P, et al. Benign carotenemia in children. Arch Dis Child. 1981;56(4):292-4.
47. Lascari AD. Carotenemia. A review. Clin Pediatr (Phila). 1981;20(1):25-9.

12

Morphological Types of Pigmentation

Biju Vasudevan, Manas Chatterjee, Rajesh Verma

Key Features

- Pigmentation can be of various morphological types ranging from simple linear patterns to complex whorled patterns.
- Certain morphological variants are characteristic of specific conditions like the flagellate and reticulate patterns, thus aiding diagnosis.
- These variants provide an insight into mosaicism and a better understanding of alignment of skin disorders.

INTRODUCTION

In the animal kingdom, the beauty of a species is usually dependent on its skin color. However in humans, pigmentation is a cue to various underlying disorders. Pigmentation is mainly of two types, diffused and localized. Most of the morphological forms of pigmentation fall into these two groups. Bizarre forms of pigmentation may also occur mainly as a result of mosaicism. This chapter will take the reader through a variety of morphological forms of pigmentation which will add color to the study of pigmentary disorders.

TYPES OF MORPHOLOGICAL PIGMENTATION

Linear Pigmentation

It is probably the most common and the most controversial morphological form of pigmentation. In fact Blaschkoid, whorled, serpentine and other morphological forms are considered many times as variants of linear pigmentation.

Linear Hypopigmentation

Linear hypopigmentation is described in conditions like hypomelanosis of Ito, nevus depigmentosus **(Fig. 1)**, focal dermal hypoplasia, lichen striatus **(Fig. 2)**, and epidermal nevi. Guttate macules in linear keratosis follicularis and linear basaloid follicular hamartoma are other causes. Linear hypopigmentation extending from site of intralesional injection of corticosteroids has been reported.[1]

Linear Hyperpigmentation

Linear hyperpigmentation has been described in Conradi-Hünermann-Happle syndrome, pigmented purpuric dermatosis, phytophotodermatitis (streaky) and focal dermal hypoplasia. Linear fixed drug eruption (FDE) to trimethoprim, linear ashy dermatosis and linear lichen planus pigmentosus **(Fig. 3)** have also been reported.[2]

Linear Erythemas

It can occur in dermatomyositis mainly on the dorsum of hands.

Whorled Pigmentation

Whorled pattern or a swirling pattern of pigmentation can be seen in epidermal nevi, hypomelanosis of Ito, linear and whorled nevoid hypermelanosis and late stages of incontinentia pigmenti.

Hypomelanosis of Ito

Hypomelanosis of Ito (HI) is a type of congenital hypo-pigmentation, occurring in a linear and whorled pattern

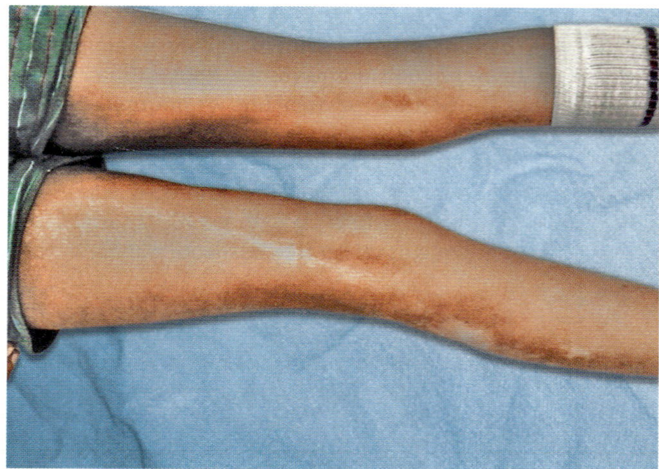

Fig. 1: Linear nevus depigmentosus

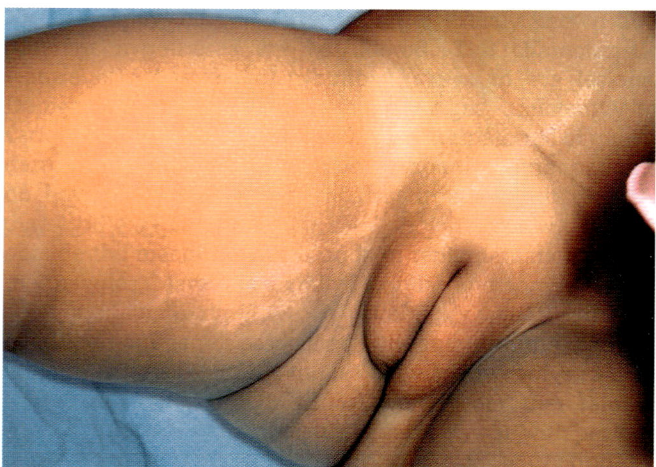

Fig. 2: Linear lichen striatus

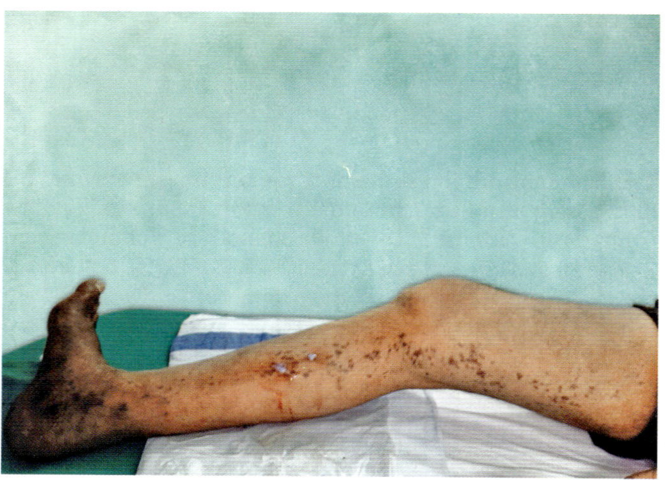

Fig. 3: Linear lichen planus pigmentosus

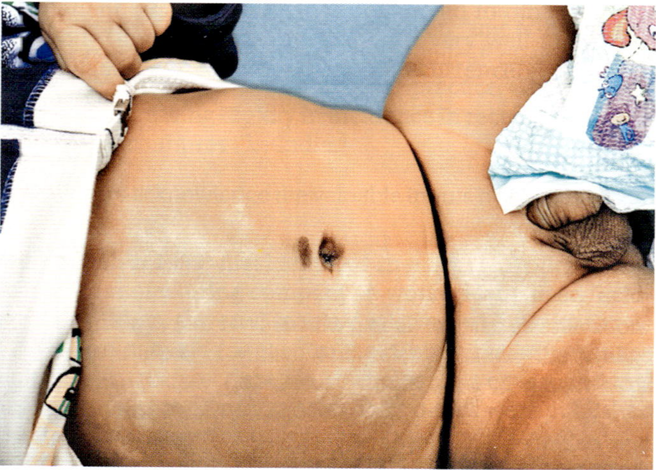

Fig. 4: Hypomelanosis of Ito

following lines of Blaschko **(Fig. 4)**. The hypopigmentation is not preceded by either vesicular or verrucous lesions. It is associated with neurologic deficits, epilepsy and asymmetrical abnormalities in other organs.

The terminology linear and whorled nevoid hypermelanosis (LWNH) was introduced by Kalter in 1988 to define a pigmentary anomaly characterized by swirls and streaks of macular hyperpigmentation which followed the lines of Blaschko **(Figs 5A and B)**.[3] Different names like zosteriform lentiginous nevus, zebra-like hyperpigmentation, zosteriform reticulate hyperpigmentation, reticulate hyperpigmentation of Iijima, progressive cribriform and zosteriform hyperpigmentation have been ascribed to this condition. The diagnostic criteria proposed by Kalter for diagnosis of LWNH include:

- Onset within few weeks of births with progression for 1–2 years before stabilizing.
- Linear and whorled hyperpigmentation following lines of Blaschko without preceding bullae or verrucae.
- Hyperpigmented areas with increased pigmentation of basal layer and prominence of melanocytes without incontinence of pigment.
- Sporadic occurrence without sex predilection.
- Sparing of mucous membranes, eyes, palms, and soles.
- Possible association with congenital anomalies.

Linear and whorled hypermelanosis resembles HI in all aspects, excepting the color of skin markings.

All of above conditions represent variants of pigmentary mosaicism.[4] This pattern of hypo- or hyperpigmentation has also been reported in *Proteus* syndrome.[5]

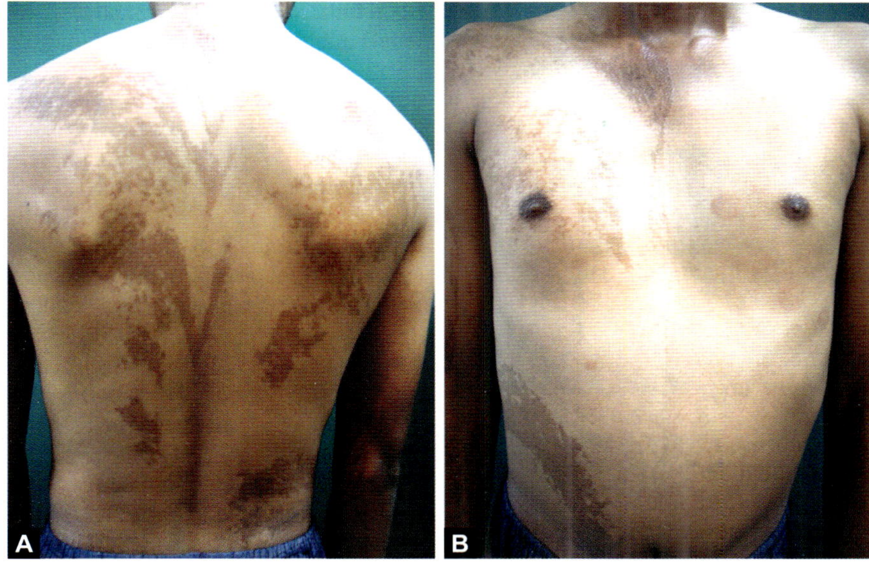

Figs 5A and B: Linear and whorled hypermelanosis

Blaschkoid Pigmentation

Alfred Blaschko (1901) described imaginary lines which correspond to the pigmentary pattern of certain nevi and dermatoses, classical of which was incontinentia pigmenti. Linear and whorled nevoid hypermelanosis, nevus spilus, café-au-lait spots, melanocytic nevi and nevus depigmentosus have all been reported in a Blaschkoid pigmented distribution. Linear pigmentary changes in Blaschkoid distribution can be seen in Conradi-Hünermann-Happle syndrome, X-linked dominant ichthyosis, lichen planus including lichen planus pigmentosus, **(Fig. 6)** lichenoid drug eruption and rarely in pityriasis versicolor.[6]

Segmental Pigmentation

Disorders which are found in a segmental pattern are as follows:

Segmented hypopigmentation: Vitiligo, nevus depigmentosus **(Fig. 7)**, ash leaf macules, hypomelanosis of Ito.

Segmental hyperpigmentation: Cafe-au-lait macule, speckled lentiginous nevus **(Fig. 8)**, linear and whorled nevoid hypermelanosis, McCune-Albright syndrome and lichen planus pigmentosus **(Fig. 9)**.

Segmental pigmented purpuric dermatoses (PPD): Lichen aureus.

Others: Segmental hypo- and hyperpigmented disorder (SHHPD): First described in 1983 by Metzker et al. in a series of 30 children, it is characterized by hypo- or hyperpigmented patches in a dermatomal distribution, with sharp delineation along the midline and less well defined on the lateral aspect. Commonly found in darker skinned infants involving the abdomen, chest and back, it can rarely be familial too. No association with systemic disorders has been found.[7] The condition is probably due to somatic mutation reflecting the disparate pigmentation properties and usually resembles the "checkerboard" pattern.[8]

Zosteriform Pigmentation

Zosteriform pigmentation has been described in lichen planus pigmentosus (LPP) **(Fig. 10)**, Beckwith-Wiedemann syndrome, lentiginous nevus, nevus spilus and multiple agminated spitz nevi.

Progressive cribriform and zosteriform hyperpigmentation (PCZH) is a distinct entity having this type of morphological pigmentation. First described by Rower et al.[9] the diagnostic criteria for PCZH includes: (i) uniform, tan cribriform pigmentation in zosteriform distribution, (ii) histologic pattern showing mild increase in basal cell melanin pigment along with complete absence of nevus cells, (iii) not secondary to any cause like injury or inflammation, (iv) onset much later after birth with gradual progression, and (v) lack of associated cutaneous or systemic abnormalities. They are localized lesions numbering one to four, occurring mainly on trunk and extremities and usually follow the lines of Blaschko. Controversy also exists whether they are Becker's melanosis without hypertrichosis.

Reticulate Pigmentation

There is a lot of ambiguity as to what actually is meant by the term "reticulate pigmentation". Various other terminologies

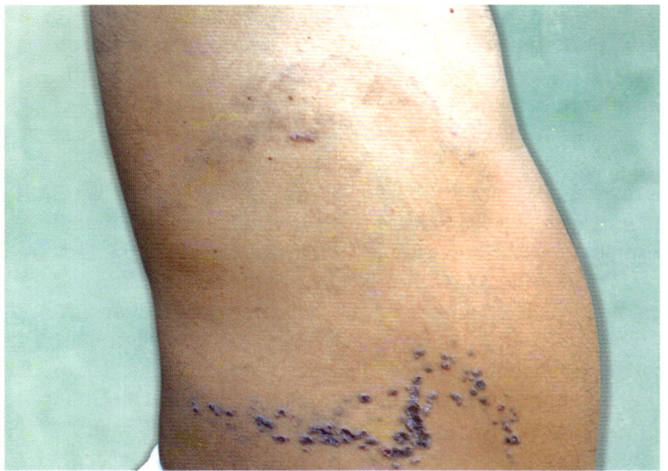

Fig. 6: Blaschkoid lichen planus pigmentosus

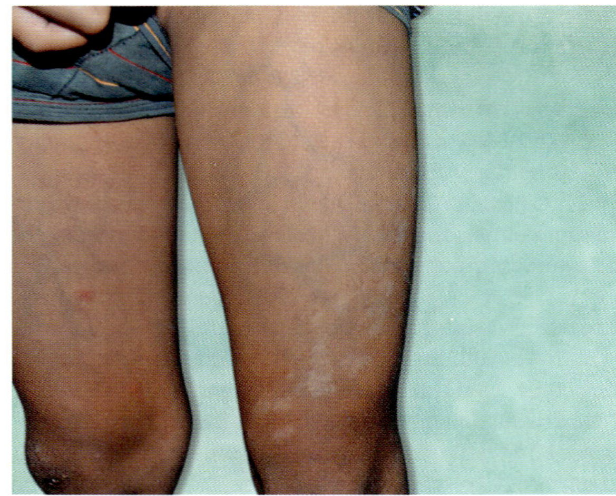

Fig. 7: Segmental nevus depigmentosus

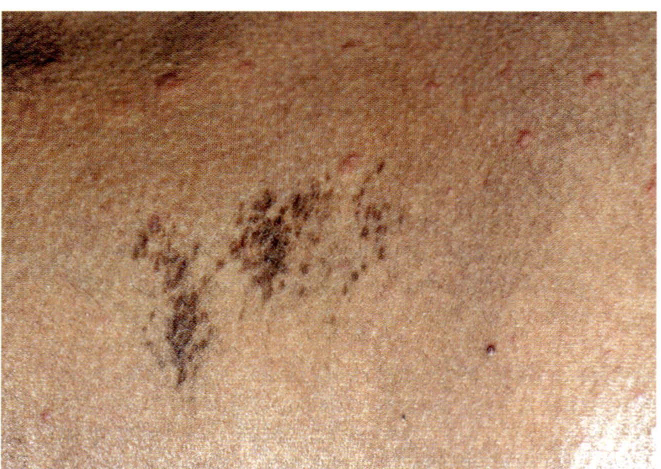

Fig. 8: Speckled lentiginous nevus

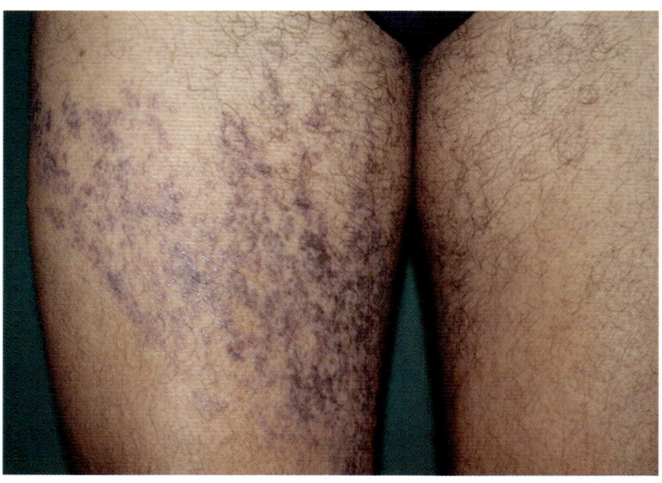

Fig. 9: Segmental lichen planus pigmentosus

which are used interchangeably with this morphological pattern are as follows:[10]

Mottled pigmentation: Polysized hypopigmented or hyperpigmented lesions in different shades leading to a blotchy appearance.

Dyschromatosis: Hypopigmented and hyperpigmented freckle like macules.

Reticular: Lacy or net like pattern, complete or partial rings regularly spaced with intervening normal skin.

Reticulate hyperpigmentation: Congenital or acquired "ephelid like" lesions with indistinct borders.

Poikilodermatous: Atrophy, macular or reticulate pigmentation and telengiectasias.

Reticulate pigmentation is most commonly found in various inherited disorders and the features are as described in **Table 1**.

Other conditions in which reticulate pigmentation is found are cutis marmorata (blue, vascular), cutis marmorata telangiectatica congenita (fixed reticulate), neonatal lupus erythematosus (extensive reticulate erythema), "chicken-wire" reticulate erythema, prodrome of hereditary angioedema, atopic dirty neck, livedo reticularis, erythema ab igne,

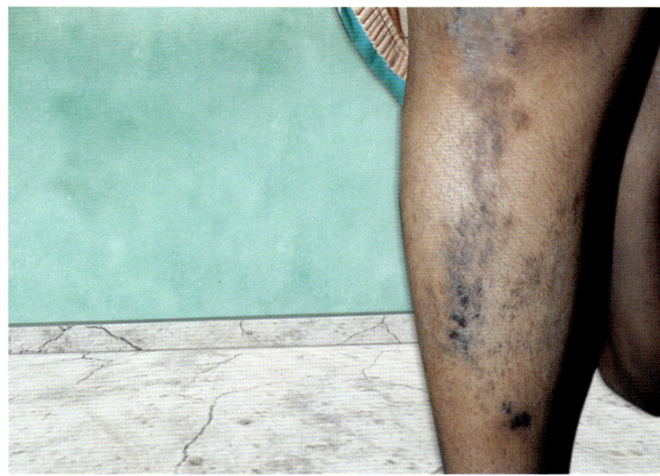

Fig. 10: Zosteriform lichen planus pigmentosus

Table 1: Disorders having reticulate pigmentation

Disease	*Genetic*	*Site predominant*
Dowling-Dego's disease **(Fig. 11)**	AD	Flexures
Reticulate acropigmentation of Dohi **(Fig. 12)**	AD	Dorsum of hands and feet, face
Reticulate acropigmentation of Kitamura	AD	Dorsum of hands, trunk
Haber's syndrome	AD	Flexural pigmentation, rosacea-like facial eruption, pitted facial scars
Dyskeratosis congenita	XLR	Neck, thighs
Rothmund-Thomson syndrome	AR	Face, hands, forearms, lower legs
Pseudoxanthoma elasticum	AR	Abdomen
Naegeli-Franceschetti-Jadassohn syndrome	AD	Neck, axillae
Dermatopathia pigmentosa reticularis	AD	Trunk
Mendes da Costa-van der Valk syndrome	XLR	Face, limbs
Hoyeraal-Hreidarsson syndrome	X linked	Neck, chest, upper extremities
Epidermolysis bullosa simplex (EBS) with mottled pigmentation	AR	Neck, upper trunk, extremities
Ankyloblepharon-ectodermal defects, cleft lip and palate (AEC) syndrome	AD	Generalized

acute graft versus host disease (GVHD), zosteriform reticulate pigmentation (four cases from Japan), prurigo pigmentosa, poikiloderma of Civatte (sides of neck), porphyria cutanea tarda, reticulate erythematous mucinosis (areas of pink, reticulate or sheet-like erythema present on the central part of the chest and back), primary localized cutaneous amyloidosis, Fanconi anemia, Opitz-Kaveggia syndrome and following use of drugs like bleomycin and fluorouracil.

Pigmentary Demarcation Lines

They are physiological lines that mark the abrupt transition between deeper and lighter pigmented skin. They are also known as Voigt's lines or Futcher's lines. They are generally more prominent in darker skin types. There are five different naturally occurring patterns of pigmentary demarcation lines that have been described and have been denoted as A–E and three more patterns on the facial skin denoted as F,G,H.[11]

A: On the lateral aspect of upper arm extending over the pectoral area
B: On the posteromedial portion of the lower limb
C: Mediosternal line, a vertical hypopigmented line in the pre and parasternal area
D: On the posteriomedial area of spine
E: Bilateral hypopigmented streaks, bands or lanceolate areas over the chest in the zone between the mid-third of the clavicle and the periareolar skin
F: "V" shaped hyperpigmented lines between the malar prominence and the temple
G: "W" shaped hyperpigmented lines between the malar prominence and the temple
H: Linear bands of hyperpigmentation from the angle of the mouth to the lateral aspects of the chin.

Rippling Pigmentation

Rippling is a type of morphological pigmentation classically seen in macular amyloidosis.[12] In macular amyloidosis, lesions are small, dusky brown/grayish pigmented macules distributed mainly over upper back, shins and arms. Rippling pigmentation is also seen in atopic dermatitis, especially on the neck, where it is termed as "dirty neck." It is also described in nephrogenic fibrosing dermopathy, frictional melanosis, variant of Dowling-Degos disease and Wilson's disease.[13]

Flagellate Pigmentation

Flagellate erythema is classically described as linear erythemato-violaceous streaks seen on trunk or shoulders following systemic or local bleomycin use.[14] It can occur due to exposure from as low doses of 14–15 units within 12–24 hours or even after 6 months and can occur after intravenous, intramuscular, intrapleural, intraperitoneal and intracutaneous injections. Factors blamed for the flagellate erythema include microtrauma after scratching

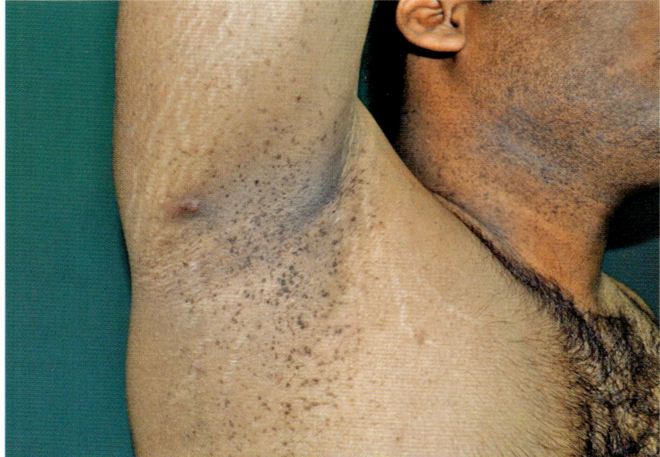

Fig. 11: Dowling-Degos' disease

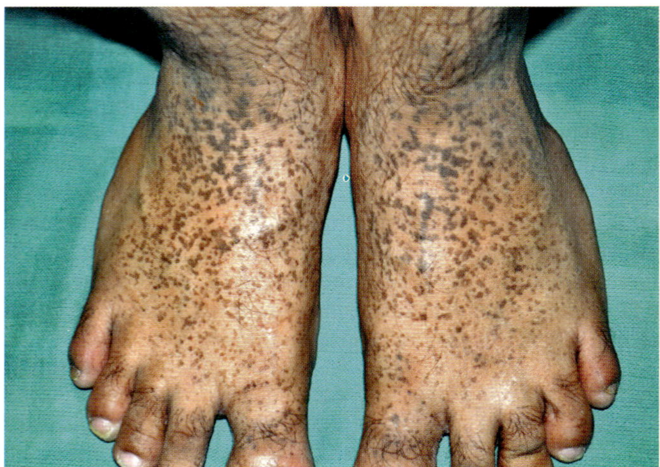

Fig. 12: Acropigmentation of Dohi

following pruritus and hyperthermia, both induced by the drug. Other drugs reported to cause this are docetaxel and bleomycin derivatives like peplomycin. It can also be seen in dermatomyositis, adult onset Still's disease and shiitake dermatitis (mushroom intake).[15]

Striated Pigmentation

Striated erythema on ears and face has been described in early stages of Rothmund-Thomson syndrome.

Serpentine Pigmentation

Persistent serpentine supravenous hyperpigmentation has been seen with combined dactinomycin and vincristine therapy. It can also be seen with Fluorouracil intravenous injections. The pathophysiology is still to be fully elucidated but may involve endothelial injury from infusion factors or autoantibodies with resultant alterations in melanin synthesis or melanosome packaging.

Stippled Pigmentation

Stippled pigmentation is classically described in talon noir as bluish black pigmented specks occurring suddenly on the back or sides of the heel. It usually occurs in sportspersons like athletes, footballers and rarely in the hands of weightlifters. Stippled pigmentation has also been described in basal cell carcinoma (BCC).

Raindrop Pigmentation

This is characteristically seen in arsenic poisoning **(Fig. 13)**. There is diffuse macular bronzy pigmentation usually on the trunk with a "raindrop appearance" caused by contrast of hyperpigmentation along with interspersed small areas of either normal or depigmented skin.[16] Pigmentation occurring in other disorders which are described as raindrop include reticulate pigmentary disorders like dyschromatosis universalis hereditaria, dyschromatosis symmetrica hereditaria, reticulate acropigmentation of Kitamura, Dowling-Degos disease and others like antimalarial-induced hyperpigmentation, biliary cirrhosis, Fanconi's anemia, dyskeratosis congenita and familial gigantic melanocytosis.[17]

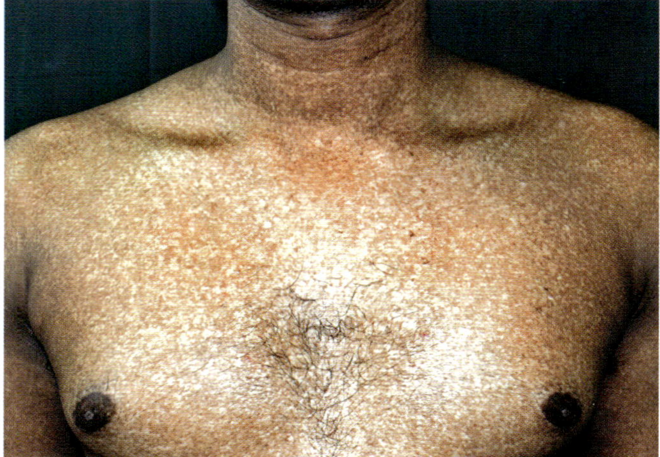

Fig. 13: Raindrop pigmentation in arsenicosis

Confetti Pigmentation

Confetti-like hypomelanosis or confetti depigmentation usually refers to small, 1–3 mm hypopigmented macules. It may results from a localized alteration in melanin production, melanin transfer or destruction of melanocytes.

Many disorders cause confetti-like hypomelanosis including tuberous sclerosis, morphea, mycosis fungoides, chemicals like hydroquinone and its monobenzyl ether, idiopathic guttate hypomelanosis, systemic sclerosis and of course vitiligo. Contact leukomelanosis in confetti-like pattern has been reported following application of steamed betel leaves.[18] Grover's disease, Darier's disease, pityriasis versicolor and melanoma can also cause confetti-like hypomelanosis. Mimicks of confetti hypomelanosis include stucco keratosis, lichen sclerosus et atrophicus and verrucae planae juveniles. Leukoderma punctatum is another such condition having confetti hypopigmentation and was first described by Falabella.[19] It commonly occurs in women being treated with 8-methoxypsoralen and sun exposure, though it has also been reported with light chamber ultraviolet A (UV-A) and topical psoralen ultraviolet A (PUVA).[20]

Lenticular Pigmentation

Characteristically described in Laugier-Hunziker syndrome wherein oval dark macules occur on the lips, oral mucosa, and nails and rarely on neck, thorax, abdomen, genitalia, perianal area, sclera, tongue and esophagus.[21] Described as small lentil like skin lesions, they are characterized by basal layer hyperpigmentation and melanocytic hyperplasia. They can occur in all the familial lentiginosis syndromes like Carney complex, LEOPARD syndrome, Peutz-Jeghers syndrome, syndrome of arterial dissections and lentiginosis (ADL) and benign familial lentiginosis.

Spotty Pigmentation

Classically described in Carney's complex which also has atrial myxomas and endocrine abnormalities,[22] this mucocutaneous pigmentation is usually centrofacial and has perioral and periorbital accentuation. The characteristic sites of pigmentation are lips, conjunctiva, inner or outer canthi, vaginal and penile mucosa. It can also be used to denote the various reticular pigmentary disorders.

Mottled Pigmentation

This can be seen in melanoleukoderma, Cockayne's syndrome, Rothmund-Thomson syndrome, reticular pigmentary disorders, photoaging, variant of Epidermolysis Bullosa Simplex (EBS), pangeria, progeria, acrogeria, systemic sclerosis **(Fig. 14)**, dysplastic nevus, Fanconi's anemia, B_{12} deficiency, Becker's syndrome, ochronosis and porphyria cutanea tarda.

Addisonian Pigmentation

Pigmentation in Addison's disease has a generalized distribution with predominance on mucosal surfaces, genital areas, sun-exposed areas, frictional areas, skin-folds, palmar creases, nipples and areas of scarring.[23] In addition, lentiginous type of pigmentation is found on oral mucosa, lips and the anogenital regions **(Fig. 15)**. Proopiomelanocortin which is the precursor for β-lipotropin, γ-melanocyte-stimulating hormone (MSH), β-MSH and α-MSH stimulates melanocyte leading to the pigmentation. Rarely Addisonian like pigmentation has been reported with malignant pheochromocytoma. Ectopic secretion of adrenocorticotropic hormone (ACTH) and its precursors by the tumor tissue is the most acceptable hypothesis.

Other causes of Addisonian pigmentation include endocrine disorders like hyperthyroidism, porphyria, hemochromatosis, nephropathies, hepatopathies like Wilson's disease, malnutrition especially B_{12} deficiency, lymphogranulomatosis, metastasizing melanoma and certain medications like

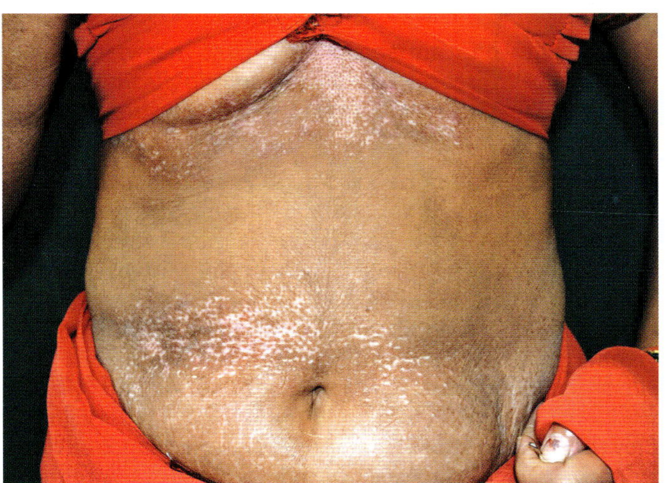

Fig. 14: Mottled pigmentation in systemic sclerosis

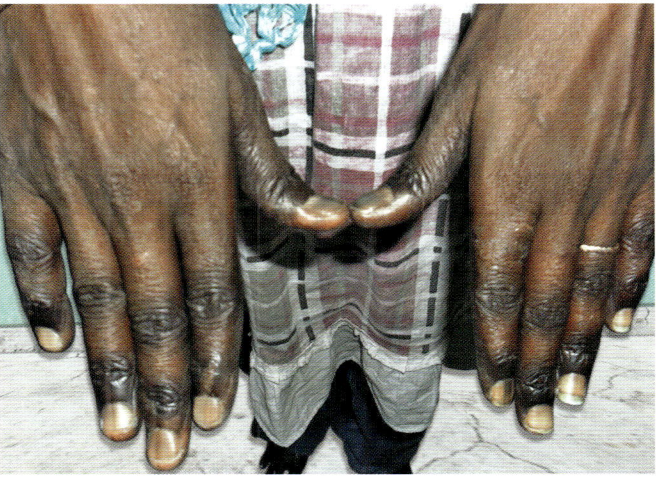

Fig. 15: Addisonian pigmentation

antimalarials, amiodarone, minocycline, antiretroviral drugs, and other chemotherapeutic agents.[24]

Sock Line Pigmentation

Linear hyperpigmentation resulting from post-inflammatory changes due to wearing of elastic bands of socks have been reported in infants and referred to as sock line pigmentation. They appear as bilateral, curvilinear hyperpigmentation, mainly of the calves and do not follow Blaschko lines. They histologically demonstrate lentiginous melanocytic hyperplasia along with basal layer hyperpigmentation.

Miscellaneous

Various types of benign transient congenital pigmentation are found in neonates and infants. Pigmentation of lips is seen in Peutz-Jeghers syndrome, Laugier-Hunziker syndrome, Addison's disease, and Hutchinson's sign. In adrenal insufficiency and thyroid dysfunction, pigmentation is accentuated at angles of lips as in Peutz-Jeghers syndrome and Laugier-Hunziker syndrome. Periungual hyperpigmentation of digits and pigmentation of lips is simultaneously seen in Laugier-Hunziker syndrome. Digital pigmentation occurs transiently as isolated melanotic hyperpigmentation of the distal digits (IMHDD).

CONCLUSION

These morphological forms of pigmentation give us an insight in understanding the process of mosaicism and pigmentary biology in general. Blaschkoid, checkerboard, phylloid, spiral and zosteriform patterns may all be manifestations of mosaic pigmentation.

REFERENCES

1. Nanda V, Parwaz MA, Handa S. Linear hypopigmentation after triamcinolone injection: a rare complication of a common procedure. Aesthetic Plast Surg. 2006;30:118-9.
2. Özkaya-Bayazit E, Baykal C. Trimethoprim-induced linear fixed drug eruption. Br J Dermatol. 1997;137:1028-9.
3. Kalter DC, Griffiths WA, Atherton DJ. Linear and whorled nevoid hypermelanosis. J Am Acad Dermatol. 1988;19: 1037-44.
4. Taibjee SM, Bennett DC, Moss C. Abnormal pigmentation in hypomelanosis of Ito and pigmentary mosaicism: the role of pigmentary genes. Br J Dermatol. 2004;151:269-82.
5. Viljoen DL, Nelson MM, de Jong G, et al. *Proteus* syndrome in Southern Africa: natural history and clinical manifestations in six individuals. Am J Med Genet. 1987; 27:87-97.
6. Kabbash C, Laude TA, Weinberg JM, et al. Lichen planus in the lines of Blaschko. Pediatr Dermatol. 2002;19:541-5.
7. Metzker A, Morag C, Weitz R. Segmental pigmentation disorder. Acta Derm Venereol. 1983;63:167-9.
8. Hogeling M, Frieden IJ. Segmental pigmentation disorder. Br J Dermatol. 2010;162:1337-41.
9. Rower JM, Carr RD, Lowney ED. Progressive cribriform and zosteriform hyperpigmentation. Arch Dermatol. 1978; 114:98-9.
10. Sardana K, Goel K, Chugh S. Reticulate pigmentary disorders. Indian J Dermatol. Venereol Leprol. 2013;79:17-29.
11. Somani VK, Razvi F, Sita VV. Pigmentary demarcation lines over the face. Indian J Dermatol Venereol Leprol. 2004; 70:336-41.
12. Lines RR, Hansen RC. A hyperpigmented, rippled eruption in a Hispanic woman. Macular amyloidosis. Arch Dermatol. 1997;133:383-6.
13. Panda S, Bandyopadhyay D, Tarafder A. Nephrogenic fibrosing dermopathy: a series in a non-Western population. J Am Acad Dermatol. 2006;54:155-9.
14. Polla BS, Merot Y, Saurat JH, et al. Flagellate pigmentation from bleomycin. J Am Acad Dermatol. 1986;14:690.
15. Centeno PG, Sanchez-Aguilar D, Pereiro M, et al. Flagellate erythema and dermatomyositis. Clin Exp Dermatol. 1998; 23:239-40.
16. Levantine A, Almeyda J. Drug induced changes in pigmentation. Br J Dermatol. 1973;89:105-12.
17. El-Darouti MA. Familial melanopathy with gigantic melanocytes. Am J Dermatopathol. 1984;6:31-4.
18. Markey AC, Black AK, Rycroft RJG. Confetti-like depigmentation from hydroquinone. Contact Dermatitis. 1989;20: 148-9.
19. Falabella R, Escobar CE, Carrascal E, et al. Leucoderma punctata. J Am Acad Dermatol. 1988;18:485-94.
20. Dogra S, Jain R, Parsad D, et al. Leukoderma punctatum following systemic PUVA therapy. Int J Dermatol. 2002;41: 922.
21. Laugier P, Hunziker N. Essential lenticular melanic pigmentation of the lip and cheek mucosa. Arch Belg Dermatol Syphiligr. 1970;26:391-9.
22. Carney IA. Carney complex: the complex of myxomas. Spotty pigmentation, endocrine overactivily and schwannomas. Semin Dermatol. 1995:14:90-8.
23. Banba K, Tanaka N, Fujioka A, et al. Hyperpigmentation caused by hyperthyroidism: differences from the pigmentation of Addison's disease. Clin Exp Dermatol. 1999; 24:196-8.
24. Hendrix JD, Greer KE. Cutaneous hyperpigmentation caused by systemic drugs. Int J Dermatol. 1992;31:458-66.

13

Pigmented Variants of Skin Disorders

Biju Vasudevan, Rajesh Verma, Ruby Venugopal

Key Features

- Pigmented variants exist for many skin disorders, and can be classified as mainly hypopigmented and hyperpigmented types.
- The pigmented variants offer various challenges to the dermatologist, especially in diagnosis.
- It is important to differentiate the pigmented benign tumors from melanoma as they offer different therapeutic challenges.

INTRODUCTION

Skin disorders distinguish themselves by captivating interest of the human mind because of the visible diagnosis and colorful images of characteristic clinical features. Pigmented variants of skin disorders are even more fascinating from the aspect that they are much more colorful, can mimic various other disorders and are diagnostically challenging. The important pigmented variants of skin disorders can be classified as given in **Table 1**.

Important features of these conditions are as follows:

HYPERPIGMENTED VARIANTS

Hyperpigmented Nevi

Pigmented Spindle Cell Nevus of Reed

It is a deeply pigmented variant of spindle cell nevus, first described in 1975.[1] It usually manifests on thighs as densely pigmented, irregularly shaped, dark isolated nodules. Histopathologically, they consist of fascicles of uniform spindle cells usually limited to epidermis and papillary dermis.

Pigmented Spitz Nevus

They are simulators of melanoma from clinical, dermatoscopic and histopathological viewpoints. They are usually larger than common nevi, have irregular outline, a scaly, crusted or eroded surface and may show variegated colors. Because these clinical features are also characteristic of congenital melancyctic nevi, they are often difficult to differentiate from each other.

Hyperpigmented Tumors

Benign

Pigmented seborrheic keratosis: About one-third of seborrheic keratoses is hyperpigmented **(Fig. 1)**. They show dendritic melanocytes containing large amount of cytoplasmic melanin, which is distributed between basaloid and squamous epithelial cells of conventional seborrheic keratosis. Heavily pigmented acanthotic seborrheic keratoses with melanocytic proliferation are termed melanoacanthomas. They are confused with malignant melanoma, melanocytic nevus, pigmented basal cell carcinoma (BCC) and angiokeratomas.

Pigmented actinic keratosis: First described in 1978 by James, pigmented actinic keratosis (PAK) have either a hyperpigmented or a reticulated appearance **(Fig. 2)**.[2] Located mainly on face, with size more than or equal to 15 mm, they usually have a brown color, smooth surface and radial spread. PAKs histologically comprises of hypertrophied melanocytes and dysplastic keratinocytes with large amounts of incontinent melanin inside the dermis making it difficult to differentiate from lentigo maligna. The hyperpigmentation of keratinocytes in PAK is probably due to melanocyte melanin transfer block or presence of melanophages in the upper corium owing to pigment incontinence.

Table 1: Classification of pigmented variants of skin disorders			
Types of pigmented variants	*Subtypes*	*Sub-subtypes*	*Disorders*
Hyperpigmented variants	Nevi	–	Pigmented spindle cell nevus Pigmented spitz nevus
	Tumors	Benign	Pigmented seborrheic keratosis Pigmented actinic keratosis Pigmented trichoblastoma Pigmented pilomatricoma Pigmented eccrine poroma Pigmented Bowen's disease Pigmented Paget's disease Pigmented dermatofibrosarcoma protruberans Pigmented neurofibroma Pigmented epitheloid melanocytoma
		Malignant	Pigmented basal cell carcinoma Pigmented squamous cell carcinoma Hyperpigmented mycosis fungoides
	Infections	–	Pigmented pityriasis versicolor Pigmented warts
	Others	–	Pigmented cosmetic dermatitis Lichen planus pigmentosus Pigmented purpuric mycosis fungoides Pigmented colloid milium Pigmented follicular cysts
Hypopigmented variants	–	–	Hypopigmented mycosis fungoides Hypopigmented sarcoidosis Leukoderma syphiliticum
Other variants	–	–	Poikilodermia mycosis fungoides

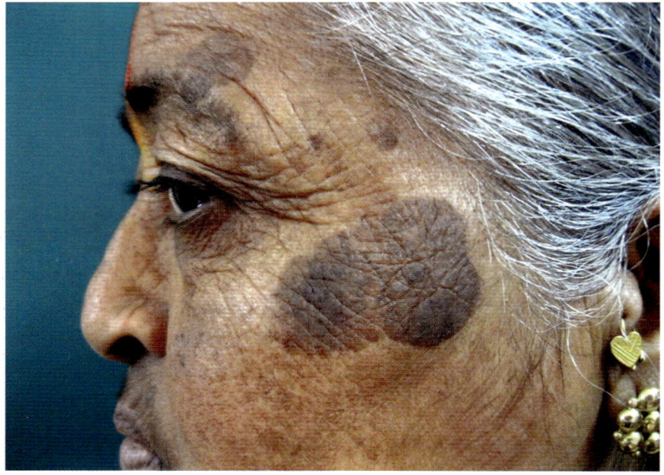

Fig. 1: Pigmented seborrheic keratosis

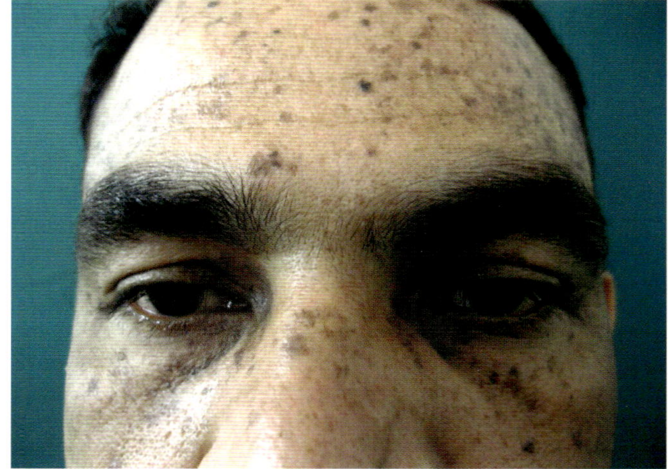

Fig. 2: Pigmented actinic keratosis

Pigmented trichoblastoma: They usually arise in nevus sebaceous, resemble malignant melanoma and are therefore referred to as "melanotrichoblastoma". They are very rare tumors with less than 10 reported cases and are usually benign. On immunohistochemistry (IHC), they show abundant dendritic melanocytes which have all the features of the hair follicle melanocytes, i.e. they express S-100 protein, gp100/HMB-45 and tyrosinase within tumor mass.[3]

Pigmented pilomatricoma: Pigmentation in a pilomatricoma is not rare and it occurs mainly due to secondary melanization of the matrical cells. Pigmented pilomatricomas do not exhibit prominent melanocytic hyperplasia while malignant melanoma exhibits a prominent proliferation of pigmented dendritic melanocyte. They give rise to appearance of "vanilla fudge cyst".

Pigmented eccrine poroma: The pigmented variant is more common in non-white races. Clinically, they are usually misdiagnosed as either malignant melanomas or pigmented BCCs.[4] In this tumor, melanin granules and melanocytes are dispersed. Melanocyte colonization of eccrine porocarcinoma has also been rarely described.[5]

Pigmented Bowen's disease: It is an unusual variant of Bowen's disease characterized by a hyperpigmented appearance and is exceedingly uncommon, representing less than 2% of reported cases of Bowen's disease.[6] It has been reported exclusively in the intertriginous areas, especially the anogenital region and is important because of its resemblance to malignant melanoma. It commonly presents as hyperpigmented, sharply marginated plaques with velvety, verrucous or flat surface. It has been linked etiologically to human papilloma virus infection. Differential diagnosis includes superficial spreading melanoma, pigmented BCC, bowenoid papulosis, melanocytic nevus and seborrheic keratosis.

In addition to features common to Bowen's disease, the pigmented form shows significant melanin within basal epidermal cells and highly dendritic non-neoplastic melanocytes within dermal melanophages.[7] Proposed mechanisms for the pigmented variant include increased temperature and natural hyperpigmentation of anogenital area where it is commonly found, neoplastic cells producing factors which induce melanocyte proliferation and stimulate melanin production. Few of them may also be arising from seborrheic keratoses. There is no difference in metastatic potential or therapeutic response in this variant.

Pigmented Paget's and extramammary Paget's disease: Pigmented Paget's disease (PD) is characterized by the presence of melanin pigment in Paget's cells or dendritic melanocytes within tumor nests and is a rare, distinct variant of PD.[8] Pigmented mammary PD was first described by Cuberson and Horn.[9] It is characterized by Paget's cells within epidermis having dusty melanin pigment along with intervening dendritic melanocytes. Paget's cells endocytose, the melanin pigment and thus distinction from malignant melanoma is very difficult without IHC aid.

Pigmented extramammary PD is characterized by intraepidermal Paget cells having melanin pigment which are surrounded by dendritic melanocytes. It is a very rare neoplasm with three documented cases so far.[10] Transfer of the melanin pigment from surrounding melanocytes to the carcinomatous cells and basic fibroblastic growth factor with other chemotactic factors which aid transfer of this pigment are blamed in the etiopathogenesis.[11] The diagnosis is confirmed by IHC through demonstration of cytokeratin expression, especially CK7, by the tumor cells.

Pigmented dermatofibrosarcoma protuberans: First described by Bednar, it is a low-grade fibrohistiocytic tumor which is indistinguishable from dermatofibrosarcoma protuberans (DFSP) except for the scattered non-neoplastic pigmented dendritic cells.[12] It accounts for fewer than 5% of all cases of DFSP and very rarely may undergo fibrosarcomatous transformation with distant metastasis.[13] It occurs in early adulthood or middle ages, predominantly affecting the trunk and proximal extremities and manifests as slow growing, firm plaques or nodules. It is also referred to as storiform neurofibroma because histologically, it is characterized by spindle-shaped cells occurring in a storiform pattern. Immunohistochemically, they are positive for CD34, negative for desmin, S-100 and factor XIIIa. There is strong evidence for a neural crest origin in the tumor cells. Mutation responsible for Bednar tumor occurs from rearrangement in chromosomes 17 and 22, producing a fusion protein which contains segments of collagen type 1 and platelet derived growth factor (COL1A1-PDGFB).

Pigmented neurofibroma: A variant of neurofibroma, it can be seen in patients with or without neurofibromatosis. It is characterized histologically by coexistence of scattered melanin-laden cells and benign spindle cells with neural differentiation. It is very difficult to differentiate it from the Bednar tumor. It is found in young adults, has a low local recurrence and is positive for S-100. Criteria proposed for pathological diagnosis of pigmented neurofibroma include: (1) low-power histopathological appearance typical of neurofibromas and (2) immunoreactivity to S-100 protein, HMB-45 antigen and CD34.[14]

Pigmented epithelioid melanocytoma: This term is used to refer to a spectrum of melanocytic tumors with metastatic potential and encompasses both animal type melanocytoma and the epithelioid blue nevus.[15] The tumor microscopically consists of three cell populations: (1) Polygonal cells with pigmented cytoplasm, (2) Epithelioid cells with melanin granules at the periphery and (3) Blue nevus like dendritic cells. These cells are positive for MART-1, HMB-45 and S-100 protein. They rarely demonstrate dermal fibrosis, cytological atypia or mitotic activity.

Some other pigmented variants of epithelial tumors described include pigmented apocrine hidrocystoma, pigmented nodular hidradenoma and Bowenoid papulosis.

Malignant Tumors

Pigmented basal cell carcinoma: This form of BCC may represent a wide range of proportion of total BCCs from

10% in Caucasians to 84% in Japanese.[16,17] Pigmentation is very unevenly distributed in pigmented BCCs on clinical examination **(Fig. 3)**. Melanocytes in this variant are large with hypertrophied dendritic processes, as evident on Fontana-Masson staining.[18] The melanocytes are morphologically active and the tumor cells do not phagocytose melanosome-containing dendrites resulting in blockage of transfer of melanosomes from the melanocytes to tumor cells. Down regulation of protease-activated receptor (PAR)-2 has been found to interrupt melanosome transfer in pigmented BCC probably by increasing secretion of melanogenic cytokines by the highly proliferating basaloid cells.[19] Endothelin-1 has also been implicated in the pigmentation process.

On dermoscopy, there is absence of pigmented network and in addition, one of the following six positive features may be present: large gray-blue ovoid nests, spoke wheel areas, multiple gray-blue globules, leaf-like areas, ulceration and arborizing "tree-like" telangiectasia.[20]

Histopathologically, it is characterized by dense melanin deposition within the melanocytes, neoplastic cells, macrophages and stroma.

Pigmented BCCs are more frequently excised with adequate margins. But, they may have a poorer therapeutic response following photodynamic therapy compared to other types.[21]

Pigmented squamous cell carcinoma in situ and squamous cell carcinoma: It is a very rare variant characterized by melanin deposition in malignant epithelial cells. It is proposed that the neoplastic epithelial cells obtain melanin granules from melanocytes like other epithelial cells. There is no difference in prognosis. A strongly positive cytokeratin stain with negative S-100 stain will help distinguishing it from melanoma.

Hyperpigmented mycosis fungoides: Hyperpigmented mycosis fungoides (MF) variant is characterized by presence of diffuse macular hyperpigmentation (like ashy dermatosis and acanthosis nigricans) **(Fig. 4)**. Histopathologically there is presence of abundant melanin in basal layer and spinous layer along with giant melanin granules in the neoplastic lymphocytes, keratinocytes, Langerhans' cells and melanocytes. The melanin granules in the Langerhans' cells are located within lysosomes or are encircled by the Langerhans' bodies, accounting for the hyperpigmentation.[22]

Hyperpigmented Variants of Cutaneous Infections

Pigmentary Pityriasis Versicolor

It refers to the hyperpigmented variety of pityriasis versicolor. In this variant, the stratum corneum is thicker and both the spores and hyphae are more numerous. Merkel cells are stimulated by the fungus to differentiate from epidermal cells and show increased activity by containing compound melanosomes along with secretory granules. Melanocytes are larger, singly distributed and usually hypertrophic. Both inflammation and increased melanocytes are blamed for the hyperpigmentation. Increased perivascular inflammation and lymphocytic infiltrate are also seen in this variant.

Pigmented Warts

It is a type of wart usually associated with the human papillomavirus types 4, 60 and 65 and is characterized by brown to black nodules or plaques **(Fig. 5)**.[23] Histologically,

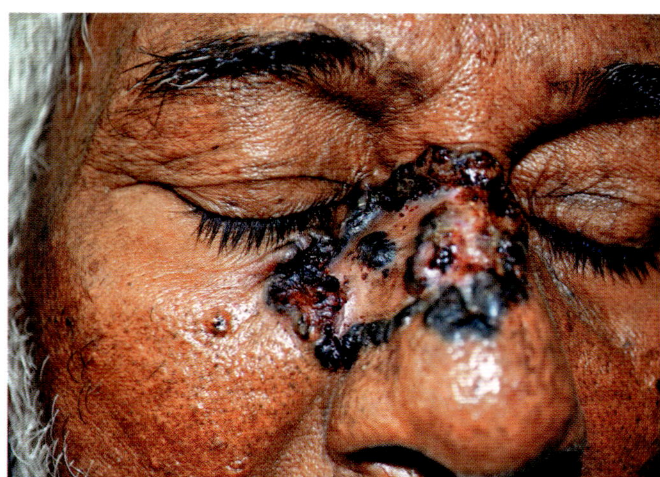

Fig. 3: Pigmented basal cell carcinoma

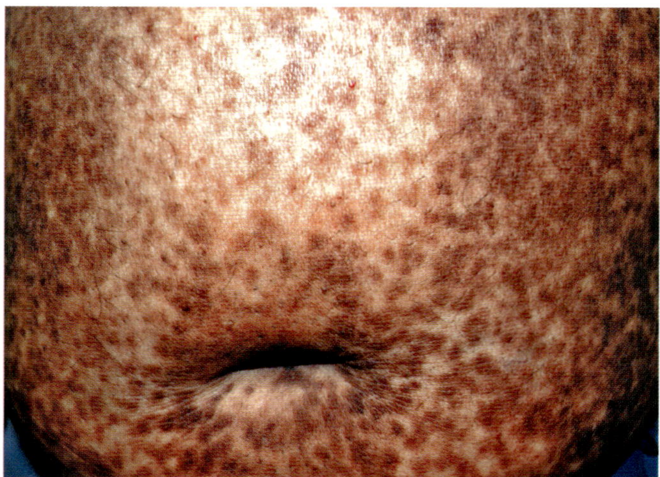

Fig. 4: Hyperpigmented mycosis fungoides

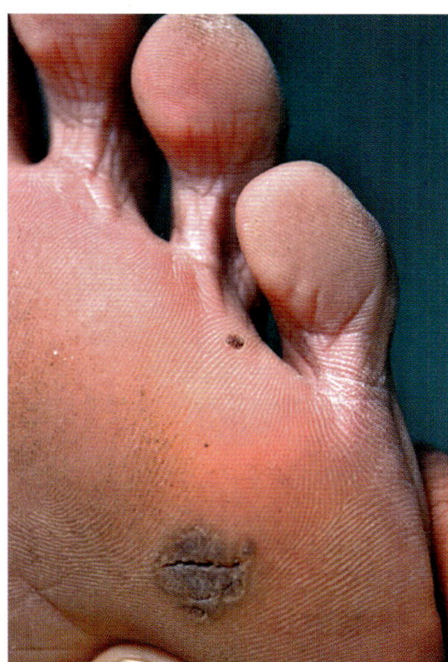

Fig. 5: Pigmented warts

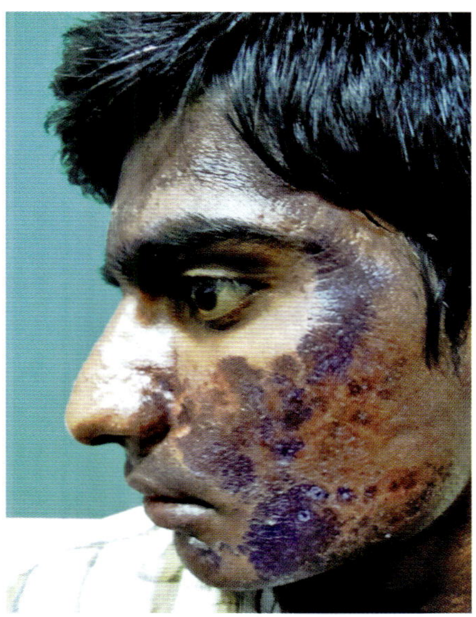

Fig. 6: Lichen planus pigmentosus

there is melanin blockade in melanocytes and also intracytoplasmic inclusion bodies, which are eosinophilic inclusion bodies inside keratinocytes. Dispersion of melanin granules in dendrites of melanocytes lead to blockade and increased melanin granules in keratinocytes may be responsible for the pigmentation in these warts. Pigmented anogenital warts resembling seborrheic keratosis have also been described.

Other Pigmented Variants

Pigmented Purpuric Mycosis Fungoides

Patients present with persistent pigmented purpuric lesions which are histologically characterized by a lichenoid band like infiltrate comprised of small cerebriform lymphocytes with substantial number of siderophages, extravasated red blood cells and few histiocytes. Majority of invading cells are CD4+ with few expressing CD8. Spongiosis and apoptosis are usually not seen.[24]

Lichen Planus Pigmentosus

Lichen planus pigmentosus (LPP), is a relatively rare variant of lichen planus (LP), characterized by the insidious onset of hyperpigmented, dark-brown macules mainly in areas exposed to the sun (especially, face and upper limbs and rarely trunk), with or without slight pruritus. It was first described by Bhutani et al. in 1974.[25] It usually starts in the third or fourth decade with a slight female predilection. Lesions initially starts as small, ill-defined, oval to round macules which later become confluent and form large areas of pigmentation, slate-gray to brown-black **(Fig. 6)**. The preauricular region (including temples and forehead) are predominantly involved first and present in almost all patients. Pigmentation is mostly diffuse or rarely reticular, linear, zosteriform, blaschkoid, perifollicular or generalized in pattern.

It is very common in Indian population. It has a chronic clinical course without pruritus or scalp, nail and mucosal involvement. Classical LP lesions accompany LPP, in about 25% of patients. LPP with predominant localization in the intertriginous areas is referred to as LPP inversus **(Fig. 7)**.[26]

Differential diagnosis include fixed drug eruption, acanthosis nigricans, erythema dyschromicum perstans, linear and whorled nevoid melanosis, incontinentia pigmenti, actinic LP, Riehl's melanosis, and other drug-related melanoses.

The characteristic histopathology findings are an atrophic epidermis, vacuolar alteration of basal cell layer, scarce lymphohistiocytic or lichenoid infiltrates in dermis along with pigmentary incontinence and presence of melanophages.[27]

In contrast to LP, the keratinocytes express focal weak immunoreaction to HLA-DR, which explains the absent or mild pruritus and minimal inflammation.

Drugs, increased sun exposure, internal malignancies, liver diseases, impaired carbohydrate metabolism, and black races, have all been proposed as pathogenesis of LPP.

Treatment is unsatisfactory in most cases. Drugs tried include, dimethylsulfoxide, topical and oral steroids, topical tacrolimus, retinoids and chloroquine with inconsistent results.

Pigmented Contact and Cosmetic Dermatitis

It was first described by Osmundsen.[28] It occurs mainly on covered areas and was first reported due to an optical whitener

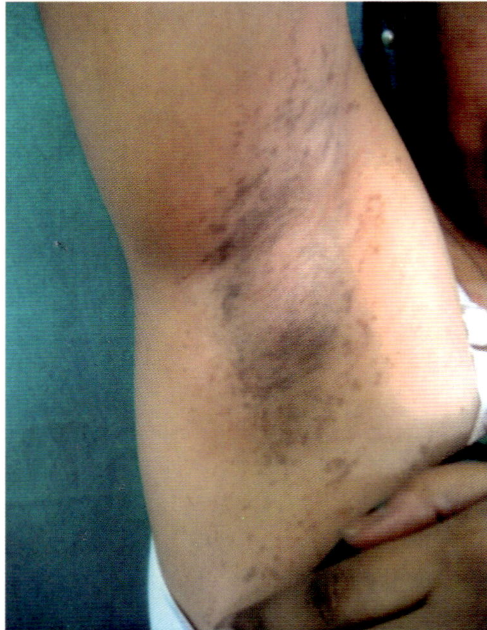

Fig. 7: Inverse lichen planus pigmentosus

used in washing powder. Other reported causes include: textile dyes, fungicides and color index blue. Pigmented cosmetic dermatitis mainly occurs in oriental women on the cheeks. Allergens associated are fragrances and soaps.[29] Pigmented cheilitis due to ricinoleic acid in castor oil used for lipsticks has been reported.[30] *Bindi* dermatitis due to *kumkum*, is another pigmented dermatitis.

Pigmented Colloid Milium

It is one among the four subtypes of adult colloid milium. It is associated with use of hydroquinone, i.e. exogenous ochronosis.[31]

Pigmented Follicular Cysts

They have predilection for the scalp and cervical areas and contain degenerated hair shafts which have turned into melanin like substance.[32]

HYPOPIGMENTED VARIANTS

HYPOPIGMENTED MYCOSIS FUNGOIDES

Hypopigmented MF is an uncommon variant of MF, first described by Ryan et al. in 1993 and seen usually in young darker skinned patients, mainly of African or Indian origin.[33,34] They present as asymptomatic or mildly itchy, nonscaling or scaly patches, with irregular borders mainly involving the trunk, especially the pelvic girdle **(Figs 8Aand B)**. They may be accompanied by typical patches, plaques or tumors of MF in few cases. They slowly progress over several years to finally involve wide areas on the body. Differential diagnosis includes: Pityriasis alba, pityriasis versicolor, vitiligo, sarcoidosis, leprosy and post-inflammatory hypopigmentation.

The histopathological findings are very similar to those of classical patch stage disease, as is the clinical course. There is marked epidermotropism when compared to the subtlety of the clinical features.

The hypopigmentation might result from decreased transfer of the melanosomes from melanocytes to keratinocytes or melanocyte degeneration as seen by electron microscopy. The neoplastic cells present in hypopigmented MF usually express CD8.[35] Suppressor CD8-positive T-lymphocytes destroy melanocytes by destabilization and there is decreased expression of CD117. IHC also reveals loss of CD7+ cells. Tumor necrosis factor-α and decreased basic fibroblast growth factor mRNA expression has also been reported.[36]

Khopkar et al. have described hypopigmented MF in a large series of 15 Indian patients wherein they found that the variant was common in males between second and fourth decades with average disease duration of 3 83 years.[37] Disproportionate epidermotropism, tagging of lymphocytes, halolymphocytes, dermal papillary fibrosis and monomorphous infiltrate were found to be characteristic of hypopigmented MF in this study.[38]

Hypopigmented MF usually has better prognosis than the conventional MF. They respond well to photochemotherapy and topical immunotherapy like nitrogen mustard and carmustine. Recurrence is, however, common. Perifollicular repigmentation may occur in response to treatment of such cases. In addition, when typical MF lesions are treated with psoralen plus ultraviolet A (PUVA), vitiligo-like lesions may occur.[39]

Hypopigmented Sarcoidosis

It is an unusual variant of cutaneous sarcoidosis characterized by macular hypopigmentation or hypopigmented areas around indurated lesions. They mainly occur on extremities and range in size from 0.2 to 1 cm. Histologically, they resemble other cutaneous sarcoid lesions. The melanocytes show degeneration under electron microscopy and the condition is unresponsive to corticosteroids. PUVA is the treatment of choice.

Leukoderma Syphiliticum

Macular syphilids are the earliest manifestations of secondary syphilis. When these macular rashes are fading, they sometimes leave a pattern consisting of depigmented spots on a hyperpigmented background. This is referred to as leukoderma syphiliticum. When such a pattern manifests itself on the back or sides of neck, it used to be referred to as the "necklace of Venus".

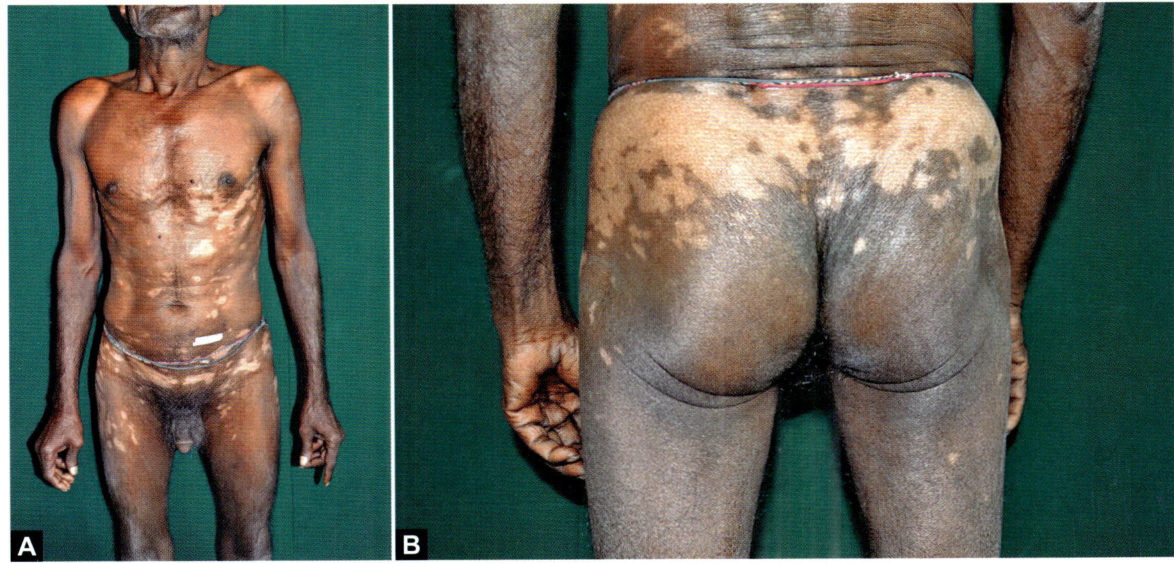

Figs 8A and B: Hypopigmented mycosis fungoides

OTHER PIGMENTARY VARIANTS

Poikilodermic Mycosis Fungoides

It usually develops in patients with otherwise typical lesions of MF and is characterized by alternating hypo- and hyperpigmentation, atrophy and telangiectasia, i.e. features of poikiloderma atrophicans vasculare. The lesions develop at sites of the pre-existing patches, especially in areas where skin is rubbed by the clothes. Generalized poikiloderma may also occur. Additional histopathological changes include epidermal atrophy with flattening and loss of rete ridges, vacuolar alteration of basal layer with pigment loss, increased melanophages in papillary and the upper reticular dermis and also dilatation of superficial blood vessels.[4]

Nonpigmenting Fixed Drug Eruption

A distinct variety of fixed drug eruption (FDE) characterized by large, symmetrical, well-defined, tender, erythematous plaques which appears and disappears on the same site has been described by Shelley and Shelley in 1987.[40] These lesions usually fade without any pigmentation over a period of 2-3-weeks. It has therefore been named as nonpigmenting FDE. It has been reported with various drugs, like paracetamol, pseudoephidrine, piroxicam, cimetidine thiopental, betahistine and cotrimoxazole and radiocontrast media.[41,42] Microscopic findings in this variant includes, a normal epidermis along with a perivascular infiltrate of lymphocytes, neutrophils and eosinophils. There is no hydropic degeneration of basal cell layer or dermal melanophages as seen in the usual pigmenting variety. So the site of drug hypersensitivity in nonpigmenting FDE may be the dermis rather than epidermis. Solitary lesions like in classic pigmenting FDE have also been described. This entity has been described as it is a rare nonpigmented variant of a pigmentary disorder.

CONCLUSION

Pigmented variants of numerous skin disorders exist both in practice and literature. It is important to distinguish them, especially the benign pigmented tumors from melanoma. These pigmented variants are not only visually fascinating, but are also diagnostically challenging and therefore are important subsets of pigmentary disorders.

REFERENCES

1. Reed RJ, Ichinose H, Clark WH, et al. Common and uncommon melanocytic nevi and borderline melanomas. Semin Oncol. 1975;2(2):119-47.
2. James MP, Wells GC, Whimster IW. Spreading pigmented actinic keratoses. Br J Dermatol. 1978;98(4):373-9.
3. Kanitakis J, Brutzkus A, Butnaru AC, et al. Melanotrichoblastoma: immunohistochemical study of a variant of pigmented trichoblastoma. Am J Dermatopathol. 2002;24(6): 498-501.
4. Mousawi A, Kibbi AG. Pigmented eccrine poroma: a simulant of nodular melanoma. Int J Dermatol. 1995;34(12):857-8.
5. Nakanishi Y, Matsuno Y, Shimoda T, et al. Eccrine porocarcinoma with melanocyte colonization. Br J Dermatol. 1998;138(3):519-21.
6. Ragi G, Turner MS, Klein LE, et al. Pigmented Bowen's disease and review of 420 Bowen's disease lesions. J Dermatol Surg Oncol. 1988;14(7):765-9.
7. Papageorgiou PP, Koumarianou AA, Chu AC. Pigmented Bowen's disease. Br J Dermatol. 1998;138(3):515-8.

8. Petersson F, Ivan D, Kazakov DV, et al. Pigmented Paget disease: a diagnostic pitfall mimicking melanoma. Am J Dermatopathol. 2009;31(3):223-6.
9. Cuberson JD, Horn RC. Paget's disease of the nipple: review of twenty-five cases with special references to melanin pigmentation of Page cells. AMA Arch Surg. 1956;72(2):224-31.
10. Chiba H, Kazama T, Takenouchi T, et al. Two cases of vulval pigmented extramammary Paget's disease: histochemical and immunohistochemical studies. Br J Dermatol. 2000;142(6):1190-4.
11. Saitoh K, Saga K, Okazaki M, et al. Pigmented primary carcinoma of the breast: a clinical mimic of malignant melanoma. Br J Dermatol. 1998;139(2):287-90.
12. Bednar B. Storiform neurofibromas of the skin, pigmented and nonpigmented. Cancer. 1957;10(2):368-76.
13. Suehara Y, Yazawa Y, Hitachi K. Metastatic Bednar tumor (pigmented dermatofibrosarcoma protuberans) with fibrosarcomatous change: a case report. J Orthop Sci. 2004; 9(6):662-5.
14. Fetsch JF, Michal M, Mittinen M. Pigmented (melanotic) neurofibroma: a clinicopathologic and immunohistochemical analysis of 19 lesions from 17 patients. Am J Surg Pathol. 2000;24(3):331-43.
15. Zembowicz A, Carney JA, Mihm MC. Pigmented epithelioid melanocytoma: a low-grade melanocytic tumor with metastatic potential indistinguishable from animal-type melanoma and epithelioid blue nevus. Am J Surg Pathol. 2004;28(1):31-40.
16. Kikuchi A, Shimizu H, Nishikawa T. Clinical and histopathological characteristics of basal cell carcinoma in Japanese patients. Arch Dermatol. 1996;132(3):320-4.
17. Betti R, Gualandri L, Cerri A, et al. Clinical features and histologic pattern analysis of pigmented basal cell carcinomas in an Italian population. J Dermatol. 1998;25(10): 691-4.
18. Maloney ME, Jones DB, Sexton FM. Pigmented basal cell carcinoma: investigation of 70 cases. J Am Acad Dermatol. 1992;27(1):74-8.
19. Sakuraba K, Hayashi N, Kawashima M, et al. Down-regulated PAP-2 is associated in part with interrupted melanosome transfer in pigmented basal cell epithelioma. Pigment Cell Res. 2004;17(4):371-8.
20. Menzies SW, Westerhoff K, Rabinovitz H, et al. Surface microscopy of pigmented basal cell carcinoma. Arch Dermatol. 2000;136(8):1012-6.
21. Kaviani A, Ataie-Fashtami L, Fateh M, et al. Photodynamic therapy of head and neck basal cell carcinoma according to different clinicopathologic features. Lasers Surg Med. 2005;36(5):377-82.
22. David M, Shanon A, Hazaz B et al. Diffuse, progressive hyperpigmentation: an unusual skin manifestation of mycosis fungoides. J Am Acad Dermatol. 1987;16(1 Pt 2): 257-60.
23. Egawa K, Honda Y, Inaba Y, et al. Pigmented viral warts: a clinical and histopathological study including human papillomavirus typing. Br J Dermatol. 1998;138(3):381-9.
24. Georgala S, Katoulis AC, Symeonidou S, et al. Persistent pigmented purpuric eruption associated with mycosis fungoides: a case report and review of the literature. J Eur Acad Dermatol Venereol. 2001;15(1):62-4.
25. Bhutani LK, Bedi TR, Pandhi RK, et al. Lichen planus pigmentosus. Dermatologica. 1974;149(1):43-50.
26. Pock L, Jelinkova L, Drlik L, et al. Lichen planus pigmentosus-inversus. J Eur Acad Dermatol Venereol. 2001;15(5):452-4.
27. Kanwar AJ, Dogra S, Handa S, et al. A study of 124 Indian patients with lichen planus pigmentosus. Clin Exp Dermatol. 2003;28(5):481-5.
28. Osmundsen PE. Contact dermatitis due to an optical whitener in washing powders. Br J Dermatol. 1969;81(11):799-803.
29. Nakayama H, Matsuo S, Hayakawa K, et al. Pigmented cosmetic dermatitis. Int J Dermatol. 1984;23(5):299-305.
30. Leow YH, Tan SH, Ng SK. Pigmented contact cheilitis from ricinoleic acid in lipsticks. Contact Dermatitis. 2003;49(1): 48-9.
31. Findlay GH, Morrison JG, Simson IW. Exogenous ochronosis and pigmented colloid milium from hydroquinone bleaching creams. Br J Dermatol. 1975;93(6):613-22.
32. Requena Caballero L, Sanchez Yus E. Pigmented follicular cyst. J Am Acad Dermatol. 1989;21(5 Pt 2):1073-5.
33. Handfield-Jones SE, Smith NP, Breathnach SM. Hypopigmented mycosis fungoides. Clin Exp Dermatol. 1992; 17(5):374-5.
34. Ryan EA, Sanderson KV, Barták P, et al. Can mycosis fungoides begin in the epidermis? A hypothesis. Br J Dermatol. 1973;88(5):419-29.
35. El-Shabrawi-Caelen L, Cerroni L, Medeiros LJ, et al. Hypopigmented mycosis fungoides: frequent expression of a CD8+ T-cell phenotype. Am J Surg Pathol. 2002;26(4):450-7.
36. Seif El Nasr H, Shaker OG, Fawzi MM, et al. Basic fibroblast growth factor and tumour necrosis factor alpha in vitiligo and other hypopigmented disorders: suggestive possible therapeutic targets. J Eur Acad Dermatol Venereol. 2013; 27(1):103-8.
37. Khopkar U, Doshi BR, Dongre AM, et al. A study of clinicopathologic profile of 15 cases of hypopigmented mycosis fungoides. Indian J Dermatol Venereol Leprol. 2011;77(2):167-73.
38. Koorse S, Tirumalae R, Yeliur IK, et al. Clinicopathologic profile of hypopigmented mycosis fungoides in India. Am J Dermatopathol. 2012;34(2):161-4.
39. Mimouni D, David M, Feinmesser M, et al. Vitiligo-like leucoderma during photochemotherapy for mycosis fungoides. Br J Dermatol. 2001;145(6):1008-14.
40. Shelley WB, Shelley ED. Non-pigmenting fixed drug eruption as a distinctive reaction pattern: examples caused by sensitivity to pseudoephedrine hydrochloride and tetrahydrozoline. J Am Acad Dermatol. 1987;17(3):403-7.
41. Galindo PA, Borja J, Feo F, et al. Non-pigmented fixed drug eruption caused by paracetamol. J Investig Allergol Clin Immunol. 1999;9(6):399-400.
42. Montoro J, Diaz M, Genis C, et al. Non-pigmenting cutaneous–mucosal fixed drug eruption due to piroxicam. Allergol Immunopathol (Madr). 2003;31(1):53-5.

14

Vitiligo and Melanocyte Reservoir

Rafael Falabella, Maria I Barona

Key Features

- Repigmentation in vitiligo is accomplished under appropriate stimulation, with topical or systemic medications and/or ultraviolet radiation. Nevertheless for an adequate response a melanocyte reservoir should be present. This reservoir has been found within the bulge, where stem cells are in a privileged location, away from immune attacks.
- The bulge, is a small protuberance located in the middle portion of the external root sheath of the hair follicle between the sebaceous gland and the insertion of the *arrector pili* muscle. Undifferentiated pigment stem cells within the bulge, when stimulated by diverse therapies, undergo cell multiplication, migration and neomelanogenesis that replenish the basal cell layer of the epidermis devoid of melanocytes damaged during vitiligo depigmentation.
- Recent findings including: (a) Stem cells related to keratinocytes found in the deep rete ridges of interfollicular skin, also present in palms and soles, (b) multipotent dermal stem cells from neonatal foreskin which may differentiate into multiple cell lineages including melanocytes expressing melanocyte markers, and (c) a common pluripotent progenitor for different cell types including melanocytes present in the early cephalic neural crest, support the concept of melanocyte stem cells present in epidermal and dermal tissues and not exclusively located in the bulge region of the hair follicle. These findings are in favor of a melanocyte reservoir as an evolving concept, still under construction.

INTRODUCTION

Destruction of melanocytes is well known in vitíligo due to the constant attack to melanocytes with autoantibodies, immune cells and multiple reactive molecules,[1] or inflammation;[2] however, depigmentation mechanisms are complex and the etiology is not completely known. The prevailing hypothesis is that genetically affected individuals are increasingly prone to damage affecting melanocytes, which evokes an immune response targeting melanocytes antigens that leads to depigmentation.[3]

The concept of a melanocyte reservoir evolved from observing that depigmented skin was able to achieve a normal pigmentation with different treatments suggesting that mature or immature melanocyte precursors should be present within anatomical structures of depigmented skin **(Figs 1 and 2)**. Because of diffused or spotted, perifollicular, or marginal repigmentation[4] occurring in vitiligo lesions, good candidates for a reservoir of melanocytes or its precursors were the epidermis or hair follicle units.

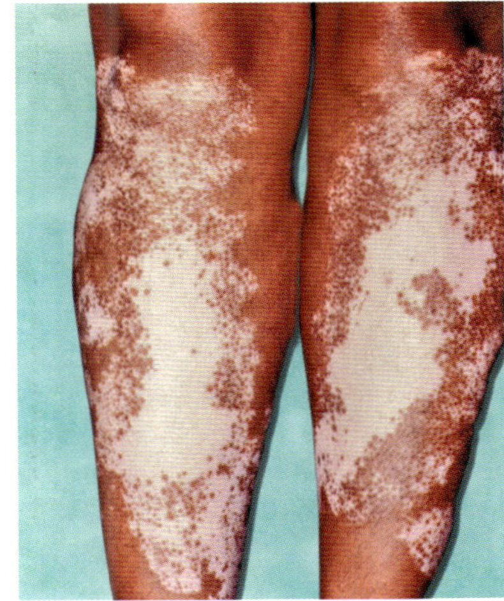

Fig. 1: Non-segmental vitiligo: A 28-year-old woman with bilateral lesions of the legs shows an early response with NB-UVB with a perifollicular pattern illustrating the role of hair follicles in repigmentation

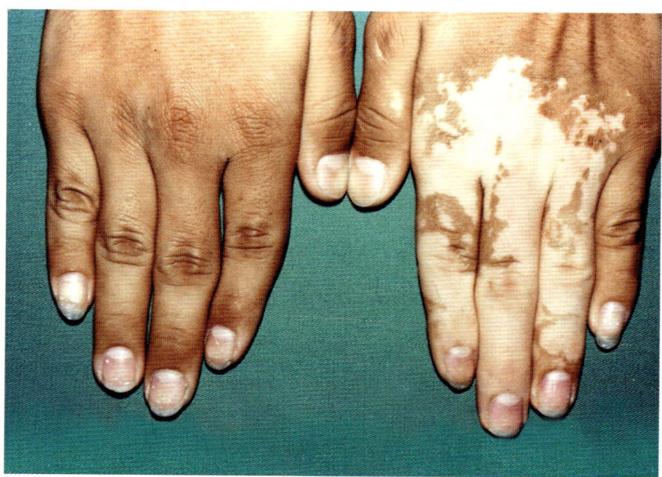

Fig. 2: Segmental vitiligo: A 34-year-old woman with segmental vitiligo of left hand discloses minimal repigmentation after treatment with targeted NB-UVB phototherapy, mostly in hairless areas.

HISTORICAL HIGHLIGHTS ON SKIN PIGMENTATION

During renaissance Andreas Vesalius (1514–1564) noticed that after producing a burn on a living subject the skin was composed of two layers.[5] Riolan the Younger (1580–1657) experimenting with a vesicant substance on the skin of a black individual separated the dark upper layer or "cuticle" (epidermis) from the lower layer or "cutis" that was as "white as snow" (dermis).[5] Marcello Malpighi (1628–1694), detached the "cuticle" (epidermis) from the "cutis" (dermis) by the putrefaction technique of a skin fragment during 4 days and found that skin color was present between the "cuticle and cutis".[5] Gaultier M in France as cited by James C Prichard (1786–1848),[6] noticed that after using a vesicant on the skin of a black subject the skin color reappeared after healing in a perifollicular pattern suggesting that hair follicles were somehow linked to repigmentation. Next, Giousue Sangiovanni (1775–1849) discovered the pigment producing cells in the squid that he labeled "chromatophores".[5] Friedrich Henle (1809–1885) confirmed the presence of such cells in human epidermis which were similar to the pigment cells in the eye.[5] Moritz Kaposi (1837–1902) observed for the first time that pigment cells were lacking in the rete pegs of vitiligo.[5] And finally, Bruno Bloch (1878–1933) described the dihydroxyphenylalanine (DOPA) reaction demonstrating the role of tyrosinase to produce melanin granules for skin pigmentation.[5] Since the beginning of Renaissance, four centuries elapsed before confirmation that a pigment producing cell was responsible for skin color, that repigmentation could arise from hair follicle units, and also that melanocytes were absent in vitiligo lesions.

CONCEPT OF A MELANOCYTE RESERVOIR

Initial Observations

From observing perifollicular and spotted repigmentation after therapy in vitiligo, investigators suspected that a source of melanocytes or related precursor cells should be present in the epidermis or hair follicles to provide pigment when pigment cell killing or senescence occurred.

During the past 5 decades up to present, significant findings about pigment cell structure, gene characterization, physiology, physiopathology, bio-molecular structure and repigmentation with diverse therapies were achieved; nevertheless in spite of this progress there are still important unknown data about the complete sequence of mechanisms that initiate and maintain melanocyte destruction in vitiligo.[7]

Melanocyte Patterns of Repigmentation

Three repigmentation patterns may be observed in vitiligo: (1) perifollicular, around each hair follicle unit with new melanocytes migrating 2–5 mm centrifugally, with remarkable repigmentation yield in relation to the very small diameter of hair follicles **(Fig. 3)**; (2) diffuse, with an even appearance or arising as small spotted islands several mm in size, unrelated to hair follicles, originating from unharmed melanocytes at random sites within vitiligo lesions **(Fig. 4)**; (3) marginal, where pigment cells spread 2–4 mm from the edges of normally pigmented skin[5] **(Fig. 5)**; these patterns have also been shown to depend upon therapy types: (a) perifollicular with topical and systemic psoralen-ultraviolet A (PUVA); (b) diffuse with topical corticosteroids and (c) marginal, with systemic PUVA and topical calcipotriol.[4] In addition, narrow band-ultraviolet B (NB-UVB) shows the best rates of perifollicular repigmentation.[8]

Searching for a Melanocyte Reservoir

Staricco in 1959 demonstrated amelanotic melanocytes located in the external root sheath of hair follicles which were interpreted as immature melanocytes migrating towards depigmented epidermis.[9] Later on, Ortonne et al. in 1979 when treating vitiligo patients with PUVA found DOPA negative, non-dendritic pigment cells on the external root sheath migrating to the epidermis and proposed the concept of a hair follicle melanocyte reservoir.[10] Cui et al. in 1991 described similar cells in the outer root sheath migrating towards the epidermis in vitiligo patients under treatment which correlated with perifollicular repigmentation.[11] Experimentally, after transplantation of the lower half of scalp follicles into depigmented vitiligo skin, DOPA positive cells in repigmented epidermis were found, suggesting a melanocyte

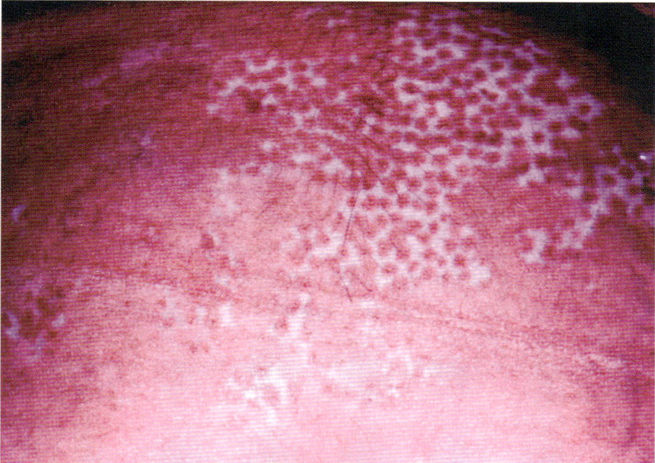

Fig. 3: Perifollicular repigmentation pattern: Numerous 4–5 mm repigmented spots around hair follicle units are seen in a patient with non-segmental vitiligo under NB-UVB therapy. Coalescence of spots will eventually repigment the entire treated area

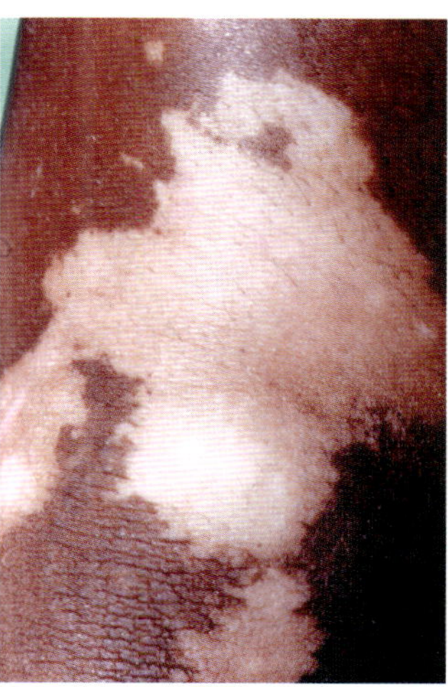

Fig. 4: Diffuse repigmentation pattern: A diffuse pigmentation on the knee of this 14-year-old girl with vitiligo vulgaris is observed 3 months after initiation of therapy with NB-UVB

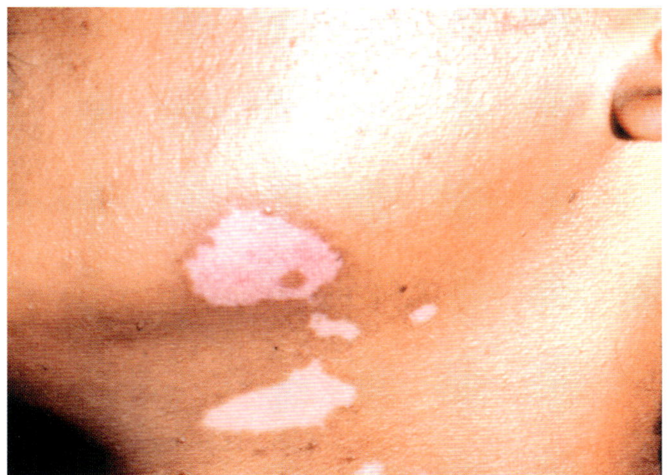

Fig. 5: Marginal repigmentation pattern: Repigmentation at the periphery of two vitiligo macules on the face and neck of this 16-year-old boy with segmental vitiligo, disclose a 3–4 mm repigmentation rim at the edge of lesions

reservoir in the lower half of the hair follicle.[12] In addition, pigment cell precursors were reported in 1996 by Grichnik et al. as numerous immature dendritic, tyrosynase negative but c-kit positive cells around the follicular ostium and to a lesser extent in the rete pegs and external root sheath, suggesting a possible source of pigment cells able to provide epidermal repigmentation when needed.[13]

HAIR FOLLICLE AND THE MELANOCYTE RESERVOIR

Histological Structure and Physiology

Hair follicles begin during the third month of embryonic life as the dermal papilla, with more than 20 different cell types and six compartments: dermal papilla with fibroblasts, connective tissue sheath, outer root sheath, inner root sheath, hair shaft and sebaceous gland.[14]

The completely developed and mature hair follicle is composed of an upper segment which remains as permanent and a lower segment that changes by remodeling its structure during hair cycles: (a) anagen, a growth stage generating the hair shaft, inner and outer root sheaths and hair matrix; (b) catagen with cell apoptosis and epithelial regression; (c) telogen, or resting stage with inactive cells.[15] Large, dendritic, tyrosynase positive melanocytes in the hair bulb provide pigmentation for hair shafts.

Bulge the Niche and Melanocyte Stem Cells

Stem cell in mammals has the ability of: (1) differentiate into specialized embryonic tissues and (2) being present in adult tissues regenerating to maintain normal cell turnover. Stem cells must be immature, self-maintaining, slow cycling and competent to regenerate their same cell progeny.[16] All stem

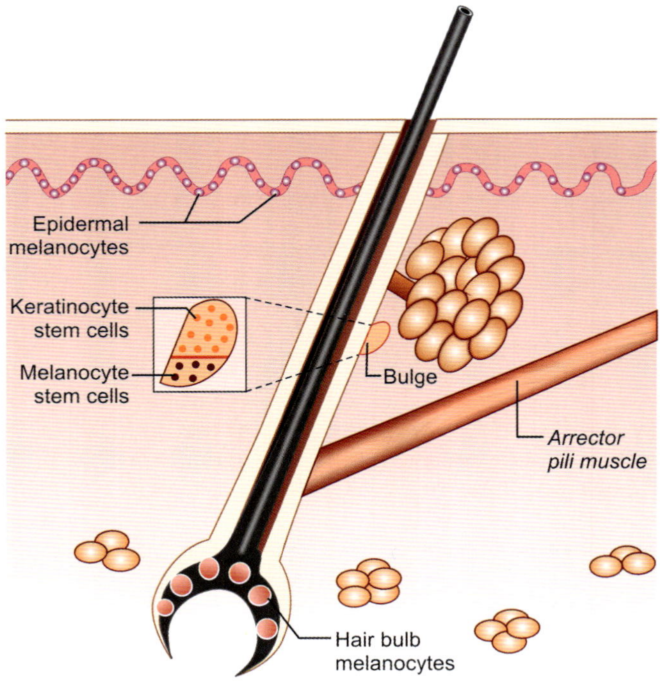

Fig. 6: The bulge and melanocyte reservoir

cell types are located within different organs in specific sites known as the "niche", providing specific signals to guide their function. The niche for melanocyte stem cells was found in the bulge, located in the outer root sheath at the insertion of the *arrector pili* muscle where epidermal stem cells also have their niche[17-19] **(Fig. 6)**, and are activated during early anagen. Stem cells in scalp hair follicles have been found in a site of relative immune privilege against autoimmune aggression;[20] this "immune sanctuary" could be the reason for finding pigmented hairs within vitiligo lesions.

Hair Cycling and Melanogenesis

Hair melanocytes located in the bulb are very active; melanogenesis and transfer of melanin granules are regulated by several enzymes, regulatory proteins, transporters, receptors and their ligands related to all physiological stages of hair follicles. During a new hair cycle melanogenesis is closely bound and coupled to the anagen stage of the hair follicle which gives rise to a normally pigmented hair until the next catagen stage begins and melanocytes undergo apoptosis remaining absent through telogen; at this time another hair cycle begins and stem cells at the niche give rise to melanocyte proliferation and migration again, a mechanism repeating periodically during each hair cycle.[21]

In addition, melanogenesis is modulated by melanocortin-1 receptor, adrenocorticotropic hormone (ACTH), melanocyte stimulating hormone (MSH), agouti protein ligands, c-Kit and endothelin receptor (ET-1).[21]

Pro-inflammatory Cytokines

During repigmentation of vitiligo two melanocyte functions are important, (1) neo-melanogenesis with production of new melanin granules and (2) melanocyte migration which requires pigment cells displacement towards the depigmented basal cell layer.[5]

Available melanocytes from a viable reservoir is a first step to initiate repigmentation; however, additional stimuli are necessary to continue this process and several cytokines have been shown *in vitro* to have important effects on melanocytes: (1) prostaglandin D2 (PGD2), leukotriene B4 (LTB4), leukotriene C4 (LTC4), leukotriene E4 (LTE4), leukotriene D4 (LTD4), thromboxane B2 and hydroxyeicosatetraenoic (HETE) produce increased dendricity and high levels of tyrosinase;[22] (2) transforming growth factor α (TGF-α), basic fibroblast growth factor (bFGF), stem cell factor (SCF) and ET-1, increase melanocyte migration;[23,24] LTB4, LTC4, ET-1, and epidermal growth factor (EGF) produce both effects. Considering this cytokine activity, it would not be surprising that these molecules would be used in the future as therapeutic tools to stimulate melanogenesis and melanocyte migration in vitiligo.[5]

Role of Ultraviolet Radiation

Two major effects with ultraviolet radiation (UVR) have been observed in vitiligo:

1. Immunosuppression, preventing destruction of melanocytes; activation of T-regulatory cells under effects of UVB and UVA may attenuate autoimmune activity;[25] NB-UVB is more effective than broad band UVB because of a higher response of natural killer cells, cytokines and lympho-proliferation.[26]
2. Stimulation of proliferation and migration of residual melanocytes in vitiligo skin or those present within follicle reservoirs by UVR via increased production of melanocyte growth factors; in a study when patients were treated with PUVA, their sera were found to contain higher levels of bFGF, SCF and hepatocyte growth factor (HGF) which may have increased melanocyte proliferation.[27] Furthermore, in vitiligo, melanocyte proliferation after UVR may occur by stimulation with ET-1 and bFGF;[28,29] in addition, a single UVB overexposure has been shown to induce melanocyte proliferation.[30] Finally, metalloproteinase 2 in culture has been shown to induce melanocyte migration under PUVA stimulation.[31]

MELANOCYTE RESERVOIR UNRELATED TO HAIR FOLLICLES

A population of stem cells related to keratinocytes was found in the deep rete ridges of interfollicular skin of breast, palms and soles;[32] moreover, differentiation of other human skin stem cells into functional melanocytes may also occur,[33] and this could explain repigmentation observed in palmar skin of some patients following NB-UVB or PUVA for vitiligo,[34] and in other areas devoid of hair follicles. In addition, multipotent dermal stem cells from neonatal foreskin which may differentiate into multiple cell lineages and also melanocytes have been described; these cells can migrate to the epidermal basement membrane where they differentiate as mature melanocytes, expressing melanocyte markers, and suggesting that dermal stem cells may become part of normal melanocytes present in the epidermis.[35] More recently, a common pluripotent progenitor for different cell types including melanocytes present in the early cephalic neural crest has been found, reinforcing the concept of a stem cell model for embryogenesis and also in adult tissues to maintain homeostasis.[36] These findings support the concept of melanocyte stem cells present in epidermal and dermal tissues and not exclusively located in the bulge region of the hair follicle.

LEUKOTRICHIA A DEPLETED MELANOCYTE RESERVOIR

White hairs within vitiligo lesions develop frequently, occurring in segmental vitiligo within a few months **(Fig. 7)** after onset as compared with vitiligo vulgaris, where it is less common although leukotrichia may also occur in long standing, widespread, progressive and persisting non-segmental lesions. Once established, leukotrichia suggests that the melanocyte

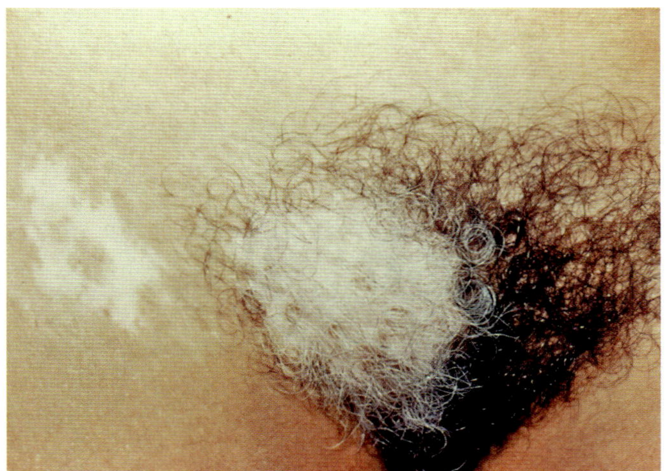

Fig. 7: Leukotrichia: A 23-year-old woman with segmental vitiligo discloses white hairs whose depigmentation occurred 4 months after vitiligo developed. Repigmentation with medical therapy is very unlikely

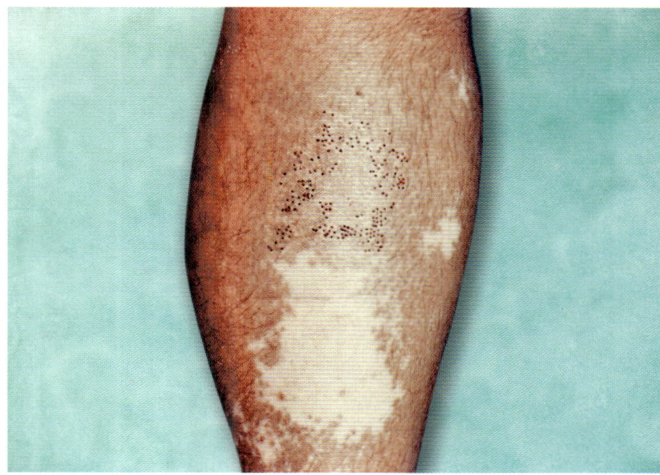

Fig. 8: Repigmentation with minigrafting: A 34-year-old woman with non-segmental vitiligo of the legs shows 50% repigmentation of depigmented areas with minigrafting after lack of response to previous medical treatment. Recently, 1.0 mm minigrafts were implanted to treat residual depigmentation

reservoir is depleted of melanocytes in which case restoration of pigmentation is very unlikely with medical therapy and melanocyte transplantation may be indicated[37,38] **(Fig. 8)**. On the contrary, the presence of pigmented hairs in vitiligo lesions is a good prognostic sign for repigmentation success with appropriate therapy. The observation of leukotrichia appearing after intense light therapy for hair removal suggests that if performed in patients with vitiligo, melanocyte reservoirs may be definitely eliminated and repigmentation may not be possible in treated areas.[39]

CONCLUSION

Repigmentation in vitiligo is dependent upon the integrity of a melanocyte reservoir; its presence within the hair follicle structure and possibly together with stem cells in the interfollicular epidermis or even in the dermis is essential, but the complementary action of UVR exposure, pro-inflammatory cytokines, growth factors and hormones are necessary to stimulate such stem cells and unharmed pigment cells in the epidermis and hair follicles to produce neo-melanogenesis and cell migration. Further studies are necessary for halting vitiligo progression and for stimulating more effectively stem cells to improve therapeutic outcomes.

REFERENCES

1. Nordlund JJ, Ortonne JP. Vitiligo vulgaris. In: Nordlund JJ, Boissy RE, Hearing VJ, King RA, Ortonne JP (Eds). The pigmentary system: Physiology and pathophysiology. New York: Oxford University Press; 1998. pp. 513-51.
2. Ezzedine K, Diallo A, Léauté-Labrèze C, et al. Multivariate analysis of factors associated with early-onset segmental

and nonsegmental vitiligo: a prospective observational study of 213 patients. Br J Dermatol. 2011;165:44-9.

3. Falabella R, Barona MI. Update on skin repigmentation therapies in vitiligo. Pigment Cell Melanoma Res. 2009;22:42-65.
4. Parsad D, Pandhi R, Dogra S, et al. Clinical study of repigmentation patterns with different treatment modalities and their correlation with speed and stability of repigmentation in 352 vitiliginous patches. J Am Acad Dermatol. 2004;50:63-7.
5. Falabella R. Vitiligo and the melanocyte reservoir. Indian J Dermatol. 2009;54:313-3177.
6. Prichard JC. Researches into the physical history of man. London: John & Arthur Arch; 1913. pp. 238-9.
7. Taïeb A. Intrinsic and extrinsic pathomechanisms in vitiligo. Pigment Cell Res. 2000;13:41-7.
8. Yang YS, Cho HR, Ryou JH, et al. Clinical study of repigmentation patterns with either narrow-band ultraviolet B (NB UVB) or 308 nm excimer laser treatment in Korean vitiligo patients. Int J Dermatol. 2010; 49:317-23.
9. Staricco RG. Amelanotic melanocytes in the outer sheath of the human hair follicle. J Invest Dermatol. 1959;33:295-7.
10. Ortonne JP, MacDonald DM, Micoud A, et al. PUVA induced repigmentation of vitiligo: A histochemical (split-DOPA) and ultrastructural study. Br J Dermatol. 1979;101:1-12.
11. Cui J, Shen LY, Wang GC. Role of hair follicles in the repigmentation of vitiligo. J Invest Dermatol. 1991;97:410-6.
12. Arrunátegui A, Arroyo C, Garcia L, et al. Melanocyte reservoir in vitiligo. Int J Dermatol. 1994;33:484-7.
13. Grichnik JM, Ali WN, Burch JA, et al. KIT expression reveals a population of precursor melanocytes in human skin. J Invest Dermatol. 1996;106:967-71.
14. Hardy MH. The secret life of the hair follicle. Trends Genet. 1992;8:55-61.
15. Stenn KS, Paus R. Controls of hair follicle cycling. Physiol Rev. 2001;81:449-94.
16. Li L, Xie T. Stem cell niche: Structure and function. Annu Rev Cell Dev Biol. 2005;21:605-31.
17. Loomis CA, Koss J, Chu D. Embriology. In: Bolognia JL, Jorizzo JL, Rapini RP (Eds). Dermatology. Spain: Elsevier; 2008. pp. 37-47.
18. Nishimura EK. Melanocyte stem cells: a melanocyte reservoir in hair follicles for hair and skin pigmentation. Pigment Cell Melanoma Res. 2011;24:401-10.
19. Wang X, Shi Y, Zhou Q, et al. Detailed histological structure of human hair follicle bulge region at different ages: a visible niche for nesting adult stem cells. J Huazhong Univ Sci Technolog Med Sci. 2012;32:648-56.
20. Meyer KC, Klatte JE, Dinh HV, et al. Evidence that the bulge region is a site of relative immune privilege in human hair follicles. Br J Dermatol. 2008;159:1077-85.
21. Slominski A, Wortsman J, Plonka PM, et al. Hair follicle pigmentation. J Invest Dermatol. 2005;124:13-21.
22. Tomita Y, Maeda K, Tagami H. Melanocyte-stimulating properties of arachidonic acid metabolites: Possible role in post-inflammatory pigmentation. Pigment Cell Res. 1992;5:357-61.
23. Morelli JG, Kincannon J, Yohn JJ, et al. Leukotriene C4 and TGF-alpha are stimulators of human melanocyte migration *in vitro*. J Invest Dermatol. 1992; 98:290-5.
24. Horikawa T, Norris DA, Yohn JJ, et al. Melanocyte mitogens induce both melanocyte chemokinesis and chemotaxis. J Invest Dermatol. 1995;104:256-9.
25. Ponsonby AL, Lucas RM, van der Mei IA. UVR, vitamin D and three autoimmune diseases-multiple sclerosis, type 1 diabetes, rheumatoid arthritis. Photochem Photobiol. 2005;81:1267-75.
26. El-Ghorr AA, Norval M. Biological effects of narrowband (311 nm TL01) UVB irradiation: A review. J Photochem Photobiol. 1997;38:99-106.
27. Wu CS, Lan CC, Wang LF, et al. Effects of psoralen plus ultraviolet A irradiation on cultured epidermal cells *in-vitro* and patients with vitiligo *in vivo*. Br J Dermatol. 2007;156:122-9.
28. Abdel-Naser MB, El-Khateeb EA, Sallam TH, et al. Endothelin-1 is significantly elevated in plasma of patients with vitiligo treated with psoralen plus ultraviolet A. Clin Exp Dermatol. 2006;31:571-5.
29. Hirobe T. Role of keratinocyte-derived factors involved in regulating the proliferation and differentiation of mammalian epidermal melanocytes. Pigment Cell Res. 2005;18:2-12.
30. van Schanke A, Jongsma MJ, Bisschop R, et al. Single UVB overexposure stimulates melanocyte proliferation in murine skin, in contrast to fractionated or UVA-1 exposure. J Invest Dermatol. 2005;124:241-7.
31. Lei TC, Vieira WD, Hearing VJ. *In vitro* migration of melanoblasts requires matrix metalloproteinase-2: implications to vitiligo therapy by photochemotherapy. Pigment Cell Res. 2002;15:426-32.
32. Kaur P. Interfollicular epidermal stem cells: Identification, challenges, potential. J Invest Dermatol. 2006;126:1450-8.
33. Gola M, Czajkowski R, Bajek A, et al. Melanocyte stem cells: biology and current aspects. Med Sci Monit. 2012;18:155-9.
34. Davids LM, du Toit E, Kidson SH, et al. A rare repigmentation pattern in a vitiligo patient: A clue to an epidermal stem-cell reservoir of melanocytes? Clin Exp Dermatol. 2009;34:246-8.
35. Li I, Fukunaga-Kalabis M, Herlyn M. Isolation and cultivation of dermal stem cells that differentiate into functional epidermal melanocytes. Methods Mol Biol. 2012;806:15-29.
36. Dupin E, Calloni GW, Le Douarin NM. The cephalic neural crest of amniote vertebrates is composed of a large majority of precursors endowed with neural, melanocytic, chondrogenic and osteogenic potentialities. Cell Cycle. 2010;9:238-49.
37. Falabella R. Surgical treatment of vitiligo: Why, when and how. J Eur Acad Dermatol Venereol. 2003;17:518-20.
38. Lahiri K. Evolution and evaluation of autologous mini-punch grafting in vitiligo. Indian J Dermatol. 2009;54: 159-67.
39. Radmanesh M, Mostaghimi M, Yousefi L, et al. Leukotrichia developed following application of intense pulsed light for hair removal. Dermatol Surg. 2002;28:572-4.

15

Clinical, Biochemical and Immunological Aspects of Vitiligo

Manoj Kumar Tembhre, Alpana Sharma, Rehan Khan, Somesh Gupta

Key Features

- Vitiligo can grossly be divided into two types, generalized and localized.
- There are three principal hypotheses for pathogenesis of vitiligo, biochemical, neural, and autoimmune. Inherent genetic predisposition plays an important role.
- Autoimmunity is the most promising theory in pathogenesis of vitiligo.

INTRODUCTION

Vitiligo is one of the most common skin depigmentary disorders affecting approximately 1–2% of population worldwide.[1] Although, not fatal, vitiligo is having cosmetically and psychologically devastating effects on affected individuals[2,3] particularly in Asian sub-continent.

CLINICAL ASPECTS OF VITILIGO

Vitiligo is characterized by patchy loss of pigmentation due to destruction of functional melanocytes from the epidermis of the skin, often overlying hair and mucous membrane. The progression of vitiligo is variable and based on the clinical presentation, i.e. the extent of involvement and distribution of the macule; vitiligo can be broadly classified into two types:

I. Generalized (non-segmental) vitiligo
II. Localized vitiligo

Generalized vitiligo is further subdivided into:

1. Acrofacial
2. Vulgaris
3. Mixed
4. Universalis

Localized vitiligo is categorized into:

1. Focal vitiligo
2. Segmental vitiligo

Generalized or symmetrical type vitiligo is characterized by a bilateral, symmetrical depigmentation which can affect the face (especially periorificial areas), neck, torso, the extensor surfaces or bony prominences of the hands, wrists, legs, axillae and also orifices or mucosal surfaces.[4] Generalized vitiligo can be further divided into acrofacial (distal parts of the extremities and face), vulgaris (scattered macules all over the body) and mixed (different types of vitiligo at the same time) types.[5] Universal type has nearly complete or complete depigmentation of the skin.[5] Localized vitiligo can further divide into focal (one or a few macules in nondermatomal distribution), segmental (one or more macules in dermatomal distribution).

Segmental type vitiligo has a dermatomal, asymmetrical distribution of depigmentation[4] and often begins in childhood. It is rarely associated with autoimmune disorders and has stable results after autologous grafting. In contrast, symmetrical vitiligo has a later age of onset, is frequently associated with autoimmunity and has unstable results with autologous grafting.[4] These contrasts have lead to speculation that symmetrical and segmental vitiligo represents two quite separate disease manifestations.[4,6]

Other unusual forms of vitiligo are trichrome, inflammatory and occupational vitiligo. Trichrome vitiligo involves macules in which there are areas of both complete and partial loss of pigment, forming a pattern of varying hues between the affected and non-affected skin.[7,8] Inflammatory vitiligo is characterized by actively spreading lesions which are inflamed, presenting a raised erythematous perilesional border.[9,10] Chemically induced occupational vitiligo can occur in workers exposed to compounds such as catechols, phenols, hydroquinone and monobenzone. The depigmentation is usually confined to the parts of the body exposed to the chemical, e.g. the hands and forearms, but can arise in areas distant from the original point of contact, suggestive of systemic exposure through percutaneous adsorption, inhalation or ingestion. The clinical classification has been changed during the years[11,12] with little modifications and there is no consensus about the phenotypic characterization among the physicians.

PATHOGENESIS OF VITILIGO

The precise etiology of vitiligo is not known. There are various hypotheses put forward such as the (i) biochemical hypothesis,[13] (ii) the neural hypothesis[14,15] (iii) the autoimmune hypothesis[16,17] (iv) defective free-radical defense[18,19] (v) a deficiency of melanocyte growth factors,[20] (vi) intrinsic defect of melanocytes adhesion[21] or (vii) inherent genetic predisposition,[22,23] were proposed to be involved in the melanocyte cytotoxicity. Furthermore, environmental factors, including psychological stress, mechanical stress injury and infections, have been proposed to contribute to vitiligo etiology.[6] This chapter has the main focus on clinical, biochemical and immunological aspects of vitiligo.

BIOCHEMICAL THEORY OF VITILIGO

The biochemical theory involves two main components, i.e. elevated catecholamine and altered antioxidant defense. The catecholamine such as norepinephrine, epinephrine, and semiquinones, i.e. dopamine, estrogens, and their metabolites[14,24-26] are reported to be produced from epidermal cells such as keratinocytes and melanocytes. The biochemical theory is supported by the clinical observation that certain chemical compounds can produce a pattern of depigmentation that is similar to idiopathic vitiligo, e.g. mercaptamines[27] and phenolic agents;[28] and treatment with antioxidants,[29] or pseudocatalase[30] leads to repigmentation in vitiligo patients. The proposed involvement of some of the biochemicals thought to contribute to vitiligo pathogenesis through melanocyte autocytoxicity. This is accomplished by the proposed process of haptenation. In this process, the most preferred target of o-quinones (endogenous or exogenous) is tyrosinase, a key enzyme in the melanin synthesis.[31] Due to structural similarity these o-quinones (haptens) competes with the natural physiological substrate of tyrosinase, i.e. tyrosine and bind covalently to the active site of the enzyme.[32,33] This binding elicits an immune response. It is proposed that this tyrosinase-o-quinone complex can be recognized as a potential autoantigen by skin Langerhans cells (LC) and carried to regional lymph node. In the lymph node LC presented the antigen to major histocompatibility complex class I (MHC I)[34] expressed on CD4+ T cells thereby stimulating the proliferation of melanocyte specific cytotoxic T cells. These autoreactive cytotoxic T cells then migrate from regional lymph node to the lesional site and mediate the selective destruction of melanocytes facilitating depigmentation process eventually leading to vitiligo. However, none of these steps have been experimentally proved. There are growing evidences like increased catecholamine concentration in serum and urine of vitiligo patients supporting this hypothesis[24,25] and it is implicated equally to both segmental and generalized vitiligo[35] that are thought to be clinically different. Besides tyrosinase, o-quinones are also reported to interact with tyrosinase related protein (TRP-1 and TRP-2) and structural melanosomal proteins, like MART1/Melan-A, Pmel17/gp100 and gp75 suggesting the possible alternative autoantigens.

Further, it has been proposed that altered antioxidant defense and disturbed redox state contributes to the biochemical hypothesis of vitiligo. Increased levels of H_2O_2 is contributed by several factors such as defect in NADPH oxidase function, deficiency of detoxifying ezymes such as catalase, superoxide dismutase (SOD) glutathione peroxidase (GPX), thioredoxin peroxidase (TrxPX), thioredoxin reductase (TrxR) and γ-glutamyl transpeptidase (γ-GT) leading to generation of free radicals.[36] Trauma to the skin, ultraviolet (UV) radiation and other sources of inflammation leads to increase in epidermal pool of H_2O_2 in a non-specific manner via NADPH oxidase stimulation. In particular, UVB induces generation of free radicals and it is reported that the effect can be ameliorated by vitamin D by upregulating expression of metallothionein (a free radical scavenger protein with photoprotective properties).[37] Further, melanogenesis is known to produce significant levels of reactive oxygen species (ROS).[38] The H_2O_2 mediated oxidative stress affects epidermal pro-opiomelanocortin (POMC) peptides and furin that have a key role in melanogenesis.[39] Accumulation of excessive H_2O_2 leads to down-regulation of microphthalmia-associated transcription factor (MITF) expression that is critical for melanogenesis and melanocyte survival.[40]

Inducible nitric oxide synthase levels in vitiligo epidermis are elevated, producing both H_2O_2 and peroxynitrite.[41] Peroxynitrite, like the hydroxyl radical, can react directly with proteins and other macromolecules resulting in lipid peroxidation.[36] Malondialdehyde (MDA) is an end-product of lipid peroxidation, and elevated serum levels of MDA have been documented in patients with vitiligo.[42-44] Ultrastructural changes indicative of lipid peroxidation have been demonstrated in melanocytes, keratinocytes and Langerhans cells in the skin of patients with vitiligo, both in affected and perilesional areas.[45] Excessive free radical generation, leading to lipid peroxidation in vitiligo, may be related to a decrease in SOD.

Therefore, the imbalance in redox homeostasis due to elevated levels of H_2O_2 may induce the Fenton-type hydroxylation processes converting tyrosine, or exogenous monophenols to the catechols.[46,47] These catechols are then oxidized into reactive o-quinones and take part in haptenation process as explained above.

IMMUNOLOGICAL ASPECTS OF VITILIGO: ROLE OF AUTOIMMUNITY

The first evidence of immune mediated pathogenesis of vitiligo came from frequent clinical association of vitiligo with diseases of an autoimmune origin such as type I diabetes mellitus, pernicious anemia, alopecia areata, Grave's disease, autoimmune polyglandular syndrome. Moreover, the presence of organ-specific autoantibodies targeting pigment cell antigens in vitiligo patients[44,48-51] also supported the autoimmune theory of vitiligo. Autoreactive T lymphocytes targeting melanocyte-specific proteins have also been identified both circulating in the blood and at the margins of advancing lesions of vitiligo patients.[52-54] Further, association of vitiligo with certain human leukocyte antigen (HLA) specificities and other immune response genes adds credence to an autoimmune hypothesis. Most of the current therapeutic treatment modalities such as psoralen with ultraviolet A radiation (PUVA),[55] topical corticosteroids[56] and topical cytotoxic drugs such as fluorouracil[57] in vitiligo is believed to mediate their action by immunosuppression of local immune reaction that damages functional melanocytes.

The studies on animal experimental model also strongly supported the autoimmune basis of vitiligo. The Smyth line chicken is best documented experimental animal model for vitiligo and expresses a genetically inherited vitiligo-like depigmentation. An increase in infiltration of T cells is seen in the feather pulp and in the circulation of Smyth chicks prior to the onset and during development of vitiligo-like depigmentation.[58,59] The anti-melanocyte antibodies has been detected in the sera of 100% of Smyth line chicks that is not found in the sera of normally pigmented birds and further confirms the autoimmune involvement.[60] Recent studies have demonstrated participation of various immune cells like regulatory T cells (Tregs), T helper (Th1, Th2 and Th17), natural killer cells and their effector cytokines in the development of vitiligo suggesting the autoimmune implication in vitiligo.[61-66] Tregs especially has gained a wide attraction as it is thought to maintained the immune system homeostasis and prevent the development of autoimmune diseases by maintaining the tolerance to self antigens. Deficiency of Tregs frequency, function and homing has been observed in active phase of vitiligo[61,62] indicating a breach in tolerance mechanism. Although, there are inconsistencies such as autoantibodies have not been observed in all vitiligo patients and there is

Flow chart 1: Network of proposed contributing factors that eventually converge and leading to melanocyte destruction. The autoimmune hypothesis is the most compelling one and likely to be at the center stage where all prevailing factors converged

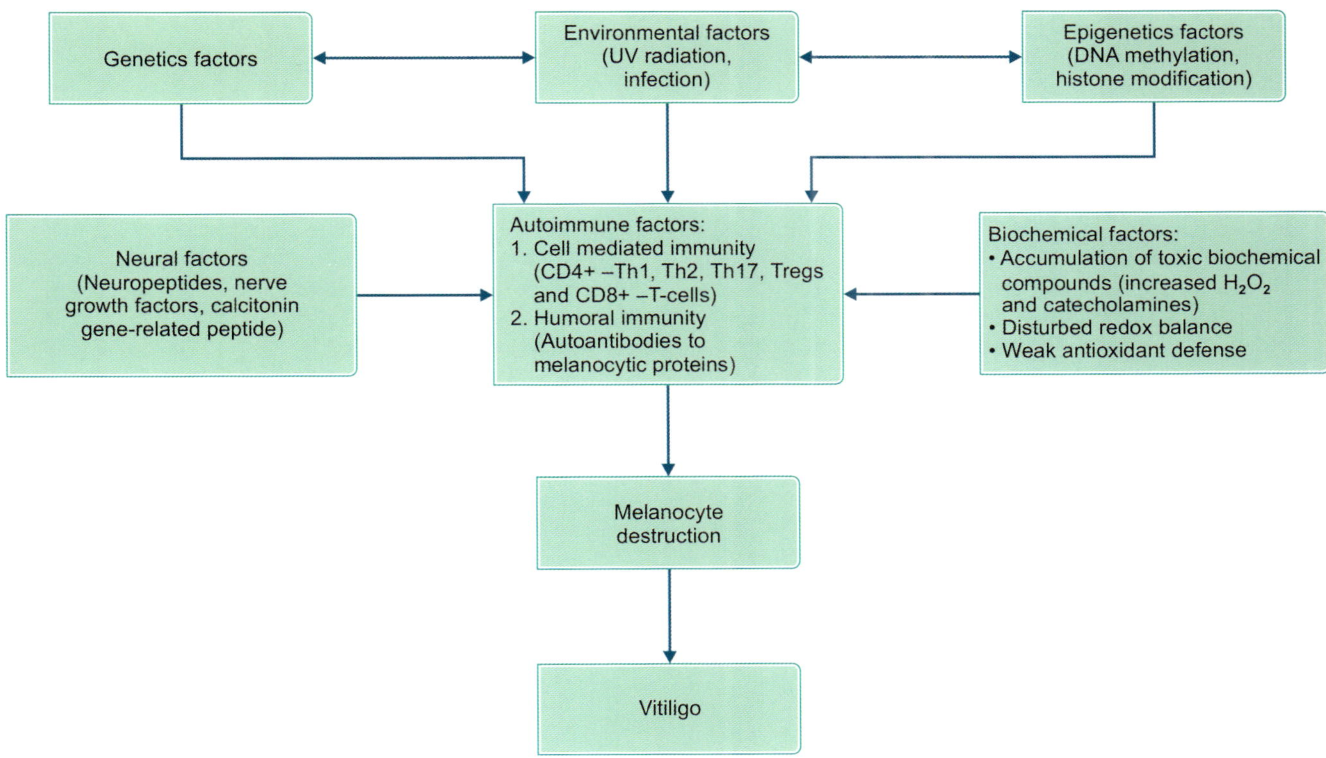

also lack of uniform positive HLA association and results are often variable. This inconcordance may be attributed to the discrepancies in clinical classification.

Further, it is possible that different pathogenic mechanisms may account for the different clinical subtypes of vitiligo. For example, associated autoimmunity is rare in patients with segmental vitiligo and, therefore, immune mechanisms might be supposed to play a lesser role as compared to the disease forms in which associated autoimmunity is more common.

CONCLUSION

Despite enough evidences it is currently not known whether autoimmunity is the primary cause of the disease or the consequence that arises as epiphenomenon resulting from the damage to the melanocytes from other intrinsic or extrinsic mechanisms, and in turn exacerbates the condition. This chapter has provided insights to the clinical, biochemical and immunological aspects of vitiligo. Collectively, there is interplay between biochemical and immunological factors resulting in formation of an environment where mealnocytes become vulnerable to survive. ROS and T-cells play a major role by acting in concert to kill or debilitate melanocytes in an environment of cytokine imbalance and oxidative stress. However, vitiligo is a complex disease and none of theory alone can define the complete etiology. It is multifactorial disorder where contributing factors are tightly interconnected and this intricate biological network **(Flow chart 1)** is difficult to decipher and remains open to speculation and need further investigations to reach to concrete conclusion.

REFERENCES

1. Howitz J, Brodthagen H, Schwartz M, et al. Prevalence of vitiligo. Epidemiological survey on the Isle of Bornholm, Denmark. Arch Dermatol. 1977;113:47-52.
2. Porter J, Beuf AH, Lerner A, et al. Response to cosmetic disfigurement: patients with vitiligo. Cutis. 1987;39:493-4.
3. Porter JR, Beuf AH, Lerner A, et al. Psychosocial effect of vitiligo: a comparison of vitiligo patients with "normal" control subjects, with psoriasis patients, and with patients with other pigmentary disorders. J Am Acad Dermatol. 1986;15:220-4.
4. Kovacs SO. Vitiligo. J Am Acad Dermatol. 1998;38(5 Pt 1):647-66; quiz 667-8.
5. Hann SK, Nordlund JJ. Clinical features of generalized vitiligo. In: Hann SK, Nordlund JJ (Eds). Vitiligo. Oxford: Blackwell Science; 2000. pp. 35-48.
6. Taieb A. Intrinsic and extrinsic pathomechanisms in vitiligo. Pigment Cell Res. 2000; 13(Suppl 8):41-7.
7. Fitzpatrick TB. Hypomelanosis. South Med J. 1964;57:995-1005.
8. Gawkrodger DJ. Vitiligo. Endocrine Autoimmunity and Associated Conditions. Weetman P (Ed). London: Kluwer Academic Publishers; 1998. pp. 269-84.
9. Grab J, Wise F. Vitiligo with raised borders. Arch Dermatol Syphilol. 1948;58:148-53.
10. Le Poole IC, vanden Wijngaard RMJGJ, Westerhof W, et al. Presence of T cells and macrophages in inflammatory vitiligo skin parallels melanocyte disappearance. Am J Path. 1996;148:1219-28.
11. Zaima H, Koga M. Clinical course of 44 cases of localized type vitiligo. J Dermatol. 2002;29:15-9.
12. Liu JB, Li M, Yang S, et al. Clinical profiles of vitiligo in China: an analysis of 3742 patients. Clin and Exp Dermatol. 2005;30:327-31.
13. Boissy RE, Manga P. On the etiology of contact/occupational vitiligo. Pigment Cell Res. 2004;17:208-14.
14. Cucchi ML, Frattini P, Santagostino G, et al. Higher plasma catecholamine and metabolite levels in the early phase of non-segmental vitiligo. Pigment Cell Res. 2000;13:28-32.
15. Lerner AB. Vitiligo. J Invest Dermatol. 1959;32:285-310.
16. Garbelli S, Mantovani S, Palermo B, et al. Melanocyte-specific, cytotoxic T cell responses in vitiligo: the effective variant of melanoma immunity? Pigment Cell Res. 2005;18: 234-42.
17. Ongenae K, Van Geel N, Naeyaert JM. Evidence for an autoimmune pathogenesis of vitiligo. Pigment Cell Res. 2003;16:90-100.
18. Dell'Anna ML, Picardo M. A review and a new hypothesis for non-immunological pathogenetic mechanisms in vitiligo. Pigment Cell Res. 2006;19:406-11.
19. Schallreuter KU. Oxidative stress in the human epidermis. G Ital Dermatol. Venereol 2005;140:505-14.
20. Moretti S, Spallanzani A, Amato L, et al. New insights into the pathogenesis of vitiligo: imbalance of epidermal cytokines at sites of lesions. Pigment Cell Res. 2002;15:87-92.
21. Gauthier Y, Cario AM, Taieb A. A critical appraisal of vitiligo etiologic theories. Is melanocyte loss a melanocytorrhagy? Pigment Cell Res. 2003;16:322-32.
22. Zhang XJ, Chen JJ, Liu JB. The genetic concept of vitiligo. J Dermatol Sci. 2005;39:137-46.
23. Quan C, Ren YQ, Xiang LH. Genome-wide association study for vitiligo identifies susceptibility loci at 6q27 and the MHC. Nat Genet. 2010;42:614-8.
24. Cucchi ML, Frattini P, Santagostino G, et al. Catechol- amines increase in the urine of non-segmental vitiligo especially during its active phase. Pigment Cell Res. 2003;16: 111-6.
25. Morrone A, Picardo M, de Luca C, et al. Catecholamines and vitiligo. Pigment Cell Res. 1992;5:65-9.
26. Schallreuter KU, Wood JM, Ziegler I, et al. Defective tetrahydrobiopterin and catecholamine biosynthesis in the

depigmentation disorder vitiligo. Biochim Biophys Acta. 1994;1226:181-92.

27. Bleehan SS. Vitiligo. In: SN Klaus (Ed.). Pigment Cell. Basel: Karger AG Publishers; 1979. p. 54.
28. Le Poole IC, Yang F, Brown TL, et al. Altered gene expression in melanocytes exposed to 4-tertiary butyl phenol (4-TBP): upregulation of the A2b adenosine receptor 1. J Invest Dermatol. 1999;113:725-31.
29. Maresca V, Roccella M, Roccella F, et al. Increased sensitivity to peroxidative agents as a possible pathogenic factor of melanocyte damage in vitiligo. J Invest Dermatol. 1997; 109:310-3.
30. Schallreuter KU. Effectiveness of pseudocatalase formulations in vitiligo. Clin Exp Dermatol. 2003;28:562-3.
31. Ito S, Kato T, Fujita K. Covalent binding of catechols to proteins through the sulfhydryl group. Biochem Pharmacol. 1988;37:1707-10.
32. Han R, Baden HP, Brissette JL, et al. Redefining the skin's pigmentary system with a novel tyrosinase Assay. Pigment Cell Res. 2002;15:290-7.
33. Brooks DW, Dawson CR. Aspects of tyrosinase chemistry. In: Peisach J, Aisen P, Blumberg WE (Eds). New York: Academic Press; 1997. pp. 343-57.
34. Rock KL, York IA, Goldberg AL. Post-proteasomal antigen processing for major histocompatibility complex class I presentation. Nat Immunol. 2004;5:670-7.
35. Picker LJ, Terstappen, LW, Rott LS, et al. Differential expression of homing-associated adhesion molecules by T cell subsets in man. J Immunol. 1990;145:3247-55.
36. Napolitano A, Crescenzi O, Pezzella A, et al. Generation of the neurotoxin 6-hydroxydopamine by peroxidase/H_2O_2 oxidation of dopamine. J Med Chem. 1995;38:917-22.
37. Palumbo A, Napolitano A, Barone P, et al. Nitrite- and peroxide-dependent oxidation pathways of dopamine: 6-nitrodopamine and 6-hydroxydopamine formation as potential contributory mechanisms of oxidative stress- and nitric oxide induced neurotoxicity in neuronal degeneration. Chem Res Toxicol. 1999;12:1213-22.
38. Brostoff J. Autoantibodies in patients with vitiligo. Lancet. 1969;2:177-8.
39. Betterle C, Del Prete GF, Peserico A, et al. Autoantibodies in vitiligo. Arch Dermatol. 1976;112(9):1328.
40. Zauli D, Tosti A, Biasco G, et al. Prevalence of autoimmune atrophic gastritis in vitiligo. Digestion. 1986;34:169-72.
41. Gilhar A, Zelickson B, Ulman Y, et al. *In vivo* destruction of melanocytes by the IgG fraction of serum from patients with vitiligo. J Invest Dermatol, 1995;105:683-6.
42. Mandry RC, Ortiz LJ, Lugo-Somolinos A, et al. Organ specific autoantibodies in vitiligo patients and their relatives. Int J Dermatol. 1996;35:18-21.
43. Ogg GS, Dunbar PR, Romero P, et al. High frequency of skin-homing melanocyte-specific cytotoxic T lymphocytes in autoimmune vitiligo. J Ex Med. 1998;188:1203-8.
44. Khan R, Satyam A, Gupta S, et al. Circulatory levels of antioxidants and lipid peroxidation in Indian patients with generalized and localized vitiligo. Arch Dermatol Res. 2009;301:731-7.
45. van den Wijngaard R, Wankowicz-Kalinska A, Le Poole C, et al. Local immune response in skin of generalized vitiligo patients. Destruction of melanocytes is associated with the prominent presence of CLA+ T cells at the perilesional site. Lab Invest. 2000;80:1299-309.
46. Schallreuter KU, Bahadoran P, Picardo M, et al. Vitiligo pathogenesis: autoimmune disease, genetic defect, excessive reactive oxygen species, calcium imbalance, or what else? Exp Dermatol. 2008;17:139-40.
47. Birlea SA, Costin GE, Norris DA. New insights on therapy with vitamin D analogs targeting the intracellular pathways that control repigmentation in human vitiligo. Medicinal Res Rev. 2009;29:514-46.
48. Riley PA. Radicals in melanin biochemistry. Ann N Y Acad Sci. 1988;55:111-20.
49. Spencer JD, Gibbons NCJ, Bohm M, et al. The Ca^{2+}-binding capacity of epidermal furin is disrupted by H_2O_2-medaited oxidation in vitiligo. Endocrinology. 2008;149:1638-45.
50. Hachiya A, Kobayashi A, Ohuchi A, et al. The paracrine role of stem cell factor/c-kit signaling in the activation of human melanocytes in ultraviolet B-induced pigmentation. J Invest Dermatol. 2001;116:578-86.
51. Salem MM, Shalbaf M, Gibbons NCJ, et al. Enhanced DNA binding capacity on up-regulated epidermal wild-type p53 in vitiligo by H_2O_2-mediated oxidation: a possible repair mechanism for DNA damage. FASEB J. 2009;23: 3790-807.
52. Jain D, Misra R, Kumar A. Levels of malondialdehyde and antioxidants in the blood of patients with vitiligo of age group 11–20 years. Indian J Physiol Pharmacol. 2008;52: 297-301.
53. Tobin DJ, Swanson NN, Pittelkow MR, et al. Melanocytes are not absent in lesional skin of long duration vitiligo. J Pathol. 2000;191:407-16.
54. Lang, KS, Caroli CC, Muhm A, et al. HLA-A2 restricted, melanocyte-specific CD8(+) T lymphocytes detected in vitiligo patients are related to disease activity and are predominantly directed against MelanA/MART1. J Invest Dermatol. 2001;116: 891-7.
55. Parrish JA, Fitzpatrick TB, Shea C, et al. Photochemotherapy of vitiligo. Use of orally administered psoralens and a high-intensity long-wave ultraviolet light system. Arch Dermatol. 1976;112:1531-4.
56. Kumari J. Vitiligo treated with topical clobetasol propionate. Arch Dermatol. 1984;120:631-5.
57. Tsuji T, Hamada T. Topically administered fluorouracil in vitiligo. Arch Dermatol. 1983;119:722-7.
58. Smyth JR. The Smyth chicken: a model for autoimmune amelanosis. CRC Crit Rev Poultry Biol. 1989;2:1-19.

59. Erf GF, Smyth JR. Alterations in blood leukocyte populations in Smyth line chickens with autoimmune vitiligo. Poult Sci. 1996;75(3):351-6.
60. Austin, LM, Boissy RE. Mammalian tyrosinase-related protein-1 is recognised by autoantibodies from vitiliginous Smyth chickens—an avian model for human vitiligo. Am J Path. 1995;146:1529-41.
61. Klarquist J, Denman CJ, Hernandez C, et al. Reduced skin homing by functional Treg in vitiligo. Pigment Cell Melanoma Res. 2010;23:276-86.
62. Dwivedi M, Laddha NC, Arora P, et al. Decreased regulatory T-cells and CD4(+)/CD8(+) ratio correlate with disease onset and progression in patients with generalized vitiligo. Pigment Cell Melanoma Res. 2013;26: 586-91.
63. Zhou L, Li K, Shi YL, et al. Systemic analyses of immunophenotypes of peripheral T cells in non-segmental vitiligo: implication of defective natural killer T cells. Pigment Cell Melanoma Res. 2012;25:602-11.
64. Wang CQ, Cruz-Inigo AE, Fuentes-Duculan J, et al. Th17 cells and activated dendritic cells are increased in vitiligo lesions. PLoS One. 2011;6:e18907.
65. Tembhre MK, Sharma VK, Sharma A, et al. T helper and regulatory T cell cytokine profile in active, stable and narrow band ultraviolet B treated generalized vitiligo. Clin Chim Acta. 2013;424C:27-32.
66. Khan R, Gupta S, Sharma A. Circulatory levels of T-cell cytokines (interleukin [IL]-2, IL-4, IL-17, and transforming growth factor-β) in patients with vitiligo. J Am Acad Dermatol. 2012;66:510-1.

16

Measuring Disease Severity in Vitiligo

Vishal Gupta, M Ramam

Key Features

- Most of the current methods of measuring vitiligo severity are aimed at measuring the area of depigmentation. However, this is clearly inadequate in a disease that affects several aspects of a person's physical, mental and social health.
- Other parameters that require assessment include disease activity, potential for repigmentation, disfigurement and psychosocial impact.
- Measures for some of these parameters are available while others need to be created. Recently, new disease-specific questionnaires have been developed to assess quality of life in vitiligo, viz. VitiQoL and Vitiligo Impact Scale.
- A comprehensive assessment of the burden of vitiligo will help focus attention on the varied effects of the disease and the effectiveness of therapeutic interventions in relieving them, both for individual patients and in clinical trials.

INTRODUCTION

There is no consensus regarding methods used to measure the disease severity in vitiligo. Most of the methods described in the literature are aimed at measuring the extent of depigmentation caused by vitiligo. There is also a lack of validated indices which can be used to compare treatment modalities.[1] The general principle is that more the area of involvement, the more severe is the disease. There is increased understanding that this may not always hold true and hence the need to develop additional ways to assess vitiligo severity. These methods include measuring the psychosocial impact, disease activity, disfigurement and potential for repigmentation.[2]

MEASURES OF EXTENT OF SKIN INVOLVEMENT AND INTENSITY OF DEPIGMENTATION

The development of techniques to measure the extent of depigmentation both at baseline and following therapeutic intervention has received considerable attention. Recently, techniques to assess the degree of whiteness and color match have also been proposed. In a comprehensive review article, Alghamdi et al classified these methods as subjective, semi-objective and objective, as microscopic and macroscopic, or morphometric versus colorimetric.[3]

Subjective methods include clinical evaluation by dermatologist and visual comparison of before and after photographs, taken under visible or ultraviolet (UV) light. Semi-objective methods include Wallace's rule of nine, hand palm rule, vitiligo area scoring index (VASI), and point-counting. Objective methods include software-based image analysis, tristimulus colorimetry, spectrophotometry and confocal laser microscopy. In an alternative classification, macroscopic morphological measurement methods included were visual assessment, photography under natural light or UV, photography with computerized image analysis, tristimulus colorimetry and spectrophotometry while the non-invasive micromorphological method described was confocal laser microscopy. The third classification was into morphometry and colorimetry: morphometry is the measurement of vitiliginous surface area and involves shape evaluation by measuring paramaters such as area, perimeter, minimum and maximum diameter. Colorimetry is a quantitative analysis of skin color changes (mean and standard deviation of gray levels, measurement of texture, etc). Most methods are concerned with morphometry except tristimulus colorimetry and spectrophotometry which assess color, also some of the image analysis softwares can assess both morphometry and colorimetry.[3]

Wallace's Rule of Nine

The Wallace rule of nine was initially developed to assess the extent of involvement in burns[4] and is commonly used to assess the extent of body surface area involvement. It divides the body into the following areas occupying 9% each: head, face and neck, upper anterior trunk, lower anterior trunk, upper posterior trunk, lower posterior trunk, each upper limb, buttocks and lower limb up to the knee and lower limb below the knee. The genitals and the perineum are assigned 1% of the body surface area. The palms and extended fingers are considered as covering 1% of the body surface area. In children however, the head is considered as 18% and the lower limbs are 13.5% each. The Vitiligo European Task Force (VETF) has used this method to assess the "extent" of vitiligo in patients. The investigators found that the inter-observer variability was acceptable.[5]

Lund-Browder Chart

The Lund-Browder chart was also devised to determine the area involved in burns but in this scoring system the body was divided into smaller segments than in the rule of nines, enabling a more accurate assessment of body surface area involved. According to many authors, the Lund-Browder chart is the most accurate method of estimating the burn extent. It can also be used for estimating the extent of vitiligo especially in children.[6] The Lund-Browder chart is theoretically better than the rule of 9 to score extent because the denominator is smaller for many body areas.[5] It has been used both for clinical records and research studies in our department.

Point Counting Method

The point counting method is a simple, practical and accurate technique which is used in the estimation of the irregularly shaped sectional surface area to obtain the volumes of organs or structures using macroscopic, microscopic or radiological images. When applied to vitiligo, the borders of the depigmented macule are marked with a pen and a piece of paper is immediately placed over the lesion so that the ink over the marked areas is transferred as a faint outline of the lesion onto the paper. For each lesion, the copied borders are enhanced by redrawing the margins with a pen. A transparent sheet that has points (+) marked on it at preset standard distances in the horizontal and vertical axes, similar to a graph paper is used to measure the area with the area of each + sign being 0.1 cm^2 in the grid. The grid sheet is superimposed on the lesion drawing and the numbers of points within and along the borders of the lesions are counted **(Fig. 1)**. The total area of each lesion is estimated by multiplying the total number of points counted for the lesion by the area of each point (0.1 cm^2). This method can also be used for measuring the size of other skin lesions such as psoriasis, ulcers, alopecia, burn wounds or scars in which accurate evaluation is essential for clinical follow-up and research.[3,7]

In a study of this method in 31 vitiligo lesions in 5 patients, Aydin et al. found significant agreement between the findings by point counting method and that obtained by digital planimetry and there was inter- as well as intra-observer reliability. It was suggested that this method can be used as a criterion for the evaluation of treatment or in follow-up of vitiligo lesions.[7]

Digital Planimetry

Planimetry means the measurement of plane areas. The area of the depigmented macules as seen on digital images can be calculated using different computer applications.

Image Pro Plus 4.5

In a study comparing the point counting method and digital planimetry using Image pro plus 4.5, a total of 31 vitiligo lesions from 5 patients were evaluated. All scanned drawings were stored in "jpeg" format with true color class and 300 × 300 pixel resolution and then converted to black and white format. In order to convert the area from pixel to cm^2, a square with 1 cm^2 area was attached and the number of pixels in vitiligo lesion was counted to calibrate the area measurement of the vitiligo lesion. Surface areas of the lesion and a 1 cm^2 drawn area were measured by image-pro plus 4.5 analysis processing program on the basis of planimetry. Three independent observers evaluated the outlined areas

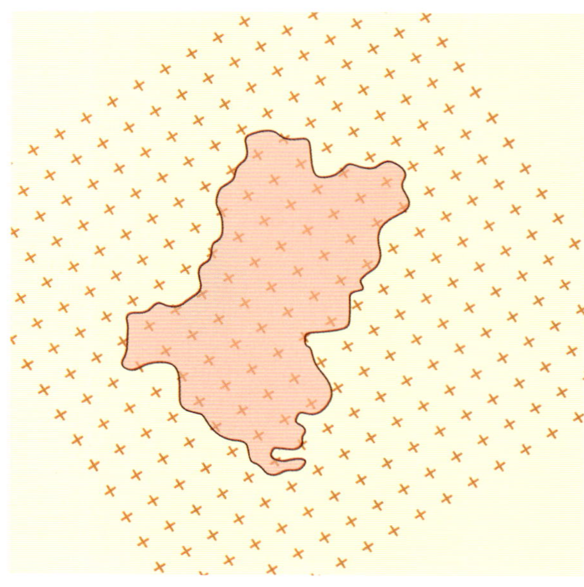

Fig. 1: Point counting method

twice using the point counting technique with an interval of 2 weeks. The same lesions were also measured by one observer applying digital planimetry. There was significant inter- and intraobserver agreement for all measurements.[7]

AutoCad 2000

Marrakchi et al.[8] designed an objective method based on the measurement of vitiligo treated areas with irregular shape using Autocad 2000. To do this, the border of the lesion was drawn on a transparent sheet tightly applied to the skin and the resulting figure either scanned or stored in the computer, or the transparent sheet applied to the screen to allow measurement of the area. For this purpose AutoCAD 2000 (Autodesk, Inc., San Raphael, CA, USA) software was used that allows the user to trace the edge profile of the vitiligo lesion on the screen either by retracing the scanned image or outlining the figure of the transparent sheet applied to the screen using the mouse. Once the outlined border of the lesion is obtained, the software allows the lesion dimensions (area and perimeter) to be determined. Some skin areas could be difficult to trace (eye sockets, ear, etc.). For these areas, the method could be improved by combining the use of AutoCad software and digital photography. However, errors that occur during the tracing of the lesion cannot be obviated.

Photoshop

Welsh et al.[9] used a morphometric based vitiligo assessment method to evaluate the repigmentation area using Photoshop. Photographs were taken with a 5 megapixel Coolpix Nikon camera at a distance of 2 meters using the same camera settings. The lesions were measured at their widest diameter at baseline and after 30 sessions of phototherapy by two independent investigators using a graduated grid (5.08 mm^2 squares) of the computer program Adobe Photoshop Elements, 1989–2001 (Adobe Systems Incorporated, San José, CA). In addition, colorimetric analysis could also be performed using Photoshop-based image analysis that uses the color information contained in each individual pixel (color hue, saturation, luminosity) and thus allows separation of colors at the levels of pixel resolution.

Corel Draw

Sanclemente et al. used both digital morphometry and digital colorimetry methods to assess repigmentation. Photographs taken with a Nikon Coolpix 4500 camera (Nikon, USA) were subjected to morphometry analysis using Corel Draw®, version 9.0 software (Corel Corporation, Ottawa, Canada). Each macule studied was delineated with a symmetrical grid and objective numbers were obtained by calculating pigmented islands that covered each square of the grid.

All the technical limitations of clinical photography apply to these methods which use digital images.

Vitiligo Area Severity Index

Vitiligo area severity index (VASI) is a quantitative tool for evaluating the extent of skin involvement and response to treatment.[1] It is a simple method analogous to the Psoriasis Area Severity Index (PASI). The body is divided into five separate and mutually exclusive regions: hands, upper extremities (excluding hands), trunk, lower extremities (excluding the feet), and feet. The axilliary and inguinal regions were included with the upper and lower extremities, respectively, while the buttocks were included with the lower extremities. One hand unit, which encompasses the palm plus the volar surface of all the digits, is approximately 1% of the total body surface area and was used as a guide to estimate the baseline percentage of vitiligo involvement of each body region. After treatment, the extent of residual depigmentation within each affected patch that had been present at baseline was estimated to the nearest of the following percentages: 0, 10%, 25%, 50%, 75%, 90% or 100%. For each body region, the VASI was determined by the product of the area of vitiligo in hand units (which was set at 1% per unit) and the extent of depigmentation within each hand unit-measured patch. The total body VASI was then calculated using the following formula by considering the contributions of all body regions (possible range, 0–100):

$$\text{VASI} = \sum_{\text{all body sites}} (\text{Hand Units}) \times (\text{extent of depigmentation})$$

Hamzavi et al. concluded that VASI is a valid quantitative clinical tool that can be used to evaluate vitiligo parametrically. The correlation with the VASI was found to be lower for patient assessment ($p = 0.05$) than for physician assessment ($p < 0.001$) but was still statistically significant.

Photography

Photographs can capture the patient's condition at an instant in time and serial photographs taken over a period can indicate the progress of the disease or the response to treatment.[10] Digital photography is a reliable and accurate method and provides a digital image record which can be analyzed and measured by investigators or by using software programs. However, a number of technical limitations may reduce the effectiveness of digital photography in vitiligo. For example, measurement precision is compromised when the distance between the camera and the surface is inconsistent. Failure to place the camera at exactly the same distance for each photograph may create the impression that the size of the lesion has changed when it has not. Similarly, the camera angle in relation to the size may affect the precision of the photographic measurement. On the other hand, the cost and amount of equipment and time required to use computer-assisted planimetry (planimetry is a technique by which the area of a two-dimension figure is measured) restricts its clinical usefulness in daily practice.[11]

Ultraviolet-light photography is based on the principle of UV rays being more selectively absorbed by melanin in the epidermis as compared with visible light. UV light photography is undertaken with a Wood's lamp which emits long wave UV radiation in a band between 320 and 400 nm with a peak at 365 nm. The light source is a high pressure mercury arc fitted with a compound filter made of barium silicate and 9% nickel oxide, the "Wood's filter". Fluorescence of tissues occurs when UV light is absorbed, and radiation of a longer wavelength, usually visible light is emitted. In depigmented skin lesions, there is reduced or no epidermal melanin and hence there is a window through which a light induced autofluorescence of dermal collagen can be seen. The lesion appears bright blue white due to autofluorescence.[12] The results of Wood light examination can be recorded through UV photography. The VETF recommends Wood's lamp examination as a diagnostic tool in evaluating vitiligo. This technique examination is less valuable in dark-skinned patients in whom hypopigmented lesions can be easily perceived by the naked eye.

Potentially Useful Newer Approaches

Diffuse Reflectance Spectroscopy

Reflectance tristimulus CIE colorimetry and narrow band reflectance spectrophotometry are used to determine skin color by measuring the intensity of reflected light of specific wavelengths using the principle of diffuse reflectance spectroscopy (DRS). The color of the skin depends mainly on its pigment content, on the spectrum of the illuminating light and on the quality of its surface. The primary chromophores in skin are melanin, oxyhemoglobin and deoxyhemoglobin. By analyzing the spectra reflected from the skin after exposure to a standardized light source, quantitative inferences can be made about these chromophores.

The components required for a DRS system are the light source, probe, analyzer, and detection device. A variety of light sources have been used including tungsten halogen lamps, xenon arc lamps and broad-band white lightemitting diodes (LEDs)[3] with the choice depending on the wavelength to be studied. Light delivery and collection is by means of a fiber optic probe providing a total delivery/collection spot diameter of 2.5 mm. Diffuse reflectance spectra are measured in the range 460–820 nm and provide quantitative information for the dominant chromophores of skin in the visible range, hemoglobin and melanin. In addition, it is promising for the study of conditions such as hyperpigmentation or hypopigmentation[13] as well as in the assessment of skin appearance.

Reflectance Tristimulus CIE Colorimetry Evaluation

Tristimulus analysis converts spectral information obtained by diffuse reflectance spectroscopy into three numbers that indicate how the color of an object appears to a human observer. This color system authorized by the CIE (Commission Internationale de l'Eclairage) is regarded as the standard for colorimetry in industrial fields.[6]

It has been used in the quantitative evaluation of UV-induced erythema and pigmentation,[14,15] the severity of irritant-induced erythema[16] and the blanching effect of topical corticosteroids.[17] Other clinical applications for colorimetry include the determination of erythema and pigmentation or depigmentation, studies on skin typology, races, anatomical distribution of pigment and to photoprotection factors, sunscreens or depigmentation agents.[15-17] This system may be useful in evaluating the degree of depigmentation in vitiligo and assessing the response to therapy.

Spectrophotometry

Reflectance spectrophotometry is used by many commercially available instruments that measure a "melanin index" (MI) (or "pigmentation index") and an "erythema index" (EI) based on reflectance measurements at selected spectral bands for melanin and hemoglobin, respectively.[6] In a study done to compare the capabilities of tristimulus colorimeter and two narrowband spectrophotometers, comparative color measurements were carried out *in vitro* on standardized color charts, *in vivo* on different skin areas in human volunteers and on skin color changes induced by various physicochemical treatments. The authors found that the *in vitro* and *in vivo* repeatability as well as the sensitivity of the three instruments was good. The instruments were able to characterize skin color and to quantify small skin color changes with moderate to high significant linear correlations between the data obtained by the different instruments.[18] This technique was employed by Tanemura et al. in a study to compare the therapeutic efficacy of sun irradiation versus narrowband UVB Phototherapy along with concomitant topical tacalcitol for vitiligo vulgaris.[19]

Reflectance Confocal Microscopy

In vivo, reflectance confocal microscopy (RCM) is a non-invasive, repetitive imaging tool that provides real-time images at nearly cellular histological resolution. A near-infrared wavelength laser beam is focussed on to specific point within the skin and reflected light is collected through a pinhole of the detector. The light source, the illuminated spot, and the pinhole are in optically conjugated focal planes, leading to the name "confocal". The illuminated spot is then scanned horizontally, producing black and white images from epidermis to the upper reticular dermis with an imaging depth of up to 250–300 microns. To visualize a larger area, a two-dimensional sequence of images are captured and stitched in software to create a mosaic that displays up to 8 × 8 mm of tissue. Highly reflective skin components including melanin, collagen and keratin appear bright (white) in RCM images. Using RCM, an increase in melanocyte size, dendricity, and number, as well as increased pigment in keratinocytes was found in UV-irradiated epidermis of guinea pigs. UVR-induced epidermal hyperplasia could also be detected and quantified.[20]

Kang et al.[21] used RCM in vitiligo and found that normal dermal papillary rings disappeared and no bright keratinocytes could be detected in the epidermis. RCM images of repigmented skin after excimer laser treatment showed dendritic melanocytes at the basal layer. Ardigo et al.[22] described changes in non-lesional skin of patients. The characteristic ring structures of healthy controls were hardly recognizable and half-rings or scalloped border-like features of the rings were observed. They suggested that this change could derive from an incomplete distribution of pigment along the basal layer because of an initial and progressive disappearance of melanocytes or to a congenital defective melanocyte distribution. This suggests that confocal microscopy might be used to estimate the risk of developing vitiligo in subjects with familial vitiligo or those exposed to chemical agents.[6] In repigmented areas 2 months after UVB narrow band therapy, the presence of activated, dendritic melanocytes in the basal layer was seen in 6 of 16 patients. These findings suggested that RCM could be used in monitoring the response to treatment and the evolution of vitiligo.

MEASURES OF DISEASE ACTIVITY/ PROGRESSION OF DISEASE/DISEASE STABILITY

It is important to know whether vitiligo is stable or progressive because the management strategies differ in each case. Although medical therapeutic modalities may be tried in both stable as well as progressive vitiligo with comparable success, surgical methods are usually reserved for stable disease. Disease activity is mainly assessed by relying on the patients' history. Information on disease activity can also be obtained by physical examination and prospectively recording the size, number of lesions and the grade of repigmentation during follow-up visits.[23] The course of vitiligo can be predicted fairly confidently for segmental disease. However, non-segmental vitiligo behaves differently in different individuals and currently there exists no method by use of which we can predict its course in a given person.[2]

Different workers have used different definitions for active vitiligo. According to Moellmann,[24] active vitiligo is the clinical stage when the lesions are enlarging in the last 6 weeks. Cui et al.[25] defined active vitiligo as the development of new lesions or the extension of previous lesions in the last 3 months while Uda et al.[26] considered vitiligo active when the lesions spread without regression over the previous 6 months. Agarwal et al. defined slowly spreading vitiligo as the development of one to five new lesions in the previous month or 6–15 new lesions in the previous 3 months.[27]

Similarly, there are a number of different definitions for stable vitiligo as well. Falabella et al.[28] defined stable vitiligo as a condition that had not been progressing for at least 2 years. Boersma et al.[29] defind stable vitiligo as disease showing neither the spread of existing lesions nor the appearance of new lesions in the previous 6 months. Kumar et al.[30] consider the disease to be stable when no progression was observed for at least 1 year. The Indian Association of Dermatologists, Venereologists and Leprologists (IADVL) task force for vitiligo surgery recommends a period of 1 year without any new lesions or extension of previous lesions as an indicator of stability.[31] It is generally said that the longer the time elapsed since the development of new lesions or the extension of previous lesions, the more stable the disease is likely to be. In effect, the past course of the disease is used to predict its future course.[2] Unpublished data from our department suggests that this assumption does not always hold true and the disease may show periods of activity even after the disease has been stable for 1 year or more.[2]

Morphological Clues to Disease Activity

Disease activity can also be assessed by clinical examination of vitiligo macules. A significant relationship was found between the clinical appearance of the vitiligo lesion and its activity in a study done of 48 patients followed-up for one year.[32] Hypomelanotic lesions with poorly defined borders corresponded to actively spreading lesions (n = 28), and amelanotic lesions with sharply demarcated borders corresponded to stable lesions (n = 20). Inflammatory vitiligo and trichrome vitiligo could also be considered as markers of activity and spreading.

The VETF recommends the use of Wood's lamp to estimate the spread of vitiligo.[5] The largest macule in a body region is first visualized under natural light, followed by examination under Wood's Lamp. A score of "0" is given if the margins are identical by both methods interpreted as no spread, "+1" if the margins under Wood's light is beyond that seen in natural light indicating progressive vitiligo (ongoing subclinical depigmentaion) and "–1" for regressive vitiligo (ongoing subclinical repigmentation). These interpretations await validation.

Vitiligo Activity Index

The vitiligo activity index (VAI) is a novel system to assess the activity of vitiligo vulgaris at a given point of time. It was proposed by Menchini and Commacchio in 2007.[33] They described the presence of small areas of depigmentation outside the main patch referred to as point depigmentation and/or presence of multiple tones of hypopigmentation surrounding the main depigmented patch as signs of on-going depigmentation. The presence of follicular repigmentation is considered to be an indicator of improvement and the presence of a sharply marginated lesion is an indicator of stability. They assigned a vitiligo activity score (VAS) ranging from +4 to -2 for these signs. The body is divided into eight regions, namely head, neck, trunk, genitals, right upper limb, left upper limb, right leg and left leg and a score of 1 is given for each involved area. The total score is called the vitiligo affected areas (VAA). The VAS is next assigned depending on signs of repigmentation/on-going depigmentation/stability on vitiligo patches over each of the affected areas. This scoring is done separately for each affected area and the total is calculated as the VAS (range: -16-32). This score divided by VAA gives the final value of vitiligo activity index, ranging from -2 to 4. A lesser value denotes less activity and vice versa. This gives a rough idea of the disease activity without taking the involved surface area into account. This index has not yet been validated.

Minigrafting Test

Falabella et al.[28] devised a method by which stable vitiligo lesions suitable for melanocyte transplantation can be identified. They evaluated the pigment spread of minigrafts when implanted within lesions of stable vitiligo as a test to identify good candidates for surgical repigmentation. Four to six minigrafts of 1.0-1.2 mm were implanted within lesions of patients with unilateral (localized) and bilateral (generalized) vitiligo. The grafted area was exposed to sunlight for 15 minutes daily for 3 months and no treatment was permitted during this test period. Pigment spread was assessed 3 months later. All the test sites were visualized under Wood's light. The test was considered positive if unequivocal repigmentation took place beyond 1 mm from the border of implanted grafts. On the other hand, if less than 1 mm or no repigmentation was observed, the test was considered negative. In this study, the authors found 95% patients with unilateral vitiligo (which is known to respond well to surgery) had a positive minigrafting test result in comparison with only 48% with bilateral vitiligo (which does not), prompting the authors to conclude that the minigrafting test is a reliable tool to identify patients with stable vitiligo who may respond to melanocyte transplantation. However, test graft positivity does not necessarily guarantee a favorable outcome in all cases even after perigraft pigmentation. Encouraging results were obtained even after grafting in some test graft negative cases.[34]

Experimentally Induced Koebner Phenomenon and Vitiligo Disease Activity (VIDA) Score

In a study conducted to find the association between vitiligo disease activity and response to treatment, the disease activity was assessed by history taking (VIDA), history of Koebner phenomenon (KP-h) and experimentally induced Koebner phenomenon (KP-e).[23] Response to therapy and VIDA scores were evaluated independently in a masked manner by 2 observers after 12 months of therapy **(Table 1)**.

Experimentally induced Koebner phenomenon: Four 2 mm punch grafts using biopsy punches were removed from a normally pigmented area. After 2 months the outcome was evaluated by two independent observers. It was scored negative when the wound healed without depigmentation and positive when the depigmentation of the biopsy scar or even beyond the biopsy margins occurred.

Table 1: Vitiligo disease activity score (VIDA-score) on a 6-point scale

Vitiligo activity	*Time period*	*VIDA score*
Active	6 weeks or less	+4
Active	6 weeks to 3 months	+3
Active	3–6 months	+2
Active	6–12 months	+1
Stable	1 year or more	0
Stable with spontaneous repigmentation	1 year or more	−1

The association between experimentally induced Koebner phenomenon, history of Koebner phenomenon, disease activity by history (VIDA score) and responsiveness to therapy was assessed in 61 patients.

There was a significant decrease in VIDA scores after therapy in treatment responders. There was a good correlation between VIDA scores and therapeutic response and experimentally induced Koebner phenomenon. But experimentally induced Koebner phenomenon did not correlate well with history of Koebner phenomenon.

The authors recommended that the presence or absence of history of Koebner phenomenon should be confirmed by inducing experimentally induced Koebner phenomenon. It was concluded that experimentally induced Koebner phenomenon may function as a valuable clinical factor to assess clinical disease activity. It may also predict responsiveness to topical steroid therapy but not to UVB. VIDA score may seem appealing for clinical use, but it needs to be validated with other patient groups.

Other Investigational Techniques

Histopathological Markers of Disease Stability

Spongiosis with microvesicle formation, clustered CD8 T lymphocytes in the epidermis and dermal melanophage deposition were associated with actively spreading vitiligo lesions while stable lesions showed rare spongiosis, rare clustered CD8 T lymphocytes in the epidermis and rare dermal melanophage deposition in a study by Benzekri et al.[32] The clinical applicability of this information is yet unclear.

Immunological Markers of Disease Stability

There is now growing evidence that a subpopulation of CD4+ T-cells, called natural Tregs, play a pivotal role in the maintenance of peripheral self-tolerance. FoxP3, a reliable marker of regulatory T cells, is a transcription factor that affects the expression of several genes and mutations of Foxp3 gene result in severe autoimmune diseases in human (e.g. IPEX syndrome) and mice. Dysfunction of Tregs has been described in several autoimmune diseases. Ben Ahmed et al.[35] demonstrated a functional defect of peripheral regulatory T lymphocytes in vitiligo patients. They found the proportion of such cells in the blood was insignificantly reduced in patients with progressive disease compared with stable disease. However, the suppressive effects of peripheral Tregs (CD4+ CD25+ T cells) on CD4+ CD25- T-cell proliferation and interferon (IFN)-gamma production were significantly reduced in vitiligo patients compared to the healthy controls. Also, the reduced suppressive effects of peripheral Tregs were correlated to the activity of the disease during the periods preceding and following the study.

In the same study, FOXP3 mRNA expression was found to be significantly higher in vitiliginous skin compared to non-lesional skin of donors. Within the perilesional skin of vitiligo patients, the quantity of FOXP3 mRNA was significantly increased in patients with progressive vitiligo compared to stable patients.

Rao et al.[36] conducted a study to determine the clinical, biochemical and immunological factors determining stability of disease in patients with generalized vitiligo. The patients were divided into three groups: Group 1 (stability > 3 months but < 1 year), Group 2 (≥ 1 year but < 2 years) and Group 3 (≥ 2 years). The authors found that the percentage of CD8 and CD45RO cells in the immunohistochemistry of a tissue biopsy is useful in the determination of stability of vitiligo and in predicting a successful outcome of melanocyte transplantation. There was no difference in the percentages of CD4, CD45RO, and CD45RA between the patients of different groups. FoxP3 levels were significantly lower in Group 1 compared with Group 2. However, the levels of FoxP3 cells were not significantly different in responders and non-responders.

The reversal of ratio of CD4:CD8 ratio in the lesional skin suggests stability of the disease.[37]

Biochemical Markers of Disease Stability

In an attempt to find a link between vitiligo and the activity of monoaminergic systems, Cucchi et al.[38] measured the plasma levels of catecholamines (norepinephrine, epinephrine, and dopamine), their precursor 3,4-dihydroxyphenylalanine (DOPA), their metabolites (3-methoxy-4-hydroxyphenylglycol, normetanephrine, metanephrine, and homovanillic acid), and 5-hydroxyindolacetic acid in vitiligo patients and controls. They found that the levels of norepinephrine, epinephrine, normetanephrine, metanephrine, homovanillic acid, and 5-hydroxyindoleacetic acid were significantly higher in patients compared to controls. The patients at an active phase of the disease showed significantly higher levels of norepinephrine, normetanephrine, 3-methoxy-4-hydroxyphenylglycol, and homovanillic acid than ones at a stable phase. The patients with progressive vitiligo and at its more recent onset (< 1 year) showed significantly increased levels of epinephrine, norepinephrine, and metanephrine in comparison with longer-term sufferers.

Various studies[39-41] suggest an increased serum levels of homocysteine in patients with active vitiligo.

In the study done by Rao et al.[36], there was no significant difference in the catalase levels in the three groups (divided on the basis of duration of disease stability). This shows that the catalase levels are independent of disease activity and that determination of catalase activity would not help in determining the stability of disease.

Currently, there are no biochemical markers that can be used in clinical practice.

MEASURES OF THE POTENTIAL FOR REPIGMENTATION

It has been suggested that the likelihood of achieving repigmentation in the vitiligo lesions may also serve as a marker of disease severity.

Type of Vitiligo

Similar to what has been observed regarding the spread of disease, even the therapeutic responsiveness can be predicted most confidently in cases of segmental vitiligo. It is known to respond well to surgical therapy, while showing none to minimal response to medical therapeutic modalities.

Anatomic Location

It is also well known that certain areas are much more resistant to attain repigmentation following therapy, such as mucosae, acral sites (hands and feet) and bony prominences. Similarly, lesions showing leukotrichia are known to be resistant to therapy.

Extent of Disease

The larger the extent of involvement, the less likely it is to achieve cosmetically significant repigmentation. Hence, the extent of body surface involvement appears to be an important factor determining the potential to achieve repigmentation.

Staging of Disease

The staging of vitiligo is based on the principle that repigmentation needs melanogenesis to be stimulated if melanocytes are still present, and further to mobilize and make them dividing from a local reservoir. This reservoir can be interfollicular when melanocytes remain in the lesion, marginal if they can migrate from its edge, and follicular from melanoblasts which can differentiate and migrate towards the interfollicular compartment.

Staging of vitiligo is based on cutaneous and hair pigmentation, and the disease is staged 0–4 on the largest macule in each body region, except hands and feet, which are assessed separately and globally as one unique area. The use of Wood's lamp is recommended by the VETF for staging of the disease. Stage 0 is normal pigmentation, Stage 1 is incomplete pigmentation (including spotty depigmentation, trichrome and homogenous pigmentation. A few white hair at this stage do not change the stage grading), Stage 2 is complete depigmentation, a few white hair at this stage do not change the stage grading, Stage 3 is partial hair whitening, less than 30%, and Stage 4 is complete hair whitening.[5] The staging of the disease indicates its prognosis and its ability to repigment.

DISFIGUREMENT

The impact of vitiligo is both external and internal. How the alteration in the physical appearance or the disfigurement caused by the disease is perceived externally by others is also an important component determining the severity of disease. This can be measured by the use of a disfigurement index.[2] Disfigurement indices have been described for a few diseases like Graves ophthalmopathy, port-wine stain, and head and neck cancers.[42-44]

Katz et al.[42] examined the validity and the inter-rater reliability of a novel nine-point observer-rated disfigurement scale in 74 head and neck cancer patients more than 6 months following treatment. Ratings of disfigurement were assigned independently by surgical and nonsurgical raters. It was found that the disfigurement was significantly related to a diagnosis of oral cancer, a history of adjunctive radiation, the type of surgical procedure performed, the degree of physical dysfunction, and the presence of postoperative complications. Observer ratings of disfigurement were significantly related to patient ratings of disfigurement indicating validity of the disfigurement scale. Inter-rater reliability of the scale was high.

In a study performed to assess the characterstics of port-wine stains in the head/neck area that contribute to disfigurement, color slides of 90 untreated port-wine stains were shown to a panel of 16 lay persons to judge the disfigurement.[43] In addition, color, patchiness, boundary, size, shape, surface structure, and hypertrophy of the underlying tissue were rated quantitatively by a panel of five professionals. By means of multiple linear regression analysis, the ratings for overall port-wine stain disfigurement (panel of lay persons) were compared with the ratings for the individual port-wine stain characteristics (panel of professionals) and the proportional contribution of each of the characteristics to overall port-wine stain disfigurement was calculated. The authors found that the size of the port-wine stain is the most important factor followed by color and boundary in contributing to disfigurement.

Terwee et al. conducted a study to determine the severity of disfigurement in patients with Graves ophthlamopathy.[44] Four separate panels each consisting of four endocrinologists, four ophthalmologists, four Graves ophthalmology patients, and four laypersons respectively, were shown standardized slides of one hundred patients of Graves' ophthlamopathy who were randomly selected from four available study populations, involving mild, moderate and severe Graves' ophthalmopathy. Panel members individually scored the disfigurement severity of each patient on a Visual Analog Scale. Agreement within a panel varied from 0.65 to 0.79 and was highest within the panel of ophthalmologists. Between-panel agreement was 0.67 and was highest between ophthalmologists and laypersons. The authors concluded that facial disfigurement severity can be measured in a reliable way using panels of evaluators.

To the best of our knowledge, a disfigurement index for vitiligo patients is not available. If developed, it is likely to be useful both in clinical trials and in routine clinical practice.[2]

PSYCHOSOCIAL IMPACT OF VITILIGO

Vitiligo is a cosmetically disturbing disease which has a major impact on the quality of life.[45,46] It has been suggested that the psychosocial burden associated with this disease does not correlate well with the clinical severity, and there is a need to measure this aspect of the disease separately.[2,47] It has been recommended that the clinician should assess the psychological and quality of life effects of vitiligo in patients and the improvement in quality of life (QoL) of patient should be made the most important outcome measure in therapeutic trials relating to vitiligo.[48] In dermatology, health-related quality of life (HRQoL) can be assessed with generic instruments (i.e. applicable in a broad range of conditions allowing for comparisons between diseases), dermatology specific instruments (i.e. applicable in all skin diseases and allowing for comparisons between skin diseases) and condition-specific instruments (i.e. use is restricted to a specific skin disease and only comparisons between patient groups with the same skin condition are possible).[49] Both generic health related and dermatology specific questionnaires have been used to measure the psychosocial burden of vitiligo. Generic instruments are useful in comparing the impact on QoL among different diseases but disease-specific instruments are more sensitive to issues related to a particular disorder. A vitiligo-specific instrument to measure health-related QoL is necessary because, unlike most other skin diseases, vitiligo is usually not associated with physical symptoms yet it causes significant psychosocial impairment. Recently, two vitiligo specific questionnaires were developed: VitiQoL[50] in the United States and vitiligo impact scale[51] in our department.

GENERIC QUALITY OF LIFE INSTRUMENTS

General measures, such as the Short Form-36 (SF-36), EuroQol-5, World Health Organization Quality of Life (WHOQoL), Willingness-to-Pay (WTP) scale and Sickness Impact Profile are designed to be used across all diseases, dermatologic as well as non-dermatologic, allowing comparison of the effect of skin disease to the effect of diseases of other systems.

SF-36

This widely used questionnaire consists of 36 items forming 8 domains or scales: physical functioning, social functioning, role physical (limitations in usual role activities because of physical problems), role emotional (limitations in usual role activities because of emotional problems), bodily pain, mental health, vitality, and general health perceptions as perceived by the patient in the previous 4 weeks.[52] It has a final score that ranges from 0 (worst) to 100 (best). SF-36 has been used to measure the HRQoL in various medical problems including vitiligo.

Homan et al. used this instrument to assess the impact of vitiligo that began in childhood in 232 adult patients and compared them with healthy subjects. The patients were also administered the Skindex-29, a dermatology specific instrument. Social and psychosexual development and generic HRQoL in young adult patients with childhood vitiligo were not different from those of healthy controls. Patients with negative childhood experiences related to vitiligo were found to have significantly poorer HRQoL in all the domains of the SF-36 and the Skindex-29.[53]

In another study, Homan et al. assessed the clinical and sociodemographic variables that adversely affect the QoL in 245 adult patients with generalized vitiligo using SF-36 and the Skindex-29. Physicians assessed sociodemographic and clinical characteristics of these patients. It was found that dark skin type, vitiligo located on the chest, and history of receiving treatment in the past appeared to have an adverse impact on the psychosocial domains of quality of life.[52]

Willingness to Pay

Willingness to pay is used to assess the burden of a disease by questioning patients about how much they are willing to pay for treatment in order to improve or heal their disease. WTP has been applied to skin diseases like psoriasis, atopic dermatitis and onychomycosis. Radtke et al. used it for vitiligo in 2009. Two closed and one open question about single and monthly WTP for complete cure of the disease were used. In addition, the patients were asked to name an unrestricted sum for a single payment. The patients' quality of life was also evaluated using dermatology life quality index (DLQI) and EuroQol. Of all patients, 9.8% were willing to make a single investment of more than 500 Euro for a cure, 22.7% would pay up to 1000 Euro, 29.4% up to 5000 Euro and 32.5% more than 5000 Euro. The Willingness to pay correlated with age, duration and extent of disease. There was significant correlation between the DLQI scores and WTP.[54]

WHOQoL-BREF

The WHOQoL questionnaire consists of 100 questions about 24 facets of general health covering physical health, psychological health, social relationships and environment. A truncated version of this questionnaire, the WHOQoL-BREF has been developed for field application consisting of 26 items, one item from each of the 24 facets contained in the WHOQoL-100 and two items for the overall QoL and general health facet.[55] Agarwal et al.[27] used this instrument along with DLQI to evaluate the change in quality of life in vitiligo patients before and after treatment with levamisole. 60 patients with slowly progressive vitiligo were randomly allocated to the levamisole or the placebo group. The results showed that there was no significant difference in the mean number of new lesions in the levamisole and placebo groups. There was a statistically significant reduction in DLQI scores in both the groups but there was no statistically significant difference between the two groups. There was no statistically significant change in the pre- and post-treatment WHOQoL-BREF scores of any of the four domains evaluated by this instrument.

Rosenberg's Self-esteem Scale

This scale consists of ten items, five items for positive self-esteem and five items for negative self-esteem with a four-point scale of responses from totally agree to totally disagree. In this ten-item four-point scale, the possible score ranges from 10 to 40. Scores from 10 to 16 indicate a poor self-esteem, scores from 17 to 33 an average self-esteem and scores from 34 to 40 indicate a high self-esteem. Kent et al.[56] used this scale in their study to test the applicability of DLQI in a non-clinic sample of vitiligo sufferers and to measure its relationship with questionnaires designed to measure a variety of psychological and demographic factors. The DLQI was completed by 614 members of the Vitiligo Society in a postal survey. The scores on DLQI were found to correlate with those of Rosenberg's self-esteem scale, apart from those of perceived stigma (a version of Ginsburg and Link's psoriasis stigma questionnaire), recent experiences, personal distress [both a symptom checklist and the 12-item General Health Questionnaire (GHQ-12)] and race.

DERMATOLOGY QUALITY OF LIFE INSTRUMENTS

There are many skin disease related quality of life instruments, e.g. the DLQI, the Skindex, the Dermatology Quality of Life Scales (DQoLS), the Dermatology-specific Quality of Life instrument, and several of them have been used in vitiligo.

Dermatology Life Quality Index

DLQI is a 10-item questionnaire to assess the impact of skin diseases in general on quality of life.[57] It was developed by Finlay and Khan in 1994 to assess the quality of life in patients with skin diseases. One hundred and twenty patients with different skin diseases were asked about the impact of their disease and its treatment on their lives and the DLQI was developed based on their answers. Items of the DLQI encompass aspects such as symptoms and feelings, daily activities, leisure, work or school, personal relationships and the side-effects of treatment. Each item is scored on a four-point Likert scale: 0, not at all not relevant; 1, a little; 2, a lot; and 3, very much. Scores of individual items (0–3) are added to yield a total score (0–30); higher scores mean greater impairment of the patient's QoL.[58] The DLQI was then completed by 200 consecutive new patients attending a dermatology clinic and 100 healthy volunteers. The mean scores of the volunteers was very low (1.6%, s.d. 3.5) compared with the mean score for dermatology patients (24.2%, s.d. 20.9). The reliability of the DLQI was examined in 53 patients using a 1 week test-retest method and was found to be high (gamma s = 0.99).

Seventeen studies describe the use of DLQI in vitiligo in a total of 1589 patients. The DLQI score ranged from 4.82 to 16.00 with a mean of 9.11.[58]

Parsad et al.[59] assessed the DLQI scores in 150 vitiligo patients and its impact on treatment outcomes. Scores on the DLQI ranged from 2 to 21 (mean ± SD 10.67 ± 4.56). There was no statistically significant difference between the DLQI scores of males and females. There were statistically significant relationships between DLQI scores and age as well as disease duration but not with other variables such as extent of disease. The mean initial DLQI score was 7.06 in patients with a successful outcome while it was 13.12 for patients with treatment failure, a difference that was statistically highly significant indicating that patients with high DLQI scores responded less favorably to therapy.

Using the DLQI, Dolatshahi et al.[60] assessed the quality of life in 100 Iranian vitiligo patients and evaluated its relation with different variables. The mean DLQI score was 8.16 ± 5.423 (range: 0–28) indicating moderate effect on QoL. There was a statistically significant relationship between DLQI score and skin phototype, marital status and disease extension. People with skin phototype V, a dark skin type had poorer scores as compared to those with lighter skin types. Married women had significantly higher DLQI scores than single women while no such difference was found in men. There was no relationship of scores with age, sex, and disease duration, visibility of the disease or the educational level of the patient.

Aghaei et al.[61] tested the reliability and validity of the 10-item Dermatology Life Quality Index (DLQI) questionnaire in 70 Iranian patients with vitiligo. Scores on the DLQI ranged from 0 to 24 (7.05 ± 5.13). There were no statistically significant differences between daily activity and personal relationship scale mean scores (domains of DLQI) in generalized versus focal-segmental involvement in sufferers (P = 0.056, P = 0.053, respectively) suggesting convergent validity. Reliability analysis showed satisfactory result (Cronbach's alpha coefficient = 0.77). The DLQI scores correlated with the extent and location of vitiligo, while no association was seen with the gender and marital status. The findings indicated that the mental health in the vitiligo patients was poor and directly correlated with the quality of life.

Borimnejad et al.[62] compared QoL in male and female patients with vitiligo in Iran using a 17-item multiple-choice questionnaire based on DLQI. A total of 77 Muslim patients with vitiligo (53 females, 24 males; mean age, 29.3 years) were included in this survey. The mean questionnaire score of 42.9 for females was significantly lower than that of 51.6 for males indicating lesser distress in females. Female patients experienced significantly greater impairment of general and psychological health, social relationships, and sexual activity than did male patients.

Kent et al.[56] assessed the applicability of DLQI in a non-clinic sample of vitiligo sufferers and to measure its relationship with questionnaires designed to measure a variety of psychological and demographic factors. The DLQI was completed by 614 members of the Vitiligo Society in a postal survey. The results supported the validity of the DLQI for this sample. DLQI scores were related to perceived stigma (a version of Ginsburg and Link's psoriasis stigma questionnaire), recent experiences, self-esteem (Rosenberg's scale), personal distress (both a symptom checklist and the 12-item GHQ) and race, suggesting that levels of disability might be reduced by interventions that target these variables.

Ongenae et al.[63] studied the burden of vitiligo in the Dutch-speaking Belgian population and compared it with the level of disability caused by psoriasis in a similarly recruited population. One hundred and nineteen patients with vitiligo and 162 patients with psoriasis were included in a postal survey that include the DLQI and additional questions related to demographic data and disease-related characteristics. The overall mean DLQI score for vitiligo (4.95) was lower than that for psoriasis (6.26) (P = 0.01). Patients with vitiligo experienced significantly less impairment of life quality from the symptoms and treatment of the disease ($p < 0.001$). The highest individual mean scores in vitiligo were found for feelings, clothing, social and leisure activities and daily routine. The interaction of disease and sex on the DLQI score was highly significant (P = 0.001). While men with vitiligo scored significantly lower than men with psoriasis ($P < 0.001$), scores were similar for both diseases in women. The number of consultations ($P = 0.005$) and severity of the disease ($P < 0.001$) were independently related to the DLQI. The authors also noted that vitiligo patients were significantly less bothered by disease symptoms and treatment leading to a lower score for vitiligo patients as compared to psoriatic patients. This led the authors to raise doubts about the suitability of DLQI in evaluating the psychosocial burden of vitiligo.

Radtke et al.[54] assessed the QoL in vitiligo patients using DLQI and the EuroQol (EQ-5D) questionnaire. Data were compared with that of 1,511 patients from a similar national survey on psoriasis. The mean DLQI in vitiligo was 7.0 (7.5 in women, 5.5 in men) compared to 8.6 in psoriasis. This value represents moderate reduction in QoL in vitiligo patients. Of the patients with vitiligo, 24.6% had a DLQI greater than 10 which indicates severe QoL impairment compared to 34.1% in patients with psoriasis. 5-Dimensional European Quality of Life Questionnaire (EQ-5D) mean score was 83.6 compared with 75.3 in psoriasis. There was a significant correlation between DLQI and EQ-5D scores. The score for women was considerably higher than that for men. Especially marked limitations in QoL were found in the DLQI for "shame" as part of the complex "symptoms and feelings" as well as for "clothing" and "daily routine", which were recorded as "daily activities". Itching was found to have little importance in the "symptoms and feelings" complex, as were "love life" and "partner and friends", which reflect the complex "personal relationships". QoL did not significantly correlate with age. Greater areas affected, visible lesions and increasing duration of disease were associated with significantly higher QoL reductions. There was a clear relationship between WTP and QoL.

Kostopoulou et al.[64] analyzed the impact of objective and psychological factors on the quality of life and self-body image of 48 patients with vitiligo in France. The objective severity was evaluated using extent, staging and spread of the disease while perceived severity was assessed by the visual analog scale. There was significant correlation between objective and perceived severity. Women were found to be significantly more depressed and anxious than men. The mean DLQI was 7.17 indicating moderate psychosocial impact of vitiligo. No or minimal effect on QoL (DLQI 0–1), mild (2–5), moderate (6–11) and severe (12–20) impairment of QoL was found in five (10%), 14 (29%), 18 (38%) and 11 (23%) patients, respectively. The mean perceived severity evaluated by the patients was 4.91 based on visual analog scale from 0 to 10. The overall mean self-body image score was 58 (range 29–82). There was no significant difference between the QoL of men and women, but women were more affected in their self body image than men. The perceived severity of the illness and personality characteristics (anxiety, depression and self-esteem) were found to be better predictors of the patients' QoL than clinical objective criteria and factors such as gender, age, disease duration and self body impairment.

Skindex

To measure the effects of skin disease on patients' quality of life, a 61-item self-administered survey instrument called Skindex was developed by Chren et al.[65] Skindex had eight scales, each of which addressed an abstract component: cognitive effects, social effects, depression, fear, embarrassment, anger, physical discomfort, and physical limitations. Item responses are standardized from 0 (no effect) to 100 (maximal effect). The instrument was validated in 201 patients with various skin diseases. Subsequently, the number of questions were pruned from 61 to 35, then to 29, then to 17 and finally to 16 with appropriate validation done at each step.[66]

In a study to determine its convergent validity and its advantage relative to a generic measure, responses of 132 dermatology patients to Skindex and the Medical Outcomes Study SF-36 were compared.[67] The patients reported their general health status to be similar to the normal population on SF-36, also SF-36 scores did not correlate with dermatologists' judgments about the severity of skin disease. On the other hand, some patients who reported that they did not suffer from any physical symptoms (37% of patients) or social effects (54%) on the SF-36, reported such effects from their skin disease on Skindex. The responses about skin-related health aspects correlated better with Skindex than SF-36 (for skin condition, mean $r = 0.42$ vs 0.28; for disfigurement, 0.38 vs 0.24). Conversely, responses concerning general health correlated more highly with SF-36 than Skindex (for self-reported health status, mean $r = 0.28$ vs 0.16; for co-morbidity, 0.48 vs 0.37).

Skindex has been used to evaluate the psychosocial impact of vitiligo by different researchers. Homan et al.[52] determined the generic and the dermatology-specific HRQoL in sociodemographically and clinically distinct subgroups of patients with generalized vitiligo using SF-36 and Skindex-29. A total of 245 patients were administered both these questionnaires and the clinical and sociodemographic characteristics of the patients were assessed. Two summary scores were calculated, the physical component summary (PCS) and the mental component summary (MCS) by adding weighted combinations of the 8 scales of SF-36. A summary score of 50 (SD 10) reflected an average quality of life of the general population. The PCS score in vitiligo was 54.4 (SD 8.6) and the MCS score was 46.3 (SD 11.2) indicating that the physical quality of life was higher but the mental quality of life was lower than that of the reference population. The mean scale scores of the Skindex-29 were 13.9 (symptoms), 35.9 (emotions), and 16.7 (functioning). These scores indicated that symptoms were mild, emotions and functioning were influenced moderately, with the most adverse impact noted on the emotional domain. Dark skin type, vitiligo located on the chest, and treatment in the past appeared to have an adverse impact on the psychosocial domains of quality of life. Surprisingly, the presence of generalized vitiligo on the face and the hands was not associated with impaired generic and dermatology-specific HRQoL. Moreover, itch was reported by 20% of the patients in this study. Measurement with the dermatology-specific Skindex-29 showed that patients with generalized vitiligo had mostly emotional problems. The severity of these emotional problems was comparable with that of patients with psoriasis, eczema, chronic hand dermatitis and acne.

Choi et al.[47] evaluated the impact of vitiligo on the quality of life and psychological adaptation in a Korean adolescent population. Fifty-seven adolescents with vitiligo aged 12–18 years were evaluated using self-report scales, namely the Skindex-29, Piers-Harris self-concept, Center for Epidemiologic Studies Depression Scale (CES-D), and Revised Children's Manifest Anxiety Scale (RCMAS). Mean Skindex-29 subscale scores were 21.8 (global), 16.3 (symptom), 18.6 (function) and 29.5 (emotion). The Piers-Harris self-concept scores showed a negative correlation with Skindex-29 scores while other psychological measures (CES-D and RCMAS) showed a positive correlation. They found that the duration of vitiligo, facial involvement, history of previous treatment and patient-assessed severity affected the Skindex-29 subscales in various ways. However, differences in Skindex-29 scores according to the type of vitiligo, extent of involvement, and family history were not observed.

Kim et al. evaluated the QoL of 133 vitiligo patients and compared it to that of 112 patients with other mild skin disorders. All participants filled the Korean version of Skindex-29. In addition, information regarding the clinical and sociodemographic characterstics was gathered. The symptom scale score of Skindex-29 was significantly lower in vitiligo patients than in controls indicating lesser distress, but the function scale and the emotion scale were higher in the vitiligo group. However, the difference in function scales between groups was statistically significant only in female patients.[68]

Zghal et al.[69] studied the quality of life in dermatological skin diseases using a Tunisian version of the Skindex-29 scale. Sixty patients (20 psoriasis, 20 vitiligo and 20 onychomycosis) were selected. The deterioration in QoL affected patients with psoriasis, vitiligo, and onychomycosis in descending order. Patients were particularly sensitive when uncovered zones were affected by disease, especially the face.

Sampogna et al.[70] evaluated the relationship between skin-related quality of life and psychiatric morbidity in 2,136 patients with different skin conditions (including 32 with vitiligo) using Skindex-29 and the GHQ-12. A cut-off threshold of 5 or more on the GHQ-12 was used to identify psychiatric morbidity. For all skin conditions, the patients had a substantially poorer score on GHQ in all three domains of quality of life: symptoms, emotions, and functioning, suggesting psychiatric morbidity was strongly associated with poorer HRQoL in the emotions and functioning scales.

Sampogna et al.[71] investigated risk factors for high quality of life impairment in patients in 181 patients with vitiligo who were asked to complete Skindex-29, GQ-12 and the 20-item Toronto alexithymia scale. It was found that the prevalence of depression (39% versus 10%; GQ-12) and alexithymia (24% vs 10%; Toronto alexithymia scale) was more in vitiligo patients as compared to the general population. Higher scores on Skindex-29 were recorded for female patients, patients older than 40 years, having moderate/severe vitiligo, and having patches on arms, legs or feet. The presence of vitiligo on the hands and on the genitalia did not seem to have an effect on QoL. Surprisingly, the presence of vitiligo lesion on the face did not lead to a significant impairment in QoL. The QoL problems most frequently experienced were worry of the disease getting worse (60%), anger (37%), embarrassment (34%), depression (31%), having social life affected (28%), and shame (28%).

In a parallel-group randomized controlled trial, 84 patients with non-segmental vitiligo were randomized to 308-nm excimer laser phototherapy twice weekly alone or in combination with topical hydrocortisone 17-butyrate cream twice daily for three periods of 3 weeks followed by a one-week steroid-free interval.[72] Seven (16.6%) patients in the excimer monotherapy arm and 18 (42.8%) patients in the combination arm showed 75% or greater reduction of vitiligo lesions at 12 weeks; this difference was statistically significant. Similarly, there was a statistically significant difference for Physician Global Assessment (PGA) scores as well. However, no difference was documented for Skindex-29.

VITILIGO SPECIFIC QUALITY OF LIFE INSTRUMENTS

Patient Defined Outcome Questionnaire

In addition to clinical efficacy, patient-defined benefit assessment has become an important outcome parameter. Recent studies of skin diseases have indicated that patient-relevant benefit can be reliably judged only by the patients themselves.

Augustin et al.[73] developed and validated a patient defined outcome questionnaire for vitiligo. A 26-item questionnaire was used to record patient-defined needs prior to therapy and to evaluate patient benefit attained after therapy. The individually perceived needs of relevant benefits were assessed at the beginning of therapy using the standardized list of the 26 items obtained in the development phase [Patient need questionnaire (PNQ)]. The PNQ showed that patients with vitiligo expect a broad spectrum of therapy benefits from treatment. For each item, a Likert scale ranging from 0 = "not at all important" or "does not apply to me" to

4 = "very important" was established. At the end of a therapy (or during its course) the degree to which these benefits were achieved was assessed by the same item list [Patient Benefit Questionnaire (PBQ)], with item scaling ranging from 0 = "treatment did not help at all" to 4 = "treatment helped a lot". QoL in patients was assessed using the DLQI to assess disease-related quality of life and the EQ-5D to assess generic quality of life. The needs prior to therapy (PNQ) and the benefits achieved by therapy (PBQ) were converted to a weighted index value, the Patient Benefit Index (PBI) with values ranging from 0 (no benefit) to 4 (maximal benefit).

$$PBI = \sum_{i=1}^{k} \frac{PNQ_i}{\sum_{i=1}^{k} PNQ_i} PBQ_i$$

Validation was based on data of 1,023 vitiligo patients. The internal consistency of PNQ was quite high (Cronbach's a 0.94). The Patient Benefit Index showed convergent and discriminant validity with respect to quality of life and patient satisfaction.

There were moderate to high correlations between the PBI and a priori selected parameters of therapeutic success but only slight correlations with DLQI and EQ-5D scores. Thus, the construct "patient benefit" is not identical to the construct 'quality of life'; rather it appears that there is a higher convergence, but not redundancy, with therapy satisfaction.

The PBI for vitiligo was found to be valid and reliable in this study. The instrument showed good usability with respect to patient acceptance and understanding. The method was found to be reliable and valid. The results show that patient-defined benefit assessed via the PBI is not identical to treatment satisfaction and also differs from simple assessments of quality of life.

VitiQoL

VitiQoL is a vitiligo-specific self-report instrument containing 16 items for measuring the QOL in patients that was developed by Lilly et al. in 2012.[50] VitiQoL, along with Skindex-16 and DLQI was administered to 90 patients with vitiligo and details of demographics, overall health, and vitiligo characteristics were recorded.

The VitiQoL items showed high internal consistency (Cronbach alpha = 0.935). Exploratory factor analysis demonstrated 3 factors: participation limitation, stigma, and behavior. Concurrent validity was shown by large correlations between self-reported severity by the patients and VitiQoL scores (r = 0.51). In the absence of an established gold standard for measuring the QOL in vitiligo patients, patients' own assessment of the severity of disease was chosen as a standard against which VitiQoL scores were measured. Known groups validity was demonstrated for the VitiQoL behavior subscale between individuals with exposed and unexposed patches (P = 0.01). There was strong correlation between VitiQoL, Skindex-16 and DLQI (Skindex-16, r = 0.82; DLQI, r = 0.83) indicating convergent validity.

The authors ensured face and content validity by developing vitiligo-specific items from in-depth open-ended interviews with 16 patients, clinical input, and literature review. Reliability (test-retest reproducibility) of the instrument was not tested. Responsiveness of the instrument was not tested because of the prolonged time course necessary to observe clinically significant change in vitiligo.

VitiQoL can be used clinically to assist the physician in the identification of aspects of HRQoL that are especially important to an individual patient. It can also provide an objective measure of disease status, burden of disease, and treatment outcome. In research, VitiQoL may be used as an end point in evaluation of new therapies or in epidemiologic studies to demonstrate need for further research.

Vitiligo Impact Scale

Vitiligo impact scale (VIS) was developed as a rating scale to assess the psychosocial impact of vitiligo in our department.[51] The study was undertaken in three broad phases: item generation, pre- and pilot testing and test administration. Items were generated mostly from a qualitative study using semi-structured interviews of the patients undertaken in the department.[45] In addition, suggestions of the faculty members from the department and relevant questions from other QoL instruments were incorporated. Face validity and content validity were assessed through pre- and pilot testing in 80 patients and the final version consisting of 27 items was administered to 100 patients who also answered the DLQI and the Skindex-16. A PGA of psychosocial impact of vitiligo in every patient was also assessed. Test-retest reliability was assessed in 20 patients.

The scale was internally consistent (Cronbach's alpha value: 0.85). There was moderately good correlation between VIS, DLQI and the Skindex (Spearman rank correlation 0.51 and 0.65 respectively). The scale was able to discriminate between patients having mild and those having moderate and severe impact as assessed by PGA. The test-retest reliability coefficient (Spearman rank correlation) was 0.80. In this study, the patients' own assessment of the psychosocial distress was not taken into account and responsiveness of the scale to therapy was not evaluated.

The VIS may be useful both in clinical practice and in therapeutic trials. It can be used in assessing and comparing the effectiveness of treatment modalities in diminishing the psychosocial burden of vitiligo. Further work is required to establish the psychometric properties of the scale and to evaluate its utility in other cultures and population groups.

CONCLUSION

So far, the emphasis has been on measuring the extent of depigmentation in assessing the severity of vitiligo. While this is important, other factors like disfigurement, psychosocial impact and potential for repigmentation should also be assessed for a comprehensive evaluation of vitiligo.

ACKNOWLEDGMENT

This chapter is excerpted from the MD thesis entitled "Validation and comparative evaluation of Vitiligo Impact Scale in assessing psychosocial burden of vitiligo" submitted by Dr Vishal Gupta to the facuty of the All India Institute of Medical Sciences in June 2013.

REFERENCES

1. Hamzavi I, Jain H, McLean D, et al. Parametric modeling of narrowband UV-B phototherapy for vitiligo using a novel quantitative tool: the Vitiligo Area Scoring Index. Arch Dermatol. 2004;140(6):677-83.
2. Ramam M, Krishna SG. Measuring the severity of vitiligo. Indian J Dermatol Venereol Leprol. 2012;78(1):5-7.
3. Alghamdi KM, Kumar A, Taïeb A, et al. Assessment methods for the evaluation of vitiligo. Journal of the European Academy of Dermatology and Venereology: JEADV; 2012.
4. Hettiaratchy S, Papini R. Initial management of a major burn: II-assessment and resuscitation. BMJ. 2004;329(7457):101-3.
5. Taïeb A, Picardo M. The definition and assessment of vitiligo: a consensus report of the Vitiligo European Task Force. Pigment Cell Res. 2007;20(1):27-35.
6. Ardigo, Muzio, Picardo, Brazzelli. Non-invasive methods for vitiligo evaluation: InVitiligo. Chapter 2.2.3.1. Springer-Verlag Berlin Heidelberg; 2010
7. Aydin F, Senturk N, Sahin B, et al. A practical method for the estimation of vitiligo surface area: a comparison between the point counting and digital planimetry techniques. Eur J Dermatol. 2007;17(1):30-2.
8. Marrakchi S, Bouassida S, Meziou TJ, et al. An objective method for the assessment of vitiligo treatment. Pigment Cell Melanoma Res. 2007;21:106-7.
9. Welsh O, Herz-Ruelas ME, Gomez M, et al. Therapeutic evaluation of UVB-targeted phototherapy in vitiligo that affects less than 10% of the body surface area. Int J Dermatol. 2009;48:529-34.
10. Aspres N, Egerton IB, Lim AC, et al. Imaging the skin. Australas J Dermatol. 2003;44(1):19-27.
11. Lagan KM, Dusoir AE, Mc Donough SM, et al. Wound measurement: the comparative reliability of direct versus photographic tracings analyzed by planimetry versus digitizing techniques. Arch Phys Med Rehabil. 2000;81: 1110-6.
12. Asawanonda P, Taylor CR. Wood's light in dermatology. Int J Dermatol. 1999;38(11):801-7.
13. Gniadecka M, Wulf HC, Mortensen NN, et al. Photoprotection in vitiligo and normal skin. A quantitative assessment of the role of stratum corneum, viable epidermis and pigmentation. Acta Derm Venereol. 1996;76(6):429-32.
14. Westerhof W, van Hasselt BA, Kammeijer A. Quantification of UV-induced erythema with a portable computer controlled chromameter. Photodermatol. 1986;3(5):310-4.
15. Seitz JC, Whitmore CG. Measurement of erythema and tanning responses in human skin using a tri-stimulus colorimeter. Dermatologica. 1988;177(2):70-5.
16. Serup J, Agner T. Colorimetric quantification of erythema—a comparison of two colorimeters (Lange Micro Color and Minolta Chroma Meter CR-200) with a clinical scoring scheme and laser-Doppler flowmetry. Clin Exp Dermatol. 1990;15(4):267-72.
17. Queille-Roussel C, Poncet M, Schaefer H. Quantification of skin-color changes induced by topical corticosteroid preparations using the Minolta Chroma Meter. Br J Dermatol. 1991;124(3):264-70.
18. Clarys P, Alewaeters K, Lambrecht R, et al. Skin color measurements: comparison between three instruments: the Chromameter (R), the DermaSpectrometer (R) and the Mexameter (R). Skin Res Technol. 2000;6(4):230-8.
19. Atsushi Tanemura, Aya Takahashi, Yuriko Ueki. Therapeutic Comparison between Sun Irradiation vs. Narrowband UVB Phototherapy along with Concomitant Topical Tacalcitol for Vitiligo Vulgaris. J Chem Dermatol Sci Appl. 2012;2: 88-91.
20. Middelkamp-Hup MA, Park H-Y, Lee J, et al. Detection of UV-induced pigmentary and epidermal changes over time using in vivo reflectance confocal microscopy. J Invest Dermatol. 2006;126(2):402-7.
21. Kang HY, Bahadoran P, Ortonne JP. Reflectance confocal microscopy for pigmentary disorders. Exp Dermatol. 2010;19(3):233-9.
22. Ardigo M, Malizewsky I, Dell'anna ML, et al. Preliminary evaluation of vitiligo using *in vivo* reflectance confocal microscopy. J Eur Acad Dermatol Venereol. 2007;21(10): 1344-50.
23. Njoo MD, Das PK, Bos JD, et al. Association of the Köbner phenomenon with disease activity and therapeutic responsiveness in vitiligo vulgaris. Arch Dermatol. 1999; 135(4):407-13.
24. Moellmann G, Klein-Angerer S, Scollay DA, et al. Extracellular granular material and degeneration of keratinocytes in the normally pigmented epidermis of patients with vitiligo. J Invest Dermatol. 1982;79(5):321-30.
25. Cui J, Arita Y, Bystryn JC. Cytolytic antibodies to melanocytes in vitiligo. J Invest Dermatol. 1993;100(6):812-5.
26. Uda H, Takei M, Mishima Y. Immunopathology of vitiligo vulgaris, Sutton's leukoderma and melanoma-associated

vitiligo in relation to steroid effects. II. The IgG and C3 deposits in the skin. J Cutan Pathol. 1984;11(2):114-24.
27. Agarwal S, Ramam M, Sharma VK, et al. A randomized placebo-controlled double-blind study of levamisole in the treatment of limited and slowly spreading vitiligo. Br J Dermatol. 2005;153(1):163-6.
28. Falabella R, Arrunategui A, Barona MI, et al. The minigrafting test for vitiligo: detection of stable lesions for melanocyte transplantation. J Am Acad Dermatol. 1995;32(2 Pt 1): 228-32.
29. Boersma BR, Westerhof W, Bos JD. Repigmentation in vitiligo vulgaris by autologous minigrafting: results in nineteen patients. J Am Acad Dermatol. 1995;33(6):990-5.
30. Singh Ajit Kumar, RC Sarin, VK Puri. Evaluation of replacement grafts and punch grafts in the treatment of Vitiligo. Indian J Dermatol Venereol Leprol. 46(3):140-5.
31. Parsad D, Gupta S. Standard guidelines of care for vitiligo surgery. Indian J Dermatol Venereol Leprol. 2008;74(Suppl): S37-45.
32. Benzekri L, Gauthier Y, Hamada S, et al. Clinical features and histological findings are potential indicators of activity in lesions of common vitiligo. Br J Dermatol. 2012.
33. Menchini G, Commacchio C. Vitiligo Activity Index, a new activity evaluation index for bilateral vitiligo vulgaris. J Plast Dermatol. 2007;3:35-9.
34. Lahiri K, Malakar S. The concept of stability of vitiligo: a reappraisal. Indian J Dermatol. 2012;57(2):83-9.
35. Ben Ahmed M, Zaraa I, Rekik R, et al. Functional defects of peripheral regulatory T lymphocytes in patients with progressive vitiligo. Pigment Cell Melanoma Res. 2012;25(1):99-109. doi:10.1111/j.1755-148X.2011.00920.x.
36. Rao A, Gupta S, Dinda AK, et al. Study of clinical, biochemical and immunological factors determining stability of disease in patients with generalized vitiligo undergoing melanocyte transplantation. Br J Dermatol. 2012;166(6):1230-6.
37. Gupta S. Stability in vitiligo: why such a hullabaloo? J Cutan Aesthet Surg. 2009;2(1):41-2.
38. Cucchi ML, Frattini P, Santagostino G, et al. Higher plasma catecholamine and metabolite levels in the early phase of nonsegmental vitiligo. Pigment Cell Res. 2000;13(1):28-32.
39. Singh S, Singh U, Pandey SS. Increased level of serum Homocysteine in vitiligo. J Clin Lab Anal. 2011;25(2):110-2.
40. Shaker OG, El-Tahlawi SMR. Is there a relationship between homocysteine and vitiligo? A pilot study. Br J Dermatol. 2008;159(3):720-4.
41. Karadag AS, Tutal E, Ertugrul DT, et al. Serum holo-transcobalamine, vitamin B12, folic acid and homocysteine levels in patients with vitiligo. Clin Exp Dermatol. 2012; 37(1):62-4.
42. Katz MR, Irish JC, Devins GM, et al. Reliability and validity of an observer-rated disfigurement scale for head and neck cancer patients. Head Neck. 2000;22(2):132-41.
43. Koster PH, Bossuyt PM, van der Horst CM, et al. Characterization of port-wine stain disfigurement. Plast Reconstr Surg. 1998;102(4):1210-6; discussion 1217-8.
44. Terwee CB, Dekker FW, Bonsel GJ, et al. Facial disfigurement: is it in the eye of the beholder? A study in patients with Graves' ophthalmopathy. Clin Endocrinol (Oxf). 2003;58(2):192-8.
45. Sehdev P. A Study of the Psychosocial Effects of vitiligo. Thesis: All India Institute of Medical Sciences, New Delhi, 2008.
46. Parsad D, Dogra S, Kanwar AJ. Quality of life in patients with vitiligo. Health Qual Life Outcomes. 2003;1:58.
47. Choi S, Kim D-Y, Whang S-H, et al. Quality of life and psychological adaptation of Korean adolescents with vitiligo. J Eur Acad Dermatol Venereol. 2010;24(5):524-9.
48. Gawkrodger DJ, Ormerod AD, Shaw L, et al. Guideline for the diagnosis and management of vitiligo. Br J Dermatol. 2008;159(5):1051-76.
49. Both H, Essink-Bot M-L, Busschbach J, et al. Critical review of generic and dermatology-specific health-related quality of life instruments. J Invest Dermatol. 2007;127(12):2726-39.
50. Lilly E, Lu PD, Borovicka JH, et al. Development and validation of a vitiligo-specific quality-of-life instrument (VitiQoL). J Am Acad Dermatol. 2012.
51. Krishna GS, Ramam M, Mehta M, et al. Vitiligo impact scale: an instrument to assess the psychosocial burden of vitiligo. Indian J Dermatol Venereol Leprol. 2013;79(2):205-10.
52. Linthorst Homan MW, Spuls PI, de Korte J, et al. The burden of vitiligo: patient characteristics associated with quality of life. J Am Acad Dermatol. 2009;61(3):411-20.
53. Linthorst Homan MW, de Korte J, Grootenhuis MA, et al. Impact of childhood vitiligo on adult life. Br J Dermatol. 2008;159(4):915-20.
54. Radtke MA, Schäfer I, Gajur A, et al. Willingness-to-pay and quality of life in patients with vitiligo. Br J Dermatol. 2009;161(1):134-9.
55. Sah Krishna G. Development of a Rating-scale to Evaluate the Psychosocial Impact of Vitiligo. Thesis: All India Institute of Medical Sciences, New Delhi, 2010.
56. Kent G, al-Abadie M. Factors affecting responses on Dermatology Life Quality Index items among vitiligo sufferers. Clin Exp Dermatol. 1996;21(5):330-3.
57. Finlay AY, Khan GK. Dermatology Life Quality Index (DLQI)—a simple practical measure for routine clinical use. Clin Exp Dermatol. 1994;19(3):210-6.
58. Basra MKA, Fenech R, Gatt RM, et al. The Dermatology Life Quality Index 1994-2007: a comprehensive review of validation data and clinical results. Br J Dermatol. 2008;159(5):997-1035.
59. Parsad D, Pandhi R, Dogra S, et al. Dermatology Life Quality Index score in vitiligo and its impact on the treatment outcome. Br J Dermatol. 2003;148(2):373-4.
60. Dolatshahi M, Ghazi P, Feizy V, et al. Life quality assessment among patients with vitiligo: comparison of married and single patients in Iran. Indian J Dermatol Venereol Leprol. 2008;74(6):700.
61. Aghaei S, Sodaifi M, Jafari P, et al. DLQI scores in vitiligo: reliability and validity of the Persian version. BMC Dermatol. 2004;4:8.

62. Borimnejad L, Parsa Yekta Z, Nikbakht-Nasrabadi A, et al. Quality of life with vitiligo: comparison of male and female muslim patients in Iran. Gend Med. 2006;3(2):124-30.
63. Ongenae K, Van Geel N, De Schepper S, et al. Effect of vitiligo on self-reported health-related quality of life. Br J Dermatol. 2005;152(6):1165-72.
64. Kostopoulou P, Jouary T, Quintard B, et al. Objective vs. subjective factors in the psychological impact of vitiligo: the experience from a French referral centre. Br J Dermatol. 2009;161(1):128-33.
65. Chren MM, Lasek RJ, Quinn LM, et al. Skindex, a quality-of-life measure for patients with skin disease: reliability, validity, and responsiveness. J Invest Dermatol. 1996;107(5): 707-13.
66. Chren MM, Lasek RJ, Sahay AP, et al. Measurement properties of Skindex-16: a brief quality-of-life measure for patients with skin diseases. J Cutan Med Surg. 2001;5(2): 105-10.
67. Chren MM, Lasek RJ, Quinn LM, et al. Convergent and discriminant validity of a generic and a disease-specific instrument to measure quality of life in patients with skin disease. J Invest Dermatol. 1997;108(1):103-7.
68. Kim DY, Lee JW, Whang SH, et al. Quality of life for Korean patients with vitiligo: Skindex-29 and its correlation with clinical profiles. J Dermatol. 2009;36(6):317-22.
69. Zghal A, Zeglaoui F, Kallel L, et al. Quality of life in dermatology: Tunisian version of the Skindex-29. Tunis Med. 2003;81(1):34-7.
70. Sampogna F, Picardi A, Chren M-M, et al. Association between poorer quality of life and psychiatric morbidity in patients with different dermatological conditions. Psychosom Med. 2004;66(4):620-4.
71. Sampogna F, Raskovic D, Guerra L, et al. Identification of categories at risk for high quality of life impairment in patients with vitiligo. Br J Dermatol. 2008;159(2):351-9.
72. Sassi F, Cazzaniga S, Tessari G, et al. Randomized controlled trial comparing the effectiveness of 308-nm excimer laser alone or in combination with topical hydrocortisone 17-butyrate cream in the treatment of vitiligo of the face and neck. Br J Dermatol. 2008;159(5):1186-91.
73. Augustin M, Gajur AI, Reich C, et al. Benefit evaluation in vitiligo treatment: development and validation of a patient-defined outcome questionnaire. Dermatology (Basel). 2008; 217(2):101-6.

17

Epidemiology of Vitiligo

Iffat Hassan, Parvaiz Rather

Key Features

- Vitiligo is a chronic relapsing disease, with considerable psychological morbidity.
- Epidemiological aspects of the disease are of prime importance, but less studied.
- This aspect of vitiligo should be evaluated on large scale basis in order to identify risk factors for a holistic approach in management with preventive and therapeutic measures.

INTRODUCTION

Vitiligo is a common disorder of pigmentation associated with psychosomatic implications because of cosmetic impairment, caused by the complex interaction between many factors in both internal and external environment of the individual. Along with extensive research for finding new treatment modalities, emphasis should be laid on identifying risk factors and establish a causal association in order that prevention of disease onset may be possible. The association may be direct or indirect. Knowledge about the epidemiology of vitiligo is important for proper integrated approach to management, which includes preventive measures at primary, secondary and tertiary levels, besides the medical and surgical treatment modalities. In this chapter, various epidemiological aspects of this distressing dermatological condition such as incidence/prevalence rate, age, sex, racial, regional, rural/urban and familial aspects will be discussed, as there is a paucity of literature available at present about this important aspect of vitiligo.

Incidence and Prevalence of Vitiligo (Magnitude of the Problem)

Incidence is the rate of occurrence of new cases over a period of time and prevalence is the total number of old and new cases at a given point of time. The incidence and prevalence figures of vitiligo worldwide are as variable as the number of clinic-epidemiological studies itself. This is expected of a disease like vitiligo, having chronic course and chances of relapse. The variation in data between different studies depends on whether it is a hospital or community based study and also on many other factors.

The incidence in the general population worldwide ranges from 0.1% to 3%, with few variations in different studies.[1-4] The estimated incidence rate varies between countries. In United states,[5] it is 1–2%, in China[6] 0.09–0.56%, in Libya[6] 0.3%, in Tanzania[6] 0.3%, in Denmark (Europe)[7] 0.38%, in French West Indies 0.5–1%,[4] in Egypt[6] 1.2% and in Saudi Arabia[8] 2.5%.

The incidence is on the rise especially in developing countries like India, which may be because of growing industrialization and exposure to environmental wastes.[9]

From the Indian subcontinent, India is amongst the countries with highest incidence rates, varying from 0.25% to 2.5%[10] to as high as 8.8% in Delhi,[11] with Gujarat and Rajasthan being high prevalence states.[12] In a previous study from India, prevalence in rural India was reported as 0.49% and that in urban areas as 1.78%.[13] This could be because of diverse ethnic, geographic and environmental conditions prevailing in different regions of the country.

Gender Considerations

There is no sex predilection for vitiligo as such and both sexes are affected equally.[1,6,10,14-17] Female preponderance found in some hospital based studies could be because of more cosmetic concern and consequent outpatient attendance among the females.[2,10,16,17] This may not hold true for frequency in population based studies.[7] Childhood vitiligo has particularly shown more incidence rates in girls.[15,18] Incidence exceptionally high in males has been rarely noted.[6,8]

Age of Involvement

Although vitiligo can develop at any age from infancy to senescence, the peak incidence is found in 10–30 years age group,[2,10] with involvement of much younger age group in India.[10] The notion that vitiligo is related to puberty and females show an earlier onset because they attain puberty earlier than males might be just a myth.[19]

There are reports of congenital vitiligo, but it usually develops in childhood or young adulthood.[14,17,20] In 25% of the cases, it starts before the age of 10-12 years.[9,18] Fifty percent cases develop vitiligo before 20 years[15,21] and 70–80% of patients develop the disease by the age of 30 years.[21] Childhood vitiligo, appearing at age less than 10–12 years, accounts for around 25% of vitiligo cases,[18] varying between different studies: 16% in Korea,[14] 24.1% in China,[20] 23.3% in North India[15]and 26% in South India.[22]

Early age of onset is associated more frequently with focal type of vitiligo especially segmental type and late onset with acrofacial type.[6,14] Early age of onset is also found in those with positive family history.[1,18]

The incidence decreases with increasing age,[5,15,23] but prevalence increases, probably because of cumulative effect and chronic course.[6] Only few studies have shown onset after 40 years of age.[7,16,17]

Racial and Regional Aspects

Vitiligo occurs worldwide but its prevalence varies between countries and among regions in a country probably because of differences in lifestyle and other environmental factors.[6] Prevalence is higher in India than other countries.[10]

All races and ethnic groups are affected,[5,24] with few exceptions. The incidence of vitiligo in those with racially pigmented skin is higher, although reliable figures are not available.[5] Fitzpatrick skin type 4 is the predominant skin type among Caucasian vitiligo patients. Black to dark brown hair and brown iris color seems more common than expected.[5] In India, the incidence of vitiligo appears to be higher in SSK (Somavamsh Sahasrarjun Kshatriya) community.[25]

Clinical types of vitiligo also differ between different populations, for example, segmental vitiligo, which is found more commonly in Koreans.[14,18]

Rural/Urban Variations

As such there is no rural-urban difference in the occurrence of vitiligo, although few studies describe different prevalence rates, with urban predominance.[6,13] This could be because of more environmental pollution in urban areas, acting as trigger factor for vitiligo.[6,13]

Risk Factors

There are many factors, modifiable and non-modifiable, which interact together in a web of causation, predisposing an individual to the development of vitiligo,[1] as displayed in **Flow chart 1**. Genetic factors have more defined role than environmental factors.[1]

Various hypotheses have been described for the development of vitiligo such as genetic theory, disturbances in autoimmune mechanism, neural theory, melanocyte

Flow chart 1: Complex interaction between multiple factors leading and development of vitiligo

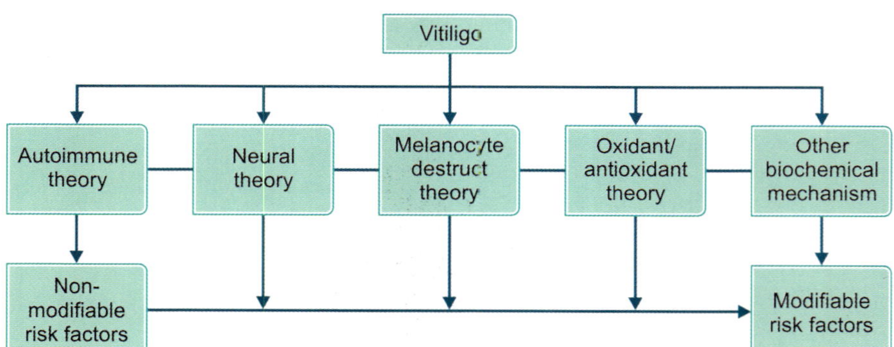

self-destruction theory, disturbed oxidant/anti-oxidant system,[5,10,11,24] the details of which are beyond the scope of this chapter. The preceding factors which actually lead to these mechanisms have seldom been studied in detail. These risk factors need to be identified and evaluated. Some of the incriminating factors are described here:

Non-modifiable Risk Factors (Constitutional Factors)

Most cases of vitiligo occur sporadically, but genetic predisposition is a documented risk factor for its development.[1] This is supported by familial occurrence of cases in the close relatives of the patient who also tend to have earlier onset of disease.[1] Childhood vitiligo also has more positive family history.[17,18]

The incidence of positive family history has variously been reported from 5% to 40% in different studies[1,2,4,6,8-10,15,16,20,24] with the exception of two Indian studies which showed a percentage of 78.29 and 90.38.[9] Positive family history is considered to be a poor prognostic factor.[10]

The mode of inheritance seems to be polygenic[10] and not simple single locus Mendelian inheritance,[1,10,13,19,24] though autosomal dominant and recessive modes have been suggested.[1,10] Various types of HLA predispose to the development of vitiligo with a consensus on type A2, DR4, DR7, CW6 in different studies.[26] The concordance in twins is only 23%,[1] suggesting that genetic factor is not the only one and other factors, like environmental, are also involved.

Modifiable Risk Factors

Emotional stress (related by the subject to some specific life event like death in family, accident, job loss), sun exposure, physical injury, major illness, surgical operation, pregnancy and other environmental factors are incriminated as precipitating factors for vitiligo.[9,11,17] Koebner phenomena may be involved in causing or precipitating vitiligo because of some of these risk factors. Precipitation of vitiligo in a susceptible host can occur by way of entry of certain noxious, melanocyte-destroying chemicals into the body through diet, consumption of preserved stale food/medicines/water contaminated by industrial waste or the air. It is presumed that all these precipitating factors disturb the immunological balance of the body, with consequent effect on patient's melanocyte system producing the lesions of vitiligo.[9,10,11,17]

ASSOCIATIONS OF VITILIGO

Vitiligo is associated with many cutaneous and systemic associations, mostly autoimmune diseases. The level of association of some of the diseases is well established. The major cutaneous associations described in various studies include leukotrichia (poliosis), premature graying of hair (canities), halo nevus, alopecia areata, lichen planus, etc. Other skin disorders are found infrequently.[11] Ocular associations include conditions like Vogt-Koyanagi-Harada syndrome, iris and retinal pigmentary abnormalities, choroidal abnormalities, iritis.[11] Auditory abnormalities may also been seen.[27] Major systemic disorders include hypo/hyperthyroidism, diabetes mellitus, Addisons' disease, pernicious anemia, lymphoma, leukemia, human immunodeficiency virus (HIV) infection, autoimmune poly-endocrinopathy, ulcerative colitis, Sjögren syndrome, giant cell myocarditis.[11]

Morbidity and Mortality Associated with Vitiligo

The mortality rate in vitiligo is practically zero and it is harmless with excellent prognosis, but psychosocial morbidity and therapy related complications may occur. Vitiligo as such does not cause physical disability or pain, but the resultant disfigurement of skin may have a substantial psychosocial impact on the patient.[28] This is particularly so in those with dark skin and lesions on visible areas of the body.[29] Adolescence or young adulthood, female gender, living alone, low socio-economic status, severe disease and co-morbid psychiatric conditions especially lead to increased psychological distress.[28] The psychiatric morbidity includes anxiety, depression, low self-esteem, poor quality of life due to social stigma and even suicidal ideation.[30] So there is a need for holistic approach with psychological intervention along with various treatment modalities to deal effectively with this dermatological condition.

CONCLUSION

In conclusion, at present, more emphasis is laid on the clinical and treatment aspects of vitiligo and little on the epidemiological aspects, knowledge of which is of prime importance for full understanding of a chronic disease like vitiligo. Need of the hour is that epidemiological studies of vitiligo, both hospital and population based, should be conducted on large scale basis to better understand the disease in order that a holistic approach in management can be adopted with emphasis on preventive measures, treatment modalities as well as addressing the psychological morbidity associated with the disease.

REFERENCES

1. Alkhateeb A, Fain PR, Thody A, et al. Epidemiology of vitiligo and associated autoimmune diseases in Caucasian probands and their relatives. Pigment Cell Res. 2003;16: 208-14.
2. Nunes DH, Esser LM. Vitiligo: epidemiological profile and the association with thyroid disease. An Bras Dermatol. 2011;86:241-8.

3. Spritz RA. Shared genetic relationships underlying generalized vitiligo and autoimmune thyroid disease. Thyroid. 2010;20:745-54.
4. Boisseau-Garsaud AM, Garsaud P, Cales-Quist D, et al. Epidemiology of vitiligo in the French West Indies (Isle of Martinique). Int J Dermatol. 2000;39:18-20.
5. Ortonne JP, Bahadoran P, Fitzpatrick TB, et al. Hypomelanosis and Hypermelanosis. In: Freedberg IM, Eisen AZ, Wolff K, Austen KF, Goldsmith LA, Katz SI, (Eds). Fitzpatrick`s Dermatology in General Medicine, 6th edn. New York: McGraw Hill; 2003. pp. 836-81.
6. Wang X, Du J, Wang T, et al. Prevalence and clinical profile of vitiligo in China: a community based study in six cities. Acta Dermatol Venereol. 2013;93:62-5.
7. Howitz J, Brodthagen H, Schwartz M, et al. Prevalence of vitiligo. Epidemiological survey the Isle of Bornholm, Denmark. Arch Dermatol. 1977;113:47-52.
8. Jarallah JS, Al-Sheikh OA, El-Shabrawy M, et al. Epidemiology and clinical pattern at King Khalid University Hospital. Ann Saudi Med. 1993;13:332-4.
9. Behl PN, Agarwal A, Srivastava G. Etiopathogenesis of vitiligo: are we dealing with an environmental disorder? Indian J Dermatol Venereol Leprol. 1999;65:161-7.
10. Shajil EM, Agrawal D, Vagadia K, et al. Vitiligo: clinical profiles in Vadodara, Gujarat. Indian J Dermatol. 2006;51:100-4.
11. Sehgal VN, Srivastava G. Vitiligo: compendium of clinico-epidemiological features. Indian J Dermatol Venereol Leprol. 2007;73:149-56.
12. Valia AK, Dutta PK. IADVL Text book and Atlas of Dermatology. Mumbai: Bhalani Publishing House; 1996. pp. 500-86.
13. Mehta NR, Shah KC, Theodore C, et al. Epidemiological study of Vitiligo in Surat area, South Gujarat. Indian J Med Res. 1973;61:145-54.
14. Cho S, Kang HC, Hahm JH. Characteristics of vitiligo in Korean children. Pediatr Dermatol. 2000;17:189-93.
15. Handa S, Dogra S. Epidemiology of childhood vitiligo: a study of 625 patients from north India. Pediatr Dermatol. 2003;20:207-10.
16. Dogra S, Parsad D, Handa S, et al. Late onset vitiligo: a study of 182 patients. Int J Dermatol. 2005;44:193-6.
17. Esfandiarpour I, Farajzadeh S. Clinical characteristics of late onset vitiligo in an Iranian population. Dermatologica Sinica. 2012;30:43-6.
18. Palit A, Inamadar AC. Childhood vitiligo. Indian J Dermatol Venereol Leprol. 2012;78:30-41.
19. Nath SK, Majumder PP, Nordlund JJ. Genetic epidemiology of vitiligo: multilocus recessivity cross-validated. Am J Hum Genet. 1994;55:981-90.
20. Hu Z, Liu JB, Ma SS, et al. Profile of childhood vitiligo in China: an analysis of 541 patients. Pediatr Dermatol. 2006;23:114-6.
21. Behl PN, Aggarwal A, Srivastava G. Vitiligo. In: Behl PN, Srivastava G (Eds). Practice of Dermatology. New Delhi: CBS Publishers; 2003. pp. 238-41.
22. Jaisankar TJ, Baruah MC, Garg BR. Vitiligo in children. Int J Dermatol. 1992;31:621-3.
23. Koga M, Tango T. Clinical features and course of type A and type B vitiligo. Br J dermatol. 1988;118:223-8.
24. Altaf H, Shah IH, Ahmad QM. Evaluation of thyroid function and presence of anti-thyroid peroxidase antibodies in patients with vitiligo. Egyptian Dermatol online J. 2010; 6:3.
25. Ramaiah A, Majumdar M, Amarnath VM. Vitiligo in SSK community of Bangalore. Ind J Dermatol Venereol Leprol. 1988;54:251-4.
26. Zhang XJ, Chen JJ, Liu JB. The genetic concept of vitiligo. J Dermatol Sci. 2005;39:137-46.
27. Akay BN, Bozkir M, Anadolu Y, et al. Epidemiology of vitiligo, associated autoimmune diseases and audiological abnormalities: Ankara study of 80 patients in Turkey. J Eur Acad Dermatol Venereol. 2010;24:1144-50.
28. Ahmed I, Ahmed S, Nasreen S. Frequency and pattern of psychiatric disorders in patients with vitiligo. J Ayub Med Coll Abbottabad. 2007;19:19-21.
29. Mattoo SK, Handa S, Kaur I, et al. Psychiatric morbidity in vitiligo: prevalence and correlates in India. J Eur Acad Dermatol Venereol. 2002;16:573-8.
30. Saleh HM, Salem SM, El-Sheshetawy RS, et al. Comparative study of psychiatric morbidity and quality of life in psoriasis, vitiligo and alopecia areata. Egyptian Dermatol Online J. 2007;4:2-28.

18

Classification of Vitiligo

Tarun Narang, Davinder Parsad

Key Features

- Vitiligo classification are based on clinical, genetic, pathobiological, epidemiological, and molecular characteristics of vitiligo.
- The Vitiligo European Task Force (VETF) classification and Bordeaux Vitiligo Global Issues Consensus Conference classification and consensus nomenclature are discussed here.
- Some unclassified conditions are mentioned.
- Vitiligo Global Issues Consensus Conference (VGICC) recently revised classification has given a comprehensive and universally accepted classification system.

INTRODUCTION

Vitiligo is an acquired skin depigmentation disorder occurring in approximately 1% of the population worldwide. Although the exact etiopathogenesis is still not completely known and various theories have been proposed but it is generally accepted to be an autoimmune process directed against the melanocytes. It is not a life-threatening disease but its association with a number of other autoimmune diseases, as well as psychosocial difficulties causes significant impairment of quality of life in patients.[1,2]

Although the clinical picture of vitiligo is similar, the etiology and pathogenesis may vary in different individuals so it is still a matter of debate as to whether vitiligo should be classified as a single disease entity or a spectrum of disorders. Vitiligo classification can be based on clinical, genetic, pathobiological, epidemiological, and molecular characteristics of vitiligo. These different classification approaches may aid clinicians to identify the most suitable treatment for each individual.[3,4] In the present scenario although there are guidelines for the management of vitiligo both surgical and non-surgical, there is still no consensus on definitions, nomenclature and disease classification which makes designing and reporting of clinical trials difficult.[4-6]

Of all the parameters that can be used to classify vitiligo the system based on clinical features is a relatively simple method which can easily be used by general practitioners as well as dermatologists and is based on objective criteria like age at onset, disease distribution, speed of spreading, lesion aspect (shape, dimension, color).

The Vitiligo European Task Force (VETF) had proposed consensus definitions for the disease,[7] **(Table 1)** but broader international consensus was lacking so the Vitiligo Global Issues Consensus guidelines were formulated by consultants representing seven regional working groups North and South Africa, North and South/Central America, Europe, Middle East, Continental Asia/Singapore, Japan/Taiwan, and the Pacific. These guidelines on classification and nomenclature have tried to address majority of the issues that were not clear in the past classifications **(Table 2)**.[8]

Clinically vitiligo has been classified into two major forms, namely, segmental vitiligo (SV) and non-segmental vitiligo (NSV), the latter including several variants (generalized vitiligo, acrofacial vitiligo, universal vitiligo).[8] NSV is characterized by depigmented macules of variable sizes often involving both sides of the body with tendency toward symmetrical distribution. In NSV the body hairs are usually spared initially; however, depigmentation may occur with disease progression.

Table 1: Vitiligo European Task Force classification of vitiligo

Types of vitiligo	*Subtypes*
• Non-segmental vitiligo (NSV)	Universal vitiligo, generalized vitiligo, acrofacial vitiligo. Mucosal vitiligo, focal vitiligo
• Segmental vitiligo (type B)	
• Mixed vitiligo (MV)	Combination of initial SV followed by the occurrence of bilateral NSV

Table 2: Bordeaux Vitiligo Global Issues Consensus Conference classification and consensus nomenclature[8]

Types	*Subtypes*
• Vitiligo/NSV	Acrofacial Mucosal (more than one mucosal site) Generalized Universal Mixed (associated with SV) Rare variants
• Segmental vitiligo (SV)	Uni-, bi-, or plurisegmental
• Undetermined/ unclassified vitiligo	Focal Mucosal (one site in isolation)

Abbreviations: NSV, non-segmental vitiligo; SV, segmental vitiligo

Non-segmental vitiligo typically evolves over time, in both distribution and extension patterns. Vitiligo is a dynamic process and the evolution of the disease cannot be predetermined like a case diagnosed as focal vitiligo, may eventually evolve into SV, into NSV, or may remain unclassifiable based on the NSV/SV classification paradigm. For NSV, the disease may be initially classified as acrofacial but will later progress to be better classified as generalized or universal. Conversely, some cases of NSV may spare the extremities (generalized non-acrofacial vitiligo). Some cases of NSV exhibit a flexural distribution and others a predilection for extensor aspects, suggesting different triggers or etiologies. Therefore, precisely reporting the involved sites is of importance.[5,8] More recently, mixed vitiligo (MV) has been defined as the combination of initial SV followed by the occurrence of bilateral NSV patches several months or, more rarely, years later.[9]

These examples represent that the concept of segmental and non-segmental is not axiomatic and these clinical reports of mixed SV and NSV as well as the evidence of inflammation in some cases of early SV, have challenged the concept that these two forms of vitiligo are distinct.[9-16]

The current classification has tried to improve some of these flaws in the past classification. The definitions for various subtypes as given by Vitiligo Global Issues Consensus Conference are:[8]

DEFINITIONS

Vitiligo/Non-segmental Vitiligo

Common Vitiligo (Formerly Referred to as Vitiligo Vulgaris)

It is the most common form of vitiligo; characterized by asymptomatic, well-circumscribed, milky-white macules involving multiple parts of the body, usually in a symmetrical pattern. The disease can start at any site of the body but the fingers, hands and face are frequently the initial sites.

Acrofacial Vitiligo

In acrofacial vitiligo, the involved sites are usually limited to face, head, hands and feet. A distinctive feature is depigmentation of the distal fingers and facial orifices. It may later include other body sites, resulting in typical generalized vitiligo.

Vitiligo Universalis

Vitiligo universalis (VU) is the most extensive form of the disease and generally occurs in adulthood. "Universalis" is generally used when depigmentation is virtually universal (80–90% of body surface), but some pigmentation may be still present. Hairs may also be partially spared. Whereas this diagnosis is straightforward in dark-skinned individuals, it may be difficult in very fair-skinned individuals. Usually, VU is preceded by generalized vitiligo that gradually evolves to complete or near complete depigmentation of the skin and hair.

Mucosal Vitiligo

Mucosal vitiligo refers to the involvement of the oral and/or genital mucosae. It may present as part of generalized vitiligo when associated with other sites of skin involvement, or as an isolated condition, which in the Vitiligo Global Issues Consensus Conference nomenclature, remains in the "unclassified" category at least 2 years of follow-up.

Mixed Vitiligo

Mixed vitiligo refers to concomitant occurrence of SV and vitiligo/NSV **(Figs 1A and B)**. Usually, SV precedes vitiligo/NSV, though not always. Criteria proposed for MV are:

- Absence of depigmented areas in a segmental distribution at birth and in the first year of life, and Wood's lamp examination excluding nevus depigmentosus
- Segmental vitiligo followed by vitiligo/NSV with a delay of at least 6 months
- Segmental vitiligo affecting at least 20% of the theoretical distribution of a dermatomal segment or presenting a definite Blaschko linear distribution
- Response to narrow-band ultraviolet B treatment in between SV (poor response) and vitiligo/NSV (good response).

Focal Vitiligo

Focal vitiligo refers to a small isolated patch that does not fit a segmental distribution, and which has not evolved into vitiligo/NSV after a period of at least 2 year. This form of vitiligo may evolve into either SV or vitiligo/NSV.

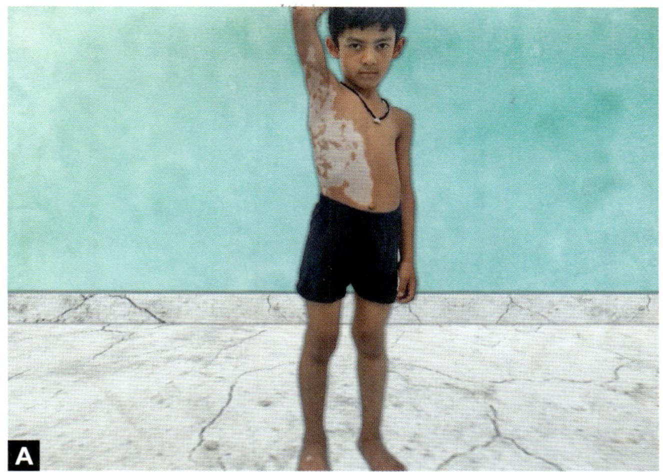
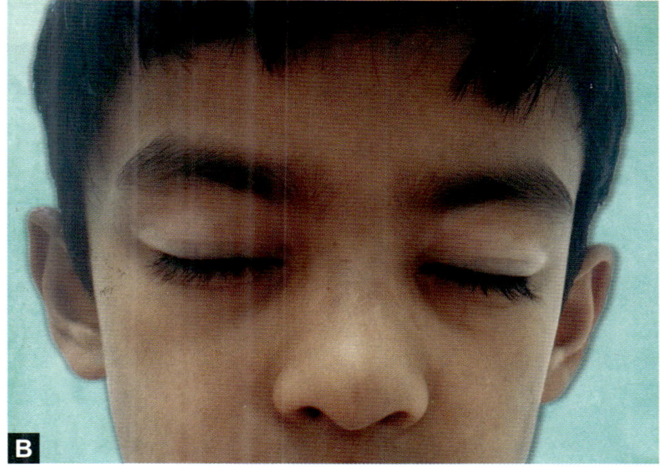

Figs 1A and B: Mixed vitiligo showing both segmental vitiligo and non-segmental vitiligo

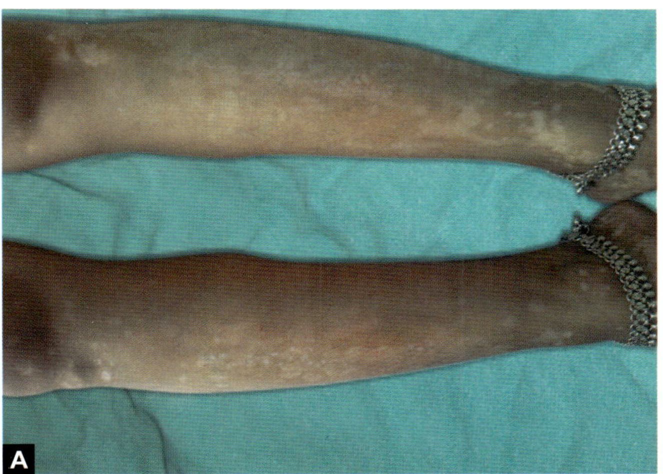
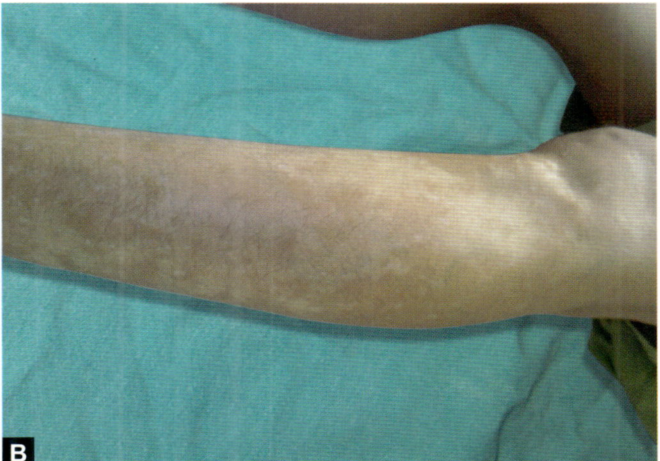

Figs 2A and B: Hypopigmented well to ill-defined lesions of vitiligo minor

Other Unclassified Conditions

Vitiligo Punctata

Lesions present as sharply demarcated depigmented punctiform 1–1.5 mm macules involving any area of the body.

Vitiligo Minor

This form of NSV is rarely reported.[17] The disease seems to be limited to dark-skinned individuals. The term "minor" does not strictly refer to the limitation of the disease to a restricted surface area but rather to the partial defect in pigmentation **(Figs 2A and B)**. The relation to true vitiligo comes from pathology and coexistence with conventional vitiligo macules. The differential diagnosis from early stage cutaneous lymphoma is of primary importance, and repeated biopsies with molecular studies of clonality may be needed.

Follicular Vitiligo

This refers to a form of generalized vitiligo seen in a young black patient that primary involved the follicular reservoir with limited skin involvement, contrasting with marked generalized hair whitening, and melanocyte loss in hair follicles.[17] Additional cases are required to further assess whether follicular vitiligo constitutes a separate form of vitiligo.

Segmental Vitiligo

Monosegmental vitiligo (one or more depigmented macules distributed on one side of the body) is considered to be the most common form of SV, **(Fig. 3)**, usually on one side of midline (although some lesions may partly cross the midline). The pathophysiology of the segmental distribution remains highly controversial. It was initially thought to be a

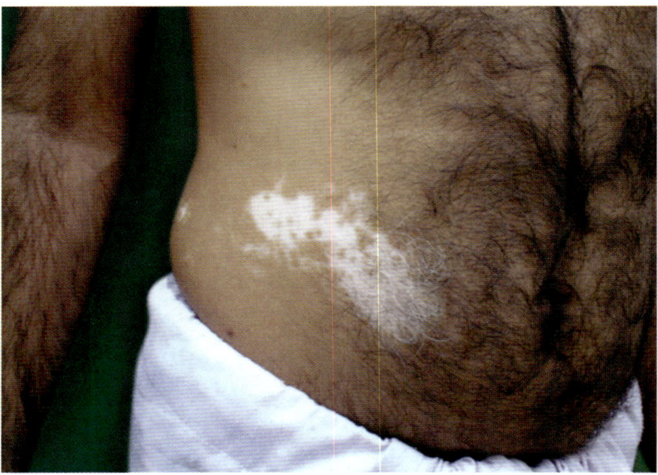

Fig. 3: Unisegmental vitiligo

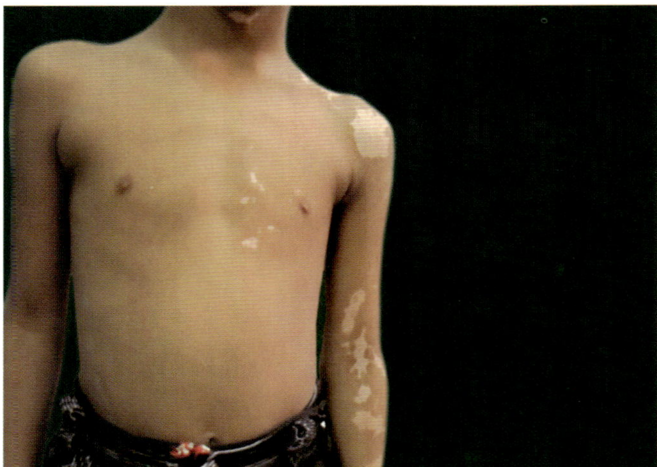

Fig. 4: Bisegmental vitiligo

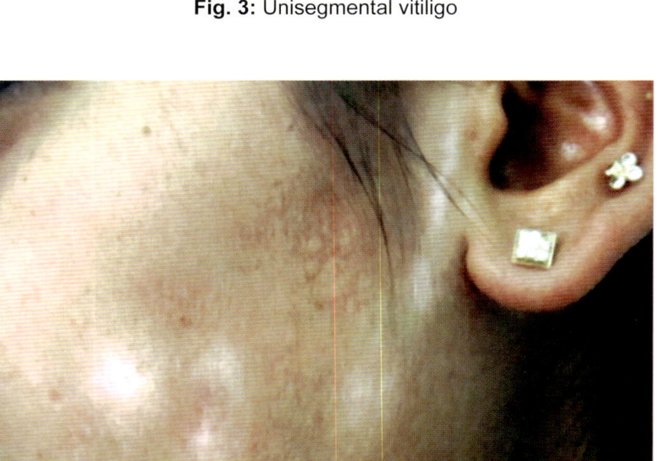

Fig. 5: Segmental vitiligo type II

non-inflammatory process; however, the recent research has proven that some degree of inflammation is seen in the initial stages.[11,12,18,19] It is characterized by early follicular involvement (leukotrichia), spreads within the segment over a period of 6–24 months and then stop; further extension is rare. Rarely, SV may involve multiple segmental lesions distributed either unilaterally or bilaterally **(Fig. 4)**. The onset of these lesions may or may not occur simultaneously. However a clear segmental distribution with midline demarcation, together with the associated features described in monosegmental cases (leukotrichia, protracted course), distinguishes it from vitiligo/NSV. SV also has earlier age of onset than NSV.[8,10,12,18,19] In addition, melanocyte autografts typically yield good results in SV patients, with stable repigmentation.

Facial segmental vitiligo: The lesions on the face do not always correspond to dermatomal distribution. Han et al.[20] classified facial SV into several distinct subtypes according to specific distributions based on long-term observations. They also suggested that such classification might be valuable for prognosis, including the likely degree and path of lesion spreading:

- *Type I-a:* Mid-level face from the forehead to the lower cheek
- *Type I-b:* Forehead and scalp hair
- *Type II:* Lower face and the neck area (mandibular area) **(Fig. 5)**
- *Type III:* Lower face and the neck area **(Fig. 6)**
- *Type IV:* Mid-level face from the forehead to the lower cheek, but selectively appeared on the right side of the face and did not cross the midline
- *Type V:* Lesions were distributed mostly around the right orbital area.

Besides the SV, NSV and MV clinical variants of vitiligo can be seen with the above subtypes. Inflammatory vitiligo **(Fig. 7)** presents with a peripheral erythematous rim. In trichrome vitiligo, three pigmentary hues are seen, with a visible gradient from depigmented to hypopigmented to normally pigmented skin. Quadrichrome vitiligo is trichrome vitiligo with the addition of perifollicular or marginal hyperpigmentation, and is more common in patients with darkly pigmented skin.

Occupational/contact vitiligo: Although the precise definition of contact vitiligo (CV) is unclear it is a distinct form of vitiligo induced by exposure to certain chemicals; commonly implicated chemicals are aromatic or aliphatic derivatives of phenols and catechols.[21,22] At the onset the depigmentation may be confined to the areas exposed to chemicals but subsequently it may extend progressively to the whole body resembling NSV.[23] These chemical agents may be considered as the environmental triggers or haptens for the induction of NSV. However, at present CV is not included in the classification of vitiligo as a separate entity.[8]

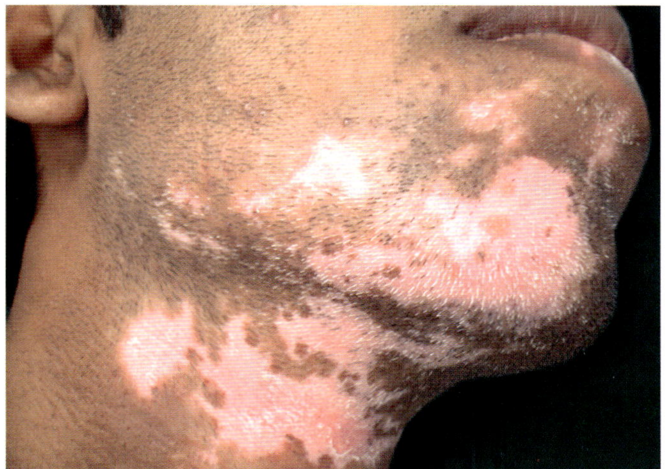

Fig. 6: Segmental vitiligo type III

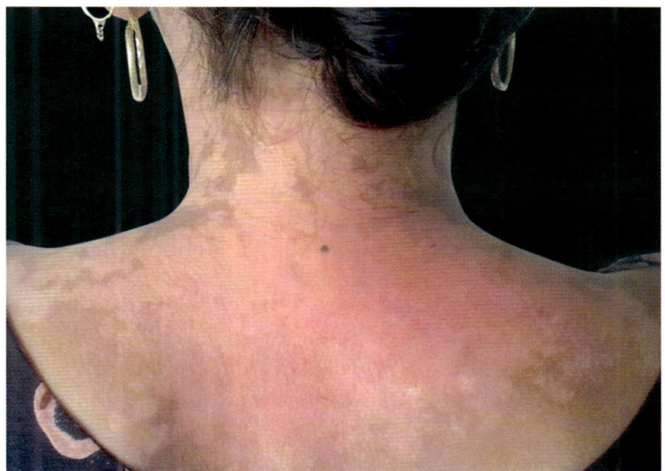

Fig. 7: Inflammatory vitiligo

Table 3: Classification of Koebner's phenomenon[8]

Koebner's type	*Assessment*
Type 1: By history	Depigmentation after trauma during last year? Types of trauma: • Physical (wound, cuts, scratching) • Mechanical (friction) • Chemical/thermal (burns) • Allergic (contact dermatitis or irritant reactions (vaccination, tattoos, etc.) • Chronic pressure • Inflammatory dermatoses • Therapeutics (radiotherapy, phototherapy, etc.)
Type 2: Clinically	• Depigmentation corresponding either to areas of repeated pressure or friction (e.g. elbows, knees) or areas of chronic friction related to cloths/accessory. • Depigmentation clearly induced by trauma (linear, punctiform, crenate) Eliciting trauma
Type 3: Experimentally induced	• Repeated pressure/friction • Superficial (epidermal) trauma • Dermoepidermal trauma

Other Proposed Criteria

Prognosis-oriented Classification

This classification will be useful to give correct information to an individual patient with respect to future expectation and prognosis, and to make a reasonable choice of therapy. Various disease characteristics that help predict the course and treatment outcome are:

Koebner Phenomenon

Koebner phenomenon (KP), also called "isomorphic response". To create a universally acceptable specific system for the evaluation of KP in vitiligo, VETF group have proposed, a new assessment and classification method for the evaluation of KP in vitiligo **(Table 3)**.

Age of Onset

Early onset versus late onset. However, at present there is no consensus about the cut off age for this type of segregation.

Halo Nevus

Sites of involvement: However, at the moment, it is impossible to predict future evolution, localization and activity of the disease.

However, no classification system in vitiligo can be deemed perfect as the disease is characterized by a number of variables and a particular phenotype may be a result of combinations and permutations of these factors. Hercogová et al.[4] proposed other schemes of classification based on genetics, pathobiology, associated multisystem organ dysfunction, triggering events and specific immunoregulatory proteins and stressed on the importance of molecular classification because a limited number of molecules play a major role in depigmentation and repigmentation of the skin, which is shared by the majority of the subjects that manifest with the same (or very similar) phenotype. However, the future is bright and considering the pace at which research on pathobiology and genetics of vitiligo is being conducted we may soon have a more accurate classification system which will be useful for guiding treatment in each individual.

CONCLUSION

Classification systems for vitiligo have been proposed for the last 50 years because it behaves in the different ways in different people or has different characteristics, response to treatment or prognosis. Vitiligo Global Issues Consensus Conference (VGICC) recently revised classification has given a comprehensive and universally accepted classification system that can be used in future studies on vitiligo. Incorporation of pathophysiology or prognosis based classifications would make this classification more useful. Other issues like distribution of the lesions, patterns of spread (along blashko's lines vs dermatomal) and association with other autoimmune diseases also need to be considered in future in refining classification systems for both SV and NSV.

REFERENCES

1. Alikhan A, Felsten LM, Daly M, et al. Vitiligo: a comprehensive overview Part I. Introduction, epidemiology, quality of life, diagnosis, differential diagnosis, associations, histopathology, etiology, and work-up. J Am Acad Dermatol. 2011; 65:473-91.
2. Krüger C, Schallreuter KU. A review of the worldwide prevalence of vitiligo in children/adolescents and adults. Int J Dermatol. 2012;51(10):1206-12.
3. Hercogová J, Schwartz RA, Lotti TM. Classification of vitiligo: a challenging endeavor. Dermatol Ther. 2012;25(Suppl 1):S10-6.
4. Bacigalupi RM, Postolova A, Davis RS. Evidence-based, non-surgical treatments for vitiligo: a review. Am J Clin Dermatol. 2012;13(4):217-37.
5. Gawkrodger DJ, Ormerod AD, Shaw L, et al. Guideline for the diagnosis and management of vitiligo. Br J Dermatol. 2008;159(5):1051-76.
6. Parsad D, Gupta S. Standard guidelines of care for vitiligo surgery. Indian J Dermatol Venereol Leprol. 2008;74(Suppl): S37-45.
7. Taïeb A, Picardo M. The definition and assessment of vitiligo: a consensus report of the Vitiligo European Task Force. Pigment Cell Res. 2007;20(1):27-35.
8. Ezzedine K, Lim HW, Suzuki T, Katayama I, Hamzavi I, Lan CC et al. Revised classification/nomenclature of vitiligo and related issues: the Vitiligo Global Issues Consensus Conference. Pigment Cell Melanoma Res. 2012;25:E1-13.
9. Ezzedine K, Gauthier Y, Léauté-Labrèze C, et al. Segmental vitiligo associated with generalized vitiligo (mixed vitiligo): a retrospective case series of 19 patients. J Am Acad Dermatol. 2011;65(5):965-71.
10. Gauthier Y, Cario Andre M, Taïeb A. A critical appraisal of vitiligo etiologic theories. Is melanocyte loss a melanocytorrhagy? Pigment Cell Res. 2003;16(4):322-32.
11. van Geel NAC, Mollet IG, De Schepper S, et al. First histopathological and immunophenotypic analysis of early dynamic events in a patient with segmental vitiligo associated with halo nevi. Pigment Cell Melanoma Res. 2010;23(3):375-84.
12. van Geel N, De Lille S, Vandenhaute S, et al. Different phenotypes of segmental vitiligo based on a clinical observational study. J Eur Acad Dermatol Venereol. 2011;25(6):673-8.
13. Mulekar SV, Al Issa A, Asaad M, et al. Mixed vitiligo. J Cutan Med Surg. 2006;10(2):104-7.
14. Schallreuter KU, Lemke R, Brandt O, et al. Vitiligo and other diseases: coexistence or true association? Hamburg study on 321 patients. Dermatology (Basel). 1994;188(4):269-75.
15. Schallreuter KU, Krüger C, Rokos H, et al. Basic research confirms coexistence of acquired Blaschkolinear Vitiligo and Acrofacial Vitiligo. Arch Dermatol Res. 2007;299(5-6): 225-30.
16. Passeron T, Ortonne JP. Generalized vitiligo. In: Picardo M, Taieb A (Eds). Vitiligo, Heidelberg: Springer Verlag; 2010. pp. 35-9.
17. Ezzedine K, Amazan E, Séneschal J, et al. Follicular vitiligo: a new form of vitiligo. Pigment Cell Melanoma Res. 2012;25(4):527-9.
18. Hann SK, Lee HJ. Segmental vitiligo: clinical findings in 208 patients. J Am Acad Dermatol. 1996; 35(5 Pt 1):671-4.
19. Taïeb A, Morice-Picard F, Jouary T, et al. Segmental vitiligo as the possible expression of cutaneous somatic mosaicism: implications for common non-segmental vitiligo. Pigment Cell Melanoma Res. 2008;21(6):646-52.
20. Kim DY, Oh SH, Hann SK. Classification of segmental vitiligo on the face: clues for prognosis. British Journal of Dermatology. 2011;164(5):1004-9.
21. Boissy RE. Vitiligo. In: Picardo M, Taieb A (Eds). Occupational vitiligo. Heidelberg: Springer Verlag; 2010. pp. 175-80.
22. Boissy RE, Manga P. On the etiology of contact/occupational vitiligo. Pigment Cell Res. 2004;17(3):208-14.
23. Cummings MP, Nordlund JJ. Chemical leukoderma: fact or fancy. Am J Contact Dermatitis. 1995;6:122-7.

19

Segmental Vitiligo

Binod K Khaitan, Sushruta Kathuria, Priyanka

Key Features

- Vitiligo is broadly divided into two types—segmental vitiligo (SV) and non-segmental vitiligo (NSV).
- Segmental vitiligo differs from NSV in several aspects including pattern and natural course.
- Segmental vitiligo show a patterned unilateral localized distribution.
- Segmental vitiligo usually does not spread to other parts of the body, it stabilizes early, responds very well to surgical methods with probably lower risk of recurrence.
- Early recognition of SV can help to counsel the patient about the natural course and treatment.

INTRODUCTION

Segmental vitiligo (SV) is a specific subtype of vitiligo with characteristic clinical features and natural course. It is localized to the "segment", and is unilateral unless more than one segment is involved, and has a specific pattern. Its clinical features, natural history and appearance is so striking that vitiligo is broadly classified into segmental (SV) and non-segmental vitiligo (NSV).[1,2]

EPIDEMIOLOGY

In World

Vitiligo, the most prevalent pigmentary disorder, occurs worldwide, with an incidence rate of 0.1–2%, irrespective of age, race, ethnic origin or skin color.[3,4] The exact incidence of SV is not well-established because different investigators report variable percentages of vitiligo patients having segmental vitligo. El-Mofty et al. reported that only 5% of patients with vitiligo had the segmental type.[5] Koga and Tango described that in their population, 27.9% had SV.[6] SV was the third most common (19.4%) type of vitiligo in 541 children under 12 years of age in a study from China.[7]

Segmental vitiligo can appear at any age, but the majority of cases occur early in life between the ages of 5 years and 30 years old. Hann and Lee reported that the mean age of onset was 15.6 years, and SV developed before 10 years of age in 41% of cases, and before 30 years of age in 87%.[8]

In India

The prevalence of vitiligo in general population in India is around 0.5%.[9] There are no population-based studies from across the country. Both sexes are almost equally affected. In a retrospective analysis on childhood vitiligo on 625 children at PGIMER, Chandigarh, India the prevalence of SV was found to be 4.6% of all vitiligo patients.[10] In another study on 90 children by Jaisankar et al.[11] SV (30%) was the second most common form. In a study from Manipal hospital, Bengaluru, SV (30%) was second most common after generalized vitiligo (31.3%) in 80 patients. Amongst them, 41 cases (51.25%) were males and 39 (48.75%) were females.[12] In a study of 450 patients of vitiligo at All India Institute of Medical Sciences (AIIMS), New Delhi, India, SV was seen in 6.7% cases.[13] In a cross-sectional study of 188 cases with SV the mean age of onset was 12 years and the sex ratio was 40.4% female versus 59.6% male.[14]

PATHOGENESIS

Vitiligo is an acquired condition caused by destruction of melanocytes. The etiology of vitiligo is multifactorial having genetic, immunological, cytological, environmental and neurological factors. People with vitiligo tend to have an intrinsic defect which predisposes their melanocytes to get destroyed. The exact pathophysiology of the SV remains highly controversial[15,16] and different hypotheses are considered.

The important feature of vitiligo is the absence of melanocytes. Many hypotheses have been proposed for the destruction of melanocytes, but the following hypotheses which are widely accepted for vitiligo:

(1) Genetic hypothesis
(2) Neural hypothesis
(3) Autoimmune hypothesis
(4) Autocytotoxic (self-destruct) hypothesis
(5) Biochemical mechanisms in pathogenesis.

Of these, the neural hypothesis has been so far most emphasized for the pathogenesis of SV. However, further insight into the SV suggests that rather than neural, it may be a manifestation of the cutaneous mosaicism.

Genetic Hypothesis

Patients with vitiligo have a genetic predisposition for the disease. In NSV, a positive family history varies from 7.5% to 27.3%,[13,17-19] while in SV, it is low varying from 9.5% to 14.9%.[14,20,21] In a retrospective study of 137 children, it was observed that SV was more common in patients with a negative family history (22.7%) than those with a positive immediate and extended family history of vitiligo (0% and 13.3% respectively).[22] In the recent Indian study, family history of vitiligo was positive in 13.2% patients having SV.[14]

There are many reports suggesting role of various genes in vitiligo such as X-box binding protein-1(XBP1),[23] SMOC2,[24] TYR[25] and TNF-α.[26] Other genes which may contribute to vitiligo susceptibility are autoimmune regulator I gene (AIRE I), cytotoxic T lymphocyte antigen 4 (CTLA 4), catalase (CAT), catechol-o-methyl transferase (COMT), light molecular weight protein (LMP), transporter associated protein (TAP), angiotensin-converting enzyme gene (ACE), melanocortin 1 receptor (MC1R), agouti signaling protein (ASIP) genes and lymphoid protein tyrosine phosphatase (PTPN 22) gene—PTPN.[27] It has been also reported that APE1-Asp148Glu polymorphism aggravates oxidative stress in human melanocytes and contributes to genetic predisposition to vitiligo in Chinese people.[28] But most of these studies do not evaluate predisposing genes specifically in SV. A relatively lower incidence of family history of vitiligo in patients with SV suggests that genetic component may not be as important in its pathogenesis as in NSV. More studies are required to clearly understand the role of genes in SV.

Neural Hypothesis

Neural hypothesis proposes that the nerves play a major role in the development of vitiligo. The basis for this hypothesis is based on facts such as: (1) the embryological origin of melanocytes and nervous system is from the neural crest, (2) the presence of hypopigmented macules in disorders affecting the nervous system like tuberous sclerosis, syphilis, leprosy and pinta, (3) occurrence of vitiligo in area supplied by nerves after brachial plexus injury, viral encephalitis, transverse myelitis and multiple sclerosis,and (4) widely accepted so-called dermatomal distribution of SV.[29] Morohashi et al. have demonstrated direct contact between free nerve endings and melanocytes.[30] An imbalance of neuropeptides, epinephrine and norepinephrine, and reduced numbers of merkel cells has been seen in vitiliginous skin and may be playing a role in pathogenesis.[31-33]

In SV, a cholinesterase-inhibitor physostigmine led to an abnormal response of sweating much more frequently as compared to generalized vitiligo.[34] On comparing stable facial SV with stable NSV, the cutaneous blood flow was three times increased in SV as compared to normal skin, but in NSV, the increase in blood flow was 1.4–1.5 times. The α- and β-adrenoceptor response of cutaneous microcirculation was also increased in segmental lesions. However, there was no difference in the level of plasma catecholamines or density of adrenoceptors on platelets between the two groups. It is possible that dysfunction of sympathetic nerves may play a role in pathogenesis of SV.[35]

Nordlund has mentioned that the association between vitiligo and nerves is based on superficial data about common origin of melanocytes and neural crest, and that the depigmented skin functions abnormally. The abnormal functioning of the skin may be explained because one of the three major epidermal cells is absent. He also categorically suggested that the distribution of SV in actuality is not dermatomal, i.e. it does not follow a specific pattern of cutaneous sensory nerves. Hence, the terms segmental and dermatomal should not be used interchangeably. The distribution of SV, according to Nordlund, does not follow innervation pattern of sympathetic or parasympathetic nerves, metameres, Blaschko's lines or other developmental patterns. The evidence, currently, is not enough to generate and sustain neural hypothesis for development of vitiligo.[36]

Autoimmune Hypothesis

This hypothesis proposes that vitiligo is an autoimmune process where antibodies are formed against the melanocytes or its components. The higher association of vitiligo with autoimmune diseases like autoimmune thyroiditis, Addison's disease, polyglandular endocrine failure, pernicious anemia, diabetes and lupus erythematosus as compared to controls supports the hypothesis.[22,36] A significantly increased frequency of organ-specific autoantibodies like antithyroglobulin, antithyroid microsomal and antiparietal cell antibodies has been found in patients with vitiligo and their first and second degree relatives as compared to normal controls.[37] Antibodies to specific melanocyte surface antigens have been found in vitiligo patients which are absent in normal individuals.[38] Inspite of evidence regarding the presence of antibodies, it is not known for sure whether these antibodies are the cause of the disease or result from destruction of melanocytes; how exactly the antibodies injure the melanocytes and whether the presence of antibodies is just an epiphenomenon.[38]

In a study conducted at AIIMS, New Delhi in 101 patients, levels of surrogate markers viz. organ-specific [anti-thyroid peroxidase (anti-TPO)] and non-organ specific autoantibodies [antinuclear antibody (ANA)] in SV and NSV were compared. It was observed that ANA were significantly more common in patients with NSV as compared to SV. TPO antibodies were more frequent in NSV; however, the difference was not statistically significant.[39]

Lin et al. observed that the CD4+ cells (helper T cells) were significantly lower and the leukocytes, lymphocytes, monocytes, CD3+ CD19– cells (total T cells), CD3– CD19+ (B cell) cells, CD16+ CD56+ natural killer T cells and HLA-DR T cells were significantly higher in SV patients as compared to healthy controls. The percentage of B cells (CD3– CD19+) was also higher as compared to controls. The percentages of CD3+ CD4+ (helper T cells) and CD3+ CD8+ (cytotoxic T cells) cells were lower in SV. Though these results show different cellular load in SV and healthy individuals, the role of T cells in the pathogenesis could not be concluded.[40] In another study by Gunduz et al. the percentage of helper T cells, CD4/CD8 ratio and activated T cells was significantly reduced in vitiligo patients as compared to controls. But, there was no significant difference between SV and NSV or stable and active vitiligo.[38]

The autoimmune hypothesis has been considered important in pathogenesis of type A (NSV) vitiligo and not in type B (SV) vitiligo by Koga and Tango.[6] A single patient case report of SV with halo nevi reports that there is an increased number of proinflammatory T cells that recognize melanocyte antigens in SV lesional skin compared with non-lesional skin and blood as has been observed in generalized vitiligo.[15] It seems that the evidence for role of autoimmunity in pathogenesis of SV is not enough.

Autocytotoxic (Self-destruct) Hypothesis

The autocytotoxic or self-destruct hypothesis is self-explanatory. It is proposed that there are some metabolites formed by the melanocytes during melanogenesis which could lead to its destruction.[41] Autocytotoxicity occurs in individuals who have a genetic susceptibility, i.e. these patients may have loss of protective genes or have genes predisposing them to autotoxicity. This theory was formulated when it was seen that phenol and its derivatives were capable of preferentially killing pigment cells.[42] Phenols and other free radicals when applied exogenously lead to destruction of melanocytes. Tyrosine and its metabolites (dopaquinone) are capable of causing destruction of melanocytes.[42,43] Melanogenesis is confined to the melanosomes to prevent disruption of other essential metabolic process. There may be an abnormality in the membrane permeability of the melanosomes which causes diffusion of toxic metabolites into the cytoplasm. So far, there are no studies which specifically investigate the role of autocytotoxic theory in the development of SV.

Biochemical Theory

The biochemical theory proposes the role of thioredoxin and pteridines in the destruction of melanocytes.[44] The catalase levels in the epidermis of patients with vitiligo are low. An alteration of the calcium transport leads to low levels of reduced thioredoxin. Due to the low levels of reduced thioredoxin and catalase, there is full oxidation of 6-tetrahydrobiopterin to 6-biopterin which can lead to a cytotoxic environment for epidermal melanocytes. Millimolar levels of H_2O_2 (hydrogen peroxide) can accumulate in the epidermis of affected individuals and consequently, there is cellular vacuolation and destruction of the melanocytes.[45] However, this hypothesis is so far not studied in the pathogenesis of SV specifically.

Cutaneous Mosaicism

A genetic mosaic is an organism composed of two or more genetically different populations of cells that originate from one zygote. By contrast, a genetic chimera is composed of cells derived from different zygotes. On the basis of phenotypic expression, mosaics can be divided into two types: (1) functional and (2) genomic mosaics. Functional mosaics are due to inactivation of one of the X chromosomes (Lyon effect) and are transmitted from mother to daughter; whereas, genomic mosaics are caused by autosomal mutations and are not inherited.[46]

Cutaneous mosaicism was first described in 1983 in a case of linear hyperpigmentation showing a trisomy 18 mosaicism.[47] Since then, it has been proven in hypomelanosis of Ito, McCune Albright syndrome, epidermal nevus (epidermolytic and non-epidermolytic type), tuberous sclerosis, acquired melanocytic nevi, generalized atrophic benign epidermolysis bullosa, neurofibromatosis I, Darier's disease, incontinentia pigmenti, CHILD syndrome and spitz nevus.[48]

Cutaneous mosaicism can have five different patterns: (1) blaschkoid, (2) checkerboard, (3) phylloid, (4) patchy and (5) lateralization pattern.[46,48] Type 1 represents blaschkoid pattern and comprises of two subtypes: type Ia is also known as narrow blaschkoid **(Figs 1A and B)** as seen in incontinentia pigmenti and hypomelanosis of Ito, type Ib has broad blaschkoid pattern **(Figs 2A and B)** as seen in McCune Albright syndrome. Type 2 or checkerboard pattern **(Fig. 3)** has alternating blocks of affected and normal skin with sharp cutoff in the midline. It is seen in systematized speckled lentiginous nevus and is also reported in SV.[14] Type 3 or phylloid pattern **(Fig. 4)** is characterized by arrangement in a leaf-like pattern. Type 1, 2 and 3 are also reported in segmental vitiligo.[1-4] Type 4 or patchy pattern without midline separation is seen in giant melanocytic

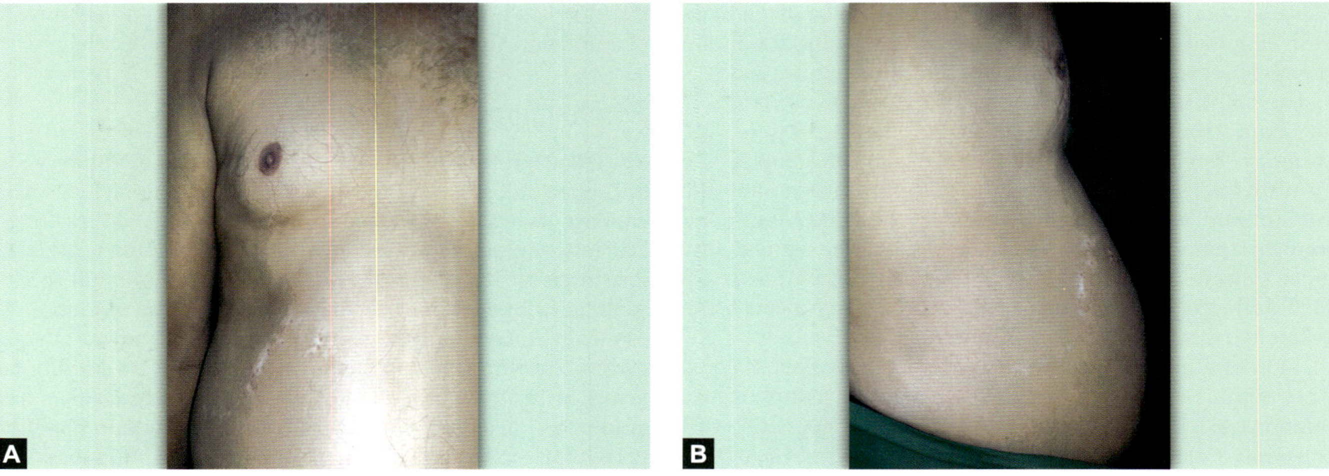

Figs 1A and B: (A) Narrow blaschkoid pattern in segmental vitiligo front; (B) Narrow blaschkoid pattern in segmental vitiligo lateral aspect

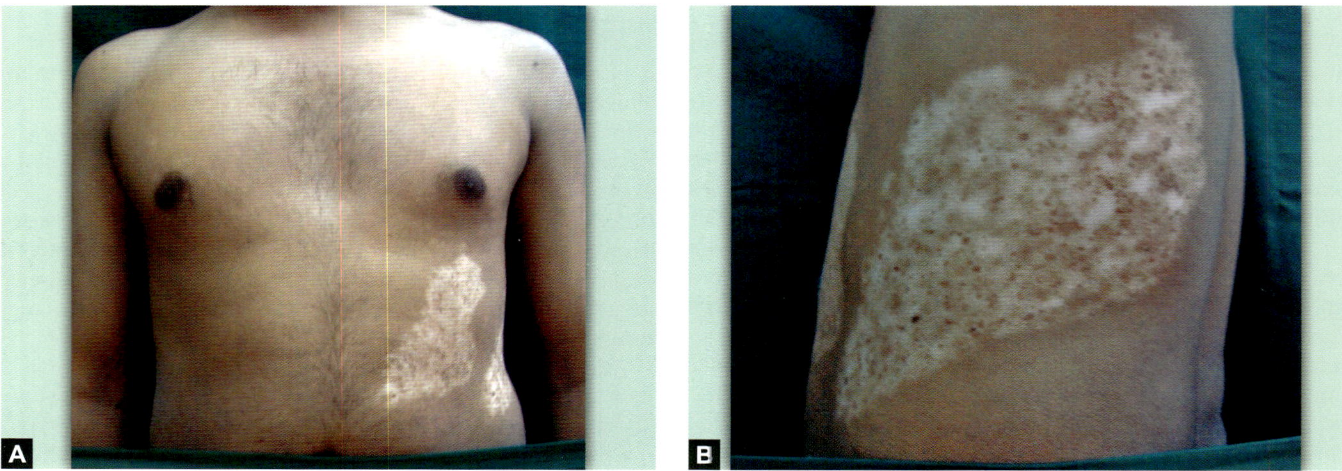

Figs 2A and B: (A) Broad blaschkoid pattern (front); (B) Broad blaschkoid pattern (lateral aspect) close up in segmental vitiligo

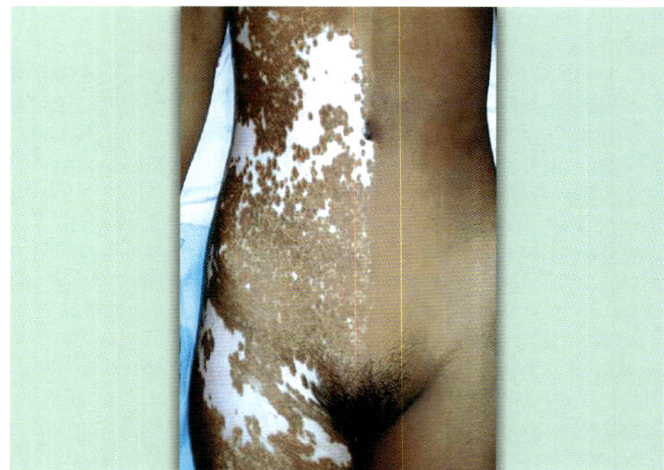

Fig. 3: Checkerboard pattern

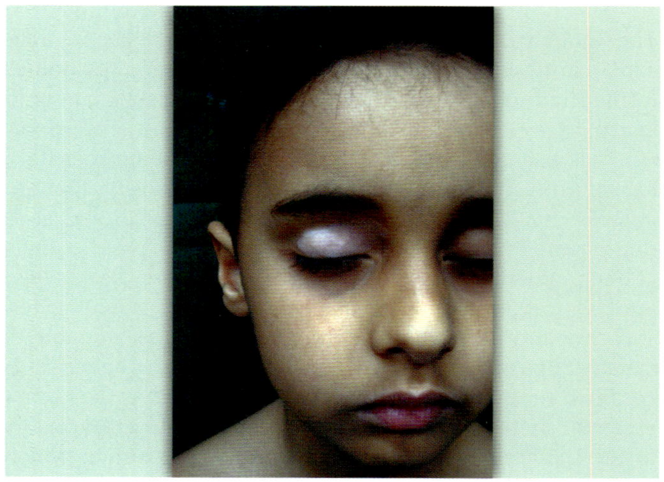

Fig. 4: Phylloid pattern

nevus or neurocutaneous melanosis. Type 5 or lateralization pattern is seen in CHILD syndrome where one half of the body is involved with sharp midline cutoff.[48]

In autosomal dominant disorders, segmental lesions can be of two types: Type 1 segmental lesions occur due to heterozygosity resulting from an early postzygotic new mutation in an otherwise healthy embryo. Here, lesions are restricted to a particular segment and have an early onset in childhood. Type 2 segmental lesions occur from early loss of the corresponding wild-type allele in a previously heterozygous embryo. Here, both segmental and non-segmental lesions are present, and segmental lesion occur early in childhood, and non-segmental lesions occur later.[49] However, concept of Type 1 should not be extended to diseases with polygenic inheritance such as vitiligo, psoriasis and lichen planus because the possibility that additional non-segmental lesions will appear later in life cannot be ruled out.[49] In cases of Type 2 segmental manifestation, monogenic diseases can be explained by loss of heterozygosity, whereas in polygenic disorders, the possibility of a postzygotic mutation giving rise to heterozygosity at an additional predisposing gene locus should be considered.[49] Also, in diseases with polygenic inheritance one cannot differentiate a healthy zygote and heterozygous zygote since there is no single determining gene. The onset of segmental lesions in diseases showing Type 2 segmental pattern with polygenic inheritance can be before non-segmental lesions. Therefore, diseases with polygenic inheritance having segmental lesions should be classified as *isolated* (when only segmental lesions are present, similar to Type 1 in diseases with monogenic inheritance) or *superimposed* (when segmental lesions and non-segmental lesions are present in same patient, similar to Type 2 in diseases with monogenic inheritance).

Bolognia has described Type B vitiligo of Koga as following blaschkoid pattern after reviewing lines of Blaschko.[50] SV is considered by many to follow cutaneous mosaicism.[16,51] In a descriptive study by Khaitan et al. on 188 patients with SV at AIIMS, New Delhi, it was observed that the pattern could be identified in 49.4% patients as blaschkoid, other definitive patterns were dermatomal (3.1%), phylloid (2%), checkerboard (0.5%), and following Voigt's lines (0.5%). However, since this characterization was clinical, in another 22 (about 12%) cases, the authors could not determine the pattern, but thought it was close to blaschkoid or dermatomal and 35% still remained to be classified in a particular pattern.[14] The affected area has developmental predisposition to melanocytic loss and this as suggested by its cutaneous distribution and success of autografting.[16] Vitiligo can be NSV, SV and mixed vitiligo (same patient having both segmental and non-segmental lesions). An interesting feature is that mixed vitiligo can start initially as segmental and then develop non-segmental lesions or vice versa. This is because vitiligo has polygenic inheritance. Hence, even though mosaicism seems very much the basis for pathogenesis of SV, it may not be attributed to loss of heterozygosity like in Type 1 and 2 segmental diseases as vitiligo has polygenic inheritance.[52]

It is a known fact that segmental lesions can occur in combination with bilateral nonlinear lesions in diseases like psoriasis (psoriasis with linear psoriasis). It has been observed that the tumors distributed in a segmental pattern tend to be more numerous and prominent than other tumors present in the same patient or his family members. Vitiligo can also present with a combination of lesions of acrofacial type or focal type with SV.[51]

Environmental Factors and Triggers

The role of external factors in pathogenesis of SV is unclear. Stress has been known to be a precipitating factor, but it is not seen in all patients. There are not many studies regarding pathogenesis of SV. In one study from China, it has been noted that stress was more commonly a precipitating factor in SV as compared to NSV.[21] In the study from AIIMS, New Delhi, however, stress or environmental factors or contact with depigmenting agent was not found as a cause for SV.[14]

CLINICAL FEATURES

Onset and Evaluation

The disease starts early in childhood with 70% having age at onset below 15 years. Even though it is a disease of childhood, late age of onset at 63 years has also been reported.[14] The lesions may start as completely depigmented macule or it may be hypopigmented initially. The lesions develop rapidly and involve an entire segment usually within 6 months to a year. However, in some patients disease may keep progressing within the segment even after a year. After that mostly the disease remains stable with occasional periods of activity within the affected segment. Segmental disease can also occur in combination with NSV (mixed vitiligo) and either can appear first. Even while the disease remains static in few patients, NSV or rarely another SV may develop.

Morphology

Apparently, the lesions in SV are in many ways similar to those of NSV. They are well-defined depigmented macules, occasionally hypopigmented, with leukotrichia. Number of segments can vary. More than 90% are having involvement of only one segment, some having two and rarely even three segments. Number of macules in the affected segment can vary from single to multiple. In a descriptive study on 188 patients,[14] predominantly completely irregular and smooth with irregular margin was present in 40.9% and 44.6% cases respectively. In the same study, complete leukotrichia within lesion and leukotrichia extending beyond margin was present

Type	Description	Frequency in 257 patients
Ia **(Fig. 5A)**	Lesion initiates from right side of forehead and crosses midline of face and spreads down to eyeballs, cheek and nose on left side	28.8%
Ib **(Fig. 5B)**	Chiefly involves the forehead and scalp	10.5%
II **(Fig. 6)**	Lesion starts from area between nose and lip and then arches to preauricular area	16%
III **(Fig. 7)**	Lesion initiates from lower lip and spreads down to chin and neck	14.4%
IV **(Fig. 8)**	Lesion originates from right side of forehead and spreads down to eyeball, nose and cheek without crossing midline	10.9%
V **(Fig. 9)**	Lesions mostly around the right orbital area	8.6%
Mixed		10.9%

Table 1: Classification of segmental vitiligo on face[54]

in 48.9% and 64.8% cases respectively. Islands of pigmented skin within lesion was seen in 65.3% cases. Hence, some of the features which are more characteristic for SV are sharp, irregular margins, prominent leukotrichia often extending beyond the margin of lesion and having islands of normal or hyperpigmented skin within the depigmented macule. These islands of pigmented skin can be present *de novo* without treatment.[14]

Distribution

Usually only a single body area is affected and there is a sharp cutoff in the midline. The single body area may be restricted to one anatomical body part such as upper limb, or may extend onto the trunk of the same side. Crossing over of lesions to opposite side may be rarely seen, but it is just a minimal spill. Head and neck is the most commonly affected site.[14,53]

Patterns

The pattern followed by SV is the most striking and intriguing feature. The pattern of the depigmented macules is one of the important features which help to differentiate for other localized vitiligo (focal vitiligo or early stage of generalized NSV). It may be assumed that if a particular configuration is being formed by the depigmented macules, then a diagnosis of SV can be made.

Despite the importance of pattern in diagnosis of SV, there is much debate about the type of pattern followed. For long, it was assumed that SV follows the dermatomal lines (as followed by herpes zoster) and that also formed the basis of neural theory in the pathogenesis of SV. But the last decade has seen a change in this concept. Many authors now believe that not all SV follow dermatomes.[14,36,50] These patterns are even more complex when observed on face. Hann et al. have recently modified their classification of SV on face into six types based on clinical observation in 257 patients with SV.[54] The six types are given in **Table 1**.

However, in the Indian study on 188 patients with SV, blaschkoid pattern, phylloid pattern and checkerboard pattern have been observed. The blaschkoid pattern **(Figs 10 and 11)** was the most common pattern (49.4%) followed by dermatomal (3.1%).[14] Some authors also feel that almost

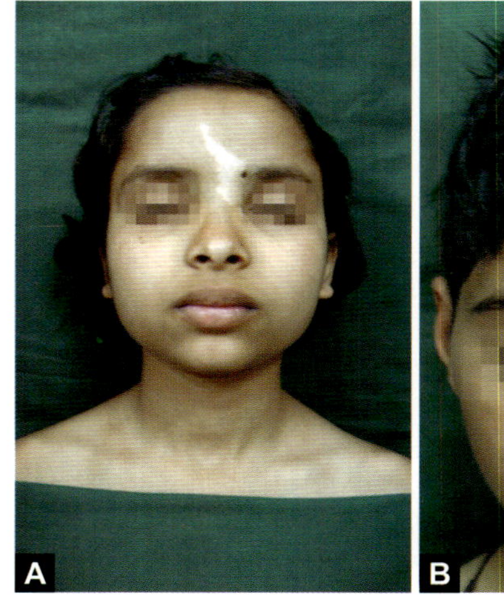

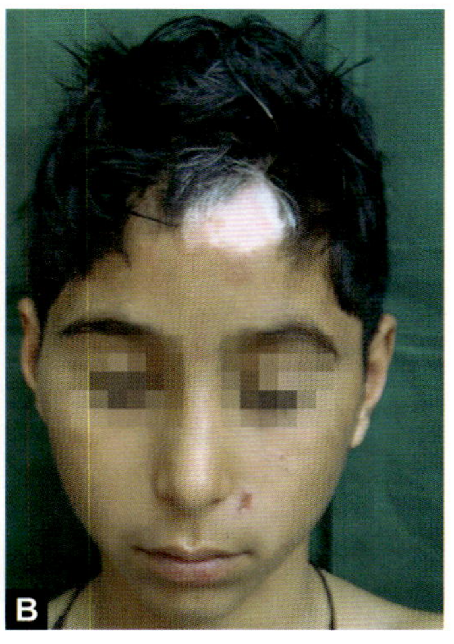

Figs 5A and B: (A) Hann type Ia; (B) Hann type Ib

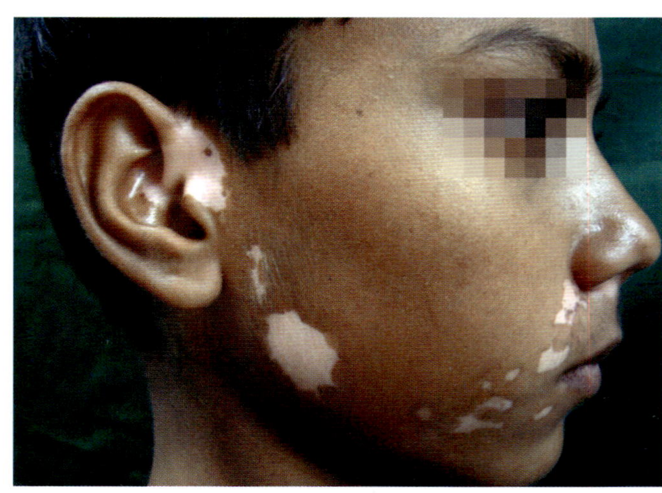

Fig. 6: Hann type II

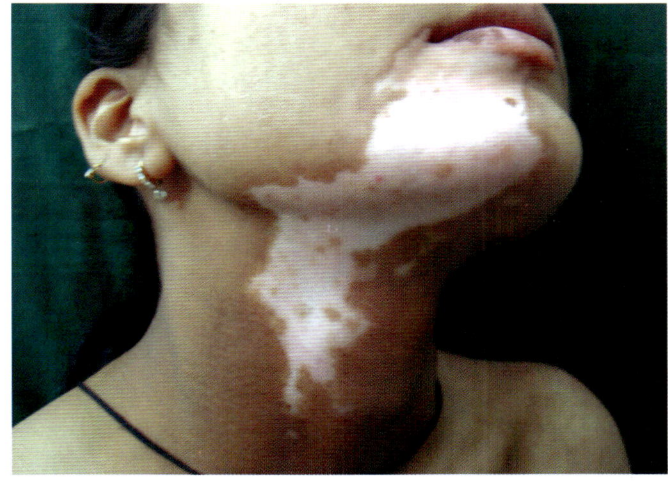

Fig. 7: Hann type III

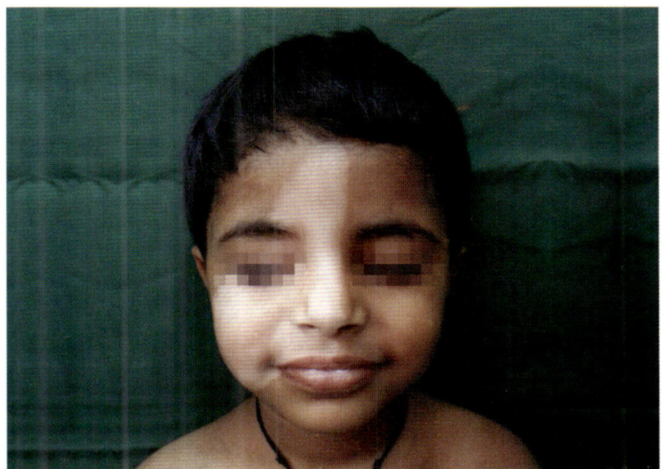

Fig. 8: Hann type IV

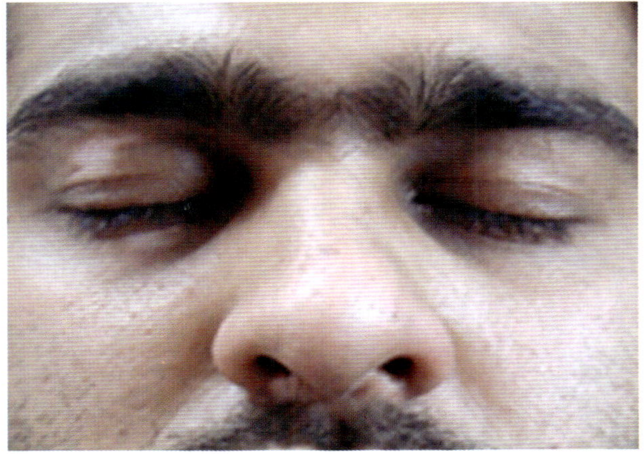

Fig. 9: Hann type V (Right periorbital)

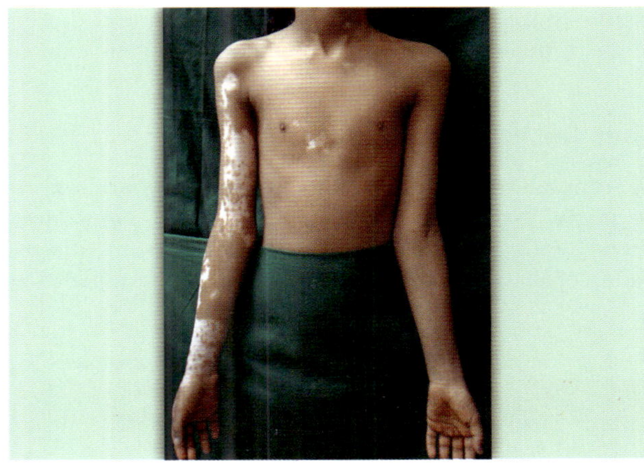

Fig. 10: Blaschkoid trunk

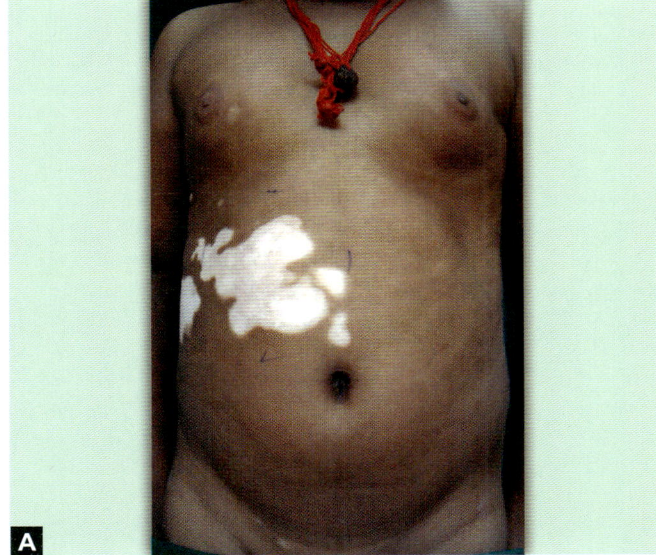

Figs 11A and B: (A) Blaschkoid pattern (front); (B) Blaschkoid pattern (right lateral aspect)

35–70%[14,53] do not follow any recognized pattern. Van Geel et al. observed that in 70% no recognizable pattern was observed and they could not ascertain dermatomal or Blaschkolinear in any.[53] They mention in their discussion that in few, the lesions did appear to be directed along Blaschkolinear pattern but did not fit in exactly, and this was probably because the Blaschko lines may not have been correctly classified till now.[53] They try to classify patterns of SV broadly and nonspecifically into focal and band like forms. Despite no consensus being available for the pattern followed, it is agreed by all that the patterns are repetitive and conspicuous.[55] Van Geel et al. compared pattern of SV with other patterned diseases such as herpes zoster, nevi, hemangioma and others. They found that there is a slight apparent resemblance to herpes zoster but when compared critically, they do not match. Also, pattern is not similar to Blaschkolinear pattern, and the best overlap was with segmental lentiginosis. Hence, they propose that it is possible that SV pattern is a distinct pattern and therefore may be termed as Type 6 pattern of cutaneous mosaicism.[55]

Other Associated Diseases

It is accepted that autoimmunity may not play an important role in SV, especially because a very small proportion of patients with SV have associated autoimmune disease.[20] Khaitan et al. have reported that none of the 188 patients with SV had early onset diabetes mellitus, thyroid abnormality or Addison's disease.[14] An interesting point was that concomitant segmental disease such as nevus depigmentosus and segmental lichen planus was seen in 3 of these 188 patients.[14] Association of segmental vitiligo with segmental lichen planus has been reported previously. However, Van Geel et al. report that autoimmune disease was seen in 7 of 90 cases of isolated vitiligo and 4 of 12 with mixed vitiligo.[53] Their list of autoimmune disease was wider including thyroid diseases, diabetes type 1, alopecia areata, pernicious anemia, rheumatoid arthritis, systemic lupus erythematosus, Addison's disease and even psoriasis, which may be the reason for an increased incidence. Immunologically, Khaitan et al. have reported that ANA are significantly more common in patients with NSV as compared to SV. Similarly, TPO antibodies are more frequent in NSV; however, the difference was not statistically significant.[39]

DIFFERENCES BETWEEN SEGMENTAL AND NON-SEGMENTAL VITILIGO

Segmental vitiligo is distinct from NSV in many aspects. SV is a single entity as compared to NSV which is a broad term encompassing focal vitiligo, mucosal vitiligo, generalized vitiligo, vitiligo vulgaris, acrofacial vitiligo, mixed vitiligo and universal vitiligo.[1] Its main differences are given in **Table 2**.

Table 2: Differences between segmental and non-segmental vitiligo

	Segmental vitiligo	*Non-segmental vitiligo*
Age of onset	Early in childhood	More common in young adults and middle aged
Natural course	Early rapid progression followed by stabilization	Variable course of progression and stability
Distribution	Unilateral with sharp cutoff in midline. Some cases may have more than one segments involved and these may be bilateral	Can be unilateral or localized but a very high proportion of patients have bilateral disease
Pattern	Repetitive conspicuous pattern suggestive of mosaic disorder	No specific pattern. Generalized vitiligo may be bilaterally symmetrical
Leukotrichia	Conspicuous, covering majority of the lesion and extending beyond the margins also	May be present but usually remains within margins of depigmented macule
Margins	Sharply irregular or partially irregular with partially smooth. If near midline then straight line.	Usually smooth or may be irregular
Islands of hyper or normal pigmented skin within lesion	Present even without treatment, but not in all cases	Not common
Response to medical treatment	Poor	Variable, lesions on hair-bearing areas and face respond better than other areas
Response to surgical treatment	Excellent	Variable
Family history	9.5–14.9%[14,20,53]	7.5–27.3%[13,17-19]
Halo nevi	Rare	Common

DIAGNOSIS

Development of Criteria for Diagnosis of Segmental Vitiligo

As SV differs from NSV in several aspects, early recognition of this subtype can help to reassure the patient that it usually does not spread to other parts of the body, it stabilizes early, responds very well to surgical methods with probably lower risk of recurrence. In most cases, it is easy to recognize SV due to its patterned unilateral distribution, however in some early and localized cases where the diagnosis is uncertain, clinical criteria to differentiate segmental and NSV are required. Till now, there is limited data regarding characterization of SV in early stages. Based on the study conducted at AIIMS on 188 patients[14] a set of criteria were developed for diagnosis and these criteria are being further validated.

The proposed clinical criteria are as follows:

Essential Criteria (Major)

- Acquired depigmented macules occurring unilaterally not crossing the midline or with minimal spill onto the opposite side
- Localized to a particular body area/site
- Patterned distribution including recognizable patterns viz. blaschkoid, dermatomal, phylloid, checkerboard, linear **(Figs 12A and B)**, oblong or any other specific type.

Additional Criteria (Minor)

- Age at onset less than 15 years
- Leukotrichia more than 50% over affected lesion
- Leukotrichia extending beyond margin
- Presence of islands of normal or hyperpigmentation within the lesion or segment without treatment
- Margins more than 50% irregular/straight line **(Figs 13A and B)**
- Stability achieved in disease progression by 1 year.

Patient fulfilling all essential and any one or more of the additional criteria are considered to have SV, while, remaining patients are considered as NSV. Currently, a study is undergoing at AIIMS, New Delhi to validate these criteria.

DIFFERENTIAL DIAGNOSIS

Differential diagnoses include other localized vitiligo such as focal vitiligo and early lesions of generalized vitiligo. SV is unilateral, localized and patterned. Features such as marked leukotrichia extending beyond the lesion and islands of hyperpigmented skin can further differentiate from localized NSV.

Other hypopigmented nevoid lesions such as nevus depigmentosus is a strong differential. Nevus depigmentosus is usually congenital or detectable in the first year of life and remains stable in size in proportion to the child's growth. It is characterized as well circumscribed, irregularly shaped, hypopigmented macules whose borders appear feathered or serrated. Hairs within but not beyond the macules may also be hypopigmented.[36] The lesion usually contains a normal or subnormal number of melanocytes compared with control perilesional skin, but the production of melanin pigment is reduced. Sun exposure may attenuate the difference in pigmentation from normal skin. In difficult cases, a biopsy may help to differentiate nevus depigmentosus from SV.[56]

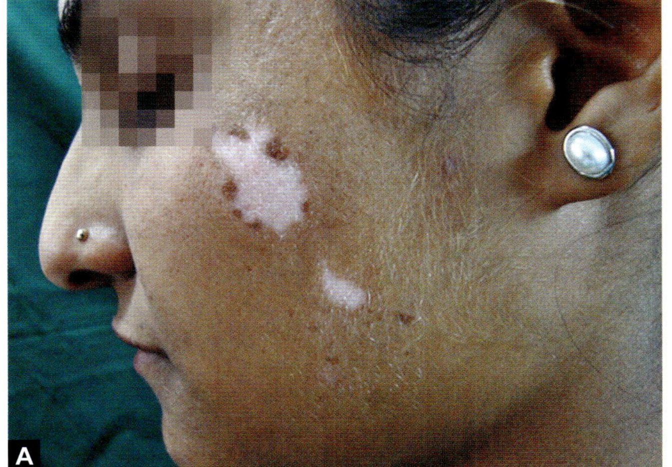

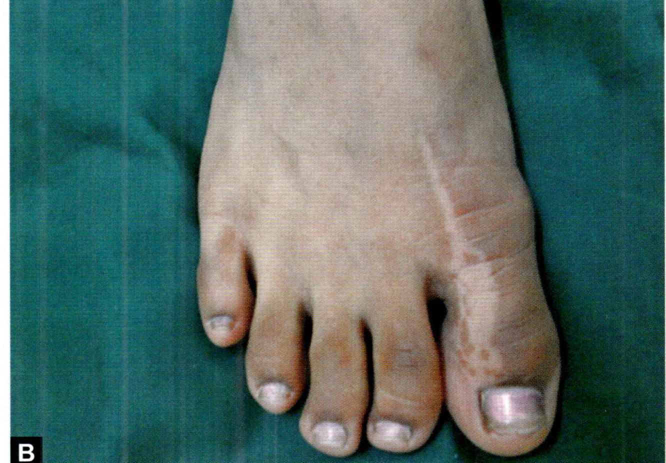

Figs 12A and B: Linear pattern

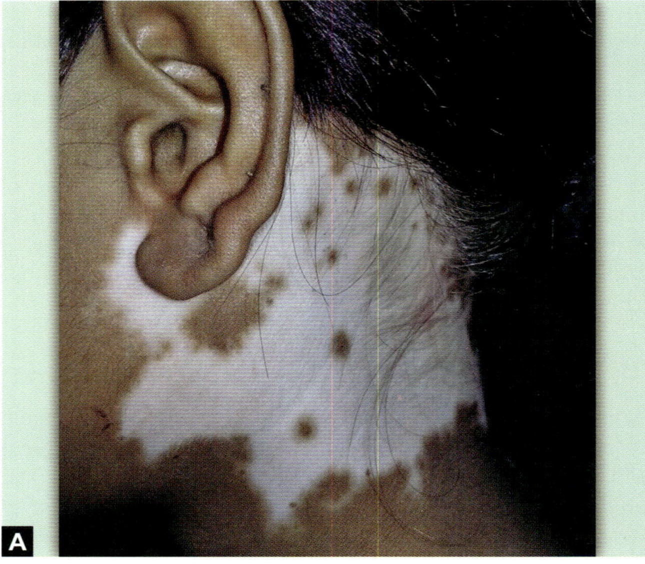

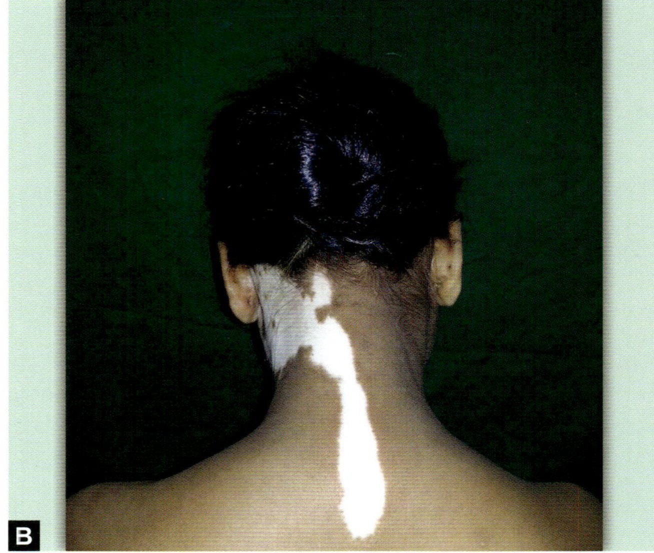

Figs 13A and B: In single lesion: (A) Irregular margin at periphery; (B) Straight margin near midline (Same patient as in A)

MANAGEMENT

Investigations

The diagnosis of SV is mainly clinical. Especially in Indian skin, the contrast between the depigmented lesions and normal skin is so marked that it is fairly easy to make the diagnosis. Skin biopsy is not very helpful in making diagnosis because the findings are nonspecific. The decrease in number of melanocytes can only be decided by comparing with normal skin tissue of same patient from same site. In Fitzpatrick Type 1 and 2 skin type, Wood's lamp may be helpful in delineating the margins of lesion, but it is rarely required in Indian skin. Leukotrichia is clearly visible in body parts such as scalp, eyebrows, eyelashes, but there may be difficulty in discerning leukotrichia of vellus hair. Lee et al. have reported use of digital portable microscope for evaluating leukotrichia in body parts having vellus hair.[57]

The association of SV with autoimmune diseases including thyroid diseases is weak. Laboratory investigations have also shown that autoantibody levels are insignificant in SV.[39] Hence, there is no role of screening for thyroid disorders or autoimmune diseases in SV.

Medical Treatment

It is well known that SV is difficult to treat with medical modalities and usually resistant to medical treatment. Various treatment modalities including topical steroids, topical immunomodulators and psoralen combined with ultraviolet A (PUVA) has been used with very little success. Because of this impression that SV usually does not respond to medical treatment, there are very few studies evaluating the response of SV to different medical therapeutic modalities. Khalid and Mujtaba assessed the efficacy of clobetasol propionate 0.05% cream applied twice daily in 40 patients with SV. After every 6 weeks, the therapy was interrupted for 2 weeks and the patients were treated with 3 such courses. In case, there was no response after 2 courses, then it was considered as treatment failure. After completion of the treatment, more than 50% repigmentation was observed in 34.2% and more than 75% repigmentation was seen in 18.4%. In 21.1% patients, no response was seen. The results were relatively better on the face. The repigmentation was significantly better in patients with disease duration of less than 1 year. Side effects like mild atrophy, telangiectasia and acneiform papules were observed but none were severe enough to require withdrawal of treatment.[58]

An Indian study by Kathuria et al. compared the efficacy and safety of 0.1% tacrolimus ointment versus 0.05% fluticasone propionate cream in 60 consecutive patients of SV. Patients were block randomized into two groups to recieve tacrolimus 0.1% ointment (29 patients) twice daily and 0.05% of fluticasone cream (31 patients) once daily for 6 months. Nineteen patients treated with tacrolimus and 21 patients treated with fluticasone completed the treatment with median repigmentation of 15% and 5%, respectively, at 6 months ($P = 0.38$). Transient side effects like burning, mild pruritus, mild erythema, etc. were observed with tacrolimus and acneiform eruption and rarely mild erythema or mild atrophy with fluticasone and these were limited to the application site.

Hence, tacrolimus and fluticasone propionate are found to produce variable but overall unsatisfactory repigmentation in SV.[59]

There are various treatment-studies in different types of vitiligo, but a seperate analysis of patients with SV is not mentioned in these.[60,61] Daily oral prednisolone has been given in actively spreading vitiligo of both segmental and non-segmental type in 81 patients in a study by Kim et al.[62] For first 2 months, prednisolone was given at 0.3 mg/kg body weight followed by half the initial dose in the 3rd month and then one-fourth the initial dose in the 4th month. The progression of disease was arrested in 87.7%, but the authors do not analyze distinguishing the results between segmental and non-segmental type. However, the repigmentation rate was higher in patients with segmental (23 out of 30, 76.7%) as compared to generalized vitiligo (27 out of 43, 62.8%). The patients with localized non-segmental lesions showed best response (7 out of 8 patients, 87.5%).[62]

Since SV is a localized disease and rarely involves large body surface areas, there are no studies showing the use of oral PUVA or narrowband ultraviolet B (UVB) exclusively in SV. However, narrowband UVB-microphototherapy has been found quite effective.[63] In this study, a phototherapy device was used which has emission spectrum between 300 nm and 320 nm with peak emission at 311 nm with 400 mW/cm^2 intensity. The advantage of microphototherapy is that only the affected area is exposed to UVB. This has an advantage of avoiding whole body irradiation, decreasing the total cumulative dose and hyperpigmentation of the surrounding normal skin. In the study by Menchini et al.[63] the irradiation was given once every 2 weeks for 12 consecutive months. The initial dose was 20% less than minimum erythema dose (MED) with 20% increments every session until the development of erythema. At the end of 1 year, 510 subjects (69.48%) out of total of 734 had achieved more than 75% pigmentation. There were 68 patients with SV. The differences in repigmentation rates between SV and NSV were not significant; however, the exact values were not mentioned separately.

Surgical Treatment

Most of the studies on surgical treatment of vitiligo have a large proportion of SV patients suggesting that once the disease activity stabilizes, surgical treatment is considered the best option.[64-67] SV responds favorably to surgical treatment modalities. Autologous minigrafting (punch grafting) was found to be successful in SV by Falabella.[68] Das and Pasricha reported pigment spread of more than 6 mm within 6 months of punch grafting in 87.5% patients and 92.9% grafts in SV.[66] Savant mentions 22 patients of SV among 62 cases of stable vitiligo who were treated with autologous miniature punch grafting but has not analyzed results of SV separately.[69] In a study by Sarkar et al. 15 Indian patients with SV were treated with autologous miniature punch grafting and 90–100% pigmentation was seen in 12 (80%) cases.[70] In a study conducted in AIIMS by Barman et al. to compare punch grafting followed by topical corticosteroid versus punch grafting followed by PUVA therapy in stable vitiligo, there were 25 (59.52%) patients of SV. The mean pigment spread at 6 months post-surgery was 2.25 mm in 11 patients treated with PUVA after punch grafting and 2.56 mm in 14 patients treated with topical fluocinolone acetonide 0.1% after punch grafting.[65] Epidermal grafting was first introduced by Falabella for achromic and granulating areas[71] and later he also used it for vitiligo.[67] Suction epidermal blister grafting is effective in SV. More than 75% repigmentation has been found in 88–91% patients of segmental/focal vitiligo.[71] Mulekar demonstrated excellent response (95–100%) in 41 out of 50 patients (84%) after autologous, noncultured melanocytes-keratinocyte cell transplantation and the pigment was retained up to 5 years.[72] Cultured autologous pure melanocytes transplantation after laser-abrasion was done by Chen et al. and it led to 95–100% repigmentation in 21 out of 25 patients. In the remaining 4 patients, 65–94% repigmentation was seen.[73] Mulekar used low-dose oral pulse betamethasone (0.1 mg/kg/week), which is similar or marginally lower dose as used by Pasricha and Khaitan in combination with autologous noncultured melanocytes-keratinocyte cell transplantation in 8 patients of SV and 6 out of 8 had an excellent response (95–100% repigmentation).[64] Among the Lasers, helium-neon laser has been found effective in producing more than 50% repigmentation in 60% patients.[73]

The details of surgical management of vitiligo are given in another chapter on this topic.

Approach to Management[74]

First Line Management

Avoidance of triggering factors and use of topical agents (corticosteroids, calcineurin inhibitors).

Second Line Management

Localized NB-UVB therapy, especially excimer monochromatic lamp or laser.

Third Line Management

Consider surgical techniques if repigmentation cosmetically unsatisfactory on visible areas.

Camouflage

Segmental vitiligo though limited in body surface area causes psychological distress to patients if present especially on exposed parts. A patterned depigmented macule can look odd especially on the face. Most studies evaluating quality of life in patients with vitiligo include all types of vitiligo, and are not exclusively conducted on SV. It is reported that lifestyle-altering interventions are selectively effective for patients with more severe quality of life impairment.[75] Camouflage techniques in vitiligo involve using a colored powder and cream combination to cover the depigmented patch. This effect is temporary and can be washed off with water. A study by Ongenae et al. showed that the dermatology life quality index (DLQI) improved after the use of camouflage and hence, recommended the use of camouflage in patients with higher DLQI scores.[76] The advantage in SV is that since affected area is localized, it is easier to apply.

Counseling

Counseling of patient includes different approaches according to the patient's needs. It includes:

Psychoeducation

Psychoeducation includes informing the patient about their disease, available treatment options and their efficacy, facts, and stigma about the disease. Through this process, the patient is encouraged to move toward openness and self-trust.

Cognitive Behavior Therapy

Cognitive behavior therapy is that it is not the stimulus itself which elicits the distress or emotional response directly but our evaluation of thought about that stimulus. In a study[77] conducted at AIIMS, New Delhi, 13 patients (> 12 years of age) of vitiligo, who presented with psychosocial distress, were given five sessions of cognitive behavior therapy full course of cognitive behavior therapy felt more relaxed, more confident and were less bothered about the identify specific problems by listening to the patient's verbalization of thoughts and feelings. The second step is to determine the goals of the therapy. The third step is to develop a hypothesis about the underlying beliefs or environmental events that stimulate, maintain or minimize these thoughts and behaviors. The fourth step is to test the hypothesis of cause and effect by altering the underlying cognitions, the behavior, the environment, or all three, and to observe the effects on the patient's dysfunctional thoughts, feelings, and actions. The fifth step is to revise the hypothesis if the desired results are not obtained or to continue the treatment.[78]

The effect of a dermatological condition penetrates much deeper than the skin. So, while treating patients, it should be realized that these conditions also affect their emotional well-being and quality of life and psychological therapies should be considered as an adjunct to therapy.

CONCLUSION

Vitiligo can be broadly divided into two types: segmental and non-segmental. SV differs from NSV in terms of clinical features, natural history as well as treatment response. The pathophysiology of the SV is not exactly known and different hypotheses are considered. The characteristic feature of SV is the distribution pattern of the lesions. Depigmented macules of SV are arranged unilaterally in various patterns including blaschkoid, dermatomal or quasi-dermatomal, phylloid and checkerboard. Some patients do have conspicuous patterns, but it is difficult to label them. Lesions of SV usually show leukotrichia within and outside the macules, with islands of repigmentation within the macules. Margin is usually irregular and sometimes its straight line if near midline. SV usually has an early onset in childhood and is not associated with autoimmune diseases in contrast to NSV. In SV, the lesions usually evolve rapidly over short span of time in a localized area and then remain stable whereas NSV has a highly variable course with periods of progression, remission, stability and/or exacerbation. SV is usually resistant to medical treatment and responds best to surgical measures. Thus, SV recognition is important as early recognition can help in reassuring and counseling the patient that it usually does not spread to other parts of the body, it stabilizes early, responds very well to surgical methods with probably lower risk of recurrence.

ACKNOWLEDGMENT

The authors acknowledge the valuable inputs by Dr M Ramam.

REFERENCES

1. Ezzedine K, Lim HW, Suzuki T, et al. Revised classification/nomenclature of vitiligo and related issues: the Vitiligo Global Issues Consensus Conference. Pigment Cell Melanoma Res. 2012;25(3):E1-13.
2. Taïeb A, Picardo M, VETF Members. The definition and assessment of vitiligo: a consensus report of the Vitiligo European Task Force. Pigment Cell Res. 2007;20(1):27-35.
3. Krüger C, Schallreuter KU. A review of the worldwide prevalence of vitiligo in children/adolescents and adults. Int J Dermatol. 2012;51(10):1206-12.
4. Ezzedine K, Diallo A, Léauté-Labrèze C, et al. Multivariate analysis of factors associated with early-onset segmental and non-segmental vitiligo: a prospective observational study of 213 patients. Br J Dermatol. 2011;165(1):44-9.
5. el-Mofty AM, el-Mofty M. Vitiligo. A symptom complex. Int J Dermatol. 1980;19(5):237-44.
6. Koga M, Tango T. Clinical features and course of type A and type B vitiligo. Br J Dermatol. 1988;118(2):223-8.
7. Hu Z, Liu JB, Ma SS, et al. Profile of childhood vitiligo in China: an analysis of 541 patients. Pediatr Dermatol. 2006; 23(2):114-6.
8. Park JH, Lee DY. Segmental vitiligo. In: Park KK (Ed). Vitiligo—Managment and Therapy. InTech; 2011. Available from http://www.intechopen.com/books/vitiligo-management-and-therapy/segmental-vitiligo.[Accessed October 2013].

9. Das SK, Majumder PP, Chakraborty R, et al. Studies on vitiligo. I. Epidemiological profile in Calcutta, India. Genet Epidemiol. 1985;2(1):71-8.
10. Handa S, Dogra S. Epidemiology of childhood vitiligo: a study of 625 patients from north India. Pediatr Dermatol. 2003;20(3):207-10.
11. Jaisankar TJ, Baruah MC, Garg BR. Vitiligo in children. Int J Dermatol. 1992;31(9):621-3.
12. Shankar DS, Shashikala K, Madala R. Clinical patterns of vitiligo and its associated comorbidities: A prospective controlled cross-sectional study in South India. Indian Dermatol Online J. 2012;3(2):114-8.
13. Khaitan BK, Pasricha JS, Sood A. Clinical Profile of 450 Indian Vitiligo Patients. American Academy of Dermatology 61st annual meeting 2003, San Francisco.
14. Khaitan BK, Kathuria S, Ramam M. A descriptive study to characterize segmental vitiligo. Indian J Dermatol Venereol Leprol. 2012;78(6):715-21.
15. Van Geel NA, Mollet IG, De Schepper S, et al. First histopathological and immunophenotypic analysis of early dynamic events in a patient with segmental vitiligo associated with halo nevi. Pigment Cell Melanoma Res. 2010;23(3):375-84.
16. Taïeb A. Intrinsic and extrinsic pathomechanisms in vitiligo. Pigment Cell Res. 2000;13(Suppl 8):41-7.
17. Tawade YV, Parakh AP, Bharatia PR, et al. Vitiligo: a study of 998 cases attending KEM Hospital in Pune. Indian J Dermatol Venereol Leprol. 1997;63(2):95-8.
18. Martis J, Bhat R, Nandakishore B, et al. A clinical study of vitiligo. Indian J Dermatol Venereol Leprol. 2002;68(2):92-3.
19. Handa S, Kaur I. Vitiligo: clinical findings in 1436 patients. J Dermatol. 1999;26(10):653-7.
20. Hann SK, Lee HJ. Segmental vitiligo: clinical findings in 208 patients. J Am Acad Dermatol. 1996;35(5 pt 1):671-4.
21. Lin X, Tang LY, Fu WW, et al. Childhood vitiligo in China: clinical profiles and immunological findings in 620 cases. Am J Clin Dermatol. 2011;12(4):277-81.
22. Barona MI, Arrunátegui A, Falabella R, et al. An epidemiologic case-control study in a population with vitiligo. J Am Acad Dermatol. 1995;33(4):621-5.
23. Ren Y, Yang S, Xu S, et al. Genetic variation of promoter sequence modulates XBP1 expression and genetic risk for vitiligo. PLoS Genet. 2009;5(6):e1000523.
24. Birlea SA, Gowan K, Fain PR, et al. Genome-wide association study of generalized vitiligo in an isolated European founder population identifies SMOC2, in close proximity to IDDM8. J Invest Dermatol. 2010;130(3):798-803.
25. Jin Y, Birlea SA, Fain PR, et al. Variant of TYR and autoimmunity susceptibility loci in generalized vitiligo. N Engl J Med. 2010;362(18):1686-97.
26. Laddha NC, Dwivedi M, Begum R. Increased tumor necrosis factor (TNF)-α and its promoter polymorphisms correlate with disease progression and higher susceptibility towards vitiligo. PloS One. 2012;7(12):e52298.
27. Shajil EM, Chatterjee S, Agrawal D, et al. Vitiligo: pathomechanisms and genetic polymorphism of susceptible genes. Indian J Exp Biol. 2006;44(7):526-39.
28. Wei C, Jian Z, Wang L, et al. Genetic variants of the APE1 gene and the risk of vitiligo in a Chinese population: a genotype-phenotype correlation study. Free Radic Biol Med. 2013;58:64-72.
29. Orecchia GE. Neural pathogenesis. In: Hann SK, Nordlund JJ (Eds). Vitiligo, 1st edn. Oxford: Blackwell Science; 2000. pp. 142-50.
30. Morohashi M, Hashimoto K, Goodman TF Jr, et al. Ultrastructural studies of vitiligo, Vogt-Koyanagi syndrome, and incontinentia pigmenti achromians. Arch Dermatol. 1977; 113(6):755-66.
31. Liu PY, Bondesson L, Löntz W, et al. The occurrence of cutaneous nerve endings and neuropeptides in vitiligo vulgaris: a case-control study. Arch Dermatol Res. 1996; 288(11):670-5.
32. Durneva SG. Changes in the content of epinephrine and norepinephrine in the blood of patients with vitiligo. Vestn Dermatol Venerol. 1973;47(10):33-6.
33. Bose SK. Probable mechanisms of loss of Merkel cells in completely depigmented skin of stable vitiligo. J Dermatol. 1994;21(10):725-8.
34. Dutta AK, Mandal SB. A study of non-nervous vasoconstrictor responses. Int J Dermatol. 1972;11(3):177-80.
35. Wu CS, Yu HS, Chang HR, et al. Cutaneous blood flow and adrenoceptor response increase in segmental-type vitiligo lesions. J Dermatol Sci. 2000;23(1):53-62.
36. Nordlund JJ, Ortonne JP, Le Poole LC. Genetic Hypomelanoses: Disorders Characterized by Acquired Depigmentation. In: Nordlund JJ, Boissy RE, Hearing VJ, King RA, Oetting W, Ortonne JP (Eds). The Pigmentary System: Physiology and Pathophysiology, 2nd edn. Oxford: Blackwell Publishing Ltd; 2006. pp. 551-98.
37. Mandry RC, Ortíz LJ, Lugo-Somolinos A, et al. Organ-specific autoantibodies in vitiligo patients and their relatives. Int J Dermatol. 1996;35(1):18-21.
38. Gunduz K, Ozturk G, Terzioglu E, et al. T cell subpopulations and IL-2R in vitiligo. J Dermatol. 2004;31(2):94-7.
39. Khaitan BK, Seshadri D, Kathuria S, et al. Prevalence of coexistent organ specific (TPO) and non-organ specific (ANA) auotoantibodies in patients with segmental vitiligo versus non-segmental vitiligo: a case-control study. Pigment Cell and Melanoma Research. 2011;24:830.
40. Lin IC, Chen YF, Li SY, et al. Imbalance of peripheral leukocyte and lymphocyte subpopulations in segmental vitiligo in Taiwanese. J Dermatol Sci. 2003;33(3):189-91.
41. Hann SK. Chun WH. Autocytotoxic hypothesis for the destruction of melanocytes as the cause of vitiligo. In: Hann SK, Nordlund JJ (Eds). Vitiligo, 1st edn. Oxford: Blackwell Science; 2000. pp. 137-41.
42. Lerner AB, Nordlund JJ. Vitiligo: the loss of pigment in skin, hair and eyes. J Dermatol. 1978;5(1):1-8.
43. Graham DG, Tiffany SM, Vogel FS. The toxicity of melanin precursors. J Invest Dermatol. 1978;70(2):113-6.
44. Schallreuter KU, Beazley WD, Wood JM. Biochemical theory of vitiligo: a role of pteridines in pigmentation. In: Hann SK, Nordlund JJ (Eds). Vitiligo, 1st edn. Oxford: Blackwell Science; 2000. pp. 151-59.

45. Schallreuter KU, Wood JM, Berger J. Low catalase levels in the epidermis of patients with vitiligo. J Invest Dermatol. 1991;97(6):1081-5.
46. Happle R. Mosaicism in human skin. Understanding the patterns and mechanisms. Arch Dermatol. 1993; 129(11): 1460-70.
47. Chemke J, Rappaport S, Etrog R. Aberrant melanoblast migration associated with trisomy 18 mosaicism. J Med Genet. 1983;20(2):135-7.
48. Happle R. Dohi Memorial Lecture. New aspects of cutaneous mosaicism. J Dermatol. 2002;29(11):681-92.
49. Happle R. Superimposed segmental manifestation of both rare and common cutaneous disorders: a new paradigm. Actas Dermosifiliogr. 2009;100(Suppl 1):77-85.
50. Bolognia JL, Orlow SJ, Glick SA. Lines of Blaschko. J Am Acad Dermatol. 1994;31(2 pt 1):157-90.
51. Taïeb A, Morice-Picard F, Jouary T, et al. Segmental vitiligo as the possible expression of cutaneous somatic mosaicism: implications for common non-segmental vitiligo. Pigment Cell Melanoma Res. 2008;21(6):646-52.
52. Happle R. Superimposed segmental vitiligo should not be categorized as "type 2 mosaicism". J Am Acad Dermatol. 2012;66(5):852.
53. Van Geel N, De Lille S, Vandenhaute S, et al. Different phenotypes of segmental vitiligo based on a clinical observational study. J Eur Acad Dermatol Venereol. 2011; 25(6):673-8.
54. Kim DY, Oh SH, Hann SK. Classification of segmental vitiligo on the face: clues for prognosis. Br J Dermatol. 2011; 164(5):1004-9.
55. Van Geel N, Speeckaert R, Melsens E, et al. The distribution pattern of segmental vitiligo: clues for somatic mosaicism. Br J Dermatol. 2013;168(1):56-64.
56. Taïeb A, Picardo M. Epidemiology, definitions and classification. In: Hann SK, Nordlund JJ (Eds). Vitiligo, 1st edition. Oxford: Blackwell Science; 2000. pp. 13-24.
57. Lee DY, Park JH, Lee JH, et al. Is segmental vitiligo always associated with leukotrichia? Examination with a digital portable microscope. Int J Dermatol. 2009;48(11):1262.
58. Khalid M, Mujtaba G. Response of segmental vitiligo to 0.05% clobetasol propionate cream. Int J Dermatol. 1998;37(9):705-8.
59. Kathuria S, Khaitan BK, Ramam M, et al. Segmental vitiligo: a randomized controlled trial to evaluate efficacy and safety of 0.1% tacrolimus ointment vs 0.05% fluticasone propionate cream. Indian J Dermatol Venereol Leprol. 2012;78(1):68-73.
60. Pasricha JS, Khaitan BK. Oral mini-pulse therapy with betamethasone in vitiligo patients having extensive or fast-spreading disease. Int J Dermatol. 1993;32(10):753-7.
61. Kanwar AJ, Dhar S, Dawn G. Oral mini pulse therapy in vitiligo. Dermatology 1995;190(3):251-2.
62. Kim SM, Lee HS, Hann SK. The efficacy of low-dose oral corticosteroids in the treatment of vitiligo patients. Int J Dermatol. 1999;38(7):546-50.
63. Menchini G, Tsoureli-Nikita E, Hercogova J. Narrow-band UV-B micro-phototherapy: a new treatment for vitiligo. J Eur Acad Dermatol Venereol. 2003;17(2):171-7.
64. Mulekar SV. Stable vitiligo treated by a combination of low-dose oral pulse betamethasone and autologous, noncultured melanocyte-keratinocyte cell transplantation. Dermatol Surg. 2006;32(4):536-41.
65. Barman KD, Khaitan BK, Verma KK. A comparative study of punch grafting followed by topical corticosteroid versus punch grafting followed by PUVA therapy in stable vitiligo. Dermatol Surg. 2004;30(1):49-53.
66. Das S Siddhartha, Pasricha JS. Punch grafting as a treatment for residual lesions of vitiligo. Indian J Dermatol Venereol Leprol. 1992;58:315-19.
67. Falabella R. Repigmentation of leukoderma by autologous epidermal grafting. J Dermatol Surg Oncol. 1984;10(2): 136-44.
68. Falabella R. Surgical therapies for vitiligo. In: Hann SK, Nordlund JJ (Eds). Vitiligo, 1st edn. Oxford: Blackwell Science; 2000. pp. 193-201
69. Savant SS. Autologous miniature punch skin grafting in stable vitiligo. Indian J Dermatol Venereol Leprol. 1992;58(5): 310-14.
70. Sarkar R, Mehta SD, Kanwar AJ. Repigmentation after autologous miniature punch grafting in segmental vitiligo in North Indian patients. J Dermatol. 2001;28(10):540-6.
71. Gupta S, Kumar B. Epidermal grafting in vitiligo: influence of age, site of lesion, and type of disease on outcome. J Am Acad Dermatol. 2003;49(1):99-104.
72. Mulekar SV. Long-term follow-up study of segmental and focal vitiligo treated by autologous, noncultured melanocyte-keratinocyte cell transplantation. Arch Dermatol. 2004;140(10):1211-5.
73. Chen YF, Chang JS, Yang PY, et al. Transplant of cultured autologous pure melanocytes after laser-abrasion for the treatment of segmental vitiligo. J Dermatol. 2000;27(7): 434-9.
74. Taieb A, Alomar A, Böhm M, et al. Guidelines for the management of vitiligo: the European Dermatology Forum consensus. Br J Dermatol. 2013;168(1):5-19.
75. Chan MF, Chua TL. The effectiveness of therapeutic interventions on quality of life for vitiligo patients: a systematic review. Int J Nurs Pract. 2012;18(4):396-405.
76. Ongenae K, Dierckxsens L, Brochez L, et al. Quality of life and stigmatization profile in a cohort of vitiligo patients and effect of the use of camouflage. Dermatology. 2005;210(4):279-85.
77. Jha A, Ramam M, Mehta M, Khaitan BK, Sharma VK. Devicing an intervention module to reduce stress in patients with vitiligo. Thesis submitted at AIIMS, June 2011 (unpublished)
78. Levenson H, Persons JB, Pope KS. Behavior therapy and cognitive therapy. In: Goldman HH (Ed). Review of General Psychiatry, 5th edn. New York: McGraw-Hill; 2000. p. 472.

20

Vitiligo in Children

Sandipan Dhar, Raghubir Banerjee, Rajib Malakar

Key Features

- About 50% of vitiligo affected patients have an onset of disease below 20 years of age.
- Vitiligo in children often starts around eyes in both boys and girls and vulva in girls.
- Associated skin and systemic diseases are not as common as in adults.
- Majority of the children do fairly well with topical steroid and tacrolimus. Children above 8 years age can be treated with PUVA therapy and NbUVB.
- Resistent patches can be treated with various types of grafting.
- Overall response to treatment and prognosis is much better in pediatric age group than in adults.
- Counseling of parents and/or older children forms the cornerstone of management.

INTRODUCTION

Vitiligo is an acquired pigmentary disorder of the skin and mucous membranes and is associated with loss of melanin and epidermal melanocytes. There is a chronic and progressive loss of melanocytes from the follicular reservoir and the epidermis. It affects 1-2% of the world population, and about 50% of affected patients have an onset of disease before the age of 20 years. There are often reports of family clustering in children and several susceptibility loci have been seen in genetic studies. Childhood vitiligo may be quoted as disease occurring with onset before the age of 12 years.

ETIOPATHOGENESIS

The condition may involve any body site, but broadly may be divided into generalized and localized (segmental) types. Several hypotheses exist regarding the pathophysiology of the disease including autoimmune, neural and autotoxic mechanisms in children who are genetically susceptible. The autoimmune theory is commonly relevant for generalized vitiligo whereas neural hypothesis is more significant for segmental variant.

The autotoxic mechanism leading to an accumulation of hydrogen peroxide due to low catalase activity could be a possible factor increasing oxidative stress leading to melanocytes destruction. Involvement of vitamin D3, melanocytes inhibition and defective adhesion theory are other possible mechanisms initiating the disease.

Melanocytes are completely absent in vitiligo lesions as seen on histology. Histological stains like DOPA or Fontana-Mason can be used to establish the entity. In early lesions the melanocytes show vacuolization and granular deposits. An inflammatory infiltrate may be seen on histology around the borders of active lesions. During repigmentation, there is migration of the cell from the follicular reservoirs.

CLASSIFICATION

Childhood vitiligo has been broadly classified as "segmental" and "nonsegmental" types. Segmental vitiligo implies appearance of depigmented macules in a dermatomal pattern, without crossing the midline, whereas in nonsegmental vitiligo, the skin lesions may be generalized (vitiligo vulgaris and universalis) or localized (focal, mucosal, acrofacial, acral). In vitiligo vulgaris, there are widely distributed depigmented lesions, whereas near-total depigmentation is coined universal vitiligo. Focal vitiligo is localized nondermatomal distribution, acral is over the extremities and with facial it defines acrofacial variant, and mucosal involves the mucous membranes.[1]

CLINICAL MANIFESTATIONS

Vitiligo in children differs from adult vitiligo in that it is more commonly seen in girls than boys, shows a higher incidence of segmental presentation, and has a lower incidence of associated autoimmune and/or endocrine diseases. Children with vitiligo have an increased incidence of autoimmune and/or endocrine diseases in immediate and extended family members. Vitiligo and leukotrichia (premature graying of the hair) are more commonly seen in family members of affected children. All races are affected but in India a higher prevalence has been reported in some studies.[2]

The morphology of a vitiligo patch is usually a well-defined ivory white asymptomatic macule. The distribution of such areas may be focal or widespread generalized pattern. The condition has been reported in infants of 4 months age and some reports of congenital disease have been documented. The localized or segmental types are common in 4–8 years age group.[3-5]

The ivory white areas are devoid of pigment and are more obvious in dark skin. Some lesions are more pronounced after sun exposure during holidays as the surrounding skin tans normally in contrast to the lesional area. Early spreading areas sometimes show a freckled pattern revealing a typical trichrome pattern. In some lesions, a hyperpigmented or an inflammatory border maybe seen.

In children, common sites are face, periorbital area, neck followed by lower limbs, trunk, and the upper extremities **(Figs 1 to 3)**. The back is usually spared with some involvement of the sacral area. The areas over the chest and abdomen reveal widespread pigmentary loss. Perineal and oral involvement in children is also a common occurrence. **Figure 4** shows chest involvement whereas the description in the text is of perineal and oral involvement. Focal involvement along the trigeminal segment has been commonly reported in children.[2,3,5,6]

Scalp involvement in children can be heralded by early appearance of leukotrichia or white hairs within the affected site. Involvement of lips and genital vitiligo is relatively common in children **(Figs 5 and 6)** and needs to be differentiated from lichen sclerosus et atrophicus when associated with burning and pruritus. Kobner phenomenon is more obvious in spreading generalized vitiligo than the segmental variety. This phenomenon is more appreciated in children as they are more active and playful in nature. The onset of Kobner phenomenon signifies active unstable nature of the disease.[2,3,5,6]

ASSOCIATED CONDITIONS

A close association is found between vitiligo and other autoimmune disorders like alopecia areata, diabetes mellitus, pernicious anemia, Addison's disease, and thyroid disorder. The association with autoimmune conditions is mostly seen with nonsegmental variant rather than the segmental type. Most studies show 1.3–3.4% children with vitiligo have associated autoimmune conditions. Thyroid studies in pediatric patients with vitiligo to rule out autoimmune thyroiditis are relevant in such cases to diagnose these associations. These endocrinopathies and autoimmune conditions are less common in children compared to adults with vitiligo.

Alopecia areata, celiac disease, urticaria and atopic disorders are some of the common associated conditions. Halo nevus is commonly appreciated in children with nonsegmental involvement as a vitiligo associated dermatosis. Although halo nevi often may precede onset of generalized vitiligo, the association is still unclear. Coexistence with psoriasis and lichen planus has been reported in some cases.

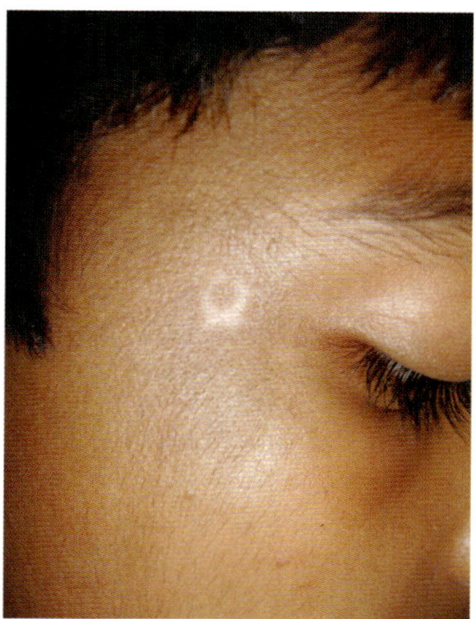

Fig. 1: Focal vitiligo (note central repigmentation)

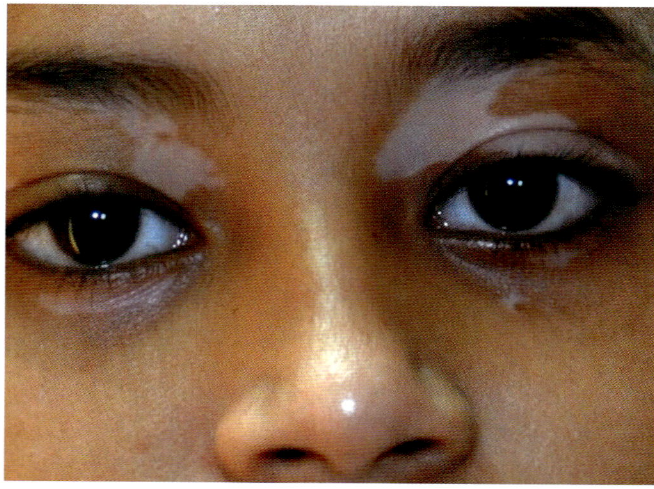

Fig. 2: Periorbital lesions (often the initial lesions in children)

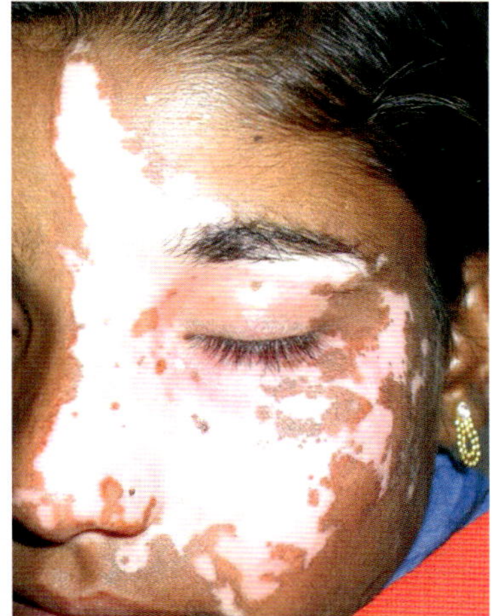

Fig. 3: Segmental vitiligo

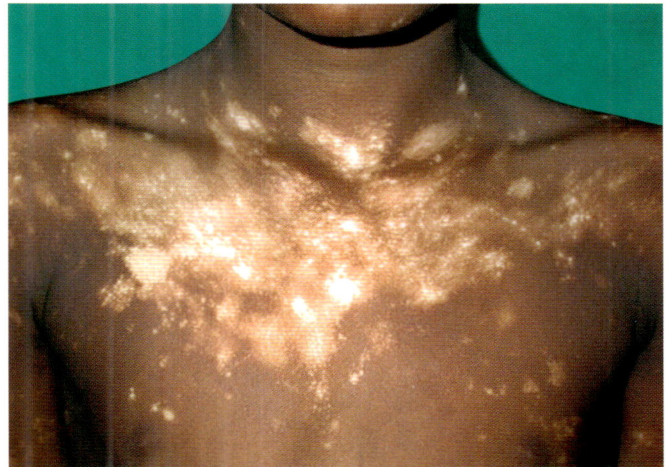

Fig. 4: Vitiligo vulgaris

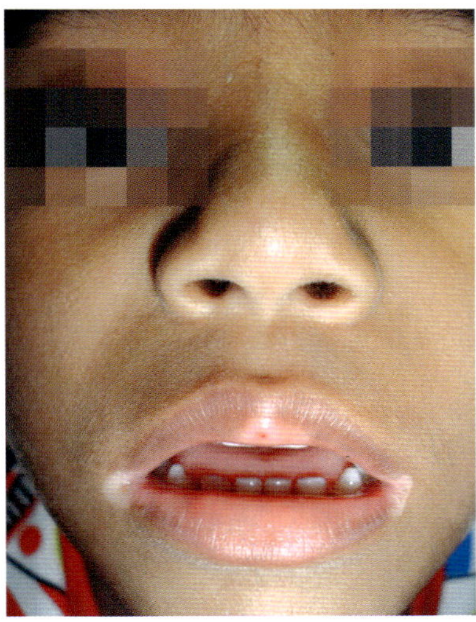

Fig. 5: Vitiligo of lip

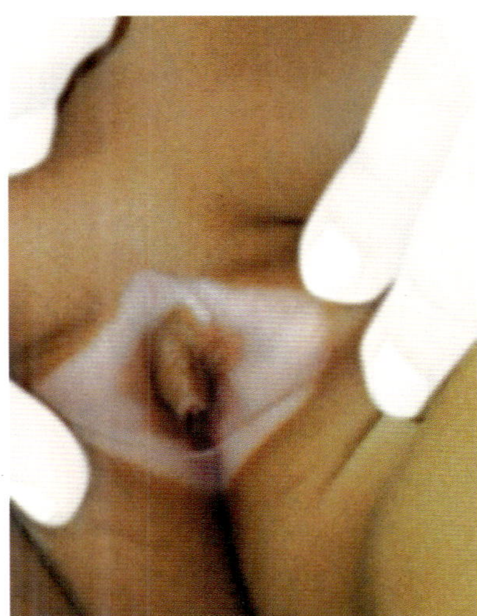

Fig. 6: Genital vitiligo in a small girl

PROGNOSIS AND OUTCOME

In generalized disease, there is a period of rapid spread for few months and then it stabilizes for a variable time frame and otherwise may slowly spread over several years. In comparison to adult disease, regression and spontaneous repigmentation is more appreciated in children with vitiligo. Repigmentation is mostly diffuse or perifollicular to start with and sometimes from the margins. Segmental variety initially has a period of activity which later on remains stable throughout.

The condition has to be differentiated from various nevoid conditions like nevus depigmentosus and anemicus, ash leaf macules and piebaldism. Linear lesions of hypomelanosis of Ito, acquired conditions like pityriasis alba and infections like pityriasis versicolor are some of the close differential diagnosis for vitiligo.

MANAGEMENT

There is no single treatment which is equally effective in all patients of vitiligo. Treatment must be individualized.

Medical Treatment[2,3,6]

Satisfactory repigmentation can be achieved in up to 70% cases of early, localized disease. Narrow band ultraviolet B

(UVB) or photochemotherapy with UVA is used extensively either alone or in combination with topical agents as the main repigmenting treatment. Use of systemic steroids and immunosuppressant or immunomodulators is controversial.

Topical Therapy

Potent to moderately potent topical corticosteroids can be used for initiation of treatment in case of localized, early disease. Repigmentation is generally rapid but unstable.

Topical pimecrolimus and tacrolimus are found to be effective in vitiligo involving head and neck used either alone or in conjunction with narrow ban ultraviolet B (NBUVB) or excimer laser.

Topical calcipotriol and tacalcitol also can be used in localized disease either alone or with NBUVB/PUVA (psoralen combined with ultraviolet).

Topical photochemotherapy with topical methoxsalen preparations are available and can be used in localized disease. Psoralen is applied on the vitiliginous patches and is exposed to UVA or solar radiation after 30–60 minutes. Photo toxicity is the most common complication, so patients should be properly educated before use.

Systemic Therapy

Narrow band UVB therapy is now used extensively in both localized and extensive disease. Vitiliginous patches are exposed to 311 nm UVB light starting with a dose of 0.21 Joule/meter square at least twice weekly on nonconsecutive days till minimum erythematic dose is reached. Approximately 50–150 treatments are necessary to produce satisfactory response.

Photochemotherapy with oral 8-methoxy psoralen or trimethylpsoralen are used along with UVA or solar radiation to achieve repigmentation. Methoxypsoralen is given at a dose of 0.4–0.6 mg/kg/day and vitiliginous patches are exposed to sun for 15–20 minutes, 2 hours after drug intake thrice weekly on nonconsecutive days. Oral photochemotherapy is associated with gastric discomfort and occasional elevation of liver enzymes and is slightly less effective than NBUVB therapy.

Pigmentation produced by both NBUVB and PUVA is slow, appears in follicular pattern but is much more stable than those produced by topical steroid therapy **(Figs 7 and 8)**.

No specific form of therapy is yet established to control progressive disease. Most commonly, systemic corticosteroids are used in daily immunosuppressive dose. But the side effect profile of long-term systemic corticosteroid precludes their regular use in children. Modified regimens of corticosteroids in weekly doses have been tried to reduce side effects but their therapeutic efficacy is not yet established. Other immunosuppressive medication like methotrexate and azathioprine have been tried but are not yet established.

Surgical Treatment[6,7]

Long-standing vitiliginous patches and those on glabrous skin tend to be resistant to treatment and occasionally do not or only partially respond to medical treatment. In these circumstances, surgical transplantation of melanocytes can be done to produce pigmentation. Several techniques are used to obtain this result, but surgery should only be tried after carefully assessing the stability of the patches. Generally, a patch is labeled stable if there is no progression of the patch or the disease for 2 years. But even then test grafting is recommended to ascertain the true nature of the disease and to ensure the success of a full procedure. The most commonly used surgical techniques are miniature punch grafting, split thickness skin grafting, suction blister grafting and cultured and noncultured melanocyte transplant.

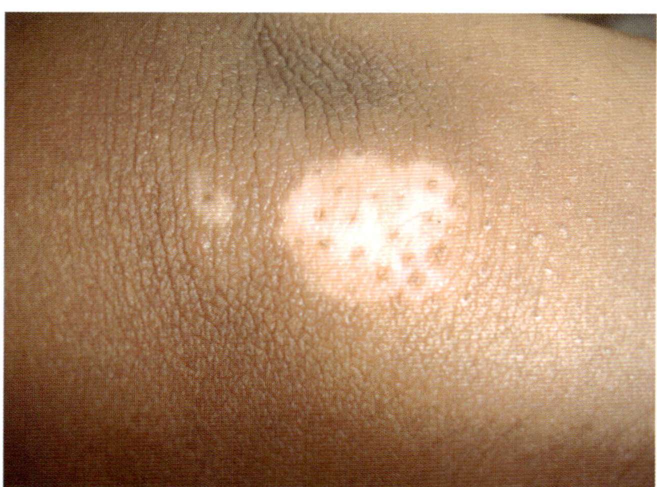

Fig. 7: Repigmenting vitiligo

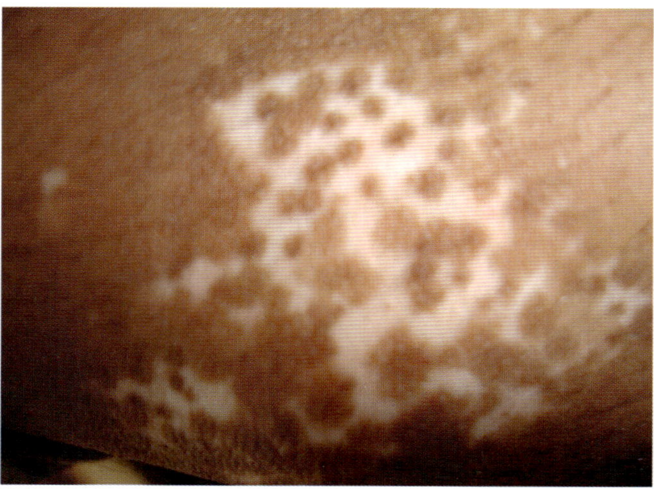

Fig. 8: Repigmenting vitiligo (close-up)

Miniature punch grafting is the most commonly practiced and easy procedure. In this technique, 1–2 mm sized full thickness cylindrical grafts are harvested from nonvitiliginous normal skin and is transplanted to pre-made recipient sites on vitiliginous patches.

In both split thickness skin grafting and suction blister grafting, thin epidermal sheets are transplanted on derma-braded recipient vitiliginous patches. The difference is in the process of harvesting the grafts. In one dermatome is used while dermoepidermal separation is achieved in the other by long-standing suction on the donor sites.[7]

Cultured and noncultured melanocyte transplant produces the best cosmetic result but is difficult and needs laboratory support. In these techniques, small amount of normal skin is taken from the donor site and is then incubated at 4°C overnight with trypsin solution to achieve cell separation. The separated cells are then either first cultured in appropriate media or installed directly in the derma-abraded recipient sites generally suspended in patient's own serum.

CONCLUSION

Vitiligo results from autoimmune destruction of the melanocytes, the exact etiology of which is still elusive. Depending on the distribution of lesions, it can be of several types: focal, segmental, vulgaris, universal, lip-tip (involvement of lips and tip of the fingers and toes) etc. The disease is often associated with other autoimmune cutaneous and systemic disorders, e.g. alopecia areata, lichen planus, psoriasis or Addison's disease, autoimmune thyroiditis, autoimmune hepatitis, pernicious anemia, diabetes mellitus, etc. Familial incidence is approximately 20–30 percent of the cases. It is not an uncommon disease in pediatric age group where segmental variant is seen more commonly, infrequently associated with autoimmune systemic disease and the response to treatment is better (cf. western literature), so also the prognosis. Repigmentation, perifollicular and at the border of patches is fairly good with topical steroid(s). Psoralen with ultraviolet A (PUVA) therapy is recommended above 8 years (according to some workers 12 years) of age only. Other drugs which may be used for extensive vitiligo in children are oral levamisole, short course of corticosteroids, cytotoxic drugs, chloroquine, topical placental extract, etc. Recently topical tacrolimus (0.03% and 0.1%) have shown promising results in the treatment of localized vitiligo.

Once the spread of vitiligo is brought under control or the stability of vitiligo is achieved, various surgical procedures which can be undertaken are micropigmentation or tattooing, punch grafting, dermabrasion, split thickness skin grafting, melanocyte transfer, etc. One must remember that there is no dietary restriction required in such patients. There is no scientific documentation in favor of avoidance of sour food/drink, vitamin C or fruit juice, etc. Lots of reassurance, explaining and counseling of children and/or parents are required in the management of vitiligo.

REFERENCES

1. Mazereeuw-Hautier J, Harper J. Vitiligo. In: Harper J, Oranje A, Prose N (Eds). Textbook of Pediatric Dermatology, 2nd edn. Oxford: Blackwell Publishing Ltd. 2006. pp. 1041-56.
2. Palit A, Inamadar AC. Childhood vitiligo. Indian J Dermatol Venereol. Leprol. 2012;78:30-41.
3. Kanwar AJ, Dhar S, Kaur S. Vitiligo in children. Ind J Dermatol. 1993;38:47-52.
4. Pajvani U, Ahmad N, Wiley A, et al. The relationship between family medical history and childhood vitiligo. J Am Acad Dermatol. 2006;55:238-44.
5. Handa S, Dogra S. Epidemiology of childhood vitiligo: a study of 625 patients from north India. Pediatr Dermatol. 2003;20:207-10.
6. Paller AS, Mancini AJ. Disorders of pigmentation. In: Paller AS, Mancini AJ, (Eds). Hurwitz clinical pediatric dermatology, 3rd edn. Philadelphia: Elsevier Saunders. 2006. pp. 265-305.
7. Malakar S, Dhar S. Treatment of stable and recalcitrant vitiligo by autologous miniature punch grafting: a prospective study with 1000 patients. Dermatology. 1999;198:133-9.

21

Concept of Stability of Vitiligo

Koushik Lahiri, Subrata Malakar

Key Features

- Stability is regarded as the most important parameter before opting for any transplantation technique to treat vitiligo.
- But, simultaneous donor site repigmentation and depigmentation of grafts at the recipient site and vice-versa has been noted.
- Successful repigmentation after regrafting in previous punch failure cases has also been reported.
- There is little consensus regarding the optimal required period of stability.
- Test grafting or Koebner phenomenon reveal the apparent clinical stability only and that may not be the true reflection of stability status of the disease at the molecular level.
- Antimelanocyte cytotoxic reactivity was observed among CD8+ TCC isolated from perilesional biopsies of patients with vitiligo.
- To clearly fathom and define stability, not merely only on clinical ground, histoenzymological analysis of the perilesional and nonlesional skin of vitiligo patients is proposed.
- Probably some growth factors which are responsible for both mitogenic and melanogenic stimulation of melanocytes should also be taken into account.
- Some serological test(s) could guide us to measure these growth factors.
- Very recently *in vivo* reflectance confocal microscopy has been applied to assess stability of vitiligo.

INTRODUCTION

Vitiligo persists to evade the researchers and patients in spite of the considerable advancement in basic understanding of the disease process and the treatment protocol over the years. Conservative medical therapy continues to be besieged with capricious and derisory outcome. When the disease becomes refractory to conventional therapy, transplantation techniques are the only options left to replenish the lost melanocytes.

Various surgical modalities and transplantation techniques have evolved during last few decades.[1-10]

But, till date none of the medical or surgical therapeutic choices could assure guaranteed success in all the cases. This is primarily because of the obscure etiopathogenesis and elusive activity profile of the disease itself. Not only with medical therapy but also with any of the surgical modus operandi deployed to achieve accomplishment, proper selection of cases is of paramount importance. The specific criteria for selection have been well defined.[6]

Any endeavor of defining norms or principles for selection is based on one single criterion, i.e. stability of the disease. It is taken as the most important parameter before opting for any transplantation technique to treat vitiligo.[9]

Stability is the decisive factor, the cornerstone of vitiligo therapy.

PERIOD OF STABILITY

Even after recognizing the significance of stability and after three decades of experience in vitiligo surgery, it is quite surprising to note the little consensus regarding the optimal required period of stability. The complete lack of unanimity can be glaring in some instances **(Table 1)**. In one study, the minimal period of stability as a prerequisite for grafting was mentioned to be as little a period as 4 months.[11] While on the other side of the spectrum in another study, it was taken as 3 years.[7]

Other variable figures, like 6 months, 1 year and 2 years, can easily be obtained from some other studies as well.[2-16]

Table 1: Minimum period of stability in different studies

Author	*Year*	*Period of stability*
Das SS, Pasricha JS[11]	1992	4 months
Boersma BR, Westerhop W[12]	1995	6 months
Jha AK, Pandey SS, Shukla VK[13]	1992	1 year
Savant SS[16]	1992	2 years
Falabella R[15]	2003	2 years
Falabella R[14]	1995	2 years
Falabella R[7]	1992	3 years

Even same author has considered different period of stability in different articles.[7,14] Unfortunately, none of these observations were based on any concrete logic/authentic proof. They were merely conceived on subjective basis and documented arbitrarily. A few years back, some unanswered questions were raised about this concept.[17] Even the 2 years time frame used to confirm whether lesions are progressive or stable has been a matter of divergence of opinion.[17] The IADVL taskforce recommendation to embark on vitiligo surgery after 1 year of inactivity is based on a similar supposition.[18] While discussing the severity of vitiligo, a recent article has also mentioned this ambiguity and cumbersome compromise.[19] Due to a dearth of a better alternative, this capricious criteria of minimal period of stability still holds good before opting for surgical procedure.

AREA BASED VARIABLE STATUS OF STABILITY

The first and foremost goal for vitiligo surgery is to induce repigmentation in depigmented part of skin. But due to some inexplicable reason, simultaneous depigmentation and repigmentation have been noticed in different areas of the same patient.[15]

Variable results were obtained over the donor site and recipient site of the same patient.[15,17,20]

Depigmentation of grafts was documented in herpes labialis-induced lip leukoderma.[21-27]

Concurrent donor site repigmentation and depigmentation of grafts at the recipient site or donor site depigmentation with complete repigmentation of the recipient area with pigment growing out from each graft have also been noticed **(Figs 1 and 2)**.

It was suggested to observe the donor site as well, to rule out koebnerization as a side effect of surgical manipulation while commenting on the stability status of the patient by minigraft test.[20]

Simultaneous perigraft spread of pigment in one area and spread of vitiligo in another area can be found in the same patient **(Figs 3 and 4)**.

Parallel concurrence of surgical repigmentation from the grafts and increase in size of an existing lesion in the same anatomical location was also observed **(Figs 5 to 7)**.

This area based variable status of stability is obviously not related to the conventional refractory behavior of vitiligo in some typical so-called resistant anatomical sites such as palm, sole, lips, nipples, areola, glans penis, and bony prominences. Neither is this related to the type of vitiligo such as unilateral (segmental/focal) or bilateral (symmetric, vulgaris, or generalized).

ASSESSMENT OF STABILITY

Before any surgical intervention or even just to have an idea about which way the disease is progressing, evaluation of stability status of vitiligo is an essential prerequisite.

Clinically, this can be judged by three simple indicators:

1. History
2. Koebner phenomenon
3. Test grafting (TG).

These were elaborated and to assess the activity status of the disease some benchmark guidelines have been proposed by Falabella.[6,14] Those are:

- Lack of progression of old lesions within the past 2 years (in unilateral vitiligo may be shorter, and in bilateral vitiligo, stability establishes after several years)
- No new lesions developing within the same period
- Absence of a recent Koebner phenomenon (either from history or experimentally produced)
- Repigmentation of depigmented areas by medical treatment or sometimes spontaneous repigmentation
- A positive minigrafting test
- Lack of Koebnerization at donor site.

On the backdrop of a pervasive incongruity about the minimal period of stability, an attempt was made for the first

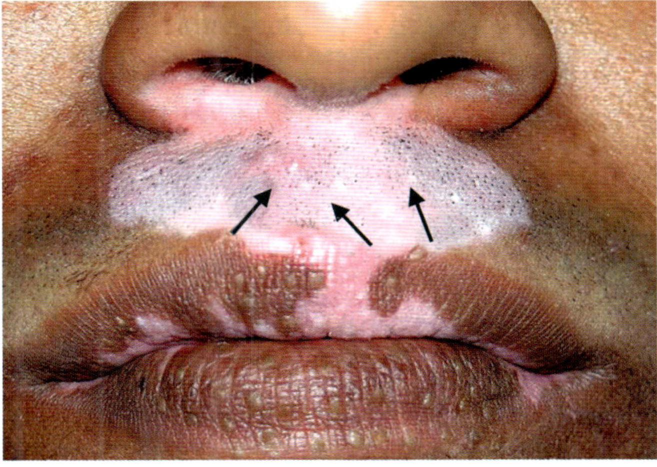

Fig. 1: Depigmentation of grafts in the recipient area of stable vitiligo (shown with arrows)

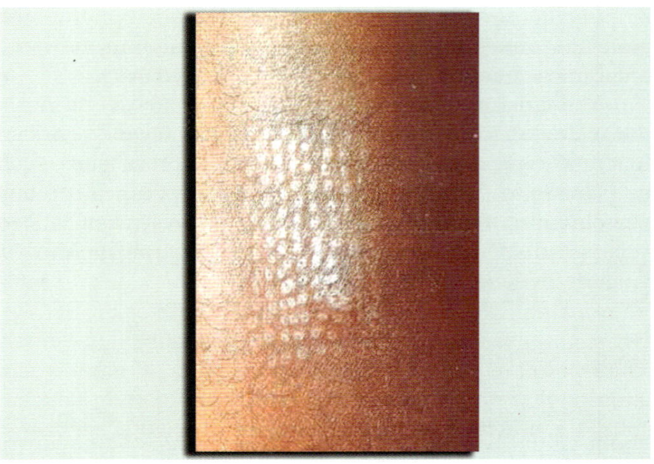

Fig. 2: Repigmentation of the donor site in the same patient

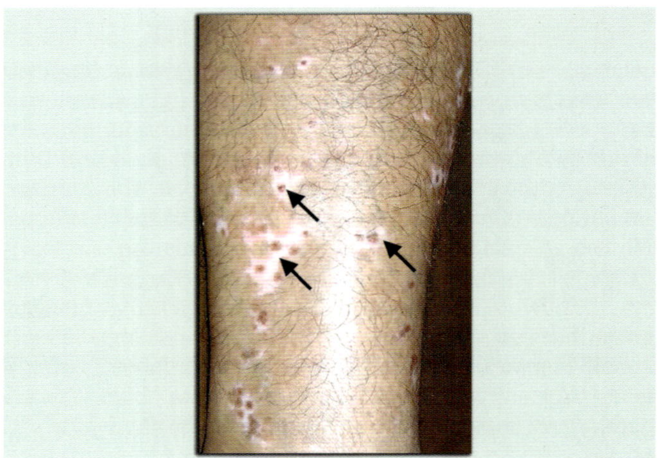

Fig. 3: Perigraft spread of pigment (shown with arrows)

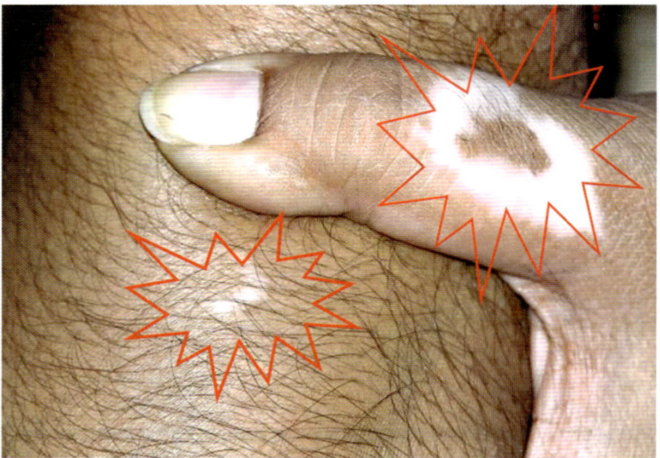

Fig. 4: Simultaneous spread of disease over thumb and knee (shown with starburst signs)

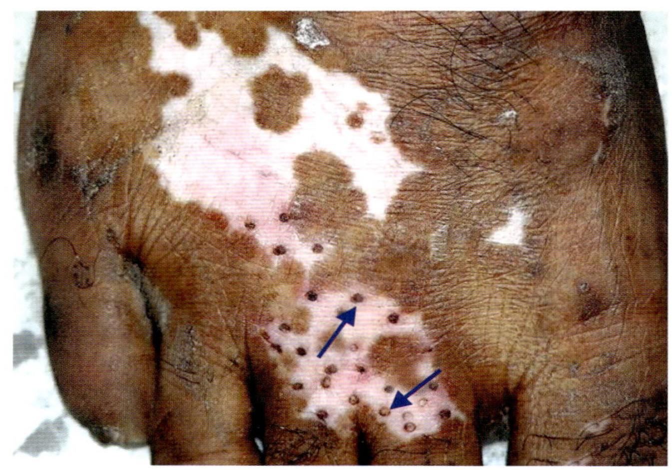

Fig. 5: Minigrafting on dorsum of foot, first session (shown with blue arrows)

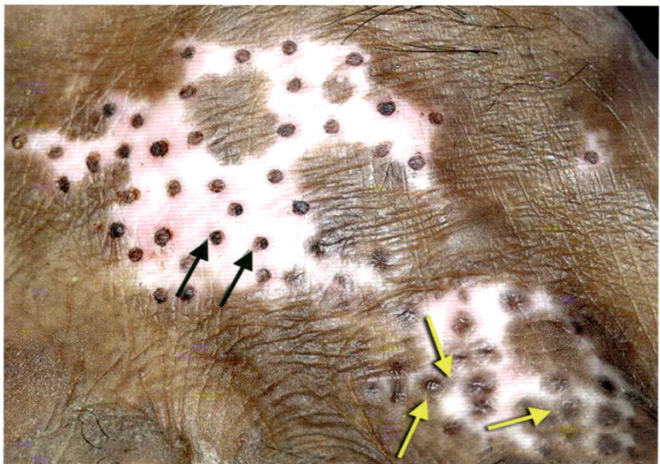

Fig. 6: Second session, perigraft repigmentation from grafts of previous session (shown with yellow arrows)

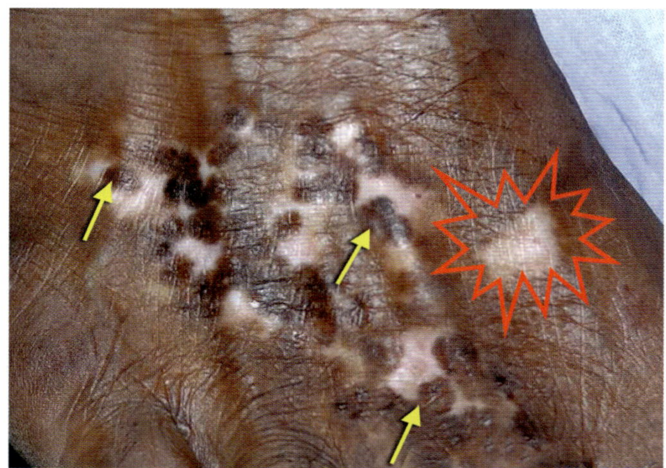

Fig. 7: Appreciable repigmentation (yellow arrows). Reactivation of disease on the same anatomical site (shown with red starburst)

time by Falabella in 1995 to fathom stability before surgery by introducing the minigrafting test.[14]

The objective of this test vowed to serve several purposes:

- Establishing the stability of the depigmenting process
- Determine a means by which patients could be selected
- Identifying patients who may respond to pigment cell transplantation
- To anticipate the response to surgical repair.

In the original suggested procedure, a few grafts (1.0–1.2 mm) were placed in the center of the depigmented lesion to be scrutinized. Dressing was done by Micropore® adhesive tape and kept for a couple of weeks. After removal of the tape, the area was exposed to sunlight for 15 minute daily for a period of 3 months. No treatment was permitted during this test period.

All test sites are visualized under Wood's light. The test was considered positive if unequivocal repigmentation takes place beyond 1 mm from the border of the implanted grafts. On the other hand, if less than 1 mm or no repigmentation was observed, the test was considered as negative.[14]

In some of the biggest series, this evaluation has been termed as "test grafting" and found this to be a more reliable exercise than the unjustified dependence on period of stability alone.[25,26,28]

Over the years, this "test" has been vindicated and acknowledged as a powerful tool for detecting stable vitiligo, which anticipates the repigmentation success in vitiligo when surgery becomes a therapeutic option.

Behl expressed some reservation while commenting on Falabella's work on minigrafting and claimed better results with thin Thiersch grafting. In a rejoinder Falabella reiterated his faith in miniature punch grafting and countered with his sets of reasons and logics in favor of punch grafting.[4,29]

But, simultaneously some valid logic of skepticism was flowing parallel to this recognition.

In the original article, no mention was there about the donor site. One of the opinions was to take the outcome of the donor site as well into consideration, concurrently along with observing the behavior of the minigrafts in the recipient site. That will give a more comprehensive idea about the status of stability.[20]

But, doubts were registered over overdependence on TG per se as that attaches a quite a few fallacies.[17,28,30]

- Test grafting positivity does not necessarily guarantee a favorable outcome in all cases even after perfect graft take up.
- Encouraging results were obtained even after grafting of a few TG negative cases.
- Simultaneous donor site repigmentation and depigmentation of grafts at the recipient site or donor site depigmentation with complete repigmentation of the recipient area are not hard to come by.

Juhlin echoed this apprehension and observed, "... neither the history nor test graft is a complete help to obtain good effect. It seems we have to wait until the method of identification and isolation of skin-homing melanocyte-specific cytotoxic T lymphocytes is available".[31]

None other than Falabella himself expressed his doubts about the comprehensiveness of minigraft test. He observed that even when the minigrafting test is positive, "depigmenting activity" may still be present and prevent satisfactory repigmentation.[7]

More recently, Njoo et al. explored the association between the experimentally induced Koebner phenomenon (KP-e) and the Koebner phenomenon by history, disease activity, and therapeutic responsiveness in vitiligo vulgaris.[32]

In the article, they proposed to measure disease activity on a 6-point scale from –1 to +4 [(vitiligo disease activity (VIDA) score] and therapy-induced repigmentation grade. But the test was lacking in application potential. The authors have observed and concluded the following:

- The VIDA score did not always predict a positive KP-e
- The KP-e may function well as a clinical factor to assess present disease activity and may also predict the responsiveness to fluticasone propionate plus UV-A therapy but not to UV-B (311 nm) therapy.

In this context, it can be concluded that overdependence on Kp or TG may be sometimes misleading in this enigmatic disease. Because what these two reveal is the apparent clinical stability only and that may not be the true reflection of stability status of the disease at the cellular level.[28]

HOW STABLE IS STABILITY?

Another important indicator is the duration of stability status of vitiligo.

It is often hard to predict how long the disease will remain stable. Similarly, difficult is to envisage when it will start to become unstable.

Repigmentation has been successfully induced in previous graft failure cases under NB-UVB (311 nm) phototherapy.[27]

It was also proposed that NB-UVB might have played the pivotal role of stabilizing the disease by promoting apoptosis of the perilesional and circulating melanocyte-specific cytotoxic CD 8 cells.[33,34]

The observation of spontaneous repigmentation of non-grafted vitiligo patches **(Figs 8 to 10)** points toward a possible release of fresh cytokines from the donor skin while stimulating the vitiliginous patches and hair follicles of the grafted sites may have played some role at the distant sites by local absorption.[35-37] Another theory was the immunogenic mechanism which was originally responsible for the development of vitiligo may have lost its antigenicity due to the autologous grafts.[34]

Successful split thickness skin graft in punch grafting failure cases further complicates the picture.[38]

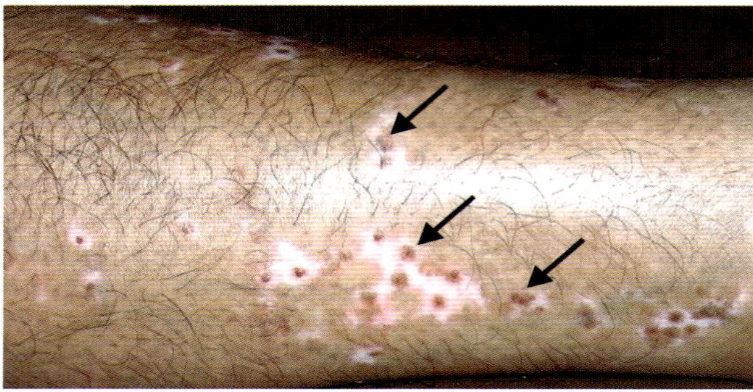

Fig. 8: Punch grafting on medial aspect of left leg

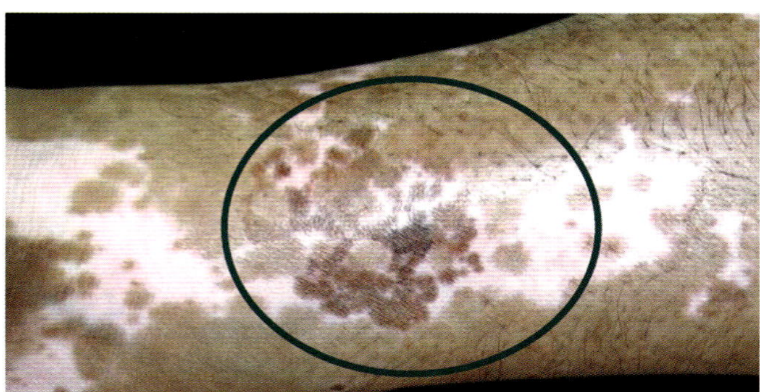

Fig. 9: Spontaneous repigmentation of medial aspect of right leg

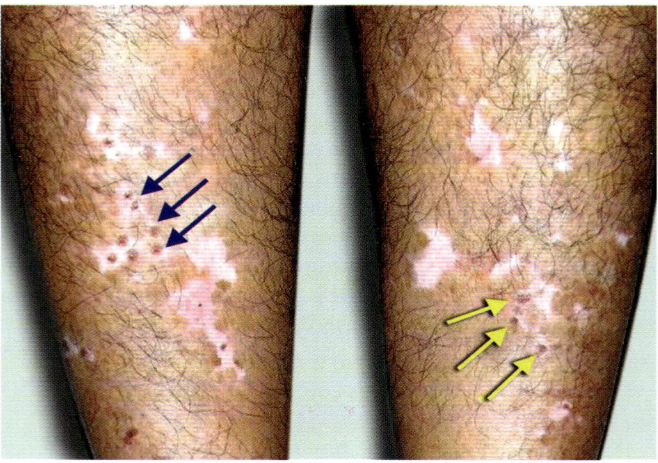

Fig. 10: Punch grafting on right leg (shown with blue arrows). Spontaneous repigmentation over left leg (shown with yellow arrows)

Period of stability of repigmentation has been proposed as 1 year. That means, to qualify as stable, the repigmentated status must be maintained for a period of not less than 1 year.[39]

UNDERSTANDING STABILITY FROM WITHIN

The exact pathomechanism of stability is as vague as the pathogenesis of the disease itself.

The incompletely understood mechanism may involve many assortments of theories and hypothesis or may be a combination various factors. The only definite and certain fact regarding the pathogenesis of vitiligo is the absence of melanocytes in the lesion. So, it can be deducted that destruction of melanocytes is the keystone for unfolding of the disease process. Classically, there have been three hypotheses to elucidate vitiligo: the neural hypothesis, the self-destruct hypothesis, and the immune hypothesis of which the last one is gaining grounds. Aberrations of both humoral and cell-mediated immunity have been noticed. Most of the patients with generalized vitiligo were found to have circulating antibodies to cell surface antigens on normal human melanocytes; these antibodies were cytotoxic to normal melanocytes and to melanoma cells in tissue culture. Perilesional and circulating T-cells strongly suggest that melanocyte-specific cytotoxic T-cells are involved. And now it is known that UVB therapy promotes this T-cell apoptosis.[33,34] Repigmentation has been successfully induced in previous graft failure cases under NB-UVB (311 nm) phototherapy.[40]

In 1986, Grimes first reported a reduction in the number of lymphocytes and helper T cells and an increase in number of natural killer cells in vitiligo patients. She also noticed decreased helper/suppressor ratios, particularly among patients with vitiligo of less than a year's duration and among those whose serum assayed positive for autoantibodies.[41]

But D'Amelio in 1990 came up with just the reverse observation. In a study of 22 patients with vitiligo stable for a year or more demonstrated high helper T-cell levels and high helper/suppressor ratios (also in 23 first-degree relatives) compared to controls. He also reported loss of circadian rhythm of helper T cells in patients with active diseases and no loss of circadian rhythm of suppressor T cell.[42]

Cui et al. observed cytotoxic antibodies more common in patients with active than with inactive disease.[43]

An attempt was made by Hann in 1994 to compare active and inactive lesion of vitiligo by immunohistochemical methods. He documented that the percentage of B cells was higher in those with disease of recent onset (under a year) than in controls (those with later onset disease). He also noticed an increase in number of CD4 lymphocytes (especially in active lesions), but not CD8 lymphocytes, in marginal skin of active lesions. As per his observation, epidermal ICAM-1 was expressed in active but not in stable epidermal lesions.[44] In the subsequent year, Hann detected decreased helper T-cell levels with a reversed helper/suppressor ratio in 1995.[45]

In the margins of lesions, Badri found increases in CD3+, CD4+, and CD8+ T cells; many were activated and expressed the cutaneous lymphocyte-associated antigen (HECA-452+) typical of infiltrating T cells; these changes were most marked within 0.6 mm of the lesional edge. He could not find any association between T-cell numbers and disease activity.[46] After that, some very interesting observations by Wankowicz-Kalinska have opened a new horizon in the basic understanding of the pathogenesis of the disease.[47]

The detection of melanocyte-reactive cytotoxic T cells in the peripheral blood of vitiligo patients and the observed correlation between perilesional T-cell infiltration and melanocyte loss *in situ* suggest the important role of cellular autoimmunity in the pathogenesis of this disease. T cells have been isolated from both perilesional and non-lesional skin biopsies of vitiligo patients, then cloned and their profile of cytokine production analyzed. Perilesional T-cell clones (TCC) derived from patients with vitiligo revealed a predominant Type-1-like cytokine secretion profile, but the degree of Type-1 polarization in uninvolved skin-derived TCC correlated with the process of microscopically observed melanocyte destruction *in situ*. Furthermore, CD8+ TCC derived from two patients also were analyzed for reactivity against autologous melanocytes. The anti-melanocyte cytotoxic reactivity was observed among CD8+ TCC isolated from perilesional biopsies of patients with vitiligo.

The theory of melanocytorrhagy and apoptosis as one of the primary defects underlying melanocyte loss was discussed later.[44] This theory proposes that non-segmental vitiligo is a primary melanocytorrhagic disorder with altered melanocyte responses to friction and possibly other types of stress, inducing their detachment and subsequent transepidermal loss. Melanocytes detachment induces apoptosis whereas adherence to basement membrane suppresses apoptosis.[48]

Very recently, a group of workers while determining the markers of the stability of vitiligo (CD 8, CD 45 RO, and FOX P3) has observed that percentage of CD8 and CD 45 RO in lesional skin biopsy may provide objective indication of lesion/area based stability. They have also observed that a higher percentage of cytotoxic CD8 cells is associated with failure of melanocyte transplantation.[49]

Very recently *in vivo* reflectance confocal microscopy has been applied to assess stability of vitiligo.[50]

CONCLUSION

So, where do we stand?

It is obvious that before any attempt to predict the outcome of any vitiligo surgery, along with the clinical stability, assessment of "cellular" stability is of paramount importance and the cellular parameters should also be taken into consideration. When these ultrastructural investigation facilities are now available, an attempt should be made to clearly fathom stability, not merely only on clinical ground but along with *in vivo* reflectance confocal microscopy and histoenzymological analysis of the perilesional and non-lesional skin of vitiligo patients. Probably some growth factors which are responsible for both mitogenic and melanogenic stimulation of melanocytes should also be taken into account. Some serological test(s) could guide us to measure these growth factors. Before embarking upon any surgical alternative no preconceived, biased and arbitrary formulae should guide us to assess stability of vitiligo.

The understanding of the area-based variable status and limited period of inertia or activity might necessitate TG at various sites at different time interval. Till those unexplored areas are charted and the cellular parameters come into existence, we should not refrain the surgical option rather we should continue surgical intervention based on logical application of our clinical knowledge.

ACKNOWLEDGMENTS

Some figures and tables used in this chapter have also been used in the following chapter and articles by me and my coauthors. With the permission of the concerned editors and publisher I would like to properly acknowledge the original source:

- Lahiri K, Malakar S. The concept of stability of vitiligo. In: Gupta S, Olsson MJ, Kanwar AJ, Ortonne JP (Eds). Surgical Management of Vitiligo, 1st edn. Oxford: Blackwell Publishing; 2007. pp. 49-55.
- Malakar S. Lahiri K. Minigrafting for vitiligo. In: Gupta S, Olsson MJ, Kanwar AJ, Ortonne JP (Eds). Surgical Management of Vitiligo. 1st edn. Oxford: Blackwell Publishing; 2007. pp. 87-95.
- Lahiri K, Malakar S, Sarma N, et al. Repigmentation of vitiligo with punch grafting and narrow-band UV-B (311 nm): a prospective study. Int J Dermatol. 2005;45(6):649-55.
- Malakar S, Lahiri K, Spontaneous repigmentation in vitiligo: why it is important. Int J Dermatol. 2006;45(4):478-9.
- Lahiri K, Malakar S. The concept of stability of vitiligo: a reappraisal. Indian J Dermatol. 2012;57:83-9.

REFERENCES

1. Orentreich N, Selmanowitz VJ. Autograft repigmentation of leukoderma. Arch Dermatol. 1972;105(5):734-6.
2. Falabella R. Repigmentation of segmental vitiligo by autologous minigrafting. J Am Acad Dermatol. 1983;9(4):514-21.
3. Halder RM, Pham HN, Breadon JY, et al. Micropigmentation for the treatment of vitiligo. J Dermatol Surg Oncol. 1989;15(10):1092-8.
4. Behl PN. Treatment of vitiligo with homologous Thiersch's Skin grafts. Curr Med Pract. 1964;8:218-21.
5. Kiistala U, Mustakallio KK. *In vivo* separation of epidermis by production of suction blisters. Lancet. 1964;1(7348): 14444-5.
6. Falabella R. Grafting and transplantation of melanocytes for repigmenting vitiligo and other types of leukodermas. Int J Dermatol. 1989;28(6):363-9.

7. Falabella R, Escobar C, Borrero I. Treatment of refractory and stable vitiligo by transplantation of *in vitro* cultured epidermal autografts bearing melanocytes. J Am Acad Dermatol. 1992;26(2 Pt 1):230-6.
8. Malakar S, Dhar S, Malakar RS. Single-hair transplant: a novel technique. Dermatology. 1999;199(4):370.
9. Olsson MJ, Juhlin L. Long-term follow-up of leucoderma patients treated with transplants of autologous cultured melanocytes, ultrathin epidermal sheets and basal cell layer suspension. Br J Dermatol. 2002;147(5):893-904.
10. Lahiri K. Evolution and evaluation of autologous mini punch grafting in vitiligo. Indian J Dermatol. 2009;54(2):159-67.
11. Das SS, Pasricha JS. Punch grafting as a treatment for residual lesions in vitiligo. Ind J Dermatol Venereol Leprol. 1992;58:315-9.
12. Boersma BR, Westerhof W, Bos JD. Repigmentation in vitiligo vulgaris by autologous minigrafting: results in nineteen patients. J Am Acad Dermatol. 1995;33(6):990-5.
13. Jha AK, Pandey SS, Shukla VK. Punch grafting in vitiligo. Ind J Dermatol Venereol Leprol. 1992;58:328-30.
14. Falabella R, Arrunategui A, Barona MI, et al. The minigrafting test for vitiligo: detection of stable lesions for melanocyte transplantation. J Am Acad Dermatol. 1995;32(2 Pt 1):228-32.
15. Falabella R. Surgical treatment of Vitiligo: Why, when and how. J Eur Acad Dermatol Venereol. 2003;17(5):518-20.
16. Savant SS. Autologous miniatures punch grafting in vitiligo. Ind J Dermatol Venereol Leprol. 1992;58:310-4.
17. Malakar S, Lahiri K, Malakar RS. How unstable is the concept of stability in surgical repigmentation of vitiligo? Dermatology. 2000;201(2):182-3.
18. Parsad D, Gupta S. IADVL Dermatosurgery Task Force. Standard guidelines of care for vitiligo surgery. Indian J Dermatol Venereol Leprol. 2008;74(Suppl):S37-45.
19. Ramam M, Krishna SG. Measuring the severity of vitiligo. Indian J Dermatol Venereol Leprol. 2012;78(1):5-7.
20. Westerhof W, Boersma B. The minigrafting test for vitiligo: detection of stable lesions for melanocyte transplantation. J Am Acad Dermatol. 1995;33(6):1061-2.
21. Malakar S, Dhar S. Rejection of punch grafts in three cases of herpes-simplex-induced lip leukoderma: caution and precaution. Dermatology. 1997;195(4):414.
22. Malakar S, Dhar S. Acyclovir can abort rejection of punch grafts in herpes-simplex induced lip leucoderma. Dermatology. 1999;199(1):75.
23. Malakar S, Lahri K. Successful repigmentation of six cases of herpes-labialis-induced lip leucoderma by micropigmentation. Dermatology. 2001;203(2):194.
24. Lahiri K, Malakar S, Sarma N. Herpes-simplex-induced lip leucoderma revisited. Dermatology. 2004;208(2):182.
25. Malakar S, Dhar S. Treatment of stable and recalcitrant vitiligo by autologous miniature punch grafting: a prospective study of 1,000 patients. Dermatology. 1999;198(2):133-9.
26. Malakar S, Lahiri K. Punch grafting for lip leucoderma. Dermatology. 2004;208(2):125-8.
27. Lahiri K, Malakar S, Sarma N, et al. Repigmentation of vitiligo with punch grafting and narrow-band UV-B (311 nm)—a prospective study. Int J Dermatol. 2006;45(6):649-55.
28. Lahiri K, Malakar S, Banerjee U, et al. Clinico-cellular stability of vitiligo in surgical repigmentation: an unexplored frontier. Dermatology. 2004;209(2):170-1.
29. Falabella R. Reply. J Am Acad Dermatol. 1995;33:1061.
30. Lahiri K. Stability in vitiligo? What's that? J Cutan Aesthet Surg. 2009;2(1):38-40.
31. Juhlin L. How unstable is the concept of stability in surgical repigmentation of vitiligo. Dermatology. 2000;201(2):183.
32. Njoo MD, Das PK, Bos JD, et al. Association of the Köebner phenomenon with disease activity and therapeutic responsiveness in vitiligo vulgaris. Arch Dermatol. 1999; 135(4):407-13.
33. Ortonne JP. Vitiligo pathogenesis: What›s new? J Eur Acad Dermatol Venereol Barcelona, Spain. 2003;17(Suppl 3):30.
34. van den Wijngaard RM, Aten J, Scheepmaker A. Expression and modulation of apoptosis regulatory molecules in human melanocytes: significance in vitiligo. Br J Dermatol. 2000;143:573-81.
35. Malakar S. Spontaneous repigmentation of vitiligo patches other than the grafted site. Indian J Dermatol. 1997;472: 68-70.
36. Malakar S, Dhar S. Spontaneous repigmentation of vitiligo patches distant from the autologous skin graft sites: a remote reverse Koebner's phenomenon? Dermatology. 1998;197(3):274.
37. Malakar S, Lahiri K. Spontaneous repigmentation in vitiligo: why it is important. Int J Dermatol. 2006;45(4):478-9.
38. Malakar S. Successful split thickness skin graft in stable vitiligo not responding to autologous miniature punch grafts. Indian J Dermatol. 1997;42:215-8.
39. Parsad D, Pandhi R, Dogra S, et al. Clinical study of repigmentation patterns with different treatment modalities and their correlation with speed and stability of repigmentation in 352 vitiliginous patches. J Am Acad Dermatol. 2004;50(1):63-7.
40. Lahiri K, Malakar S. Inducing repigmentation by regrafting and phototherapy (311 nm) in punch failure cases of lip vitiligo-a pilot study. Indian J Dermatol Venereol Leprol. 2004;70(3):156-8.
41. Grimes PE, Ghoneum M, Stockton T, et al. T cell profiles in vitiligo. J Am Acad Dermatol. 1986;14(2 Pt 1):196-201.
42. D'Amelio R, Frati C, Fattorossi A, et al. Peripheral T-cell subset imbalance in patients with vitiligo and in their apparently healthy first-degree relatives. Ann Allergy. 1990;65(2):143-5.
43. Cui J, Arita Y, Bystryn JC. Cytolytic antibodies to melanocytes in vitiligo. J Invest Dermatol. 1993;100(6):812-5.

44. Ahn SK, Choi EH, Lee SH, et al. Immunohistochemical studies from vitiligo—comparison between active and inactive lesions. Yonsei Med J. 1994;35(4):404-10.
45. Hann SK, Kim JB. Detection of antibodies to human melanoma cell in vitiligo by western blot analysis. Yonsei Med J. 1995;36(5):457-61.
46. Badri AM, Todd PM, Garioch JJ, et al. An immunohistological study of cutaneous lymphocytes in vitiligo. J Pathol. 1993; 170(2):149-55.
47. Wankowicz-Kalinska A, van den Wijngaard RM, Tigges BJ, et al. Immunopolarization of CD4+ and CD8+ T cells to Type-1-like is associated with melanocyte loss in human vitiligo. Lab Invest. 2003;83(5): 683-95.
48. Kumar R, Parsad D. Melanocytorrhagy and apoptosis in vitiligo: connecting jigsaw pieces. Indian J Dermatol Venereol Leprol. 2012;78(1):19-23.
49. Rao A, Gupta S, Dinda AK, et al. Study of clinical, biochemical and immunological factors determining stability of disease in patients with generalized vitiligo undergoing melanocyte transplantation. Br J Dermatol. 2012;166(6):1230-6.
50. LI W, Wang S, XU Ae. Role of *in vivo* reflectance confocal microscopy in determining stability in vitiligo: a preliminary study. Indian J Dermatol. 2013;58:429-32.

22

Phototherapy in Vitiligo

Prescilia N Isedeh, Iltefat Hamzavi

Key Features

- The use of ultraviolet radiation, also known as phototherapy, is a form of medical management in the treatment of vitiligo.
- Narrowband ultraviolet B (NB-UVB), psoralen plus ultraviolet A (PUVA) and targeted phototherapy with monochromic excimer laser or light are the three most commonly used phototherapy modalities.
- NB-UVB is the gold-standard medical option to treat generalized and nonsegmental vitiligo.

INTRODUCTION

Vitiligo can have a direct impact on the patient, both physically and psychologically, which can have a negative impact on the patient's quality of life (QoL). While vitiligo is a challenging disease to treat, proper management can greatly affect ones overall QoL. Currently, vitiligo can be managed medically and surgically. Medical management consists of topical or oral medications as well as phototherapy. Phototherapy employs the use of ultraviolet radiation (UVR) in the treatment of generalized and nonsegmental vitiligo. Although modern psoralen plus ultraviolet A (PUVA) therapy was first introduced in 1948,[1] it was discovered more than 3,000 years ago when plant extracts such as *Psoralea corylifolia* Linnaeus and *Ammi majus* Linnaeus were used as oral and topical treatments in India and Egypt, respectively, to treat vitiligo.[2-5] For a long period of time, PUVA was the mainstay treatment of vitiligo until narrowband ultraviolet B (NB-UVB) was introduced in 1997.[6] Since its introduction, NB-UVB serves effectively as the first line medical treatment for patients with generalized and nonsegmental vitiligo.[6-11] In recent years, targeted phototherapy, such as excimer laser or light, have been shown to be effective in the treatment of localized vitiligo. Excimer laser targets only the depigmented areas, which gives it an advantage over NB-UVB, which irradiates both normal and depigmented skin.[12] This chapter will review all of these phototherapy modalities in the treatment of vitiligo in adults and children.

PSORALEN PLUS ULTRAVIOLET A THERAPY

Psoralen plus ultraviolet A is a form of photochemotherapy, where a photosensitizer called psoralen is given, either in an oral or a topical form, to a patient approximately 2 hours before total body irradiation with UVA (320–400 nm) two to three times a week on nonconsecutive days. The most common oral photosensitizer used for generalized vitiligo is 8-methoxypsoralen (8-MOP), generally at a dose of 0.6 mg/kg body weight.[5,13-15] For all oral PUVA protocols, the initial dose should be based on the patient's skin phototype and can vary from 0.25 J/cm^2 to 2.5 J/cm^2 with incremental increases based on patient's response.[4,5,7,14,16-19] Topical PUVA, using 8-MOP (0.1% or less) is a good therapeutic option in adults and children over the age of 2 who have localized vitiligo because of a lower cumulative UVA dose and insignificant systemic absorption.[5] Topical psoralen is applied 30 minutes before UVA exposure with a dose of 0.12 J/cm^2 to 0.25 J/cm^2, which is gradually increased, according to the patient's skin phototype, until mild erythema is achieved in the depigmented areas.[5,14]

The mechanism of action of psoralen is unclear, but it is known to have a biochemical reaction with DNA to stimulate melanogenesis. The greatest repigmentation response with PUVA is seen on the face and neck, with moderate response to the trunk and proximal extremities and little to no repigmentation to the hands and feet.[16,17,20-22] PUVA combined with fluticasone or calcipotriene, a vitamin D$_3$ analog, has been found to increase repigmentation rate as well as reduce the number of UVR sessions, respectively.[23,24] With regard to the QoL, Parsad et al.[25] who treated 141 adults with PUVA in combination with pulsed systemic corticosteroids, or oral levamisole, found that the mean Dermatology Quality of Life Index (DQLI) scores were lower when compared with mean DQLI scores before treatment in subjects who failed treatment.

Psoralen plus ultraviolet A is known to have many systemic side effects. Short-term side effects of oral PUVA include cutaneous phototoxicity, ocular phototoxicity such as cataracts, and gastrointestinal irritation.[5,11,14,21,26] Long-term side effects of PUVA are dose related. These long-term side effects are photoaging, nonmelanoma skin cancer such as squamous cell carcinoma (SCC) and basal cell carcinoma, and melanoma skin cancer.[5,27-29] There is a strong correlation in patients with lower skin types and the development of nonmelanoma skin cancer, mainly SCC.[30] Recommended skin cancer prevention include limiting the number of yearly treatments, limiting maintenance treatments and performing a yearly clinical full body skin examination for patients that exceed the number of recommended sessions.[5,31,32] Other preventive measures against short-term and long-term side effects include ultraviolet (UV) protective goggles worn during treatment and UV protective glasses worn 12–24 hours after treatment and protection of male genitalia with a shield since these areas have an increased susceptibility to skin cancer. Sunscreens can be used on vitiligo areas and patients should be counseled on the avoidance of sunlight after treatment.[5]

NARROWBAND ULTRAVIOLET B

For many decades, PUVA was considered the treatment of choice for generalized and nonsegmental vitiligo, but in recent years, NB-UVB (311–313 nm) has become the first line medical therapy for these types of vitiligo. In 1997, Westerhof and Nieuweboer-Krobotova[6] first reported the efficacy of NB-UVB. In this interventional study, comparing NB-UVB and topical PUVA, treating 78 patients with NB-UVB and 28 patients with topical PUVA, they found that 67% of the patients who received NB-UVB treatments experienced repigmentation more frequently than 46% of the patients who received PUVA after 4 months of treatment.[6] There have since been several more studies who have reported the efficacy and superiority of NB-UVB over PUVA in the treatment of generalized and nonsegmental vitiligo.[7,16-18]

The initial dose of NB-UVB is between 150 mJ/cm^2 and 250 mJ/cm^2, as it is believed that vitiligo patients, in terms of photosensitivity, behave as skin type I.[4,5] Additionally, starting doses can be based on phototesting results, using 70% of the minimal erythema dosing (MED), which is defined as the minimum dose of light that causes barely perceptible visible erythema.[4,5,33] The treatment can be given two to three times a week on nonconsecutive days with subsequent dosage increase by 10–20% increments, according to the maximum erythema that occurred since the previous treatment.[4,6,7,16-18,34] A few studies have indirectly compared the twice a week and three times a week dosing of NB-UVB and have found that thrice weekly dosing led to a rapid onset of repigmentation as well as maintenance of repigmentation.[8,9]

Narrowband ultraviolet B stimulates melanocyte production and melanogenesis as well as induces local immunosuppression.[8,21,23,35] Like PUVA, repigmentation occurs in a perifollicular fashion as well as in the periphery of the depigmented lesions with the best repigmentation response occurring on the face and neck **(Figs 1A and B)** and poor repigmentation noted in the hands and feet.[6,16-18,21,22] The predictors of patients who will have a good response to NB-UVB are those patients who have a lesser duration of the disease, anatomic sites of depigmentation such as the face and neck, smaller areas of depigmentation, those with an

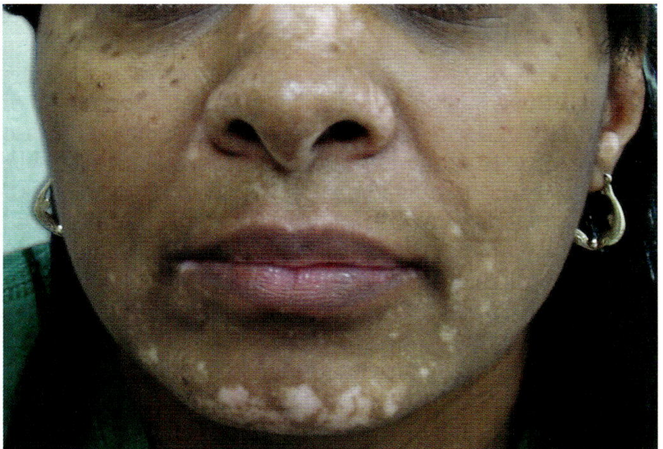

Fig. 1A: Vitiligo located on the nose and chin. Before narrowband ultraviolet B treatments

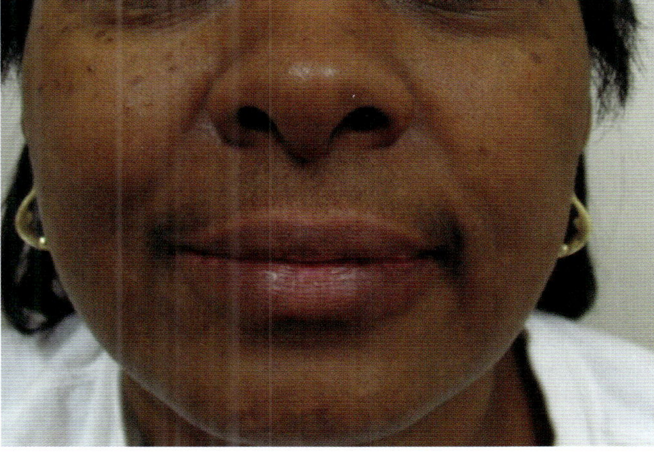

Fig. 1B: After 9 months of narrowband ultraviolet B treatments

early response to treatment, and those with dark skin types such as III–V.[5,36-38]

Patients should expect approximately 50% repigmentation of their vitiligo within 6 months of initiation of NB-UVB in nonacral areas.[33] In general, treatment should be discontinued, if no repigmentation is observed within 3 months or after 6 months if there is minimal repigmentation, such as less than 25% repigmentation.[5] In some instances, when the repigmentation is slow, treatment may be discontinued and then resumed after 2 months as it is thought that "intermittent irradiation" might stimulate a more effective melanogenesis.[5] An important concept to keep in mind when counseling patients is the concept of photoadaptation as it can have an effect on dosing. Photoadaptation is a phenomenon that occurs when increasing subsequent radiation doses are required to cause the same effect on the skin after the initial treatment. In a study by Hexsel et al.[39] two-thirds of patients receiving NB-UVB for vitiligo were photoadapters as they reported higher MED after treatments than before treatments. The group noted a mean change of 49% in their MED, while one-third of these patients were non-photoadapters which had no change in their MED. Also it was noted that darker skin types have a greater capacity to photoadapt because of the ability to tolerate a higher initial UVR dose.[39] In the authors experience non-photoadaptors should not have dose increases but can still repigment.

Narrowband ultraviolet B does not have as many side effects as PUVA, thus making it a more desirable therapy. However, there are patients who seem to have a better response to PUVA than NB-UVB based upon the author's experience. Thus far the predictors of this subgroup have not been described. The most acute side effect is phototoxicity with occasional transient hyperpigmentation.[5,22,26] The long-term risk as well as carcinogenicity of NB-UVB remain unclear. Long-term follow-up, with patients who have been treated with NB-UVB, is crucial in order to determine the exact carcinogenic risk of this form of phototherapy.

Combination therapy with NB-UVB and other topical treatments may enhance repigmentation response. Some studies have reported, which was similarly reported with PUVA, a reduced number of treatment sessions and an overall lower cumulative irradiation dosage needed for repigmentation when calcipotriene is added to NB-UVB,[40] while other studies did not show this same benefit.[41,42] Additionally, a few studies[43,44] showed improved repigmentation rates when topical tacrolimus was added to NB-UVB while the opposite was found in an isolated study.[45] Oral pulse dose of steroids have been found to achieve the highest repigmentation rate when compared to other conventional phototherapy.[46] One retrospective QoL study by Tijoe et al.[47] reported the results of a nonvalidated modified DQLI survey of 30 patients treated with NB-UVB. They found that 70% reported an improvement in QoL, while 26.7% reported a worsening of their health-related QoL. Additionally, 23.3% noticed that their vitiligo had less influence on their leisure activity, but 30% of the patients had to spend more time camouflaging than 10% who spent less time.[47]

TARGETED PHOTOTHERAPY

In the early 2000s, targeted phototherapy, which utilizes light or laser, was developed for the treatment of localized and nonsegmental vitiligo. These new therapeutic devices are capable of emitting light with higher irradiance[48] and selectively treating the depigmented lesions while sparing normal skin. There are several types of targeted phototherapy: monochromatic excimer (308 nm) laser or light or lamp (MEL), Helium-Neon laser (632.8 nm), bioskin or microphototherapy.[4,5,10,14,26] Bioskin is a device developed in Italy that transmits focus 311 nm UVB phototherapy.[21]

The mechanism of action of all targeted phototherapy is unclear, but like NB-UVB, they may promote repigmentation by stimulating melanogenesis, stabilization and maintenance of vitiligo through immunosuppression and immunomodulation.[21,49] MEL treatment sessions occur two to three times a week on nonconsecutive days with the initial doses determined by either between 100 mJ/cm^2 and 200 mJ/cm^2 or MED, increasing the dose by 50 mJ/cm^2 in the absence of erythema.[49] The predictors of a good response to MEL are: location of the vitiligo such as the face **(Figs 2A and B)**, darker skin types, smaller lesions, newer vitiligo areas and age of patient as children are known to respond better than adults.[49] Additionally, the repigmentation rate is thought to be associated with the total number of sessions and not to the frequency of treatment sessions.[50] The side effects are erythema, blistering or perilesional pigmentation.[49,51]

Monochromatic excimer laser or light or lamp is the most commonly used laser therapy for vitiligo. Spencer et al.[52] in 2002 conducted the first study using MEL. In this pilot study, 18 patients with a total of 29 patches of vitiligo were treated with 308 nm xenon-chloride excimer laser three times a week for a total of 12 treatments while untreated vitiligo patches served as control sites.[52] The result of this study showed that the 23 vitiligo patches from 12 patients, who received six treatments, reported repigmentation in 57% of the treated areas while 11 depigmented areas that received all 12 treatments resulted in some repigmentation in 82% of the treated areas.[52] There has since been other studies using MEL that have found that it produces faster repigmentation rates than any other medical therapy in the treatment of localized and segmental vitiligo.[53-56] It may require 11–22 MEL treatments before observing repigmentation.[57,58]

When MEL was compared to NB-UVB, MEL was found to have better clinical outcomes and quicker repigmentation.[12,59] Casacci et al.[12] conducted a 6 month long randomized multicenter study comparing the effectiveness of NB-UVB and MEL using a half-side comparison design in 21 patients who received twice-weekly treatments of NB-UVB to one side and MEL twice-weekly for 6 months to the other side of the

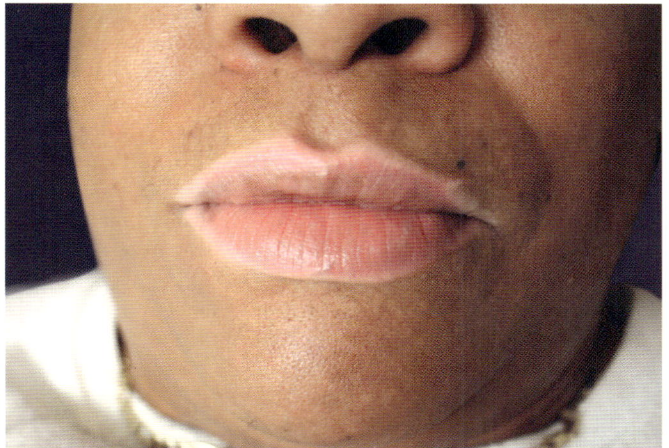

Fig. 2A: Vitiligo along the vermillion border of the month. Before treatment with monochromatic excimer (308 nm) laser

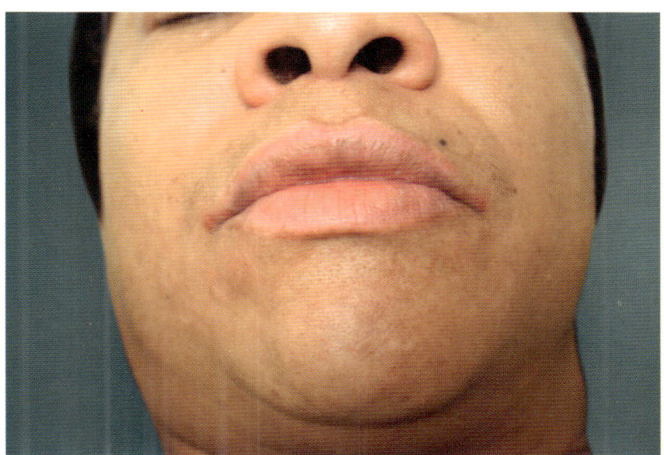

Fig. 2B: After 30 treatments with monochromatic excimer laser

body. Their results showed six vitiligo areas (37.5%) treated with MEL and one (6%) treated with NB-UVB achieved excellent repigmentation (between 76% and 100%) while four lesions (25%) treated with MEL and five lesions (31%) treated with NB-UVB showed good repigmentation (between 51% and 75%).[12]

Combining MEL with topical medications, such as hydrocortisone or tacrolimus 0.1%, resulted in an increase in repigmentation.[60-62] Patients who received split-skin grafting and had MEL treatments had excellent repigmentation during their 12-month follow-up visit. When MEL was compared with NB-UVB after miniature punch grafting, there was no significant difference in repigmentation after 12 weeks.[63] Patient satisfaction was noted with more with NB-UVB than with MEL, but there was a 71.4% decrease in the cumulative dose with MEL. Lan et al.[48] have suggested that irradiance is a more important factor than fluence in upregulating surrogate markers of pigmentation. These experiments were done *in vitro* but might explain why MEL produces faster results than NB-UVB.

ADJUVANT THERAPY WITH PHOTOTHERAPY

Khellin Plus UVA

Khellin is a furanochromone, which is derived from the *Ammi visnaga* plant seed and has similar functions as psoralen.[5,21,64] The mechanism of action is unclear, but it is thought to facilitate repigmentation through stimulation of melanogenesis and melanocyte proliferation.[5,21,64] Systemic and topical khellin plus UVA have been found to be as effective as PUVA.[65-68] Side effects of systemic khellin include transaminitis and nausea. Khellin forms fewer crosslinks in DNA, making it less carcinogenic than psoralen.

L-Phenylalanine Plus UVA

Phenylalanine is an essential amino acid that is an important step in melanogenesis initiation. L-phenylalanine (L-phe) gives rise to L-tyrosine, which is crucial to melanin production. Patients with vitiligo have a decreased calcium dependent melanocyte uptake of L-phe thus leading to impaired turnover of L-phe. L-phe is not phototoxic, but when combined with UV light, L-phe stimulates the migration of melanocytes resulting in repigmentation.[5,21] L-phe plus UVA have been shown to produce varying repigmentation rates between 50% and 100%.[69,70] Side effects are minimal, but therapy is contraindicated in patients with phenylketonuria.[5,21]

PHOTOTHERAPY IN CHILDREN

Vitiligo, beginning during childhood, can have a negative impact on the child's self-esteem affecting their QoL. The initial onset of depigmentation occurs in approximately half of vitiligo patients before the age of 20.[71,72] NB-UVB is thought to be an effective treatment option for patients with generalized and nonsegmental vitiligo.[73-75] Njoo et al.[73] was the first to conduct an open trial to study the efficacy of NB-UVB in the treatment of 51 children with generalized vitiligo. They found that 53% of the patients had more than 75% repigmentation and 80% of the patients had stabilization of their disease.[73] As a general rule, NB-UVB should not be used longer than 12 months in children and if no response is seen after 6 months. MEL has also been found to be more effective in children than in adults.[73] Oral PUVA is contraindicated in children.[5] The effects of phototherapy on QoL have been documented.

Njoo et al. used a validated Dutch version of the Children's Dermatology Life Quality Index (CDLQI) tool to measure QoL before and after treatment and found that patients with 26-75% repigmentation or more than 75% repigmentation vitiligo showed a significant decrease in CDLQI scores, which correlated with an improvement of their QoL after a successful treatment.[73]

CONCLUSION

Phototherapy is an important medical therapy in the treatment of vitiligo. This therapeutic modality results in repigmentation as well as stabilization of the disease. NB-UVB is considered the first-line therapy, over PUVA, for the treatment of generalized and nonsegmental vitiligo. In recent years, targeted phototherapy with MEL has been found to be effective in the treatment of localized depigmented vitiligo areas while sparing normal skin. When these above-mentioned phototherapy modalities improve the patient's outward appearance, it has been show to improve their overall QoL.

REFERENCES

1. Monem El Mofty A. A preliminary clinical report on the treatment of leucodermia with *Ammi majus* Linn. J Egypt Med Assoc. 1948;31(8):651-65.
2. McKenna WB. *Ammi majus* Linn in the treatment of vitiligo. Scott Med J. 1957;2(2):69-70.
3. Benedetto AV. The psoralens: an historical perspective. Cutis. 1977;20(4):469-71.
4. Hamzavi IH, Lim HW, Syed ZU. Ultraviolet-based therapy for vitiligo: what's new? Indian J Dermatol Venereol Leprol. 2012;78(1):42-8.
5. Pacifico A, Leone G. Photo (chemo) therapy for vitiligo. Photodermatol Photoimmunol Photomed. 2011;27(5):261-77.
6. Westerhof W, Nieuweboer-Krobotova L. Treatment of vitiligo with UV-B radiation vs topical psoralen plus UV-A. Arch Dermatol. 1997;133(12):1525-8.
7. Yones SS, Palmer RA, Garibaldinos TM, et al. Randomized double-blind trial of treatment of vitiligo: efficacy of psoralen-UV-A therapy vs Narrow-UV-B therapy. 2007; 143(5):578-84.
8. Scherschun L, Kim JJ, Lim HW. Narrow-band ultraviolet B is a useful and well-tolerated treatment for vitiligo. J Am Acad Dermatol. 2001;44(6):999-1003.
9. Kanwar AJ, Dogra S, Parsad D, et al. Narrow-band UVB for the treatment of vitiligo: an emerging effective an well-tolerated therapy. Int J Dermatol. 2005;44(1):57-60.
10. Forschner T, Buchholtz S, Stockfleth E. Current state of vitiligo therapy-evidence-based analysis of the literature. J Dtsch Dermatol Ges. 2007;5(6):467-75.
11. Njoo MD, Spuls PI, Bos JD, et al. Nonsurgical repigmentation therapies in vitiligo. Meta-analysis of the literature. Arch Dermatol. 1998;134(12):1532-40.
12. Casacci M, Thomas P, Pacifico A, et al. Comparison between 308-nm monochromatic excimer light and narrowband UVB phototherapy (311-313 nm) in the treatment of vitiligo: a multicentre controlled study. J Eur Acad Dermatol Venereol. 2007;21(7):956-63.
13. Roelandts R. Photo (chemo) therapy for vitiligo. Photodermatol Photoimmunol Photomed. 2003;19(1):1-4.
14. Falabella R, Barona MI. Update on skin repigmentation therapies in vitiligo. Pigment Cell Melanoma Res. 2008: 22(1):42-65.
15. Singh S, Khandpur S, Sharma VK, et al. Comparison of efficacy and side-effect profile of oral PUVA vs oral PUVA sol in the treatment of vitiligo: a 36-week prospective study. J Eur Acad Dermatol Venereol. 2012.
16. Sapam R, Agrawal S, Dhali TK. Systemic PUVA vs narrowband UVB in the treatment of vitiligo: a randomized controlled study. Int J Dermatol. 2012;51(9):1107-15.
17. Parsad D, Kanvar AJ, Kumar B. Psoralen-ultraviolet A vs narrowband ultraviolet B phototherapy for the treatment of vitiligo. J Eur Acad Dermatol Venereol. 2006;20(2):175-7.
18. Bhatnagar A, Kanwar AJ, Parsad D, et al. Comparison of systemic PUVA and NB-UVB in the treatment of vitiligo: an open prospective study. J Eur Acad Dermatol Venereol. 2007;21(5):638-42.
19. Bhatnagar A, Kanwar AJ, Parsad D, et al. Psoralen and ultraviolet A and narrowband ultraviolet B in inducing stability in vitiligo, assessed by vitiligo disease activity score: an open prospective comparison study. J Eur Acad Dermatol Venereol. 2007;21(10):1381-5.
20. Mofty ME, Zaher H, Esmat S, et al. PUVA and PUVB in vitiligo: are they equally effective? Photodermatol Photoimmunol Photomed. 2001;17(4):159-63.
21. Felsten LM, Alikhan A, Petronic-Rosic V. Vitiligo: a comprehensive overview Part II: treatment options and approach to treatment. J Am Acad Dermatol. 2011;65(3):493-514.
22. Syed ZU, Hamzavi IH. Role of phototherapy in patients with skin of color. Semin Cutan Med Surg. 2011;30(4): 184-9.
23. Westerhof W, Nieuweboer-Krobotova L, Mulder PG, et al. Left-right comparison study of the combination of fluticasone propionate and UV-A vs either fluticasone propionate or UV-A alone for the long-term treatment of vitiligo. Arch Dermatol. 1999;135(9):1061-6.
24. Ermis O, Alpsoy E, Cetin L, et al. Is the efficacy of psoralen plus ultraviolet A therapy for vitiligo enhanced by concurrent topical calcipotriol? A placebo-controlled double-blind study. Br J Dermatol. 2001;145(3):472-5.
25. Parsad D, Pandhi R, Dogra S, et al. Dermatology Life Quality Index score in vitiligo and its impact on the treatment outcome. Br J Dermatol. 2003;148(2):373-4.
26. Grimes PE. New insights and new therapies in vitiligo. JAMA. 2005;293(6):730-5.
27. El Mofty M, Mostafa WZ, Hegazy R. What's New in Photobiology and Phototherapy. J Egypt Women Dermatol Soc. 2009;6:43-50.

28. Seo SL, Kim IH. Squamous cell carcinoma in a patient with generalized vitiligo. J Am Acad Dermatol. 2001;45(6 Suppl):S227-9.
29. Takeda H, Mitsuhashi Y, Kondo S. Multiple squamous cell carcinomas *in situ* in vitiligo lesions after long-term PUVA therapy. J Am Acad Dermatol. 1998;38(2 Pt 1):268-70.
30. Morison WL, Honigsmann H. Psoralen photochemotherapy. In: Lim HW, Honigsmann H, Hawk JLM (Eds). Photodermatology. New York: Informa Healthcare; 2007. pp. 348-58.
31. British Photodermatology Group guidelines for PUVA. Br J Dermatol. 1994;130(2):246-55.
32. Guidelines of Care for Phototherapy and Photochemotherapy. American Academy of Dermatology Committee on Guidelines of Care. J Am Acad Dermatol.1994;31(4):643-8.
33. Hamzavi I, Jain H, McLean D, et al. Parametric modeling of narrowband UV-B phototherapy for vitiligo using a novel quantitative tool: the Vitiligo Area Scoring Index. Arch Dermatol. 2004;140(6):677-83.
34. Anbar TS, Westerhof W, Abdel-Rahman AT, et al. Evaluation of the effects of NB-UVB in both segmental and non-segmental vitiligo affecting different body sites. Photodermatol Photoimmunol Photomed. 2006;22(3):157-63.
35. Ibbotson SH, Bilsland D, Cox NH, et al. An update and guidance on narrowband ultraviolet B phototherapy: a British Photodermatology Group Workshop Report. Br J Dermatol. 2004;151(2):283-97.
36. Njoo MD, Westerhof W, Bos JD, et al. The development of guidelines for the treatment of vitiligo. Clinical Epidemiology Unit of the Istituto Dermopatico dell'Immacolata-Istituto di Recovero e Cura a Carattere Scientifico (IDI-IRCCS) and the Archives of Dermatology. Arch Dermatol. 1999;135(12):1514-21.
37. Brazzelli V, Antoninetti M, Palazzii S, et al. Critical evaluation of the variants influencing the clinical response of vitiligo: study of 60 cases treated with ultraviolet B narrowband phototherapy. J Eur Acad Dermatol Venereol. 2007;21(10):1369-74.
38. Nicolaidou E, Antoniou C, Stratigos AJ, et al. Efficacy, predictors of response, and long-term follow-up in patients with vitiligo treated with narrowband UVB phototherapy. J Am Acad Dermatol. 2007;56(2):274-8.
39. Hexsel CL, Mahmoud BH, Mitchell D, et al. A clinical trial and molecular study of photoadaptation in vitiligo. Br J Dermatol. 2009;160(3):534-9.
40. Goktas EO, Aydin F, Senturk N, et al. Combination of narrow band UVB and topical calcipotriol for the treatment of vitiligo. J Eur Acad Dermatol Venereol. 2006;20(5):553-7.
41. Arca E, Tastan HB, Erbil AH, et al. Narrowband ultraviolet B as monotherapy and in combination with topical calcipotriol in the treatment of vitiligo. J Dermatol. 2006;33(5):338-43.
42. Hartmann A, Lurz C, Hamm H, et al. Narrowband UVB311 nm vs broadband UVB therapy in combination with topical calcipotriol vs placebo in vitiligo. Int J Dermatol. 2005;44(9):736-42.
43. Fai D, Cassano N, Vena GA. Narrowband UVB phototherapy combined with tacrolimus ointment in vitiligo: a review of 110 patients. J Eur Acad Dermatol Venereol. 2007;21(7):916-20.
44. Esfandiarpour I, Ekhlasi A, Farajzadeh S, et al. The efficacy of pimecrolimus 1% cream plus narrowband ultraviolet B in the treatment of vitiligo: a double-blind, placebo controlled clinical trial. J Dermatolog Treat. 2009;20(1):14-8.
45. Mehrabi D, Pandya AG. A randomized, placebo-controlled, double-blind trial comparing narrowband UV-B plus 0.1% tacrolimus ointment with narrowband UV-B plus placebo in the treatment of generalized vitiligo. Arch Dermatol. 2006;142(7):927-9.
46. Rath N, Kar HK, Sabhnani S. An open labeled, comparative clinical study on efficacy and tolerability of oral minipulse of steroid (OMP) alone, OMP with PUVA and broad/narrow band UVB phototherapy in progressive vitiligo. Indian J Dermatol Venereol Leprol. 2008;74(4):357-60.
47. Tjioe M, Otero ME, van de Kerkhof PC, et al. Quality of life in vitiligo patients after treatment with long-term narrowband ultraviolet B phototherapy. J Eur Acad Dermatol Venereol. 2005;19(1):56-60.
48. Lan CC, Yu HS, Lu JH, et al. Irradiance, but not fluence, plays a crucial role in UVB-induced immature pigment cell development: new insights for efficient UVB phototherapy. Pigment Cell Melanoma Res. 2013;26(3):367-76.
49. Alhowaish AK, Dietrich N, Onder M, et al. Effectiveness of a 308-nm excimer laser in treatment of vitiligo: a review. Lasers Med Sci. 2012;28(3):1035-41.
50. Taneja A, Trehan M, Taylor CR. 308-nm excimer laser for the treatment of localized vitiligo. Int J Dermatol. 2003;42(8):658-62.
51. Park KK, Liao W, Murase JE. A review of monochromatic excimer light in vitiligo. Br J Dermatol. 2012;167(3):468-78.
52. Spencer JM, Nossa R, Ajmeri J. Treatment of vitiligo with the 308-nm excimer laser: a pilot study. J Am Acad Dermatol. 2002;46(5):727-31.
53. Shen Z, Gao TW, Chen L, et al. Optimal frequency of treatment with the 308-nm excimer laser for vitiligo on the face and neck. Photomed Laser Surg. 2007;25(5):418-27.
54. Leone G, Iacovelli P, Paro Vidolin A, et al. Monochromatic excimer light 308 nm in the treatment of vitiligo: a pilot study. J Eur Acad Dermatol Venereol. 2003;17(5):531-7.
55. Ostovari N, Passeron T, Zakaria W, et al. Treatment of vitiligo by 308-nm excimer laser: an evaluation of variables affecting treatment response. Lasers Surg Med. 2004;35(2):152-6.
56. Hadi SM, Spencer JM, Lebwohl M. The use of the 308-nm excimer laser for the treatment of vitiligo. Dermatol Surg. 2004;30(7):983-6.
57. Al-Otaibi SR, Zadeh VB, Al-Abdulrazzaq AH, et al. Using a 308-nm excimer laser to treat vitiligo in Asians. Acta Dermatovenerol Alp Panonica Adriat. 2009;18(1):13-9.

58. Hofer A, Hassan AS, Legat FJ, et al. The efficacy of excimer laser (308 nm) for vitiligo at different body sites. J Eur Acad Dermatol Venereol. 2006;20(5):558-64.
59. Hong SB, Park HH, Lee MH. Short-term effects of 308-nm xenon-chloride excimer laser and narrow-band ultraviolet B in the treatment of vitiligo: a comparative study. J Korean Med Sci. 2005;20(2):273-8.
60. Sassi F, Cazzaniga S, Tessari G, et al. Randomized controlled trial comparing the effectiveness of 308-nm excimer laser alone or in combination with topical hydrocortisone 17-butyrate cream in the treatment of vitiligo of the face and neck. Br J Dermatol. 2008;159(5):1186-91.
61. Kawalek AZ, Spencer JM, Phelps RG. Combined excimer laser and topical tacrolimus for the treatment of vitiligo: a pilot study. Dermatol Surg. 2004;30(2 Pt 1):130-5.
62. Passeron T, Ostovari N, Zakaria W, et al. Topical tacrolimus and the 308-nm excimer laser: a synergistic combination for the treatment of vitiligo. Arch Dermatol. 2004;140(9): 1065-9.
63. Linthorst Homan MW, Spuls PI, Nieuweboer-Krobotova L, et al. A randomized comparison of excimer laser versus narrow-band ultraviolet B phototherapy after punch grafting in stable vitiligo patients. J Eur Acad Dermatol Venereol. 2012;26(6):690-5.
64. Patel NS, Paghdal KV, Cohen GF. Advanced treatment modalities for vitiligo. Dermatol Surg. 2012;38(3):381-91.
65. Hofer A, Kerl H, Wolf P. Long-term results in the treatment of vitiligo with oral khellin plus UVA. Eur J Dermatol. 2001;11(3):225-9.
66. Ortel B, Tanew A, Hönigsmann H. Treatment of vitiligo with khellin and ultraviolet A. J Am Acad Dermatol. 1988;18(4 Pt 1):693-701.
67. Valkova S, Trashlieva M, Christova P. Treatment of vitiligo with local khellin and UVA: comparison with systemic PUVA. Clin Exp Dermatol. 2004;29(2):180-4.
68. Carlie G, Ntusi NB, Hulley PA, et al. KUVA (khellin plus ultraviolet A) stimulates proliferation and melanogenesis in normal human melanocytes and melanoma cells *in vitro*. Br J Dermatol. 2003;149(4):707-17.
69. Schulpis CH, Antoniou C, Michas T, et al. Phenylalanine plus ultraviolet light: preliminary report of a promising treatment for childhood vitiligo. Pediatr Dermatol. 1989;6(4):332-5.
70. Siddiqui AH, Stolk LM, Bhaggoe R, et al. L-phenylalanine and UVA irradiation in the treatment of vitiligo. Dermatology. 1994;188(3):215-8.
71. Halder RM. Childhood vitiligo. Clin Dermatol. 1997;15(6): 899-906.
72. Jaisankar TJ, Baruah MC, Garg BR. Vitiligo in children. Int J Dermatol. 1992;31(9):621-3.
73. Njoo MD, Bos JD, Westerhof W. Treatment of generalized vitiligo in children with narrowband (TL-01) UVB radiation therapy. J Am Acad Dermatol. 2000;42(2 Pt 1):245-53.
74. Percivalle S, Piccinno R, Caccialanza M, et al. Narrowband ultraviolet B phototherapy in childhood vitiligo: evaluation of results in 28 patients. Pediatr Dermatol. 2012;29(2):160-5.
75. Kanwar AJ, Dogra S. Narrow-band UVB for the treatment of generalized vitiligo in children. Clin Exp Dermatol. 2005;30(4):332-6.

23

Medical Management of Vitiligo

Torello Lotti, Angelo Massimiliano D'Erme

Key Features

- The therapy of vitiligo is particularly challenging for every physicians. With an appropriate and prompt management, a lot of patients can ameliorate disease progression, achieve repigmentation, and obtain cosmetically pleasing results.
- Recently some multicenter papers have been published in order to give some more insights in the management of the different forms of vitiligo. These researches also reported evidence-based and expert-based recommendations in order to help physicians in the normal practice in the vitiligo.
- Several trials have demonstrated that combined treatments improve the overall effectiveness and the time needed to achieve repigmentation reducing the potential side effects.

INTRODUCTION

Vitiligo is an acquired depigmentary skin disorder of unknown etiology affecting 0.5% of the world population without any sex or racial differences. The prevalence ranges from less than 0.1% to greater than 8% worldwide.[1-3] Vitiligo can appear at any time during the life affecting all age groups and impair the patients' quality of life. Due to the poor understanding of its etiopathogenic mechanisms the progress in the management and treatment has hold back.[1-4]

Recently some papers have been published, either multicenter (Lotti et al.)[4,5] or national (e.g. Saudi Arabia,[6] Indian[7] or American[8,9]) or European viewpoint (Vitiligo European Task Force)[10,11] in order to give some more insights in the management of the different forms of vitiligo. These studies have also reported an evidence-based and expert-based recommendations in order to help physicians in the normal practice in the vitiligo management.

CLASSIFICATION OF VITILIGO

Recently vitiligo has been divided in localized (focal, unilateral/segmental, mucosal) generalized (vulgaris, acrofacialis and mixed), and universal (including also special forms such astrichrome vitiligo, quadrichrome vitiligo and inflammatory vitiligo).[12] Segmental vitiligo (SV) is characterized by unilateral distribution that matches totally or partially with one dermatome. It is often characterized by rapid onset and involvement of the hair follicle pigmentary system. The non-segmental vitiligo forms (NSV) do not reflect a distinct nature, but they are often associated to a systemic involvement.

Differences exist between SV and NSV in terms of management, prognosis and treatment.[3,8,12,13]

CLINICAL MANAGEMENT

Since NSV, that is the most frequent form, is associated to a systemic involvement, it is important to face patient with vitiligo as a patient affected by a systemic diseases. Hence, it is necessary to consider several aspects of the disease such as patients' features like prototypes, ethnic, age of onset presence or previous or family history of autoimmune disease. Due to the long period treatment, patients are frequently frustrated by the failure of previous ones and psychological stress is common.[1,3,8,14-16] Moretti et al (2012)[17] have demonstrated that there is a higher incidence of obsession and phobia among vitiligo patients especially in those presenting markers of autoimmune diseases.

Regarding the literature data, treatment efficacy is considered the proportion of treated patients in whom a specified degree of repigmentation is achieved. A repigmentation more than 50% or more than 75% is considered a good response.[3] These values are debatable insofar as complete repigmentation, especially in visible areas, may be needed for a high degree of satisfaction on the patient's part.[3,10]

An evaluation of autoimmunity markers, if a patient suffers from NSV has been advised. In particular the thyroid function and thyroid autoimmune disorders should be checked because the thyroid comorbidities are the most frequent endocrinologic ones.[1,3,8,10]

If the patient's history or routine laboratory parameters suggest additional autoimmune disorders, further investigations and an endocrinologist/immunologist consultation (e.g. in the case of autoimmune polyglandular syndrome) are strongly suggested.[8,10,15]

THERAPEUTICAL MANAGEMENT

In the choosing a treatment, the evaluation of disease features such as the duration and the opinion of the patient on the disease status are critical for developing a treatment protocol. Lastly, the affected area influences the prognosis and the rate of repigmentation success. Patients with a recent onset of disease, young, darker skin types, involvement of face, neck, and trunk tend to achieve the best response to the therapy.[1,3,8,10]

On the other hand, mucosal involvement, family history of vitiligo, non-segmental vitiligo, acral lesions are associated with worse prognosis and response to the treatment.[8,9] In a correct therapeutic management, the evaluation of types and durations of the previous treatments by which the patient has undergone and his opinion on each of them has to be taken in account. Lastly, in choosing therapy, it must be remembered that some therapies are not licensed for vitiligo and can only be prescribed "off-label"[12]

The treatment of vitiligo remains challenging for every physician. The etiopathogenic mechanisms of vitiligo are still poorly understood, and this has held back progress in diagnosis and treatment. Thanks to the new discoveries, several methods are available to stimulate repigmentation, ranging from topical to systemic therapy, from physical to surgical therapy.[1,3,8,10,18,19]

Since there is no definitive cure for vitiligo, new studies need to better define the first silent immune-mediated inflammatory phase of vitiligo, when the lesions progress. When, in a next phase, the lesions are stable, new therapeutic agents must be addressed toward the regeneration of achromic areas by hair follicle or form reserve population of amelanotic melanocytes. The treatment has to be discussed with and has to satisfy the patient in order to achieve a high level of compliance.[1,12,14,16]

MEDICAL TREATMENT

Several treatments are available; some of these are described in details in other chapters.

Topical Therapies

Topical therapies, as corticosteroids, calcineurin inhibitors, and vitamin D analogs, may be effective in cases of localized non-segmental or segmental vitiligo.[1,3,9,10]

Topical corticosteroids (TCS) can be used in adult and in children as first line. Their use can be advised for patients with limited, extrafacial involvement for a period not too long (not longer than 3 months).[12]

Topical calcineurin inhibitors (TCI) can be considered in adults and children with vitiligo as an alternative to topical steroids for new, actively spreading lesions on thin skin. The European guidelines, evaluating the limited data from double-blind placebo-controlled studies, suggest their use restricting it to selected areas, as the head and neck region. Vitamin D3 analogs are considered inferior to TCS. It can be adjunct to TCS but the association with light therapy is not recommended.[1,3,8,10,19]

Indications of Topical Therapy

Topical corticosteroids and TCI represent the first line treatment alone or in combination with systemic therapy. Topical monotherapy represent a first choice for children, adults who present limited skin areas involved. Since the topical treatment can be not sufficient either for the widespread of the lesions or for the stability/resistance, a combinatorial treatment has been suggested.[1,3,8,10,19]

Phototherapy

The narrow band (NB) ultraviolet B (UVB) or ultraviolet A/psoralen ultraviolet A (UVA/PUVA) are indicated for generalized NSV.

Especially NB-UVB is suggested for vitiligo lesions involving more than 15–20% of the body area or for lesions (>3% of body area) that are active spreading on the body.

Oral PUVA is currently used in adult patients with generalized vitiligo as a second-line therapy. Compared with NB-UVB it has the disadvantage of lower efficacy and higher short- and long-term risks, especially the increase of incidence of both melanoma and non-melanoma skin cancer.[1,3,8,10,20]

Targeted Phototherapies

Targeted phototherapies, such as micro-phototherapy BIOSKIN (311NM)® or monochromatic excimer laser (308 nm), can have a wide spread of indication. They allow us to treat localized vitiligo resistant to treatment, in alternation or in combination with topical therapy. They can represent the first choice for localized vitiligo and in particular for small lesions of recent onset and childhood vitiligo. They have the advantage to avoid to the patient aging and risk of skin cancer associated with total body irradiation. In particular, they are suitable for patients with higher Fitzpatrick skin types. More randomized controlled studies assessing the efficacy and safety of these approaches are needed.[1,3,8,10,20,21]

The optimum treatment duration of NB-UVB, PUVA or targeted phototherapy are discussed above.

Systemic Treatment

The use of systemic corticosteroids can be taken into consideration in order to halt disease progression and induce repigmentation; however the lack of efficacy study and their well known side effects limit their use for long time.

In the literature there is not enough data to recommend the use of immunosuppressant or biologics in vitiligo, as first line.

Systemic and topical antioxidant can be useful for the vitiligo patients especially in those who are under phototherapy. The rationale of their use is the protection of melanocytes from reactive oxygen species. Further confirmation by large studies is needed. Due to their few and mild side effects and the possibility to combine with topical and systemic treatment they have the advantage to be easy and safe to use.[1,3,6,8,10]

Surgical Therapy

The melanocytes transplant techniques including suction blister grafting, split-thickness grafting, punch grafting, and melanocyte suspension, can be a very good option for resistant patients with segmental vitiligo or non-segmental with a stable form and negative history of Koebner phenomenon. It is not without risks: scarring, graft failure, Koebnerization, infection, and variegated pigmentation can occur.[1,3,7,8,10,22]

Camouflage

Self-tanning agents in gel, cream, lotion or spray, highly pigmented cover creams, dermal pigmentation, cosmetic tattoos can be evaluated with the patient.[1,3,8,10]

Depigmenting Agents

This technique can be evaluated as one of the last ones in the cases of extensive vitiligo. Potent depigmenting agent as monobenzone or hydroquinone and laser as Q-switched ruby laser, alone or in combination with methoxyphenol can be used.[1,3,8,10,23]

Psychological Interventions

The quality of life of the patient with vitiligo is severely compromised. An association with psychiatric diseases has been reported. A psychologically evaluation support is always recommended in order to evaluate the impact of the disease on quality of life and to identify patients for whom the psychological support may be useful.[1,3,8,10,17]

Combination Therapy

Several trials have demonstrated that combined treatments improve the overall effectiveness and the time needed to achieve repigmentation reducing the potential side effects.

Combination therapies are often considered when there has been no response to phototherapy, as well as an acceleration of the response or reduction to the UV exposure has requested.[1,3,8,10]

The therapies more used are topical steroids with phototherapy, including TCS and UVB source either NB-UVB or laser therapy and topical calcineurin inhibitors and UVB sources. Regarding the latter, the combination of these two treatments is promising and provides better results than the two treatments used alone. This combination seems to be safe, but long-term data on carcinogenicity are still lacking. A possible higher risk of skin cancers promoted by this combination needs to be taken into consideration.

Vitamin D analogs can be combined with other topical therapies, mainly TCS. The benefit of use in combination with UV radiation is very limited and for that it is not recommended. Phototherapy can also be used in combination with oral antioxidant, after surgery, with topical pseudocatalase, with ablative laser (fractional CO_2 or erbium-YAG), with autologous transplanted epidermal cell suspensions, or azathiopine even they are supported by preliminary data and have to be considered and reserved in non-respondent/resistant cases. Likewise, the topical steroid with surgery.[1,3,8,10]

MANAGEMENT ALGORITHM

Recently, the Vitiligo European Task Force has proposed a therapeutical algorithm for segmental and non-segmental vitiligo **(Table 1)**.[10]

Table 1: Therapeutic option and recommendation in vitiligo in adults. From Taieb et al. (2012), modified[10]

Vitiligo
• Segmental or limited NSV (<2–3% body surface involvement) – *First treatment:* Avoiding triggering factor. Local therapies. TCS and TCI – *Second line:* Combination of topical therapy with localized UVB therapy – *Third line:* Surgical techniques
• Non-segmental (>3% body-surface involvement) – *First line:* Stabilize with NB-UVB for at least 3 months. Combination with topical therapies – *Second line:* If there is an extension of lesions under UVB therapy: systemic corticosteroids or immunosuppressive agents (recommendation supported by few studies) – *Third line:* Surgical technique – *Fourth line:* Depigmentation techniques, when the extension is over 50% or a high visible area is affected.

This algorithm is applicable for adults. In children younger than the age of 7 years, the phototherapy is not recommended (for cutaneous side effects and organizational problem). Also surgical techniques are rarely proposed before puberty.

In children the vitiligo has a better prognosis but if persist could have important physical and psychological repercussion.[1,3,8,10,24]

CONCLUSION

The therapy of vitiligo is particularly challenging for every physicians. It is noteworthy to underline that with an appropriate and prompt management; a lot of patients can ameliorate disease progression, achieve repigmentation, and obtain cosmetically pleasing results.[1,3,6-8,10]

When a patient comes to a physician, he/she is often sad, low compliant and with an important repercussion on his quality of life. Hence, it is important to face all these problems in order to achieve a high compliance to the therapy and to check the presence/absence of comorbidities.

Moreover given the importance of charlatanism in the vitiligo field, it is important the patients to avoid some therapies of dubious efficacy that could worsen the vitiligo and its comorbidities. It is crucial to personalize the therapy on the patient. At the onset of disease, a correct and aggressive anti-inflammatory therapy is recommended. Then, when there is a loss of melanocytes a repigmentation therapy must be used.

A psychological support, educational programs, and the use of cosmetics, may be vital to the patient's quality of life at all stages of treatment.

REFERENCES

1. Lotti T, Hercogovà J. Vitiligo. Problems and solutions. New York: Marcel Dekker, Inc; 2004.
2. Whitton ME, Pinart M, Batchelor J, et al. Interventions for vitiligo. Cochrane Database Syst Rev. 2010; 1:CD003263.
3. Taieb A, Picardo M. Clinical practice: vitiligo. N Engl J Med. 2009;360:160-9.
4. Lotti TM, Hercogová J, Schwartz RA, et al. Treatments of vitiligo: what's new at the horizon. Dermatol Ther. 2012;25 (Suppl 1):S32-40.
5. Lotti TM, Berti SF, Hercogova J, et al. Vitiligo: recent insights and new therapeutic approaches. G Ital Dermatol Venereol. 2012;147(6):637-47.
6. Ismail SA, Sayed DS, Abdelghani LN. Vitiligo management strategy in Jeddah, Saudi Arabia as reported by dermatologists and experienced by patients. J Dermatolog Treat; 2012.
7. Parsad D, Gupta S. IADVL Dermatosurgery Task Force. Standard guidelines of care for vitiligo surgery. Indian J Dermatol Venereol Leprol. 2008;74(Suppl):S37-45.
8. Alikhan A, Felsten LM, Daly M, et al. Vitiligo: a comprehensive overview Part I. Introduction, epidemiology, quality of life, diagnosis, differential diagnosis, associations, histopathology, etiology, and work-up. J Am Acad Dermatol. 2011;65(3):473-91.
9. Felsten LM, Alikhan A, Petronic-Rosic V. Vitiligo: a comprehensive overview Part II: treatment options and approach to treatment. J Am Acad Dermatol. 2011;65(3):493-514.
10. Taieb A, Alomar A, Böhm M, et al. Guidelines for the management of vitiligo: the European Dermatology Forum consensus. Br J Dermatol. 2013;168(1):5-19.
11. van Geel N, Speeckaert R, Taieb A, et al. Koebner's phenomenon in vitiligo: European position paper. Pigment Cell Melanoma Res. 2011;24(3):564-73.
12. Hercogová J, Schwartz RA, Lotti TM. Classification of vitiligo: a challenging endeavor. Dermatol Ther. 2012;25(Suppl 1): S10-6.
13. Lahiri K, Malakar S. The concept of stability of vitiligo: a reappraisal. Indian J Dermatol. 2012;57(2):83-9. doi: 10.4103/0019-5154.94271.
14. Lee BW, Schwartz RA, Hercogová J, et al. Vitiligo road map. Dermatol Ther. 2012;25(Suppl 1):S44-56.
15. Pietrzak A, Bartosińska J, Hercogová J, et al. Metabolic syndrome in vitiligo. Dermatol Ther. 2012;25(Suppl 1): S41-3.
16. Valle Y, Lotti TM, Hercogova J, et al. Multidisciplinary approach to R&D in vitiligo, a neglected skin disease. Dermatol Ther. 2012;25(Suppl 1):S1-9.
17. Moretti S, Arunachalam M, Colucci R, et al. Autoimmune markers in vitiligo patients appear correlated with obsession and phobia. J Eur Acad Dermatol Venereol. 2012;26(7): 861-7.
18. Buggiani G, Tsampau D, Hercogovà J, et al. Clinical efficacy of a novel topical formulation for vitiligo: compared evaluation of different treatment modalities in 149 patients. Dermatol Ther. 2012;25(5):472-6.
19. Kathuria S, Khaitan BK, Ramam M, et al. Segmental vitiligo: a randomized controlled trial to evaluate efficacy and safety of 0.1% tacrolimus ointment vs 0.05% fluticasone propionate cream. Indian J Dermatol Venereol Leprol. 2012;78(1):68-73.
20. Leone G, Iacovelli P, Paro Vidolin A, et al. Monochromatic excimer light 308 nm in the treatment of vitiligo: a pilot study. J Eur Acad Dermatol Venereol. 2003;17(5):531-7.
21. Lotti T, Buggiani G, Troiano M, et al. Targeted and combination treatments for vitiligo. Comparative evaluation of different current modalities in 458 subjects. Dermatol Ther. 2008;21(Suppl 1):S20-6.
22. Lahiri K. Evolution and evaluation of autologous mini punch grafting in vitiligo. Indian J Dermatol. 2009;54(2):159-67.
23. Gupta D, Kumari R, Thappa DM. Depigmentation therapies in vitiligo. Indian J Dermatol Venereol Leprol. 2012;78(1): 49-58.
24. Kanwar AJ, Kumaran MS. Childhood vitiligo: treatment paradigms. Indian J Dermatol. 2012;57(6):466-74.

24

Oral and Systemic Corticosteroids in Management of Vitiligo

Binod K Khaitan, Sushruta Kathuria

Key Features

- The usual approach to the treatment of vitiligo has been to regain pigment in vitiliginous areas rather than controlling the disease process.
- The priority for the treatment of vitiligo should be first to control the disease process, and then taking measures to repigment existing lesions.
- Corticosteroids suppress autoantibody formation and also induce apoptosis of cytotoxic. T-cells: The autoimmune hypothesis still prevails in the pathogenesis of non-segmental vitiligo. In progressive disease, there is continuous assault on melanocytes.
- Systemic corticosteroids are the first-line treatment when a patient presents with rapidly progressive vitiligo. It helps not only in halting progression of the disease but also induces repigmentation as normal melanocytes from the periphery of the lesions or perifollicular areas take over, once the process of melanocyte destruction is arrested.
- Because of the nature of the disease, treatment of vitiligo is known to be long-term, hence the question of long-term safety of systemic corticosteroids is an important consideration. To reduce long-term complications of corticosteroids, oral mini-pulse (OMP) therapy was introduced in 1989 and was established in 1993, where instead of daily oral corticosteroids, a long-acting corticosteroid was given on two consecutive days of the week for 6 months or longer.
- Since then, systemic corticosteroids are used in day-to-day practice in extensive and progressive vitiligo. Most studies indicate that systemic corticosteroids are helpful in halting disease progression in rapidly spreading vitiligo and inducing spontaneous repigmentation. However, their role in static vitiligo is not well documented. Areas that require further research are the risk of osteoporosis with corticosteroids and the efficacy of calcium supplementation. Studies with longer follow-up periods are required to evaluate the potential for relapse.
- Head-to-head comparative studies between betamethasone, prednisolone and deflazacort may be useful for determining the optimal agent for treatment.
- The issue of relapse after achieving arrest of disease activity in long-term is not yet studied. Currently, for relapsed cases, the approach in clinical practice is to repeat OMP therapy as episodic treatment for 8–12 weeks or even longer to aim control of the disease activity.
- There seems to be a definite role for systemic corticosteroids in the treatment of certain types of vitiligo:
    - Rapidly progressing vitiligo
    - Slowly progressing vitiligo with extensive involvement and frequent exacerbation
    - Frank inflammatory vitiligo
    - Patients with direct or indirect evidence of autoimmune disease (e.g. high titers of thyroid autoantibodies)
    - Long-term recalcitrant static vitiligo with sudden exacerbation.
- Although daily or alternate day, oral corticosteroids may be treatment options, OMP therapy seems to be the best regimen for long-term use with minimal side effects. The duration of OMP therapy should be at least 6 months or longer and tapering to discontinuation should be slow and stepwise.
- Systemic corticosteroids should not be considered for universal vitiligo, segmental vitiligo or focal limited vitiligo.

INTRODUCTION

Vitiligo is an acquired disorder of pigmentation characterized by depigmented or hypopigmented macules. It also involves hair and mucosa. Its prevalence worldwide is 0.1–2% and varies from country to country.[1] It is associated with variable psychosocial impact and dysfunction, particularly in darker skin types where the contrast between normal and depigmented skin is highly pronounced.[2,3] The usual approach to the treatment of vitiligo has been to regain pigment in vitiliginous areas rather than controlling the disease process. This is akin to treating the effects of the disease rather than treating the disease itself. Such an approach frequently results in frustration because patients can continue to develop disease progression as new lesions at other sites or extension of existing lesions, even while some of those existing lesions are repigmenting, or the disease may be reactivated at a later stage even after achieving a fair degree of therapeutic success.[4] Therefore, the priority for the treatment of vitiligo should be first to control the disease process, and then taking measures to repigment existing lesions.

Systemic corticosteroids are widely used in various dermatological and non-dermatological conditions. Corticosteroids, both topical and systemic, have been used in vitiligo for over four decades with some concern about its efficacy as well as its known or expected adverse effects. Further research may provide more evidence that systemic corticosteroids may be an important modality for the treatment of vitiligo particularly progressive vitiligo.

HISTORY

In 1967, oral corticosteroids were used for the first time in vitiligo. Triamcinolone orally was found to have a synergistic effect with methoxypsoralen as compared to methoxypsoralen alone.[5] In 1976, adrenocorticotropic hormone (ACTH) was found to be effective in inducing repigmentation in patients who had previously not responded to photochemotherapy with psoralen followed by ultraviolet light A (PUVA) exposure.[6] In another study in the same year, a mixture of prednisolone, betamethasone, paramethasone acetate and methylprednisolone given orally was effective in producing satisfactory repigmentation in one-third of patients studied, thus confirming the efficacy of corticosteroids in vitiligo.[7] Because of the nature of the disease, treatment of vitiligo is known to be long-term, hence the question of long-term safety of systemic corticosteroids is an important consideration. To reduce long-term complications of corticosteroids, OMP therapy was introduced in 1989 and was established in 1993, where instead of daily oral corticosteroids, a long-acting corticosteroid was given on two consecutive days of the week.[8,9] Since then, systemic corticosteroids are used in day-to-day practice in extensive and progressive vitiligo.

STRUCTURE AND CLASSIFICATION OF SYSTEMIC CORTICOSTEROIDS

The structure of corticosteroids consists of three hexane rings and one pentane ring known as the cyclopentanoperhydrophenanthrene. The different systemic corticosteroids are variations of this basic structure. Systemic corticosteroids are classified according to their half-lives. There are other parameters pertaining to efficacy and side effects based on which different molecules are preferred by the treating physicians **(Table 1)**.

The structure, mechanism of action and pharmacokinetic profile of various systemic corticosteroids are very similar.

Table 1: Classification of corticosteroids[10,11]

Corticosteroid	*Equivalent dose (mg)*	*Glucocorticoid potency*	*Mineralocorticoid potency*	*Plasma half-life (minutes)*	*Biological half-life (hours)*
Short acting					
Cortisone	25.00	0.80	2+	30–90	8–12
Hydrocortisone	20.00	1.00	2+	60–120	8–12
Deflazacort	6.00	3.30	0	90–120	<12
Intermediate acting					
Prednisone	5.00	4.00	1+	60	24–36
Prednisolone	5.00	4.00	1+	115–212	24–36
Methyl prednisolone	4.00	5.00	0	180	24–36
Triamcinolone	4.00	5.00	0	78–188	24–36
Long acting					
Dexamethasone	0.75	20.30	0	100–300	36–54
Betamethasone	0.6–0.75	20–30	0	100–300	36–54

The main difference is in their glucocorticoid and mineralocorticoid effects and biological half-life. Hence, the choice of corticosteroid is decided by the duration of action needed, the dosing schedule to be used, and the clinical profile of the patient. Having a working knowledge of equivalent dosing helps in dose conversion when one corticosteroid is switched to another. However, the calculation of equivalence may not necessarily work all the time.

MECHANISM OF ACTION OF CORTICOSTEROIDS IN VITILIGO

Vitiligo is considered to be primarily an autoimmune condition that results in the loss of melanocytes. Melanocytes are lost in vitiligo due to the destruction by humoral or intrinsic cellular mechanisms.[12] Humoral mechanisms involve destruction of melanocytes by pathogenic autoantibodies directed against melanocytes and the tyrosinase enzyme. Cellular mechanisms are perhaps more important as humoral in destroying melanocytes. Biopsies from vitiligo lesions show mild mononuclear infiltrate in the margins of lesional skin in active vitiligo with or without basal vacuolization. Active lesions show increased numbers of CD4+ T-cells and increased epidermal expression of intercellular adhesion molecule-1 (ICAM-1).[13] Peripheral T-cell activation is also seen in non-segmental vitiligo and T-cell dysregulation is not only limited to the lesions.[14] The peripheral blood of vitiligo patients express more of the cutaneous lymphocyte-associated antigen positive melanocyte-specific cytotoxic T-lymphocytes indicating that there is recruitment of T-cells in the circulation to the skin.[15] Both the CD4+ and CD8+ T-cells from perilesional and non-lesional skin in vitiligo show polarization towards the Type 1 cytokine profile which parallels depigmentation.[16] The melanocyte-specific cytotoxic T-cells found in perilesional biopsies have the ability to infiltrate normal skin and destroy the melanocytes.[17] Besides cytotoxic T-cells, regulatory T-cells (T regs) also have a role in vitiligo. The T reg population is not decreased in the peripheral circulation; however, these T regs are not able to settle in the skin and this defect seems to be crucial in the observed perpetual anti-melanocyte reactivity in progressive disease.[18] Cytokines also play an important role, e.g. IL-6 (inhibitor of melanocyte proliferation) is increased in vitiliginous skin.

Corticosteroids suppress autoantibody formation and also induce apoptosis of cytotoxic T-cells. The autoimmune hypothesis still prevails in the pathogenesis of non-segmental vitiligo, and the autoimmune process is not always limited to the skin. In progressive disease, there is continuous assault on melanocytes. Topical corticosteroids, tacrolimus or any other topical agent may suppress autoimmune dysfunction at the site of a vitiligo lesion, but for obvious reasons these do not have any effect on the disease process beyond the lesion. Photochemotherapy and phototherapy stimulate melanocytes to cause repigmentation and have minimal immunomodulatory action on T-lymphocytes, but may not halt the rapid destruction of melanocytes. Systemic corticosteroids act not only on lesional immune activity, but also on the T-cells in peripheral circulation. Besides modulating cell-mediated immunity, corticosteroids also suppress autoantibody formation. The serum of actively spreading vitiligo patients who received oral corticosteroids and showed improvement had a decrease in complement-mediated cytotoxicity by melanocyte autoantibodies and a reduced antibody titer to the melanocyte surface antigen.[19]

Indications

Systemic corticosteroids are the first-line treatment when a patient presents with rapidly progressive vitiligo. It helps not only in halting progression of the disease, but also induces repigmentation as normal melanocytes from the periphery of the lesions or perifollicular areas take over, once the process of melanocyte destruction is arrested. Assessment of treatment response is important. Since the patient is not always sure whether new lesions have appeared or not since corticosteroid initiation, a baseline photographic record must be taken before starting treatment and periodically throughout treatment, preferably at 4-week intervals. The time taken for disease activity to stop is variable and may range from a few weeks to months. Once stability is achieved clinically (defined as no new lesion formation and no extension of existing lesions), one must consider tapering the dose of corticosteroids slowly and add other modalities for augmentation of repigmentation.

Patients with extensive slowly progressive vitiligo (body surface area more than 10% with the continuous appearance of new lesions or slow extension of existing lesions) may also benefit from systemic corticosteroids as this suggests "simmering" autoimmune activity that may be long-term.

After stoppage of systemic corticosteroids, episodic treatment for another round of same duration or a minimum of 8–12 weeks at a time can also be added whenever there is a relapse.

Systemic corticosteroids can also be added to photochemotherapy or phototherapy when there is transient fluctuation or worsening of disease activity.

It is not advisable to use corticosteroid monotherapy in segmental vitiligo because segmental vitiligo is known to stabilize after some time. The initial period of progression within the segment may be rapid in segmental vitiligo, but nearly all lesions stabilize and remain confined to one part of the body. Hence use of corticosteroids may not be advisable. However, it can also be an adjuvant to surgery in both segmental and non-segmental vitiligo.[20,21] Patients with stable vitiligo will also not benefit from corticosteroids because they are not simply repigmenting agents; rather their efficacy comes from their effects on active disease. Universal or near universal vitiligo is also not an indication for the use of corticosteroids since treatment is usually depigmentation of residual pigmented areas.

The total duration of treatment varies in different patients. However, a minimum period of 3–6 months of treatment with systemic corticosteroids is usually required. Some patients may require even longer duration of treatment for control of the disease activity. Therefore, periodic assessment and fine-tuning of the dosage schedule and monitoring of the side effects are must and after optimizing the use of systemic corticosteroids, addition of other modalities should also be considered.

Modes of Administration

Systemic corticosteroids given orally are effective in halting progression of vitiligo and producing variable repigmentation. However, the long treatment duration required in vitiligo raises concern about the long-term cumulative side effects of corticosteroids. Daily doses or alternate day dosing is thereby avoided in vitiligo. Therefore, OMP therapy is preferred for the planned long-term maintenance therapy for 6 months or beyond.[9] OMP therapy refers to giving a higher than the usual daily dose of corticosteroid on two consecutive days a week and leaving the remaining 5 days treatment-free. A long-acting corticosteroid is preferred so that the effect lasts for about 3 days at a time. Corticotropin and cortisol levels fall rapidly after the second dose of drug, but returns to baseline before the next oral dexamethasone pulse.[22] Hence, it is preferred to give a long-acting corticosteroid on two consecutive days in a week rather than once in 3 days to give the hypothalamic-pituitary-adrenal axis (HPA) reference time to revert back to normal before the next dose. The standard regimen is to give oral betamethasone 5 mg (five of the 1 mg betamethasone tablets) after breakfast on Saturday and Sunday (or any other two consecutive days) every week.[9] Dexamethasone pulse has been used in doses of 5 mg or 10 mg in this manner.[22,23] Betamethasone pulse has been given as an adjunct with surgery.[24] Besides this standard regimen, there can be variations in OMP therapy. If no response is seen, the dose can be increased from 5 mg up to 7.5 mg. In children, dose is reduced from 5 mg to 2.5–4 mg. Additional immunosuppressants, for example, cyclophosphamide and azathioprine, may also be added to the therapeutic regimen.

Methylprednisolone[25] has been used intravenously as high dose pulse therapy given on three consecutive days in a month but should not be considered as first-line treatment. Daily low dose prednisolone has also been used in tapering doses to discontinuation.[26,27] The intramuscular route is not preferred as it is painful, and the level of drug in the circulation is unpredictable and good results are achieved by oral administration. Monitoring of weight, fasting blood sugar and blood pressure every month are necessary for any patient on systemic corticosteroids. Baseline and periodic photographs should also be done to monitor treatment response and repigmentation.

Table 2: Side effects of systemic corticosteroids[10]

System affected	*Side effects*
HPA axis	Steroid withdrawal syndrome, Addisonian crisis
Metabolic	Hyperglycemia, increased appetite and weight gain, hypertension, congestive heart failure, hypokalemia, hypertriglyceridemia, cushingoid changes, menstrual irregularities
Bone	Osteoporosis, osteonecrosis, hypocalcemia
Gastrointestinal	Peptic ulcer disease, bowel perforation, fatty liver changes, esophageal reflux, nausea, vomiting
Ocular	Cataracts, glaucoma, infections
Psychiatric	Psychosis, agitation, depression
Neurological	Pseudotumor cerebri, peripheral neuropathy
Muscular	Myopathy
Cutaneous	Delayed wound healing, acneiform eruption, purpura, cutaneous infections, telogen effluvium, hirsutism, acanthosis nigricans

Side Effects and Contraindications

Systemic corticosteroids are known to have a variety of adverse effects. The predominant side effects are described in **Table 2**. However, these adverse effects also depend on dose, duration of treatment and individual susceptibility. All patients do not develop the same adverse effects. Therefore, clinical evaluation and monitoring is the best way to ascertain whether adverse effects are minimal or serious, and reversible or irreversible. Minimal and reversible side effects are acceptable for continuing treatment.

The primary consideration in treating vitiligo with systemic corticosteroids is careful patient selection in order to maximize response to vitiligo while minimizing adverse effects. The other concern is determination of proper dose and dosing schedule. Side effects can be dose-dependent or duration-dependent. Dose-dependent side effects of corticosteroids are hyperglycemia, hyperlipidemia, peptic ulcer disease and psychosis. Duration-dependent changes are hypertension, cushingoid changes, growth impairment in children, osteoporosis, osteonecrosis and opportunistic infections.[10] Steroid withdrawal syndrome is observed when systemic corticosteroids given at high doses are abruptly stopped and it presents as vague symptoms of lethargy, generalized weakness and myalgia. Abrupt withdrawal of the corticosteroid may not give enough time for the suppressed HPA axis to recover. It is observed with doses higher than

20–30 mg of prednisolone. Duration of treatment is not a predictable causative factor.[28,29] High doses of corticosteroid for prolonged period can also lead to extreme suppression of adrenals (Addisonian crisis) manifesting as hypotension and extreme weakness. Intermittent dosing schedules are likely to produce fewer side effects including HPA axis suppression. Cushingoid changes occur with long-term treatment and present as puffiness of face, moon facies, buffalo hump, striae, increased hair growth on face, skin atrophy, increased abdominal girth with thin extremities and others. Growth impairment and opportunistic infections can be decreased by avoiding daily administration either by using alternate day dosing or OMP therapy. OMP therapy has fewer side effects (e.g. moon facies, weight gain, acne) compared to daily dosing as reviewed in a meta-analysis.[30]

Betamethasone and dexamethasone can be used interchangeably as the potency and half-life are almost same. When compared to other corticosteroids, deflazacort is considered to have relatively fewer cases of growth retardation in children, osteoporosis, weight gain and HPA axis suppression.[11] However, deflazacort is a short-acting corticosteroid.

Absolute contraindications to use of systemic corticosteroids are very few, and include such conditions as systemic fungal infections and herpes simplex keratitis. Relative contraindications are congestive heart failure, human immunodeficiency virus (HIV), psychosis, active peptic ulcer disease, active tuberculosis, and septicemia. Well-controlled diabetes and hypertension are not contraindications, but lower doses of corticosteroids may be used and the concomitant disease must be adequately treated, and the patient should be monitored more frequently.

There are various approaches to minimize the side effects of corticosteroids. First is to give corticosteroids only as long as disease activity is present and then taper it slowly (over a period of 3–6 months) when no indication of new lesions are present. The OMP therapy regimen has significantly less side effects compared to typical daily dosing of corticosteroids. An important finding is the lack of prolonged HPA axis suppression with OMP therapy.[22] Furthermore, higher doses of dexamethasone (10 mg) do not seem to provide any additional benefit to 5 mg betamethasone.[9,22] Choosing corticosteroids with less risk of mineralocorticoid-type effects (i.e. dexamethasone, betamethasone) or one with supposedly fewer side effects (i.e. deflazacort) can be beneficial for all patients. Calcium supplementation, salt restriction, proper diet, daily exercise and use of antacids can minimize risk of side effects. Regular monitoring of weight, fasting blood sugar and blood pressure will help in early detection of side effects if they occur. It is recommended to give calcium and vitamin D (800 IU daily) supplementation for prevention and treatment of steroid-induced osteoporosis in all patients (American College of Rheumatology Guidelines, 2011).

Safety in Children and Pregnancy

The decision to treat progressive vitiligo in children below 4 years of age can be rather difficult as limited data is available for this population. It is suggested that OMP therapy be modified (i.e. 1 mg of dexamethasone or betamethasone given for every 10 kg) and used.

Corticosteroids have been safely used in pregnancy and are classified as category C drugs (animal reproduction studies have shown an adverse effect on the fetus and there are no adequate and well-controlled studies in humans, but potential benefits may warrant use of the drug in pregnant women despite potential risks). However, it is best to reserve its use in pregnancy when the benefits of treatment outweigh the risk of side effects. Pregnancy is known to precipitate and aggravate vitiligo. However, vitiligo being a non-life threatening condition, a pregnant patient should defer any type of systemic treatment, including corticosteroids.

EFFICACY OF CORTICOSTEROIDS IN VITILIGO

Worldwide, there are only few studies published documenting the efficacy and safety of corticosteroids in vitiligo. The available reports are primarily case series and till now there is a lack of well validated randomized controlled trials.

Oral Mini Pulse Therapy

Pasricha et al. evaluated the effect of five different regimens in causing repigmentation and stopping disease activity for 4 months and noted that regimens using corticosteroids were superior to those excluding corticosteroids. The improvement observed was 87.5%, 85% and 90.9% respectively with the regimens comprising of 3 mg betamethasone orally on alternate days combined with levamisole and topical fluocinolone; 2 mg betamethasone orally alternating with 20 mg 8-methoxypsoralen and sun exposure, and OMP consisting of 5 mg betamethasone orally twice a week combined with 50 mg cyclophosphamide daily orally. Two other regimens having levamisole had different results. Levamisole 150 mg orally two consecutive days a week showed improvement in 53.8%. Addition of topical fluocinolone acetonide to levamisole showed better response in 81.8%.[8] However, a number of patient in various regimens in this study were small.

In a study on 40 patients by Pasricha and Khaitan, 5 mg betamethasone as a single oral dose after breakfast on two consecutive days per week was found effective in halting disease progression in 89% patients within 1–3 months and inducing variable spontaneous repigmentation in patients with extensive and rapidly progressive disease.[9] Only 2 patients did not show response initially, but once the dose was increased from 5 mg to 7.5 mg, there was notable improvement. Side effects were seen in 23% (17) patients, such as weight gain (5), mild headache (2), transient general weakness (2), bad taste in mouth (3), acne (2) and mild puffiness, perioral dermatitis, as well as herpes zoster, glaucoma and amenorrhea, all of which were reported in 1 patient each. Kanwar et al.[23]and Radakovic-Fijan et al.[22] also reported efficacy of dexamethasone OMP therapy in arresting progression of rapidly spreading vitiligo in 43.8% and 88% respectively. The difference in response in the study by Kanwar et al. and the one conducted by Pasricha and Khaitan could be because of the higher proportion of patients with segmental vitiligo and shorter duration of treatment in the study by Kanwar et al. In the study by Radakovic-Fijan et al. from Vienna, OMP therapy was used in higher dose (10 mg dexamethasone on two consecutive days every week) for 24 weeks. The results and side effects were almost similar as observed by Pasricha and Khaitan; however, Radakovic-Fijan et al. further observed the safety that sustained suppression of endogenous cortisol production does not occur with OMP therapy.

OMP therapy has been found to be effective in patients with unstable generalized and acrofacial vitiligo in a randomized double-blind placebo-controlled randomized prospective study.[31] Prednisolone has been used as once a week oral dose of 2 mg/kg in 50 patients with extensive and rapidly spreading vitiligo. The disease progression was arrested in 93% and repigmentation observed in 88% with only 3 patients developing side effects.[32] Methylprednisolone 0.8 mg/kg given as OMP therapy along with topical fluticasone in children for 6 months was safe and effective in arresting disease in 90% and producing variable repigmentation in 65%.[33] OMP therapy in combination with other standard vitiligo treatments has also been studied. Betamethasone has been used as an adjunct to surgery for treatment of stable vitiligo patches in patients who did not respond to their first surgical procedure.[24] It has also been combined with phototherapy and photochemotherapy. Dexamethasone OMP therapy has been found effective and safe with psoralen with solar ultraviolet light (PUVAsol) in fast spreading vitiligo.[31] OMP therapy has been safely used in children and was more effective than 8-methoxypsoralen alone.[34] Combination of narrowband-ultraviolet B (NB-UVB) with OMP therapy has been compared with PUVA photochemotherapy with OMP therapy. Disease progression is arrested in both, but repigmentation was better and earlier with NB-UVB.[35]

Other immunosuppressants can also be added to OMP therapy. A comparative study of three regimens: (1) OMP therapy with daily cyclophosphamide, (2) a 3-day dexamethasone-cyclophosphamide pulse given monthly and (3) daily cyclophosphamide and dexamethasone-cyclophosphamide pulse given only on 1 day in a month showed that disease activity was arrested by all three modalities but repigmentation up to 75% was seen in 71%, 62% and 53% respectively. The higher response with OMP therapy may be because weekly dosing may provide better immunosuppression in the context of vitiligo as compared to monthly dosing in pulse therapy.[36] Weight gain was more frequent with OMP therapy, but otherwise all three regimens had a similar frequency of side effects.[36] In a recent retrospective study by Kanwar et al. from Chandigarh, it has been observed that even low-dose OMP dexamethasone (2.5 mg) therapy is a good option for arresting progressive unstable vitiligo with minimal adverse effects.[37]

In the recent guidelines for the management of vitiligo by the European Dermatology Forum, it was noted that overall, OMP therapy with either betamethasone or dexamethasone can arrest, without inducing repigmentation, the progression of vitiligo. During fast spreading vitiligo, phototherapy is usually commenced after this intervention. However, there are no randomized clinical trials confirming that either speed or magnitude of response to phototherapy and photochemotherapy might be potentiated by concomitant administration of OMP therapy.[38]

Daily Corticosteroids

In everyday practice, corticosteroids are primarily administered daily at doses individualized for each specific patient. Published studies are based on prednisolone given at 0.3 mg/kg as a single oral dose after breakfast initially for the first 2 months. The dosage is then reduced to half the initial dose during at the third month and halved again at the fourth month of treatment. With this regimen, Kim et al. noted that disease progression was halted in 87.7% of patients and in 70.4%, repigmentation was also seen.[26] In a study by Banerjee et al. disease progression was arrested in 90% and repigmentation was seen in 76%.[27] The side effects observed in both studies were not serious, and did not warrant a change in dose or dosing schedule. Disease was also reported to completely subside after discontinuing treatment in addition to other positive observations; this suggests that low dose corticosteroids given for 4 months may be reasonably safe and effective treatment option.

Intravenous Pulse Therapy

Methylprednisolone (8 mg/kg) given intravenously on three consecutive days a month was used in a study as pulse therapy in 14 patients with generalized vitiligo. Eighty-five percent of the patients who presented with progressive disease showed cessation of disease progression and 71% of these patients had repigmentation. None of the 6 patients presenting with static disease showed any repigmentation. The therapy was well tolerated in all but 1 patient who developed intermittent arterial hypertension during therapy.[39]

Lee et al. evaluated the efficacy and safety of combination therapy with intravenous methylprednisolone and PUVA. In 36 patients with vitiligo, intravenous methylprednisolone for 3 days was followed by PUVA twice weekly. After 6 months, vitiligo lesions on the face were reduced in size by 57.5%, on the upper extremities by 34.5%, on the trunk by 30.4% and on the lower extremities by 26.3%. Overall, improvement was seen in 13 patients (36.1%), with more than 50% repigmentation. Side effects were mild and transient.[40]

CONCLUSION

Most studies indicate that systemic corticosteroids are helpful in halting disease progression in rapidly spreading vitiligo and inducing spontaneous repigmentation. However, their role in static vitiligo is not well documented. As of now, corticosteroids can be recommended for rapidly spreading vitiligo for a short duration to halt disease activity, but it should not be used for repigmentation in static vitiligo, even if disease is extensive. Areas that require further research are the risk of osteoporosis with corticosteroids and the efficacy of calcium supplementation. Studies with longer follow-up periods are required to evaluate the potential for relapse. Deflazacort needs to be evaluated as a relatively safer corticosteroid option for vitiligo since its use in vitiligo is very limited as compared to betamethasone/dexamethasone. Head-to-head comparative studies between betamethasone, prednisolone, and deflazacort may be useful for determining the optimal agent for treatment. The issue of relapse after achieving arrest of disease activity in long-term is not yet studied. Currently, for relapsed cases, the approach in clinical practice is to repeat OMP therapy as episodic treatment for 8–12 weeks or even longer to aim control of the disease activity. There seems to be a definite role for systemic corticosteroids in the treatment of certain types of vitiligo:

- Rapidly progressing vitiligo
- Slowly progressing vitiligo with extensive involvement and frequent exacerbation
- Frank inflammatory vitiligo
- Patients with direct or indirect evidence of autoimmune disease (e.g. high titers of thyroid autoantibodies)
- Long-term recalcitrant static vitiligo with sudden exacerbation
- Rescue therapy.

Systemic corticosteroids should not be considered for universal vitiligo, segmental vitiligo or focal limited vitiligo. Although daily or alternate day oral corticosteroids may be treatment options, OMP therapy seems to be the best regimen for long-term use with minimal side effects. The duration of OMP therapy should be at least 6 months or longer and tapering to discontinuation should be slow and stepwise, e.g. a patient receiving 5 mg betamethasone in OMP therapy regimen should be tapered off monthly over next 4 months by reducing the dose by 1 mg each month. When a patient is on any regimen that includes systemic corticosteroids, regular and periodic monitoring must be done to assess the risk-to-benefit ratio of treatment and to evaluate efficacy. Further study is needed to provide more definitive evidence for systemic corticosteroid use in vitiligo as well as the long-term implications of treatment.

ACKNOWLEDGMENTS

A major part of this chapter is taken from the chapter by the same authors, i.e. "Khaitan BK, Kathuria S Systemic corticosteroids in vitiligo. In: Kyung Hwa K, Murase JE (Eds). Vitiligo: Management and Therapy. InTech Open Access Publisher; 2011. pp. 108-16." *Authors sincerely thank the editors and the publisher.*

Authors would also like to pronounce their gratitude and record the contribution of Dr JS Pasricha, whose pioneer work in this field encouraged several dermatologists including authors to work further.

Also, our sincere thanks to Dr Ameet Valia for some useful discussion on this topic.

REFERENCES

1. Krüger C, Schallreuter KU. A review of the worldwide prevalence of vitiligo in children/adolescents and adults. Int J Dermatol. 2012;51:1206-12.
2. Pahwa P, Mehta M, Khaitan BK, et al. The psychosocial impact of vitiligo in Indian patients. Indian J Dermatol Venereol Leprol. 2013;79:679-85.
3. Linthorst Homan MW, Spuls PI, de Korte J, et al. The burden of vitiligo: patient characteristics associated with quality of life. J Am Acad Dermatol. 2009;61:411-20.
4. Pasricha JS, Khaitan BK. Drugs for Vitiligo. New Delhi: New Age International (P) limited; 1996. pp. 37-43.
5. Farah FS, Kurban AK, Chaglassian HT. The treatment of vitiligo with psoralens and triamcinolone by mouth. Br J Dermatol. 1967;79:89-91.
6. Gokhale BB, Gokhale TB. Corticotrophin and vitiligo (preliminary observations). Br J Dermatol. 1976;95:329.
7. Imamura S, Tagami H. Treatment of vitiligo with oral corticosteroids. Dermatologica. 1976;153:179-85.
8. Pasricha JS, Seetharam KA, Dashore A. Evaluation of five different regimes for the treatment of vitiligo. Indian J Dermatol Venereol. 1989;55:18-21.
9. Pasricha JS, Khaitan BK. Oral mini-pulse therapy with betamethasone in vitiligo patients having extensive or fast-spreading disease. Int J Dermatol. 1993;32:753-7.
10. Wolverton SE. Systemic corticosteroids. In: Wolverton SE (Ed). Comprehensive Dermatologic Drug Therapy, 2nd edition. Philadelphia: Saunders Elseviers; 2007. pp. 127-61.
11. Joshi N, Rajeshwari K. Deflazacort. J Postgrad Med. 2009;55: 296-300.
12. Abdel-Naser MB, Krüger-Krasagakes S, Krasagakis K, et al. Further evidence for involvement of both cell mediated and humoral immunity in generalized vitiligo. Pigment Cell Res. 1994;7:1-8.

13. Ahn SK, Choi EH, Lee SH, et al. Immunohistochemical studies from vitiligo: comparison between active and inactive lesions. Yonsei Med J. 1994;35:404-10.
14. Abdel-Naser MB, Ludwig WD, Gollnick H, et al. Nonsegmental vitiligo: decrease of the CD45RA+ T-cell subset and evidence for peripheral T-cell activation. Int J Dermatol. 1992;31:321-6.
15. Ogg GS, Rod Dunbar P, Romero P, et al. High frequency of skin homing melanocyte-specific cytotoxic T lymphocytes in autoimmune vitiligo. J Exp Med. 1998;188:1203-8.
16. Wańkowicz-Kalińska A, van den Wijngaard RM, Tigges BJ, et al. Immunopolarization of CD4+ and CD8+ T cells to Type-1-like is associated with melanocyte loss in human vitiligo. Lab Invest. 2003;83:683-95.
17. van den Boorn JG, Konijnenberg D, Dellemijn TA, et al. Autoimmune destruction of skin melanocytes by perilesional T cells from vitiligo patients. J Invest Dermatol. 2009;129:2220-32.
18. Klarquist J, Denman CJ, Hernandez C, et al. Reduced skin homing by functional Treg in vitiligo. Pigment Cell Melanoma Res. 2010;23:276-86.
19. Hann SK, Kim HI, Im S, et al. The change of melanocyte cytotoxicity after systemic steroid treatment in vitiligo patients. J Dermatol Sci. 1993;6:201-5.
20. Lee DY, Choi SC, Lee JH. Generalized vitiligo treated by combination therapy of epidermal graft and systemic corticosteroid. Clin Exp Dermatol. 2009;34:838.
21. Lee DY, Lee KJ, Choi SC, et al. Segmental vitiligo treated by the combination of epidermal grafting and systemic corticosteroids. Dermatol Surg. 2010;36:575-6.
22. Radakovic-Fijan S, Fürnsinn-Friedl AM, Hönigsmann H, et al. Oral dexamethasone pulse treatment for vitiligo. J Am Acad Dermatol. 2001;44:814-7.
23. Kanwar AJ, Dhar S, Dawn G. Oral mini pulse therapy in vitiligo. Dermatology. 1995;190:251-2.
24. Mulekar SV. Stable vitiligo treated by a combination of low-dose oral pulse betamethasone and autologous, non-cultured melanocyte-keratinocyte cell transplantation. Dermatol Surg. 2006;32:536-41.
25. Seiter S, Ugurel S, Pföhler C, et al. Successful treatment of progressive vitiligo with high-dose intravenous methylprednisolone 'pulse' therapy. Dermatology. 1999;199: 261-2.
26. Kim SM, Lee HS, Hann SK. The efficacy of low-dose oral corticosteroids in the treatment of vitiligo patients. Int J Dermatol. 1999;38:546-50.
27. Banerjee K, Barbhuiya JN, Ghosh AP, et al. The efficacy of low-dose oral corticosteroids in the treatment of vitiligo patient. Indian J Dermatol Venereol Leprol. 2003;69:135-7.
28. Daly JR, Myles AB, Bacon PA, et al. Pituitary adrenal function during corticosteroid withdrawal in rheumatoid arthritis. Ann Rheum Dis. 1967;26:18-25.
29. Kumrah L, Ramam M, Shah P, et al. Pituitary-adrenal function following dexamethasone-cyclophosphamide pulse therapy for pemphigus. Br J Dermatol. 2001;145:944-8.
30. Njoo MD, Spuls PI, Bos JD, et al. Non-surgical repigmentation therapies in vitiligo. Meta-analysis of the literature. Arch Dermatol. 1998;134:1532-40.
31. Paul M, et al. OMP steroid therapy in the treatment of unstable vitiligo: a double blind placebo controlled randomized prospective study. Presented at 26th Annual Conference of IADVL, 1998.
32. Gupta RR. Modified oral mini pulse steroid therapy in unstable vitiligo: A novel once a week regimen. Presented at 29th Annual Conference of IADVL, 2001.
33. Majid I, Masood Q, Hassan I, et al. Childhood vitiligo: response to methylprednisolone OMP therapy and topical fluticasone combination. Indian J Dermatol. 2009;54:124-7.
34. Nigam PK. Clinical and oral mini pulse therapy evaluation in childhood vitiligo. Presented at 32th Annual Conference of IADVL, 2004.
35. Rath N, Kar HK, Sabhnani S. An open labeled, comparative clinical study on efficacy and tolerability of oral mini pulse of steroid (OMP) alone, OMP with PUVA and broad/narrow band UVB phototherapy in progressive vitiligo. Indian J Dermatol Venereol Leprol. 2008;74:357-60.
36. Singh YL, Khaitan BK, Ramam M, et al. A comparative study of the effect of three regimens comprising of corticosteroids and cyclophosphamide for the treatment of vitiligo. Thesis submitted to AIIMS, 1999 (unpublished).
37. Kanwar AJ, Mahajan R, Parsad D. Low-dose oral mini-pulse dexamethasone therapy in progressive unstable vitiligo. J Cutan Med Surg. 2013;17:259-68.
38. Taieb A, Alomara, Bohm M, et al. Guidelines for the management of vitiligo; the European Dermatology Forum consensus. Br J Dermatol. 2013;168:5-19.
39. Seiter S, Ugurel S, Tilgen W, et al. Use of high-dose methylprednisolone pulse therapy in patients with progressive and stable vitiligo. Int J Dermatol. 2000;39:624-7.
40. Lee Y, Seo YJ, Lee JH, et al. High-dose prednisolone and psoralen ultraviolet: a combination therapy in 36 patients with vitiligo. Clin Exp Dermatol. 2007;32:499-501.

25

Topical Treatment of Vitiligo: New Insights, New Trends

Ahmad Reza Hossani-Madani, Rebat M Halder

Key Features

- Vitiligo is a worldwide depigmenting skin disorder for which topical therapies have been a mainstay of treatment. Traditional topical therapy includes topical corticosteroids. However, with the advent of calcineurin inhibitors, vitamin D analogs and pseudocatalase, the practitioner's armamentarium has expanded and has allowed for the counteracting of suspected pathogenetic defects in vitiliginous skin.
- Certain combination therapies that include topical agents have been shown to be more effective than monotherapy in the repigmentation of vitiliginous skin.
- If repigmentation is ineffective or involvement is disfiguring or widespread, depigmentation remains a viable option.
- More randomized trials examining similar clinical endpoints are necessary to further investigate newer topical monotherapy and combination approaches.

INTRODUCTION

Vitiligo is a depigmenting skin disorder with a worldwide prevalence of 0.5–1% and incidence from 0.1 to 8.8% or greater of the population.[1] There is no racial, gender or age predilection, although two-thirds of patients with vitiligo are diagnosed before the age of 30.[1] Many theories have been proposed about the pathogenesis of vitiligo, but no single theory adequately explains all of the clinical manifestations.

There are many topical treatments that have been used for vitiligo. In this chapter, randomized trials involving established topical treatments for repigmentation of vitiligo will be reviewed. We review topical monotherapy and combination therapies involving topical modalities. Lesser used or ineffective modalities have not been included nor have topicals in the early stages of use. Topical monotherapies will begin and then proceed to a discussion of combination topical treatment approaches in vitiligo.

TOPICAL TREATMENT OF VITILIGO

Topical Monotherapy

Corticosteroids

Betamethasone valerate 0.1% in 50% isopropyl alcohol: Kandil[2] conducted one of the earliest randomized, controlled studies evaluating the use of betamethasone valerate 0.1% in 50% isopropyl alcohol against placebo for the treatment of vitiligo. Nineteen patients were enrolled for twice daily treatment, in a left-right manner, over a 4-month-period. Seventeen patients completed the trial, with 35.3% achieving greater than 90% repigmentation and 17.6% reaching 25–90% repigmentation. No patients developed repigmentation on the placebo-treated side of the body. Adverse events included hypertrichosis in 12% of patients and an acneiform eruption in 18% of patients.

Betamethasone dipropionate 0.05% cream: Two studies, Kumaran[3] and Sanclemente[4], investigated the use of topical betamethasone 0.05% cream against either calcipotriol 0.005% ointment or topical catalase/superoxide dismutase cream, respectively.

Kumaran[3] randomized 49 patients, 10–60 years old, to one of three groups: (1) betamethasone 0.05% cream twice daily, (2) calcipotriol 0.005% ointment twice daily or (3) combination of betamethasone 0.05% cream in morning and calcipotriol 0.005% ointment in the evening. Patients included those with localized and non-segmental, non-mucosal, non-acral and stable vitiligo. Forty-five patients completed the 3 months trial, with results revealing greater than 75% repigmentation occurring in none of the three groups. Adverse events included: (1) betamethasone group: lesional soreness, atrophy, dryness and hypertrichosis occurring in 47%, (2) calcipotriol group: irritant reaction and lesional soreness in 13% and (3) betamethasone/calcipotriol combination group: hypertrichosis and dryness of the skin in 13%.

The second study compared the use of topical betamethasone 0.05% cream twice daily against topical catalase/superoxide dismutase cream twice daily. This randomized, double-blind, match-paired, non-placebo-controlled, left-right trial enrolled 25 patients aged 12–74 years old. Treatment continued for 10 months with mean repigmentation being evaluated with digital morphometry and colorimetry. Patients were advised to expose treated areas for 15 minutes between 10:30 a.m. and 2:00 p.m. They found that mean repigmentation in the betamethasone group was 18.5% ± 93.14% and 12.4% ± 59% in the catalase/superoxide dismutase group, which was not statistically significant. One patient in the catalase/superoxide dismutase group experienced a mild, erythematous papular rash that self-resolved.

Betamethasone 0.05% cream did not perform better than calcipotriol 0.005% ointment or catalase/superoxide dismutase cream in eliciting clinically significant repigmentation for vitiligo. The study of Sanclemente[4] also had topical therapy confounded by the recommendation to add patient-directed sunlight exposure for 15 minutes daily. In the study of Kumaran, there were a greater number of adverse events (almost three-fold) in association with topical betamethasone monotherapy as compared with topical calcipotriol or combination therapy.

Fluticasone propionate 0.05% cream: Westerhof[5] and Kathuria[6] both investigated the use of topical fluticasone 0.05% cream with comparison to either ultraviolet A (UVA) or tacrolimus 0.1% ointment, respectively.

Westerhof[5] divided 135 patients randomly into three left-right groups: (1) fluticasone 0.05% cream at bedtime, (2) UVA 10 J/cm^2 twice weekly or (3) fluticasone 0.05% cream at bedtime plus UVA 10 J/cm^2 twice weekly (with the combination group consisting of two subgroups: fluticasone on both sides and UVA on only one side, and UVA on both sides with fluticasone applied to only one side). Bilaterally symmetrical, stable or active lesions on the arms, legs or trunk in patients aged between 18 and 80 years of age were treated. After 9 months of treatment, 96 patients completed the trial, with results revealing greater than 75% repigmentation in 3% and 4.4% of lesions in the fluticasone and UVA monotherapy groups, respectively, and 14.9% and 11.8% of lesions in the fluticasone plus UVA and UVA plus fluticasone groups, respectively. The results were statistically significant and revealed an approximately three-fold difference between the monotherapy and combination therapy groups, but with comparable rates in the fluticasone and UVA monotherapy groups. There were no clinically evident adverse events in any of the groups. However, skin biopsy samples from two symmetrical lesions in the UVA and UVA plus fluticasone groups, at the end of 9 months, revealed mild atrophy, while no atrophy was noted in the fluticasone or fluticasone plus UVA groups.

A more recent study by Kathuria[6] compared the use of fluticasone 0.05% cream daily with tacrolimus 0.1% ointment twice daily in 60 patients with segmental vitiligo (SV), aged between 5 and 55 years of age. Patients were evaluated clinically monthly and photographically every 2 months during the 6 month treatment period. Forty patients completed the trial with greater than 75% repigmentation being achieved in 9.5% of patients in the fluticasone group and 0% of patients in the tacrolimus group. P values were not calculated secondary to low patient numbers in the groups. Side effects included burning (3.8%), mild pruritus (7.6%), dryness (3.8%), mild erythema (7.6%), atrophy (7.6%), telangiectasia (7.6%) and acneiform lesions (12%) in the fluticasone group; and burning (12%), mild pruritus (15%), mild erythema (27%), atrophy (3.8%) and pyoderma localized to the lesion (3.8%) in the tacrolimus group.

Both studies found greater than 75% repigmentation in 3–9.5% of lesions/patients, with neither study finding either UVA or tacrolimus to be more effective than fluticasone. UVA performed comparably to fluticasone for generalized vitiligo, while tacrolimus performed worse than fluticasone for SV.

Clobetasol propionate 0.05% cream/ointment: Four studies investigated the use of clobetasol 0.05% cream or ointment versus placebo (1 study), tacrolimus 0.1% ointment (two studies) and topical psoralen plus ultraviolet A sunlight (PUVAsol) (1 study). Three of the four studies involved only patients less than 18 years of age. We will turn our attention to them in that order.

One of the earliest randomized studies involving the use of topical clobetasol is that of Clayton.[7] His study compared twice daily application of clobetasol 0.05% cream against twice daily application of the cream base in a left-right trial of 25 patients of undisclosed ages. After 4 months, two patients did not complete the trial and two other patients admitted to using clobetasol bilaterally. Greater than 75% repigmentation was achieved in 8.7% of patients on the clobetasol treated side and 8.7% of patients on the cream base side. Adverse events included dermal atrophy in all patients on the clobetasol treated side.

The second study is that of Ho,[8] in which he randomized 100 children (2–16 years old) with both facial and non-facial vitiligo to three groups: (1) clobetasol 0.05% ointment twice daily for 2 months, petroleum jelly twice daily for 2 months and a final 2 months of clobetasol 0.05% ointment twice daily, (2) tacrolimus 0.1% ointment twice daily for 6 months or (3) petroleum jelly twice daily for 6 months. Vitiligo types examined were predominantly non-segmental types (84%), but segmental vitiligo was also included (16%). Ninety patients completed the trial with 4 withdrawing for personal/

family reasons, 1 due to spontaneous repigmentation prior to commencement of the study, 3 for loss to follow-up and 4 due to concern over the "black box" warning in the US for tacrolimus. They defined a successful response as greater than 50% repigmentation and subdivided groups into facial and non-facial groups. In the facial groups, greater than 50% partial repigmentation was achieved by 58% of those in the clobetasol group and 58% of those in the tacrolimus group. In the non-facial group, greater than 50% partial repigmentation was achieved by 39% of those in the clobetasol group and 29% of those in the tacrolimus group. Complete repigmentation occurred in 22% of those in the clobetasol group and 11% in the tacrolimus group in facial locations. Complete repigmentation in non-facial areas occurred in 13% of those in the clobetasol group and 10% in the tacrolimus group. In the placebo group, greater than 50% partial repigmentation occurred in 16.7% of patients in the facial group and 0% in non-facial areas. Complete clearance did not occur in the placebo group in facial or non-facial areas. Results between the clobetasol and tacrolimus were not significant in either facial or non-facial areas. Both groups individually performed significantly better than placebo. Adverse events included irritation seen most commonly in the placebo group and folliculitis, occurring in 1 patient in the clobetasol group and 1 in the tacrolimus group. No significant difference was seen between adverse events in between the groups.

Lepe[9] conducted a randomized, non-placebo controlled, left-right trial comparing clobetasol 0.05% cream to tacrolimus 0.1% ointment, both used twice daily. Twenty patients with localized vitiligo (excluding segmental or mucosal types), less than 18 years of age, were enrolled. After 2 months, they found that 20% of lesions in both the clobetasol and tacrolimus groups demonstrated greater than 75% repigmentaton, which was not statistically significant. Adverse events included atrophy (15%) and telangiectasia (10%) in the clobetasol group, and burning (10%) in the tacrolimus group. They concluded that tacrolimus ointment proved almost as effective as clobetasol ointment in the repigmentation of children with vitiliginous skin, without the adverse side effect of atrophy.

The last study is that of Khalid,[10] comparing clobetasol 0.05% cream twice daily to topical psoralen and exposure with sun light (PUVAsol) (8-methoxypsoralen 0.1% in white petrolatum applied 45 minutes prior to sunlight exposure of 1–10 minutes duration thrice weekly). Fifty children, aged less than 12 years, with localized, non-segmental or mucosal vitiligo, were enrolled for 6 months. They found that 40.9% patients in the clobetasol group and 8.7% patients in the topical PUVAsol group achieved greater than 75% repigmentation. Whitton[11] recalculated their data and found significantly better repigmentation in the clobetasol group, as compared with those exposed to topical PUVAsol (Risk Ratio: 4.70; 95% CI: 1.14–19.39). Adverse events included mild atrophy (18%), telangiectasia (9%), acneiform eruption (9%) and hypertrichosis (4.5%) in the clobetasol group and blistering reactions requiring discontinuation of therapy for 1 month in 8.7% of patients in the PUVAsol group.

Clobetasol did not seem to be more effective than the cream base in achieving greater than 75% repigmentation in the study of Clayton, but did perform significantly better than placebo in Ho's study. Clobetasol and tacrolimus seemed to have similar efficacy in children, however, with less risk of side effects associated with tacrolimus. Lastly, clobetasol was significantly more effective than PUVAsol in the treatment of childhood vitiligo.

Meta-analysis: Njoo[12] conducted a meta-analysis, in which data was pooled from randomized controlled trials for the treatment of localized and generalized vitiligo. He examined the use of topical class 3 and 4 steroids in the treatment of localized vitiligo, finding that class 3, (56%; 95% CI, 50–62%) followed by class 4, corticosteroids (55%; 95% CI, 49–61%) had the highest percentage of patients achieving greater than 75% repigmentation [compared with intralesional steroids, khellin plus ultaviolet A (KUVA) and PUVA]. Pooled side effects included atrophy, occurring more commonly with class 4 steroids (14%; 95% CI, 10–18%) than class 3 steroids (2%; 95% CI, 1–5%), and less commonly telangiectasia, acne and hypertrichosis.

Calcineurin Inhibitors

Tacrolimus 0.1% ointment: Three randomized trials were conducted comparing either tacrolimus to placebo, differing dosing frequencies of topical tacrolimus or with tacrolimus to topical clobetasol 0.05% cream. We have already reviewed the study comparing tacrolimus to clobetasol[9] in the corticosteroid section above. Therefore, we will now turn our attention to the studies comparing tacrolimus to placebo and differing frequencies of tacrolimus.

Twenty patients were enrolled by Lubaki,[13] in a randomized, controlled, left-right trial, to receive treatment with either tacrolimus 0.1% ointment or placebo petrolatum twice daily. Patients were aged 14–68 years old and received treatment for 7 months, with evaluation of repigmentation every 4 weeks. They found that no patients in either group achieved greater than 75% repigmentation. However, 35% of treated lesions achieved greater than 25% repigmentation in the tacrolimus group versus 20% in the placebo group. In the tacrolimus group, 20% of patients experienced transient pruritus.

Radakovic[14] investigated the use of once versus twice daily dosing of tacrolimus 0.1% ointment. They enrolled 17 patients aged 10–61 with generalized vitiligo for 6 months of treatment. Fifteen patients with 40 target lesions completed the study. Greater than 75% repigmentation was found in 0% of patients in the once daily group and 13% of patients in the twice daily group. There was no mention of adverse events.

Pimecrolimus 1% cream: Dawid[15] and Farajzadeh[16] both conducted randomized studies using topical pimecrolimus cream versus placebo or the use of topical pimecrolimus preceded by microdermabrasion.

Dawid examined the efficacy of 1% pimecrolimus cream versus placebo cream. They randomized 20 patients in a left-right, double-blinded manner to receive treatment twice daily for 6 months. Four patients did not complete the study due to: personal reasons (1 patient), presumed lack of efficacy (2 patients) and loss to follow-up (1 patient). Pimecrolimus cream resulted in no significant change in mean target lesion size and no patient achieved repigmentation greater than 25%. No adverse effects were noted.

Farajzadeh randomized 65 patients, aged 2–18 years old, with 3 stable vitiligo lesions to treatment with either: 1% pimecrolimus cream (Lesion A), microdermabrasion on day one followed by 1% pimecrolimus cream (Lesion B), or placebo cream (Lesion C). Patients in the microdermabrasion group received additional silver 1% sulfadiazine cream and all lesions were covered by a dressing. Recommendation was made to apply sunscreen to the treated areas of spf 30 or higher. Pimecrolimus cream or placebo was applied under occlusion daily for 10 days. A blinded investigator evaluated the lesions at 3 months. Sixty patients completed the 3 months study period, with 5 patients lost to unspecified reasons unrelated to treatment. Greater than 75% repigmentation was achieved in 21.7% lesions treated with 1% pimecrolimus cream, 43.4% lesions treated with microdermabrasion and pimecrolimus, and 1.7% of lesions in the placebo group. There were statistically significant differences between the three arms of the study after three months. Response rates were found to be significantly inversely related to disease duration, with those having a longer duration of disease demonstrating a lower response rate. Adverse effects included a mild burning sensation with microdermabrasion in 30% of patients. The authors conclude that microdermabrasion may have an additive effect in the treatment of vitiligo lesions.

Dawid[15] found no significant repigmentation versus placebo in their study, while Farajzadeh[16] found a significant difference between pimecrolimus and placebo groups. Additionally, the combination of microdermabrasion improved repigmentation rates in conjunction with pimecrolimus.

Vitamin D Analogs

Calcipotriol 0.005% ointment: Investigation of the use of calcipotriol 0.005% ointment versus topical betamethasone 0.05% cream monotherapy or a combination of calcipotriol/betamethasone was carried out by Kumaran.[3] This study has been reviewed in the betamethasone dipropionae 0.05% cream section above and will not be repeated here. The conclusion of that study was that there was no clinically significant repigmentation in any of the treatment arms.

Pseudocatalase

There are no known randomized articles examining the use of pseudocatalase [otherwise known as manganese-ethylenediaminetetraacetic acid (Mn-EDTA)] monotherapy against other modalities, despite its clinical use to potentially halt the progression of vitiligo.

Depigmentation Therapy

Despite a lack of randomized controlled studies investigating the use of depigmentation therapy for vitiligo, we felt it important to make mention of this modality due to its utility and widespread use in vitiligo. Topicals used in this regard include twice daily use monobenzyl ether of hydroquinone or 4-methoxyphenol (also known as ρ-hydroxyanisole, monomethyl ether of hydroquinone or mequinol). Indications for their use include extensive involvement with unlikely repigmentation, greater than 50% body surface area involvement with therapeutic resistance or disfiguring facial involvement.[17] Side effects of monobenzyl ether of hydroquinone include dermatitis, pruritus, xerosis, conjunctival melanosis, corneal pigmentation and satellite depigmentation,[17] while side effects of 4-methoxyphenol include mild burning or itching.[18] Patients must be thoroughly advised as to the risks of incomplete depigmentation, inability to tan and the psychosocial ramifications of depigmentation therapy.

Topical Combination Therapy

Corticosteroid Combinations

There are six randomized controlled trials investigating the use of corticosteroid combination therapy in vitiligo. These studies include the use of fluocinolone acetonide 0.1% cream, fluticasone propionate 0.05% cream, hydrocortisone 17-butyrate cream, betamethasone cream and clobetasol propionate 0.05% cream in addition to another modality.

Fluocinolone acetonide 0.1% cream combination: One study investigated the use of punch grafting followed by fluocinolone acetonide 0.1% cream daily versus punch grafting followed by the use of PUVA twice weekly.[19] Fifty patients, aged 13–60 years, were enrolled (with stable, segmental vitiligo, vitiligo vulgaris and acrofacial vitiligo with a residual limited number of lesions) to receive treatment 4 weeks after punch grafting. Measuring mean pigment spread, they found that after 6 months, those in the punch grafting and fluocinolone group had an average of 6.94 mm, while those in the punch grafting plus PUVA group had 6.38 mm on average, which was not statistically significant. Side effects in the punch graft plus fluocinolone group included 20% of patients with a polka-dot appearance, 16% with cobblestoning and atrophy of the grafted area, 12% with graft depigmentation, and 4% with infection, perilesional hypopigmentation, and erythema. In the punch grafting plus PUVA group the side effects included: 41% of patients with nausea and vomiting, 35% with cobblestoning, 24% with erythema and depigmentation of the graft, 5.8% with a pyogenic infection, and 5.8% with perilesional hypopigmentation, itching, scaling, and thickening of the skin.

Fluticasone propionate 0.05% cream combination: Westerhof[5] investigated the use of the following treatment groups (1) fluticasone 0.05% cream at bedtime, (2) UVA 10 J/cm^2 twice weekly or (3) fluticasone 0.05% cream at bedtime plus UVA 10 J/cm^2 twice weekly. This study has been reviewed in the fluticasone section above and will not be repeated here. To summarize their conclusions, they found the combination group to produce a statistically significant three-fold greater difference as compared with either monotherapy group, but with comparable rates in the fluticasone and UVA monotherapy groups.

Hydrocortisone 17-butyrate cream combinations: Combinations involving hydrocortisone 17-butyrate cream were examined in two studies: Sassi[20] and Bayoumi.[21] One compared addition of hydrocortisone 17-butyrate cream to 308 nm excimer and the other added narrowband ultraviolet B (NB-UVB) ± dermabrasion.

Eighty-four patients, aged 18–75 years, were randomized to one of two groups by Sassi.[20] Patients received either 308 nm excimer laser monotherapy twice weekly or 308 nm excimer laser twice weekly plus hydrocortisone 17-butyrate 0.1g/100 g cream twice daily for 12 weeks. The steroid was given for 3 periods of 3 weeks, followed by a subsequent 1 week steroid-free interval. In the monotherapy group, 14% of patients were lost to: consent withdrawal (7.1%) patients), side effects (4.8%), and non-compliance (2.4%). In the combination group, 4.8% of patients were lost to withdrawal of consent. Of those that remained, from an intention-to-treat or perprotocol standpoint, 16.6% patients in the monotherapy group and 42.8% patients in the combination group achieved greater than 75% repigmentation, which was statistically significant. Adverse events included: moderate to severe erythemal reaction requiring temporary withdrawal of treatment (78% of patients in monotherapy and 55% of patients in combination therapy groups) and hyperpigmentation (2.8% of patients in the monotherapy and 13% of patients in the combination therapy group).

Bayoumi[21] conducted a randomized, left-right trial on patients aged 18–85 years of age with non-segmental vitiligo on resistant locations (bony prominences and/or extremities). One side of the body was randomized to receive dermabrasion using a 2940 nm erbium laser with application of hyaluronic acid cream for the first 2 days of treatment. Both sides of the body subsequently received treatment with hydrocortisone 17-butyrate cream daily for 3 months (3 cycles of 3 weeks with steroid and 1 week steroid-free) and 12 weeks of concurrent NB-UVB twice weekly. One month after ending treatment, results revealed greater than 75% repigmentation in 16.7% of patients in the dermabrasion plus steroid plus UVB group and 0% in the steroid plus UVB group, which was significant. Side effects only occurred only on the dermabrasion side, with patients experiencing delayed healing, edema lasting 2–15 days when extremities were treated and hypertrophic scars (2 patients).

Betamethasone cream combination: Akdeniz[22] compared the following three treatment groups in their study: (1) betamethasone cream, calcipotriol ointment and NB-UVB, (2) calcipotriol and NB-UVB, and (3) NB-UVB monotherapy. Forty-five patients, aged 13–55 years old, were randomized to receive treatment. They found that the percentage of pigment recovery in the above groups was 63.33 ± 7.55%, 60.67 ± 5.75% and 46.67 ± 7.98%, respectively. The only statistically significant difference was found between group 1 and group 3 ($p = 0.0048$), above.

Clobetasol propionate 0.05% cream combination: Yaghoobi[23] investigated the combination of topical clobetasol propionate 0.05% cream in isopropyl alcohol preparation (for the body) and triamcinolone acetonide 0.1% cream (face and flexures) twice daily versus topical steroid, as just mentioned, plus oral zinc sulfate daily (400 mg for adults and 10 mg/kg in capsule or syrup formulation for children). Thirty-five patients, 11–57 years old, with non-segmental vitiligo, were randomized for treatment over a 4-month-period. Blood zinc levels were drawn at 1 and 3 months after treatment commencement. They found that mean response was 21.43% ± 11.6% in the steroid group and 24.7% ± 11.0% in the steroid plus oral zinc group, which was not significant. Serum zinc levels between the groups were also not statistically significant. Lastly, 13.3% of patients in the combination steroid and oral zinc group experienced tolerable gastric burning.

Calcineurin Inhibitor Combinations

Tacrolimus plus narrowband ultraviolet B: Mehrabi[24] randomly assigned 9 patients with bilaterally symmetric vitiligo to treatment with either placebo or tacrolimus 0.1% ointment twice daily, followed by NB-UVB three times weekly for 12 weeks. Patients were examined every 4 weeks during the treatment period. They found that both sides had improved repigmentation overall. However, there was no statistically significant difference between the two groups (NB-UVB plus placebo: 41.28% improvement versus, NB-UVB plus tacrolimus: 49.24% improvement). The authors stated that common adverse effects reported by the 9 patients included redness (78%) and itching (89%). Less frequent complaints included nonspecific blistering (44%) and a burning sensation (44%). Slight vesicle formation was noted on examination of 2 patients, resulting in withholding of 1 light treatment each and in the reduction of the next treatment dose by 10%.

The second study to investigate the use of tacrolimus plus NB-UVB was that of Nordal.[25] They randomized 40 patients with bilaterally symmetrical vitiligo to treatment with tacrolimus 0.1% ointment on one side of the body and placebo ointment nightly on the other side of the body plus whole body NB-UVB twice or thrice weekly. Phototherapy was continued for 3 months. Forty patients, aged 23–69 with Fitzpatrick phototypes II-VI, completed the study. Patients had an average of 46 (range: 17–68) NB-UVB treatments and 148 (range: 33–221) topical treatments. The average duration of treatment was 177 days (range: 89–252) and the average follow-up time was 138 days (range: 42–297). They found that the median reduction in the target lesion areas was 42.1% on the tacrolimus side and 29% on the placebo side, which was statistically significant. There was a correlation between percent reduction in target lesion size and the number of tacrolimus applications, but not the number of NB-UVB treatments. Side effects included perioral dermatitis in vitiliginous skin, more pronounced on the tacrolimus side, in 1 patient and several patients found the ointment to be too greasy.

Tacrolimus plus excimer laser or monochromatic excimer light: Three studies were identified that examined the use of topical tacrolimus and excimer laser or monochromatic excimer light, those of Kawalek,[26] Passeron[27] and Nistico.[28]

Kawalek[26] conducted the first study, a randomized, left-right trial of 8 patients (with 24 symmetric vitiligo patches on elbows and knees), aged 31–51 years old. Treatment included 0.1% tacrolimus ointment on one side of the body and placebo on the other side, twice daily. 308 nm xenon chloride lasers were done on the whole body up to three times weekly for 24 treatments or 10 weeks (whichever came first). Photographs were taken at baseline and bi-weekly thereafter. Non-treated patches served as controls. Two patients were excluded from the (due to treatment non-adherence), leaving twenty lesions from 6 patients for final analysis. Greater than 75% repigmentation was achieved in 50% of lesions in the excimer/tacrolimus side, as opposed to 20% of lesions in the excimer/placebo side, which was statistically significant. Patches on the excimer/tacrolimus side achieved repigmentation faster than the excimer/placebo side, an average of 13 treatments as opposed to 16 treatments, respectively. Adverse effects included: lesional/perilesional hyperpigmentation (50% in the excimer/tacrolimus group), mild to moderate erythema (all patches), and tingling sensation and burning (80% excimer/tacrolimus group versus 30% excimer/placebo group).

Passeron[27] randomized 14 patients, aged 12–63 years, to treatment with twice weekly 308 nm excimer laser (or a total of 24 sessions) to the whole body and topical 0.1% tacrolimus ointment twice daily on one side of the body. Each side also had an untreated control lesion. All patients completed the study. They found that a repigmentation rate of 75% or more was obtained in 70% of the excimer/tacrolimus lesions and in 20% of excimer monotherapy lesions, which was statistically significant ($P < 0.001$). UV-resistant areas showed statistically greater repigmentation with combination treatment than laser monotherapy ($P < 0.002$), as opposed to UV-sensitive areas ($P = 0.61$). The average onset of repigmentation was observed at session number 10 versus 12 in the excimer/tacrolimus group and excimer monotherapy groups, respectively. Adverse events included: moderate to severe erythema (seen in all patients), localized bullous eruptions (2 lesions in combination and 2 in excimer monotherapy), and stinging (5 patients in combination group versus 0 in excimer monotherapy group).

In the third study, Nistico[28] divided 52 patients into three groups for 12 weeks of treatment: (1) monochromatic excimer light twice weekly plus oral vitamin E, (2) monochromatic excimer laser twice weekly plus tacrolimus 0.1% ointment once daily and oral vitamin E, and (3) vitamin E monotherapy. Results revealed excellent repigmentation in 25% of patients in group 1, 30% of patients in group 2 and 0% of patients in group 3. They felt that the treatments in all groups were safe, effective and well-tolerated.

Pimecrolimus plus narrowband ultraviolet B: Esfandiarpour[29] recruited 68 patients, aged 15–72 years, and randomized them to NB-UVB thrice weekly plus either pimecrolimus 1% cream or placebo (petrolatum cream) twice daily for 3 months. A blinded investigator examined lesions at baseline, 6 and 12 weeks. Fifty patients completed the study (25 in each group), with 18 patients lost to non-compliance and slow treatment response. After 12 weeks, they found that facial lesions responded significantly better to the pimecrolimus/NB-UVB, as compared with the placebo/NB-UVB (64.3 versus 25.1%; $p < 0.05$). After 12 weeks, 8% of patients in the pimecrolimus/NB-UVB group and 4% in the placebo/NB-UVB combination group achieved greater than 75% repigmentation. Side effects included erythema and pruritus that did not require cessation of treatment.

Pimecrolimus plus excimer laser: One study was identified that examined the use of the combination of pimecrolimus and the excimer laser in children (aged 6–14 years old), that of Hui-Lan.[30] Forty-nine patients, with bilaterally symmetrical lesions, were left-right randomized to receive treatment with the 308 nm excimer laser twice weekly plus 1% pimecrolimus cream twice daily on one side and 308 nm excimer laser monotherapy twice weekly on the other side. After 30 treatments, they found that 43.75% lesions in the combination group and 27.1% of lesions in the monotherapy group showed greater than 75% repigmentation, which was statistically significant. The average number of treatments to achieve greater than 75% repigmentation was 27.1 in the combination group and 25.4 in the monotherapy group. Lesions on the face showed a statistical superior repigmentation in the combination group, while lesions on the trunk and fingers were not statistically different between groups. Adverse effects in the combination group included: slight burning after first excimer treatment in 16.7%, blisters in 36.25%, and itching in 14.6%. Adverse events in the excimer monotherapy group included burning in 12.5% and blistering in 6.25%.

Vitamin D Analog Combinations

Calcipotriol cream:

Calcipotriol plus narrowband ultraviolet B: Arca[31] investigated the use of topical calcipotriol 0.05% ointment twice daily plus NB-UVB thrice weekly versus NB-UVB monotherapy thrice weekly. Forty patients with stable, non-segmental vitiligo were enrolled, with 37 patients completing the study and being included in the final analysis. After 30 treatment sessions, they found that both groups had statistically significant reductions in body surface area affected by vitiligo (NB-UVB: 27.21 ± 10.41% to 16.25 ± 8.54%, $p < 0.001$; NB-UVB plus calcipotriol: 23.35 ± 6.5% to 13.23 ± 7.05%, $p < 0.001$). However, comparison of the reduction in repigmentation rates between the two groups showed no statistically significant difference ($P > 0.05$), with 50–100% repigmentation being achieved for 46% of patients in the NB-UVB plus calcipotriol group and 41.67% of patients in the NB-UVB group. Adverse events in those who completed the study included mild, transient itching or erythema.

The combination of calcipotriol, betamethasone and NB-UVB, conducted by Akdeniz,[22] was described in the steroid combination therapy section above and will not be repeated here.

Calcipotriol plus psoralen ultraviolet A or psoralen with exposure of sun light: The combination of calcipotriol and PUVA/PUVAsol was investigated in two studies: Ermis[32] and Parsad.[33]

Ermis[32] wanted to examine the effectiveness of concurrent calcipotriol with oral PUVA. They enrolled 35 patients, greater than 16 years old, with bilaterally symmetrical vitiligo to twice weekly treatment with 0.5–0.6 mg/kg of oral 8-methoxypsoralen followed in hour by UVA. Additional placebo or calcipotriol 0.05 mg/g cream was applied to either side of the body, 1 hour before UVA. Treatment continued until cosmetically acceptable repigmentation occurred or there was arrest of repigmentation. They found that PUVA plus calcipotriol led to earlier initial repigmentation than PUVA plus placebo (9.33 ± 0.65 vs 12.00 ± 0.81 treatments) in a larger number of patients (81% vs 7%), with most cases between 4 and 8 weeks of treatment. Complete repigmentation also occurred earlier in the PUVA/calcipotriol side than the PUVA/placebo side (27.4 ± 1.47 vs 30.07 ± 1.34 treatments), with a larger number in the PUVA/calcipotriol group, (63% vs 15%). Cumulative UVA dosage was lower on the PUVA/calcipotriol side as compared with the PUVA/placebo group when comparing initial repigmentation (52.52 ± 6.10 vs 78.20 ± 7.88 J/cm^2) and complete repigmentation (232.79 ± 14.79 vs 259.93 ± 13.71 J/cm^2). All results were statistically significant. Side effects include 2 patients on the calcipotriol side and 3 patients on the placebo side with xerosis, erythema, and itching.

Parsad[33] also investigated the use of topical calcipotriol 50 µg/g cream on one side of the body and placebo on the other, twice daily in addition to thrice weekly oral 8-methoxypsoralen (0.6 mg/kg) 2 hours prior to sunlight exposure. Nineteen patients, aged 14–39 years of age, were randomized to treatment for 18 months. At the end of 18 months of treatment, 76.5% patients in the PUVA plus calcipotriol group and 52.9% patients in the PUVA plus placebo group achieved greater than 75% repigmentation, which was not statistically significant. Side effects included mild irritation on application of calcipotriol in 17.6% patients.

Calcipotriol plus excimer laser: Goldinger[34] randomly assigned 10 vitiligo patients, aged 24–60 years old, to a single-blinded, left-right trial. Treatment groups included those receiving 308 nm xenon chloride excimer laser monotherapy thrice weekly on one side of the body and 308 nm xenon chloride excimer laser thrice weekly plus topical calcipotriol 0.005% ointment twice daily on the other side of the body. After 8 weeks (24 treatments), there was a mean repigmentation of 23% (range: 1.2–33.6) on the calcipotriol combination side versus 22% (range: 6.6–31.5) on the excimer monotherapy side, which was not statistically significant. No new lesions occurred during the treatment period and no serious adverse events were observed.

Tacalcitol cream:

Tacalcitol plus heliotherapy: Rodriguez-Martin[35] investigated the efficacy of tacalcitol plus sunlight exposure in non-segmental vitiligo. Eighty adults, aged 18–72 years, were randomly assigned to one of two treatment groups: (1) placebo plus 30 minutes of sunlight daily and (2) tacalcitol 4 µg/g ointment plus 30 minutes of sunlight daily. After 4 months of treatment, 3.1% of patients in the placebo group and 0% of patients in the tacalcitol group obtained greater than 75% repigmentation, with all patients in the tacalcitol group achieving less than 25% repigmentation. There was no statistically significant difference in repigmentation between groups at the end of treatment. Adverse events included itching (15 patients in placebo group and 12 in tacalcitol group), mild contact dermatitis (4 patients in placebo and 7 in tacalcitol groups, photosensitivity (1 patient in placebo group) and mild to moderate transient erythema (14 patients in the placebo group and 26 patients in tacalcitol group).

Tacalcitol plus narrowband ultraviolet B: Leone[36] randomly assigned 32 subjects, aged 18–54, with generalized vitiligo and symmetrical lesions, to treatment with twice weekly NB-UVB or twice weekly NB-UVB plus tacalcitol 4 µg/g cream daily. NB-UVB therapy consisted of twice weekly treatments for up to 6 months, starting with 70% of the minimal erythema dose. The study showed that lesions treated in the tacalcitol/NB-UVB combination group showed significantly higher repigmentation scores than those with NB-UVB alone ($p < 0.0005$) at the end of the study. At the end of 6 months of treatment 50% of lesions in the combination group versus 0% were scored as greater than 80% pigmentation. Lastly, those lesions in the combination group showed quicker onset of repigmentation as compared with those in the NB-UVB group in those classified as "good responders" (55 ± 25 days vs 130 ± 39 days). No patients were lost to follow-up and the combination treatment was generally well-tolerated, with side effects limited to mild erythema and itching. Mild irritation and desquamation following ointment application also occurred in 12 subjects treated on the face with combination treatment.

Tacalcitol plus excimer laser or monochromatic excimer light: Lu-yan[37] enrolled 38 patients, aged 6–65 years old, to a randomized trial on bilaterally symmetrical lesions on the arms, hands, trunk, neck and face. Two treatment groups were devised: (1) 308 nm monochromatic excimer light once weekly plus placebo twice daily and (2) 308 nm monochromatic excimer light once weekly in addition to tacalcitol 2 μg/g cream twice daily for 12 treatments. Greater than 75% repigmentation was achieved in 25.7% patients in the tacalcitol group and 5.7% of patients in the placebo group, which was statistically significant ($P < 0.05$). Lesions on the face and neck responded better than those on trunk, hands and extremities. Significant initial pigmentation was obtained earlier in lesions treated in the tacalcitol group than in the placebo group (4.52 ± 0.49 vs 5.3 ± 0.52 treatments), with most occurring within 4–8 weeks of treatment. Lastly, a significantly lower cumulative MEL dosage at initial pigmentation occurred in the tacalcitol group compared to the placebo group (3.93 ± 0.59 vs 4.99 ± 0.68 J/cm^2). Adverse effects included mild to moderate erythema, xerosis, and itching in 3 patients, 2 in tacalcitol group, and 1 in placebo group.

High concentration tacalcitol 20 μg/g at bedtime was combined with the 308 nm xenon chloride excimer laser twice weekly in the study of Oh.[38] For comparison, they also included a tacalcitol 20 μg/g nightly monotherapy group and a 308 nm xenon chloride excimer laser twice weekly monotherapy group. After 16 weeks, 16 of 20 patients with non-segmental vitiligo (aged 15–60) completed the trial. Repigmentation was graded by quartiles from 0 to 4, with no patient achieving greater than 50% repigmentation. Repigmentation scores were significantly different between both the combination and excimer monotherapy groups versus the tacalcitol monotherapy group, but not significant between the combination and excimer monotherapy groups. There was no significant difference between groups for time to initial repigmentation. Side effects included itching in all but one patient in the tacalcitol group. Of note, serum calcium levels remained within normal limits from baseline to the conclusion of the study.

Pseudocatalase Combinations

One study examined the use of pseudocatalase as combination therapy, that of Bakis-Petsoglou.[39] Trial groups applied pseudocatalase cream or placebo to the entire body and then received NB-UVB 10–30 minutes later thrice weekly. Twenty-five patients with at least acrofacial vitiligo completed the trial. Analysis revealed no statistically significant difference between treatment groups on digital photography of the face and hands. There was a significant difference from baseline to the end of treatment, within groups, for the pseudocatalase group on the left and right face ($P = 0.0001$ and $P = 0.005$, respectively) and placebo group ($P = 0.003$ and $P = 0.01$), as assessed by the investigator. The most common treatment related adverse events were: pruritus, increased sweating, and thermal burns secondary to NB-UVB.

CONCLUSION

Randomized trials for treating vitiligo involving the use of topical monotherapies and combination therapies have been described in this chapter. Topical steroids examined included betamethasone valerate 0.1% in 50% isopropyl alcohol, betamethasone dipropionate 0.05% cream, fluticasone propionate 0.05% cream, clobetasol propionate 0.05% cream/ointment and meta-analysis data. Betamethasone valerate 0.1% in 50% isopropyl alcohol outperformed the unmedicated base. Betamethasone 0.05% cream did not perform better than calcipotriol 0.005% ointment or catalase/superoxide dismutase cream in eliciting clinically significant repigmentation for vitiligo. Both studies investigating fluticasone propionate 0.05% cream found that neither UVA nor tacrolimus was more effective than fluticasone. With clobetasol propionate 0.05% cream, it did not seem to be more effective than the cream base in achieving greater than 75% repigmentation in the study of Clayton, but did perform significantly better than placebo in Ho's study. Clobetasol and tacrolimus seemed to have similar efficacy in children, however, with less risk of side effects associated with tacrolimus. Lastly, clobetasol was significantly more effective than PUVAsol in the treatment of childhood vitiligo. Lastly, the meta-analysis of Njoo showed that class 3 steroids induced greater repigmentation than class 4 steroids, as compared with intralesional steroids, KUVA and PUVA.

Topical monotherapy with calcineurin inhibitors included tacrolimus and pimecrolimus. Three studies, Lubaki, Radakovic and Lepe, investigated the use of tacrolimus versus placebo or differing frequencies of tacrolimus dosing or versus clobetasol. The first two studies showed a trend toward better repigmentation in the tacrolimus group or twice daily tacrolimus dosing group, but no groups obtained greater than 75% repigmentation. There was no difference found between the tacrolimus and clobetasol groups in Lepe's study. Pimecrolimus was also investigated in two studies, comparing it to placebo or using prior microdermabrasion and then using pimecrolimus, with comparison to placebo. One study found no significant difference in repigmentation between pimecrolimus and placebo, while the other found a significant difference between pimecrolimus and placebo groups. Additionally, the combination of microdermabrasion improved repigmentation rates in conjunction with pimecrolimus. Despite variability in effectiveness, calcineurins have a safer side effect profile as compared with topical steroids.

One study investigated the use of topical vitamin D analog monotherapy. They compared calcipotriol with betamethasone dipropionate 0.05% cream. The study found no difference between any of the groups. No studies investigated pseudocatalase monotherapy for repigmentation in vitiligo. Also, there were no randomized trials investigating the use of topical depigmentation therapy.

Steroid combinations were investigated in 6 studies using fluocinolone acetonide 0.1% cream, fluticasone propionate 0.05% cream, hydrocortisone 17-butyrate cream, betamethasone cream and clobetasol propionate 0.05% cream. Mean pigment spread after punch grafting was not different with postoperative fluocinolone or PUVA. Fluticasone combined with UVA created a three-fold greater repigmentation than either modality alone. Hydrocortisone 17-butyrate cream in combination with 308 nm excimer laser produced significantly greater repigmentation than 308 nm excimer laser monotherapy. The combination of hydrocortisone 17-butyrate, dermabrasion and NB-UVB produced greater repigmentation than betamethasone and NB-UVB.

Betamethasone cream, calcipotriol ointment and NB-UVB combination performed better than NB-UVB monotherapy. Lastly, the combination of topical clobetasol and oral zinc sulfate did not outperform clobetasol monotherapy.

Seven studies investigated combination treatments with topical calcineurin inhibitors. Combinations included tacrolimus plus NB-UVB, excimer laser or monochromatic excimer light and pimecrolimus plus NB-UVB or excimer laser. Two studies looked at the use of tacrolimus or placebo plus NB-UVB, with one showing no significant difference between groups and the other showing significant repigmentation. In the groups comparing tacrolimus plus excimer laser/light, two out of three studies showed greater repigmentation with the combination versus excimer monotherapy groups. For facial lesions, pimecrolimus/NB-UVB combinations responded significantly better as compared with placebo/NB-UVB. Lastly, pimecrolimus/excimer combination therapy produced greater repigmentation than excimer monotherapy, with greater facial repigmentation.

Vitamin D analog combination therapy was utilized in 9 randomized trials. Combinations included: calcipotriol plus NB-UVB, PUVA, PUVAsol and excimer laser and tacalcitol plus heliotherapy, NB-UVB, and excimer laser and monochromatic excimer light. Calcipotriol plus NB-UVB was not better than NB-UVB for repigmentation, while the combination of calcipotriol ointment, betamethasone cream, and NB-UVB was better than NB-UVB. Also, the combination of calcipotriol plus PUVA did perform better than UVA monotherapy, while calcipotriol plus PUVAsol did not outperform PUVAsol plus placebo. Excimer plus calcipotriol was not statistically better than excimer monotherapy. With regard to tacalcitol and heliotherapy, there was no difference between groups as compared with placebo plus heliotherapy. Tacalcitol plus NB-UVB did do better than NB-UVB monotherapy. Lastly, tacalcitol plus monochromatic excimer light performed better than monochromatic excimer light plus placebo, but tacalcitol plus excimer laser did not perform better than excimer laser (but did against tacalcitol monotherapy).

Pseudocatalase combination therapy was examined in one study, where pseudocatalase plus NB-UVB was compared with NB-UVB monotherapy. No significant difference was found on analysis of repigmentation between the groups.

REFERENCES

1. Sehgal VN, Srivastava G. Vitiligo: compendium of clinico-epidemiological features. Indian J Dermatol Venereol Leprol. 2007;73(3):149-56.
2. Kandil E. Treatment of vitiligo with 0.1 percent betamethasone 17-valerate in isopropyl alcohol—a double-blind trial. Br J Dermatol. 1974;91(4):457-60.
3. Kumaran MS, Kaur I, Kumar B. Effect of topical calcipotriol, betamethasone dipropionate and their combination in the treatment of localized vitiligo. J Eur Acad Dermatol Venereol. 2006;20(30):269-73.
4. Sanclemente G, Garcia JJ, Zuleta JJ, et al. A double-blind, randomized trial of 0.05% betamethasone vs. topical catalase/dismutase superoxide in vitiligo. J Eur Acad Dermatol Venereol. 2008;22(11):1359-64.
5. Westerhof W, Nieuweboer-Krobotova L, Mulder PG, et al. Left-right comparison study of the combination of fluticasone propionate and UV-A vs. either fluticasone propionate or UV-A alone for the long-term treatment of vitiligo. Arch Dermatol. 1999;135(9):1061-6.
6. Kathuria S, Khaitan BK, Ramam M, et al. Segmental vitiligo: A randomized controlled rial to evaluate efficacy and sefety of 0.1% tacrolimus ointment vs. 0.05% fluticasone propionate cream. Indian J Dermatol Venereol Leprol. 2012;78(1):68-73.
7. Clayton R. A double-blind trial of 0.05% clobetasol proprionate in the treatment of vitiligo. Br J Dermatol. 1977;96(1):71-3.
8. Ho N, Pope E, Weinstein M, et al. A double-blind, randomized, placebo-controlled trial of topical tacrolimus 0.1% vs. clobetasol propionate 0.05% in childhood vitiligo. Br J Dermatol. 2011;165(3):626-32.
9. Lepe V, Moncada B, Castanedo-Cazares JP, et al. A double-blind randomized trial of 0.1% tacrolimus vs 0.05% clobetasol for the treatment of childhood vitiligo. Arch Dermatol. 2003;139(5):581-5.
10. Khalid M, Mujtaba G, Haroon TS. Comparison of 0.05% clobetasol propionate cream and topical Puvasol in childhood vitiligo. Int J Dermatol. 1995;34(3):203-5.
11. Whitton ME, Ashcroft DM, Barrett CW, et al. Interventions for vitiligo. Cochrane Database Syst Rev. 2006;25(1): CD003263.

12. Njoo MD, Spuls PI, Bos JD, et al. Nonsurgical repigmentation therapies in vitiligo. Meta-analysis of the literature. Arch Dermatol. 1998;134(12):1532-40.
13. Lubaki LJ, Ghanem G, Vereecken P, et al. Time-kinetic study of repigmentation in vitiligo patients by tacrolimus or pimecrolimus. Arch Dermatol Res. 2010;302(2):131-7.
14. Radakovic S, Breier-Maly J, Konschitzky R, et al. Response of vitiligo to once- vs. twice-daily topical tacrolimus: a controlled prospective, randomized, observer-blinded trial. J Eur Acad Dermatol Venereol. 2009;23(8):951-3.
15. Dawid M, Veensalu M, Grassberger M, et al. Efficacy and safety of pimecrolimus cream 1% in adult patients with vitiligo: results of a randomized, double-blind, vehicle-controlled study. J Dtsch Dermatol Ges. 2006;4(11):942-6.
16. Farajzadeh S, Daraei Z, Esfandiarpour I, et al. The efficacy of pimecrolimus 1% cream combined with microdermabrasion in the treatment of nonsegmental childhood vitiligo: a randomized placebo-controlled study. Pediatr Dermatol. 2009;26(3):286-91.
17. Drake LA, Dinehart SM, Farmer ER, et al. Guidelines of care for vitiligo. American Academy of Dermatology. J Am Acad Dermatol. 1996;35(4):620-6.
18. Njoo MD, Vodegel RM, Westerhof W. Depigmentation therapy in vitiligo universalis with topical 4-methoxyphenol and the Q-switched ruby laser. J Am Acad Dermatol. 2000;42(5 pt 1):760-9.
19. Barman KD, Khaitan BK, Verma KK. A comparative study of punch grafting followed by topical corticosteroid versus punch grafting followed by PUVA therapy in stable vitiligo. Dermatol Surg. 2004;30(1):49-53.
20. Sassi F, Cazzaniga S, Tessari G, et al. Randomized controlled trial comparing the effectiveness of 308-nm excimer laser alone or in combination with topical hydrocortisone 17-butyrate cream in the treatment of vitiligo of the face and neck. Br J Dermatol. 2008;159(5):1186-91.
21. Bayoumi W, Fontas E, Sillard L, et al. Effect of a preceding laser dermabrasion on the outcome of combined therapy with narrowband ultraviolet B and potent topical steroids for treating nonsegmental vitiligo in resistant localizations. Br J Dermatol. 2012;166:208-11.
22. Akdeniz N, Yavuz IH, Gunes Bigil S, et al. Comparison of efficacy of narrow band UVB therapies with UVB alone, in combination with calcipotriol, and with betamethasone and calcipotriol in vitiligo. J Dermatolog Treat. 2013.
23. Yaghoobi R, Omidian M, Bagherani N. Original article title: "Comparison of therapeutic efficacy of topical corticosteroid and oral zinc sulfate-topical corticosteroid combination in the treatment of vitiligo patients: a clinical trial". BMC Dermatol. 2011;11:7.
24. Mehrabi D, Pandya AG. A randomized, placebo-controlled, double-blind trial comparing narrowband UV-B Plus 0.1% tacrolimus ointment with narrowband UV-B plus placebo in the treatment of generalized vitiligo. Arch Dermatol. 2006;142(7):927-9.
25. Nordal EJ, Guleng GE, Ronnevig JR. Treatment of vitiligo with narrowband-UVB (TL01) combined with tacrolimus ointment (0.1%) vs. placebo ointment, a randomized right/left double-blind comparative study. J Eur Acad Dermatol Venereol. 2011;25(12):1440-3.
26. Kawalek AZ, Spencer JM, Phelps RG. Combined excimer laser and topical tacrolimus for the treatment of vitiligo: a pilot study. Dermatol Surg. 2004;30(2 pt 1):130-5.
27. Passeron T, Ostovari N, Zakaria W, et al. Topical tacrolimus and the 308-nm excimer laser: a synergistic combination for the treatment of vitiligo. Arch Dermatol. 2004;140(9):1065-9.
28. Nistico S, Chiricozzi A, Saraceno R, et al. Vitiligo treatment with monochromatic excimer light and tacrolimus: results of an open randomized controlled study. Photomed Laser Surg. 2012;30(1):26-30.
29. Esfandiarpour I, Ekhlasi A, Farajzadeh S, et al. The efficacy of pimecrolimus 1% cream plus narrow-band ultraviolet B in the treatment of vitiligo: a double-blind, placebo-controlled clinical trial. J Dermatolog Treat. 2009;20(1):14-8.
30. Hui-Lan Y, Xiao-Yan H, Jian-Yong F, et al. Combination of 308-nm excimer laser with topical pimecrolimus for the treatment of childhood vitiligo. Pediatr Dermatol. 2009;26(3):354-6.
31. Arca E, Tastan HB, Erbil AH, et al. Narrow-band ultraviolet B as monotherapy and in combination with topical calcipotriol in the treatment of vitiligo. J Dermatol. 2006;33(5):338-43.
32. Ermis O, Alpsoy E, Cetin L, et al. Is the efficacy of psoralen plus ultraviolet A therapy for vitiligo enhanced by concurrent topical calcipotriol? A placebo-controlled double-blind study. Br J Dermatol. 2001;145(3):472-5.
33. Parsad D, Saini R, Verma N. Combination of PUVAsol and topical calcipotriol in vitiligo. Dermatology. 1998;197(2):167-70.
34. Goldinger SM, Dummer R, Schmid P, et al. Combination of 308-nm xenon chloride excimer laser and topical calcipotriol in vitiligo. J Eur Acad Dermatol Venereol. 2007;21(4):504-8.
35. Rodriguez-Martin M, Garcia Bustinduy M, Saez Rodiguez M, et al. Randomized, double-blind clinical trial to evaluate the efficacy of topical tacalcitol and sunlight exposure in the treatment of adult nonsegmental vitiligo. Br J Dermatol. 2009;160(2):409-14.
36. Leone G, Pacifico A, Iacovelli P, et al. Tacalcitol and narrow-band phototherapy in patients with vitiligo. Clin Exp Dermatol. 2006;31(2):200-5.
37. Lu-yan T, Wen-wen F, Lei-hong X, et al. Topical tacalcitol and 308-nm monochromatic excimer light: a synergistic combination for the treatment of vitiligo. Photodermatol Photoimmunol Photomed. 2006;22(6):310-4.
38. Oh SH, Kim T, Jee H, et al. Combination treatment of non-segmental vitiligo with a 308-nm xenon chloride excimer laser and topical high-concentration tacalcitol: a prospective, single-blinded, paired, comparative study. J Am Acad Dermatol. 2011;65(2):428-30.
39. Bakis-Petsoglou S, Le Guay JL, Wittal R. A randomized, double-blinded, placebo-controlled trial of pseudocatalase cream and narrowband ultraviolet B in the treatment of vitiligo. Br J Dermatol. 2009;161(4):910-7.

26

Alternative Treatment for Vitiligo

Torello Lotti, Angelo Massimiliano D'Erme

Key Features

- Even with an appropriate therapeutic management, many patients cannot contrast the disease progression and achieve pleasing result in repigmentation.
- In medicine, the use of complementary and alternative medicine has become very popular.
- Vitiligo is a chronic and resistant disease; patients may need a complementary therapy and they often use alternative medicine such as homeopathic after the failure of the conventional one or as a first approach to the disease.

INTRODUCTION

Even with an appropriate therapeutic management, many patients cannot contrast the disease progression and achieve pleasing result in repigmentation.[1]

Often current vitiligo treatments are not satisfactory for both patients and physicians.[2-5] Vitiligo can persist at least in part, and causes physical and psychological problems. For these reasons the introduction of combination therapies in the vitiligo management have allowed us to obtain better results than that ones with a single agent. Moreover, research on novel efficacious products is mandatory to improve the therapeutic possibilities and the safety of the treatment.[1,3,6]

In medicine, the use of complementary and alternative medicine has become very popular in Europe and abroad with an increase of 20–50%.[7] Globally, these treatments have recognized more from the Governments and they could be combined with conventional cure.[8]

Vitiligo patients often use alternative medicine such as homeopathic, either after the failure of the conventional treatments or as a first approach to the disease.

Studies have shown that this preference seems to be uninfluenced or few influenced by sex, type and initial site of disease, and literary and socioeconomic status.[7] The looking for an alternative treatment is due to the expectation of complete cure proposed from these remedies and to the influence of family and friends. The stigma associated to vitiligo, linked to the social pressure, is well known and led to search for a complete and definitive cure.[7]

Several treatment options have been added to a well-known armamentarium of established treatment either topical or systemic as well as non-pharmacological one.

It is not easy to understand the efficacy of complementary/alternative treatment option for vitiligo as nearly 10% of patients with vitiligo can present spontaneous repigmentation.

ANTIOXIDANT

Recently, the role of oxidative stress has been pointed out to be implicated in the pathogenesis of vitiligo. An increase of reactive oxygen species (ROS) and a decrease of scavengers and antioxidant system has been shown in vitiligo lesions. ROS can cause membrane lyses through lipid peroxidation reactions and bleach melanin. Thus, melanocytes result more sensitive to oxidative stress causing greater cell death.[9]

Prignano et al. (2009)[10] have shown that keratinocytes from perilesional vitiligo skin also present features of damaged cells. The mitochondrial of these keratinocytes presents damages that are associated with an increase in ROS production. These cells also present high levels of activated p38, NF-κB p65 subunit, p53 and Smac/DIABLO proteins. They can have an important role in the pathogenesis of vitiligo because they can represent the area from where melanocyte death is initiated. Moreover, when keratinocytes were treated with antioxidants drugs, such as curcumin and capsaicin, an inhibition of apoptosis, an increase of total antioxidant capacity, and an improved mitochondrial activity were shown.[11] More studies need to understand all the processes of the oxidant damage. Since antioxidants might represent a complementary approach to face the vitiligo progression, it is worthy to prescribe to the patients a cure of antioxidant therapy based on vitamin E, vitamin C, alpha-lipoic acid, ginkgo biloba, curcumin, capsaicin, superoxide dismutase, polypodium leukotomos and minerals (zinc, selenium).[5,10,12] Nowadays, their use is become frequent among physicians, even their efficacy and safety has still to be defined. Their indication can benefit especially in patients that are undergoing to UV-phototherapy treatment.[5,13] The UV irradiation or photosensitizing agents causes on human epidermis an increase of ROS levels and significant depletion of skin enzymatic and non-enzymatic antioxidants. These problems may be prevented by the use of antioxidants. For instance, the assumption of polypodium leucotomos reduces the cutaneous phototoxicity of phototherapies, either UVB or psoralen ultraviolet A (PUVA).[4,5,14] Some studies have shown that vitamin E may improve the responses to PUVA preventing an oxidative distress. More studies need to confirm these data and to carry out recommendation regarding the correct use of antioxidants.

Transient erythema, pruritus and peeling are the most common side effects when these products are applied topically.[5,15] However, more research is required to define their doses, efficacy and side effect profiles.

L-PHENYLALANINE

Phenylalanine improves the action of sunlight in stimulating the migration of melanocytes and the production of melanin. For these reasons, it can be used in vitiligo. Several studies have shown the benefits of this treatment either in monotherapy or in combination with other treatments.[1,5,16] A recent open observational study evaluated the efficacy and safety in vitiligo lesions of a topical gel composed by phenylalanine, acetyl cysteine, and cucumis melo extract, in 12 weeks treatment, given alone or in combination with 311-nm narrow band microphototherapy.[3] When it was given alone, its efficacy was inferior to clobetasol propionate 0.005% ointment or 311-nm narrow band microphototherapy alone, even the side effects caused by clobetasol were noted. The association of this gel with microphototherapy led to good results in terms of repigmentation, safety and patient's compliance confirming the useful combination between topical phenylalanine therapy and phototherapy.[3]

When assumed orally, it is well tolerated. Sometimes a mild nausea can follow the assumption.[1]

KHELLIN

Khellin is a furanochromone derivative isolated from Ammi visnaga, a Mediterranean plant. Due to its chemical structure, resembling that of psoralen family, it has photobiological effect when it is activated by UVA or UVB.[1,17] However, the research regarding the use of khellin remains inconclusive and sometimes contradictory. The rationale of its use in vitiligo is that khellin seems to have similar efficacy to psoralen, but less side effects as phototoxic and mutagenic.[17] It can be administered either systemically (100 mg 2–5 hours before UV exposure) or topically (2% in acetone).[1]

New topical formulation, khellin at a concentration of 0.005% encapsulated in phosphatidylcholine liposomes, stabilized with L-phenylalanine 0.1%, has been studied recently in combination with UV phototherapy. This treatment can be followed by surgery in case of refractory cases.[17]

It seems to be safe, a part of hyperpigmentation of healthy skin. When assumed orally, a mild increase of level of transaminases for hepatotoxic side effects has been noted.[17]

HOMEOPATHY AND AYURVEDIC MEDICINE

Homeopathy considers vitiligo as an external reflection of inner pigment disorders. In fact vitiligo is not retained as skin disease but a disease of whole body. A patient suffers from vitiligo is unique and homeopathy has to treat the whole body and not only the skin.[1]

Vitiligo is one of the most common skin disorders treated in the homeopathic hospitals. These patients, often representing "effectiveness gaps" for conventional medical treatment, search to solve their disease after the available conventional treatments were not fully effective. A lot of patients reported improvement in health affecting their daily living.[18]

Ayurveda can be presently described as a humoral medical model, where humors are defined as air, phlegm, blood and bile.[1]

Instability and diseases are determined by misbalance of these humors. Vitiligo is fully described and studied in Ayurveda medicine.

Ayurveda classifies in sub-varieties of disease, even within the same patient, and attributes them to imbalances and dominance of *kapha*, when there are large or multiple lesions, *vatha*, when there are xerotic lesions, or *pitta* when there are red lesions.[2,8]

The achievement of repigmentation of vitiligo is made by the balance of the humors starting from diet. In fact, a lot of therapies focus on the gastrointestinal tract, especially on purgation. Usually vegetarian products, such as fruits, radishes or barks, are suggested. The treatment has to be followed for at least 3 months. The combination therapy with sunlight or UV exposure is not mandatory.

A lot of people can benefit from these alternative approaches, but large and double-blind studies are missing.[1,8]

PSYCHOTHERAPY

It is well known the burden on the quality of life caused by vitiligo in patients with vitiligo. In these patients, among the dermatology life and quality index (DLQI) scores the highest one were found for feelings, clothing, social and leisure activities and daily routine. Moreover patients report emotional stress and low self-esteem and tend to suffer more from anxiety and depression disorders.[5,6,19]

It is worthy to remember that a high incidence of vitiligo occurs during the second and third decades of life that are critical period for the growth of the patients and for their creation of intimate relationship. The management of vitiligo should also include education, acceptance of the disease, cosmetic correction and psychotherapy in some cases.[5,6,19]

It has been shown that the cognitive-behavioral therapy can help to improve the quality of life, self-esteem and perceived body image. There is not enough evidence that the cognitive-behavioral therapy can interfere with the progression of the disease but it represents a very important complementary treatment.[20,21]

CLIMATOLOGICAL AND BALNEOLOGICAL THERAPIES

Patients with vitiligo can benefit from heliotherapy and sanus per aquam (SPA) treatment. A lot of studies derived from the evaluation of heliotherapy and mineral spring water in patients undergoing Dead Sea climatotherapy. In these places, the mineral content of the water and ozone composition allow maximum natural UV light exposure without phototoxicity, and this led a lot of benefits to vitiligo.[1]

Some studies have shown the benefit of climatotherapy in healing vitiligo lesions. Dead Sea climatotherapy seems to have comparable or also better results to these obtained with narrowband UVB phototherapy, as reported in the literature.[21] The results seem to preserve and continue to increase after leaving the SPA.[21] For these reasons studies demonstrated that Dead Sea climatotherapy is an effective treatment modality for vitiligo, with relatively few side effects. Severity and duration of the disease, as well as length of treatment are parameters to take in account for the response to the treatment.[21]

CONCLUSION

Despite the remarkable progresses, the treatment of vitiligo remains challenging. Some patients with vitiligo can be resistant to common treatment and have benefitted from complementary and alternative treatment. Most governments recognize "pluralistic systems of health care" even large studies have still been carried out. These can be a complementary treatment to the conventional ones.

REFERENCES

1. Holíková Z, Massi D, Lotti T, et al. Insight into the pathogenesis of sporadic basal cell carcinoma. Vitiligo: problems and solutions. Int J Dermatol. 2004;43(12):865-9.
2. Lotti TM, Hercogová J, Schwartz RA, et al. Treatments of vitiligo: what's new at the horizon. Dermatol Ther. 2012;25(Suppl 1):S32-40.
3. Buggiani G, Tsampau D, Hercogovà J, et al. Clinical efficacy of a novel topical formulation for vitiligo: compared evaluation of different treatment modalities in 149 patients. Dermatol Ther. 2012;25(5):472-6.
4. Alikhan A, Felsten LM, Daly M, et al. Vitiligo: a comprehensive overview Part I. Introduction, epidemiology, quality of life, diagnosis, differential diagnosis, associations, histopathology, etiology, and work-up. J Am Acad Dermatol. 2011;65(3):493-514.
5. Felsten LM, Alikhan A, Petronic-Rosic V. Vitiligo: a comprehensive overview Part II: treatment options and approach to treatment. J Am Acad Dermatol. 2011; 65(3):473-91.
6. Taieb A, Alomar A, Böhm M, et al. Guidelines for the management of vitiligo: the European Dermatology Forum Consensus. Br J Dermatol. 2013;168(1):5-19.
7. Bhalla M, Thami GP. Factors predicting the preference of complementary and alternative systems of medicine in treatment of vitiligo. Indian J Dermatol Venereol Leprol. 2010;76(6):705-7.
8. Narahari SR, Ryan TJ, Bose KS, et al. Integrating modern dermatology and ayurveda in the treatment of vitiligo and lymphedema in India. Int J Dermatol. 2011;50(3):310-34.
9. Zhou Z, Li CY, Li K, et al. Decreased methionine sulphoxide reductase A expression renders melanocytes more sensitive to oxidative stress: a possible cause for melanocyte loss in vitiligo. Br J Dermatol. 2009;161:504-9.
10. Prignano F, Pescitelli L, Becatti M, et al. Ultrastructural and functional alterations of mitochondria in perilesional vitiligo skin. J Dermatol Sci. 2009;54(3):157-67.
11. Becatti M, Prignano F, Fiorillo C, et al. The involvement of Smac/DIABLO, p53, NF-κB, and MAPK pathways in apoptosis of keratinocytes from perilesional vitiligo skin:

protective effects of curcumin and capsaicin. Antioxid Redox Signal. 2010;13(9):1309-21.
12. Jalel A, Soumaya GS, Hamdaoui MH. Vitiligo treatment with vitamins, minerals and polyphenol supplementation. Indian J Dermatol. 2009;54(4):357-60.
13. Dell'Anna ML, Mastrofrancesco A, Sala R, et al. Antioxidants and narrow band-UVB in the treatment of vitiligo: a double-blind placebo controlled trial. Clin Exp Dermatol. 2007;32:631-6.
14. Gonzalez S, Pathak MA, Cuevas J, et al. Topical or oral administration with an extract of polypodium leucotomos prevents acute sunburn and psoralen-induced phototoxic reactions as well as depletion of Langerhans cells in human skin. Photodermatol Photoimmunol Photomed. 1997;13:50-60.
15. Sanclemente G, Garcia JJ, Zuleta JJ, et al. A double-blind, randomized trial of 0.05% betamehasone vs. topical catalase/dismutase superoxide in vitiligo. J Eur Acad Dermatol Venereol. 2008;22:1359-64.
16. Rojas-Urdaneta JE, Poleo-Romero AG. Evaluation of an antioxidant and mitochondria-stimulating cream formula on the skin of patients with stable common vitiligo. Invest Clin. 2007;48:21-31.
17. de Leeuw J, Assen YJ, van der Beek N, et al. Treatment of vitiligo with khellin liposomes, ultraviolet light and blister roof transplantation. J Eur Acad Dermatol Venereol. 2011;25(1):74-81.
18. Thompson EA, Mathie RT, Baitson ES, et al. Towards standard setting for patient-reported outcomes in the NHS homeopathic hospitals. Homeopathy. 2008;97(3):114-21.
19. Ongenae K, Van Geel N, De Schepper S, et al. Effect of vitiligo on self-reported health-related quality of life. Br J Dermatol. 2005;152(6):1165-72.
20. Picardi A, Abeni D. Can cognitive-behavioral therapy help patients with vitiligo? Arch Dermatol. 2001;137(6):786-8.
21. Czarnowicki T, Harari M, Ruzicka T, et al. Dead Sea climatotherapy for vitiligo: a retrospective study of 436 patients. J Eur Acad Dermatol Venereol. 2011;25(8):959-63.

27

Surgical Management of Vitiligo

T Salim

Key Features

- Surgical therapy of vitiligo is the gold standard in the management of resistant areas and residual lesions.
- Grafting techniques include both tissue grafts and cellular grafts. Tissue grafts are useful in managing smaller areas.
- Cellular grafting techniques have revolutionized the management of vitiligo. It is possible to treat very large areas using small donor area. It yields faster, uniform, normal textured, natural pigmentation.

INTRODUCTION

Surgical methods have a well-documented and established role in the management of resistant cases of vitiligo. These methods are gaining importance in the management of vitiligo as many patients fail to respond to medical and physical modalities of treatments. The medical management of vitiligo is dependent upon the presence of reservoir melanocytes and is effective only in 60–70% of cases. Certain types of vitiligo like segmental, mucosal, acral and leukotrichea fail to respond well to medical treatments at all and in those cases that respond, resistant lesions do persist. Moreover the severe stigma attached to the disease in the colored skinned; has a major impact on self-confidence and fear of social ostracization. Hence active surgical management is of great importance in these situations.

The surgical techniques have undergone a quantum of refinement during past one decade. The newer methods can be utilized to treat very large areas without compromising the quality of repigmentation in terms of texture, uniformity of pigmentation and cosmetic color match. This chapter will deal with overall surgical methods in the management of vitiligo other than mini grafting and mesh grafting which are dealt in other chapters.

HISTORY

Vitiligo surgeries have come up a long way from exchange skin grafts to cellular grafts.[1,2] The progressive development from one technique to the other is always in a quest for the best. Different corrective surgical methods have evolved during the last 4 decades. Transplantation of autologous pigmented skin grafts and blister roofs were the first attempts in vitiligo surgeries.[3]

Behl in 1964 described the use of thin dermo-epidermal grafts in the treatment of vitiligo.[4] Suction blister grafting by Falabella in 1971 and punch grafting by Orenteich, in 1972 were two major landmarks the surgical treatments.[1,5] Other mile stones in historic evolution of vitiligo surgeries are; minipunch grafting,[6] cultured melanocyte transplantation[7,8] non-cultured melanocyte transplantation,[9,10] Follicular melanocyte transplantation[11] and many modifications of non-culture melanocyte transplants by various authors. The current focus is on cellular transplantations as "surgical bio-therapies".

PRINCIPLE OF SURGICAL TREATMENTS

All grafting techniques rely on the basic principle of repopulating depigmented lesions with functional melanocytes arising from normal epidermis or outer root sheath (ORS) and bulge areas of the hair follicle. The transplanted melanocyte will establish and function as epidermal melanin unit and the cells survive and function if the stability has been achieved.

The objective of surgical therapies is to produce cosmetically acceptable repigmentation of the vitiliginous lesions.

INDICATIONS FOR SURGERY AND PATIENT SELECTION

Proper case selection is of paramount importance for any surgical method to yield good results. Stability of vitiligo should be the primary consideration while opting for any transplantation methods.

Type of Vitiligo

Surgery is indicated for all types of stable vitiligo including segmental, generalized and acrofacial types that do not respond to medical treatment. However the best of the results are obtained in segmental vitiligo. The chance of reactivation is much lower in segmental variants in comparison with other types of vitiligo. Moreover in a segmental vitiligo accompanied by leukotrichia, it may be considered as a first line of therapy as the reservoir of melanocyte is lacking.

Area of Involvement

Non-hair bearing areas and mucosal surfaces are resistant to medical treatments. As the reservoir is lacking in these areas surgeries may be considered to replenish with cells to regain pigment. With the development of cellular grafting techniques larger areas can be treated in a single session. Tissue grafts can be considered in small to medium sized lesions and cellular grafts for larger lesions. Very extensive depigmenations are difficult to restore by grafting techniques. Even smaller patches might require more than one session to obtain acceptable cosmetic results.

Stability

Stability indicates absence of new lesions and arrest of spreading of the existing lesions. The stability status of vitiligo is the single, most important prerequisite in case selection. Parameters for establishing stability of vitiligo include; absence of new lesions, or extension of old lesions, no Koebner phenomenon and a successful test grafting.[12] The recommended period of stability in different studies has varied from four months to three years **(Table. 1)**.[13-20] The recent consensus recommendations by IADVL Task Force regarding stability is that, vitiligo can be considered as being stable if a patient is presenting with no new lesions, no progression of existing lesions, and absence of Koebner phenomenon during the past one year.[20] A test graft may be considered whenever there is a doubt about the stability, or the patient is unable to give a clear history on stability.

Njoo et al.,[21] proposed the Vitiligo Disease Activity Score (VIDA) as another method of establishing objective criteria for stable case selection. It is a six-point scale on which the activity of the disease is evaluated by the appearance of new vitiligo lesions or the enlargement of the pre-existing lesions, gauged during a period ranging from less than 6 weeks to one year. It is suggested that surgery for vitiligo may be performed only in patients with VIDA scores of -1 or 0. Spontaneous repigmentation, presence of well defined borders and spotty pigmentation are considered as favorable signs for vitiligo surgery.

Age of the Patient

There is no uniformly accepted opinion concerning the minimum age for surgery. Even though the progress of the disease is difficult to predict in children, studies have suggested that results of transplantation procedures were better in younger individuals than in older ones.[22] The author is of the opinion that surgeries can be of great help in pediatric population with stable segmental vitiligo unresponsive to medical treatments. The physicians should exercise their judgment after taking all aspects of the individual patient into consideration.

CONTRAINDICATIONS

Bleeding disorders, active vitiligo and keloidal tendency are the absolute contraindications for vitiligo surgeries.

PREOPERATIVE COUNSELING

The surgical outcome and further chance of reactivation vary greatly between different types of vitiligo. Hence the patient should be given detailed counseling regarding the limitations of the procedures, possible reactivation of the disease and further treatment needed for optimal outcome. The nature of the disease, type of procedure, expected outcome and

Table 1: Minimum period of stability in different studies

Author	*Year*	*Period of stability*
Das SS, Pasricha JS[13]	1992	4 months
Falabella[14]	1992	3 years
Savanth[15]	1992	2 years
Jha et al.[16]	1992	1 year
Boersma and Westerhof[17]	1995	6 months
Falabella[18]	1989	2 years
Falabella[19]	2003	2 years
Parsad D, Gupta S[20]	2008	1 year

Table 2: Surgical therapy of vitiligo	
Grafting techniques	*Non-grafting techniques*
• *Tissue grafts* – Minipunch grafting – Suction blister epidermal grafting – Thin split thickness grafting – Other techniques like; hair follicle graft, smash grafts, mesh grafts, seed grafts and flip top grafts	• Micropigmentation • Excision and closure • Dermabrasion • Chemabrasion • Lasers and lights -excimer laser, excimer light, targeted phototherapy
• *Cellular grafts* – Noncultuerd epidermal cell suspension – Noncultured follicular cell suspension – Cultured melanocyte/ keratinocyte grafts	

possible complications should be clearly explained to the patient. As mandatory in any interventional procedures; an informed consent describing the procedure and possible complications should be signed by the patient before surgery.

METHODS OF SURGERY

Surgical methods in the management of vitiligo include autologous grafting and non-grafting techniques. **Table 2** enumerates the currently available surgical treatment methods.

Grafting techniques which are commonly used include both tissue grafts and cellular grafts. Search for an ideal surgical method which should provide complete repigmentation, in the shortest possible time, with no or minimal discomfort to the patient and have least side effects is continuing. A major breakthrough in the surgical treatment of vitiligo is the development of noncultured cellular transplantation. This technique has revolutionized the scenario of the surgical therapy of vitiligo. Very large area can be treated by this technique yielding cosmetically acceptable results in a short period of time.

Non-grafting techniques are used in limited situations. These include:

- Micropigmentation (Tattooing) in the form of introduction of artificial pigments into the lesions for permanent camouflage. It is recommended as a suitable method in vitiligo involving the angle of the mouth which is resistant to most of the grafting techniques.
- Therapeutic wounding of vitiliginous patch to stimulate the melanocytes from the periphery and the hair follicles to proliferate, migrate and repigment the lesion. This can be achieved by therapeutic dermabrasion, laser ablation, cryosurgery (liquid nitrogen spraying), needling, and chemabrasion by application of phenol or trichloroacetic acid.[23] These methods are used in lesions on hairy areas to produce pigmentation as adjuvant to phototherapy. This is very cost effective therapy inducing faster follicular repigmentation.
- Removal of the depigmented areas forever by excision with primary closure.

Choice of surgery depends on the type of vitiligo, extent and site of lesion, the availability of equipments and surgical skill of the treating cutaneous surgeon.

Tissue Grafts

Suction Blister Epidermal Grafting

Suction blister epidermal grafting (SBEG) is grafting technique where an ultrathin split thickness graft consisting of only epidermis is obtained by inducing a physiological split at the dermoepidermal junction. Pure epidermal cells in the absence of donor dermal tissue adopt most of the characteristics of recipient area. Hence this technique results in good color match with the surrounding skin and better esthetic outcome.

The epidermis is separated from dermis by prolonged suction at a negative pressure of -200 to -500 mm of Hg to the donor site followed by transplanting the roof of the blister to a dermabraded vitiliginous recipient site. This technique is indicated primarily for small lesions of localized stable vitiligo over skin and mucosal surfaces like lips, areola, genitals, etc.

Instruments: Suction apparatus with cups may be replaced by syringe method using disposable syringes of 20 cc and 50 cc with three way connector for induction of blisters, in resource limited setting. Other instruments required are diamond fraise dermabrader or Carbon dioxide laser, iris scissors or corneal scissors, non-toothed forceps, artery forceps and tulle dressings **(Fig. 1)**.

Technique: The suction blister can be raised by maintaining a negative pressure of -200 to -500 mm of Hg for 90 to 120 minutes using suction apparatus or by syringe technique.[24,25] Syringe suction requires 10 or 20 cc syringes to be placed as suction cups and 50 cc syringe connected via a three way connector to expel the air to create negative pressure. The bases of syringes are coated with vaseline and are applied on the donor site and air is aspirated using a 50 mL syringe and a three-way-cannula **(Fig. 2)**. A single unilocular non-hemorrhagic blister is the best result **(Figs 3A and B)**. In case of smaller blisters, one can either increase the negative pressure in the syringe by another 5 mL or intradermally inject saline into the blister to expand it.[26]

The recipient site is dermabraded by using either a manual or a motorized dermabrader, depending on the size and site of the lesion. Other techniques used to prepare recipient site include laser ablation, phototoxic separation

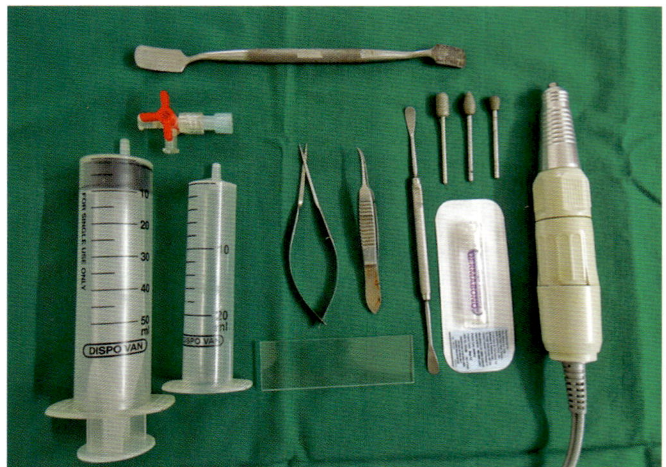

Fig. 1: Equipment required for SBEG

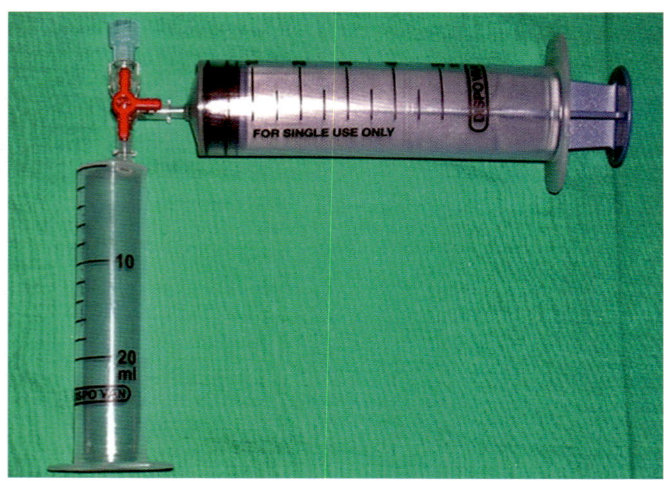

Fig. 2: Syringe and a three-way-cannula for raising suction blister

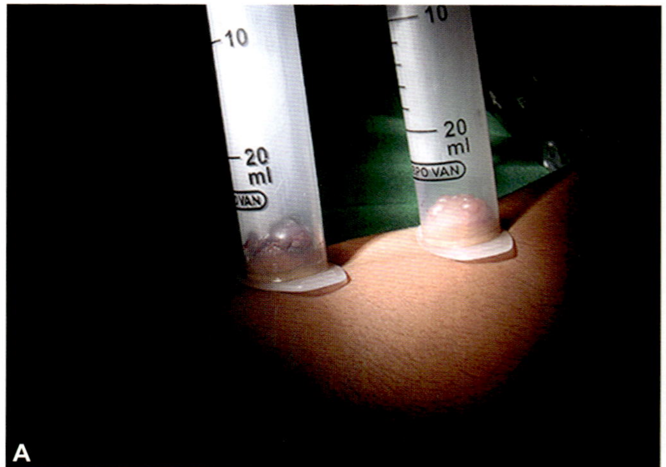

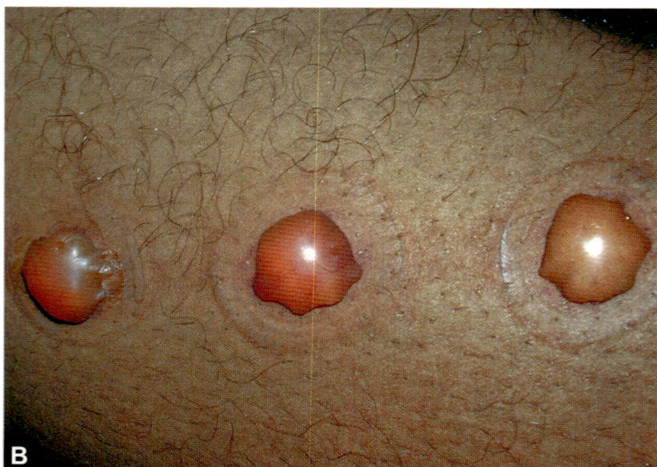

Figs 3A and B: (A) Blister being formed in syringe under negative pressure; (B) Blisters formed after 90 minutes

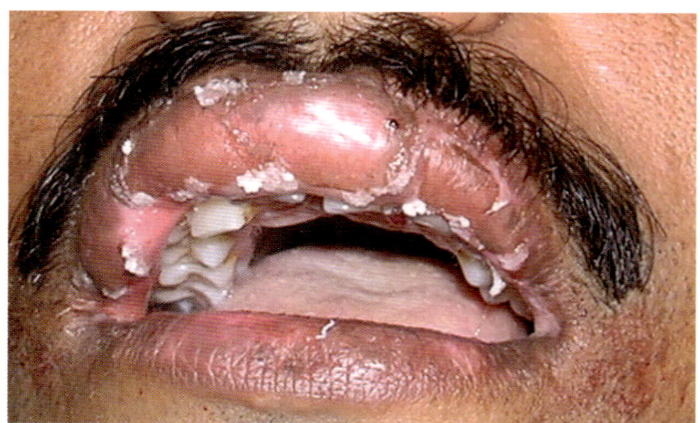

Fig. 4: Grafts secured in position with cyanoacrylate tissue adhesive

by methoxsalen and ultraviolet A, cryoblistering, suction blistering and radiofrequency ablation.[20,27,28]

Thin grafts are applied to the dermabraded recipient site. The grafts are secured in position by applying cyanoacrylate tissue adhesive on the edges of the graft **(Fig. 4)**. Primary dressing is done with framycetin tulle, followed by sterile gauze, and adhesive bandage.

Surgical outcome: The melanocyte transfer takes place within 48–72 hours to the underlying dermal surface. The dressings are removed after 5–7 days. The dried up graft comes out after the dressing removal and complete repigmentation is expected in 2–3 months time **(Figs 5 and 6)**. SBEG is an excellent technique to treat smaller vitiliginous patches. Mucosal surface like lips, areola, genitals, etc. are ideal sites for SBEG. It probably yields the best cosmetic results among

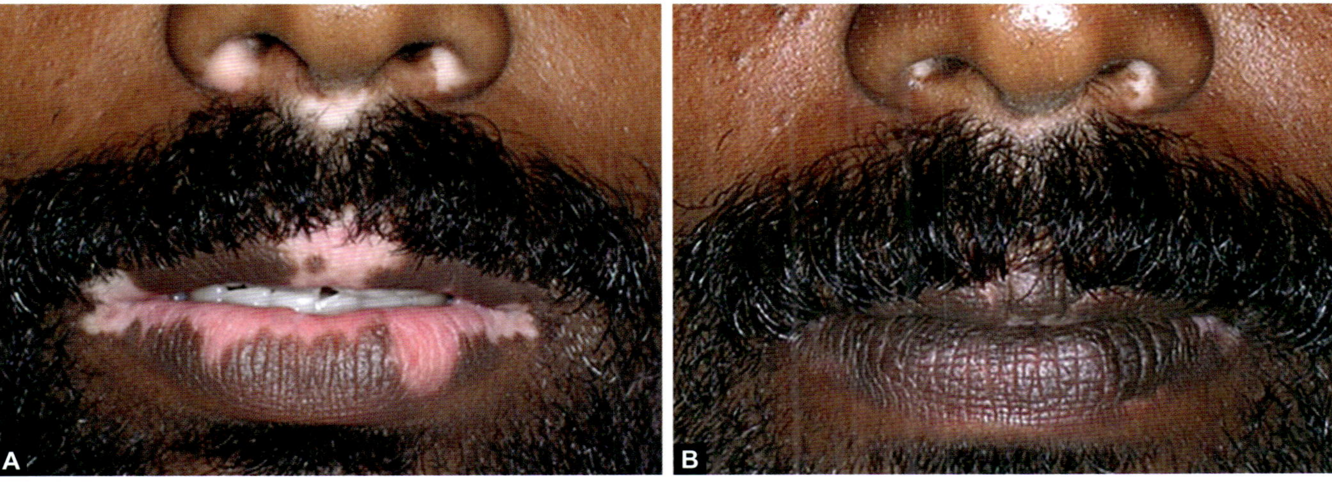

Figs 5A and B: (A) Lip vitiligo before suction blister epidermal grafting; (B) Complete repigmentation after 6 months

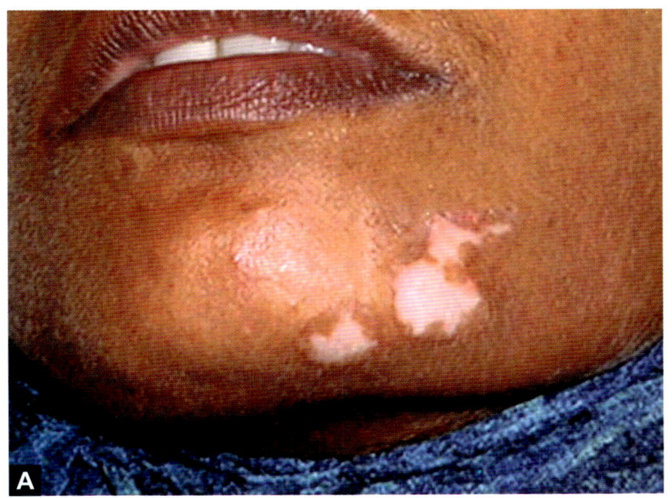

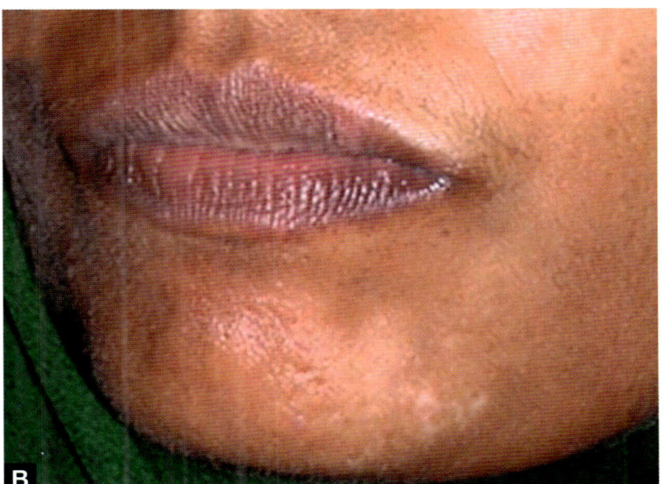

Figs 6A and B: (A) Before suction blister epidermal grafting; (B) After 3 months

Table 3: Advantages and disadvantages of suction blister epidermal grafting

Advantages
• Simple, safe and inexpensive • Excellent cosmetic results as the graft is very thin • Chances of scarring at the donor or recipient sites are minimal • Suitable for treating mucosal surfaces
Disadvantages
• Large area cannot be treated • Time consuming • Blister may not be formed if the pressure is inadequate • Partial graft take-up can lead to cosmetic disfigurement

the tissue grafts. **Table 3** enumerate various advantages and disadvantages of SBEG.

Complications: Commonly encountered immediate complications include infection, ecchymosis, and hematoma formation and partial or complete graft rejection. Hyperpigmentation, perilesional halo of recipient site and pigmentary changes at the donor sites occur occasionally.

Split-thickness Skin Grafting

Split-thickness skin grafting (STSG) is the simplest and most cost-effective surgical method which requires a fair amount of surgical skill to perform. Spit thickness skin grafting involves transfer of epidermis and often uppermost part of superficial

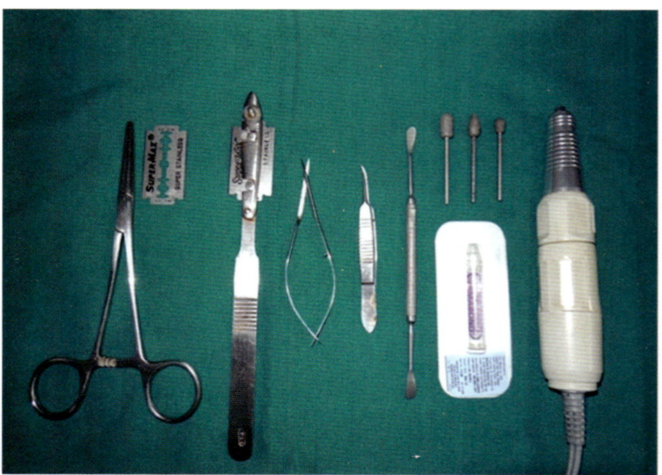

Fig. 7: Equipment required for STSG

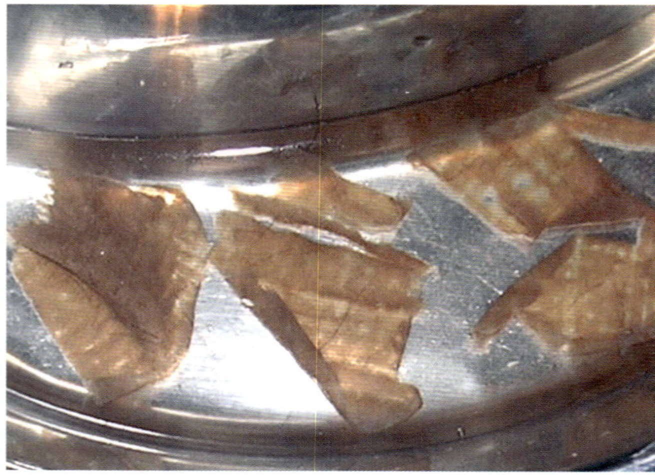

Fig. 8: Harvested graft in normal saline

Table 4: Advantages and disadvantages of split-thickness skin grafting

Advantages
• Grafted area appears skin colored immediately after the operation • Uniform pigmentation • Cost-effective procedure. No reagents and laboratory facilities required • Less time consuming procedure compared with other vitiligo surgeries
Disadvantages
• Surgical skill required to harvest adequate sized, thin grafts • Very large area cannot be treated • Color mismatch: Hyperpigmentation seen over exposed areas especially in dark skinned individuals • Milia formation • Perigraft halo • "Stuck-on" or "tire patch" appearance with thicker grafts • Cannot be used in areas like joints, tips, palms and soles • Donor site scarring

dermis to achieve transfer of melanocytes and keratinocytes to donor graft to underlying dermabraded vitiliginous area.[29] The thickness of graft ranges from 0.1 mm to 0.7 mm and different harvesting techniques are used.[30]

Instruments: Skin grafting knife in the form of Hamby's knife, Silver's knife, straight artery forceps with razor blade or Padget's, Zimmer's or Davol's dermatome can be used for harvesting. Other equipments include dermabraders, graft spreading spatulas, iris scissors, sterile petri dishes, cyanoacrylate tissue adhesive, tulle dressing **(Fig. 7)**.

Technique: The procedure is carried out under local anesthesia (for localized lesions) or general anesthesia (for extensive lesions). Preoperative preparation in the form of shaving of the recipient and donor area is important. This will prevent the lifting up of the graft and there by rejection. Use of chemical depilators and plucking of hair after administration of local anesthesia is advocated by some authors.[29]

Motorized dermatomes such as Padgett's or Zimmer's dermatomes may be used to obtain ultra-thin, split-thickness grafts, which may give cosmetically superior results compared to those with manual dermatomes. Expertise is required to obtain a uniformly thin graft especially when you use a manual dermatome. While harvesting the graft, the blade is held parallel to the skin surface and a sliding to and fro movement is employed to cut tangentially throughout the upper dermis. The thin translucent graft obtained is transferred to a petridish containing normal saline **(Fig. 8)**. The donor site is dressed using conventional occlusive or semi-occlusive dressings.

The recipient area is dermabraded including 2-3 mm of normal skin to prevent development of perilesional halo postoperatively. The graft is trimmed according to the recipient area and placed dermal side facing downwards and spread using a graft spreading spatula. Multiple small punctures are made on the graft prior to placement in order to prevent serum accumulation. This can be secured using cyanoacrylate tissue adhesive or by applying 5-0 prolene sutures. Proper immobilization is of utmost importance postoperatively and care should be taken to prevent wrinkling and beading of graft.

Surgical outcome: The first dressing change is done preferably after 24 hours to check for formation of seroma or hematoma underneath the graft. The final dressing is removed after 7 days. Repigmentation is faster in comparison with other techniques. Split-thickness skin grafting achieved the highest mean success rate ranging from 87% to 91% among the autologous transplantation methods in a systematic review.[31] The Advantages and disadvantages of STSG are given in **Table 4**.

Cellular Grafting Techniques

Tissue grafts can treat only a small area and have the limitations that large amount of donor skin is needed as there is no cell expansion in these methods. Therefore cellular grafts are preferred over tissue grafts when large area is to be treated. Cellular grafts include different methods such as, transplantation of non-cultured basal cell enriched epidermal suspension (NCES), hair follicle outer root sheath cell suspension (HFCS) and cultured melanocytes (CM) or cultured epidermis (CE).[32-36]

Noncultured Epidermal Cell Suspension

This technique has revolutionized the scenario of the surgical therapy of vitiligo helping to treat very large area utilizing a donor skin of one tenth area of recipient site. The limitations of culture expanded cells were sorted out with the introduction of the non-cultured cellular grafting techniques in 1992 by Gauthier and Surleve-Bazeille[9] and followed by several other vitiligo surgery groups. The cold trypsinization technique of Gauthier[9] was further modified by Olsson[37] there by significantly reducing the duration of the procedure.

Noncultured epidermal cell suspension (NCES) yields cosmetically acceptable results in a short period of time. More recently noncultured epidermal cell suspension have come out of tissue culture lab to operating theatre settings These techniques have become more practitioner friendly, more widely used and almost an office procedure now. The consumables and instruments required for NCES is given in **Table 5** and the principle of the procedure in **Figures 9A to F**.

Technique: The technique involves 3 steps.

1. Harvesting of donor skin.
2. Preparation of Melanocyte rich basal layer cell suspension.
3. Dermabrasion followed by application of the cells over the recipient area.

Donor site: Usually one-fifth to one-tenth the size of the recipient area is harvested from lateral aspect of the gluteal region. After cleaning with povidone iodine and alcohol; a superficial skin sample is obtained using a skin grafting knife under local anesthesia or topical anesthesia. The donor site is then covered with tulle dressing.

Table 5: Equipment and consumables for noncultured epidermal cell suspension
• Trypsin-EDTA solution of 0.25%
• Trypsin inhibitor, to neutralize excess trypsin
• Dulbecco's modified eagle's medium (DMEM)
• Centrifuge
• Aerobic incubator
• Micromotor diamond fraise dermabrader or a CO_2 laser
• A manual or electric dermatome
• Two pairs of fine pointed non-toothed forceps
• Pasture pipette or calibrated micropipette
• Centrifuge tubes, petri dishes
• Collagen dressings

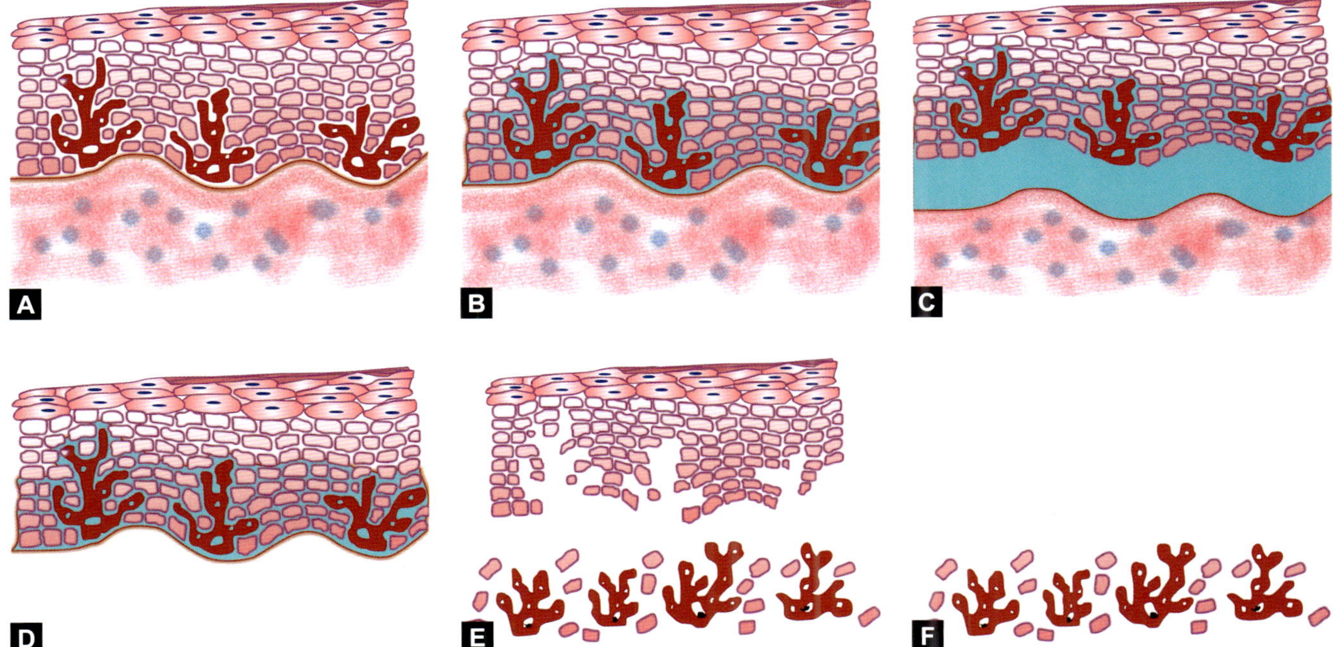

Figs 9A to F: Principle of noncultured melanocyte-keratinocyte cellular grafting. (A) Normal skin showing dermoepidermal junctions and basal melanocytes; (B) Trypsin enzyme (blue) enters and dissolve the intercellular bridges; (C) Dermis is then separated; (D to F) Dermis is separated and discarded

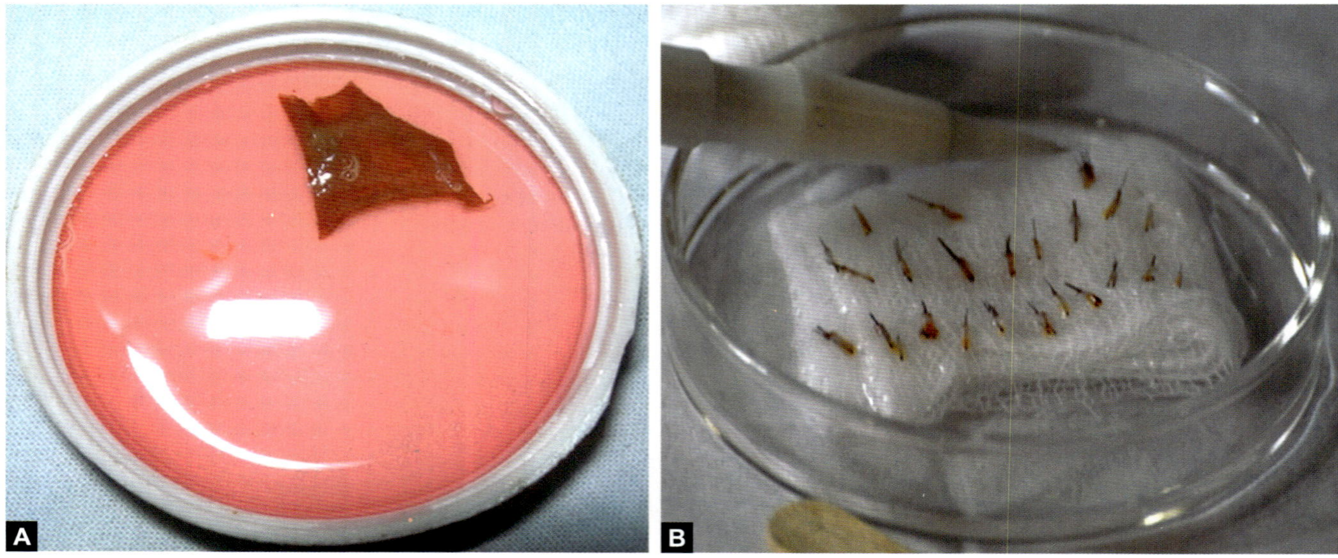

Figs 10A and B: (A) Skin samples in petri dish containing 0.25% Trypsin- EDTA solution; (B) Follicular grafts in Trypsin – EDTA solution

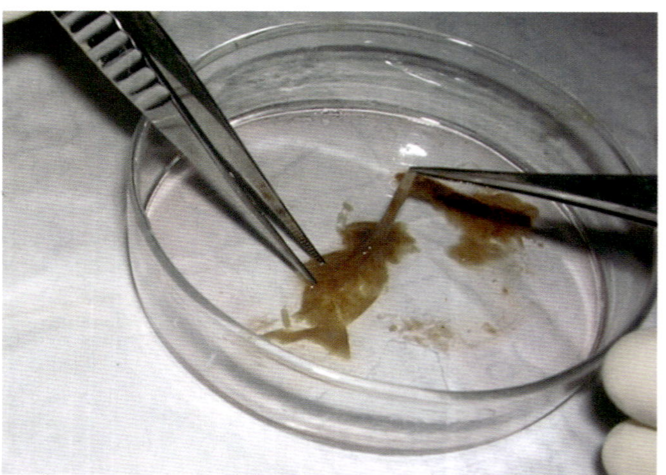

Fig. 11: Separation of epidermis and dermis

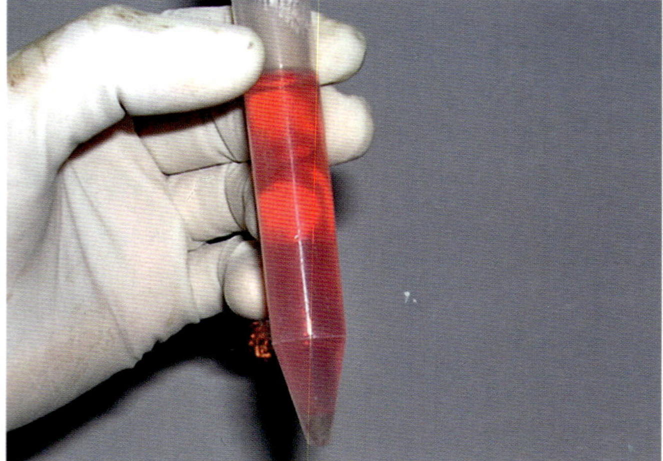

Fig. 12: Basal cell rich cell pellet formed at the bottom of the tube

Preparation of cell suspension: The skin sample is immediately transferred into a Petri dish containing 8 mL of 0.25% trypsin-EDTA solution (Sigma, St Louis, Mo,USA) **(Figs 10A and B)**. Ensure complete contact with the solution by turning the sample back and forth. It is finally placed epidermis facing upwards. Sample is then incubated in an ordinary aerobic incubator at 37°C for 50 minutes. After incubation excess of trypsin-EDTA solution is removed and about 5 mL of trypsin inhibitor (Sigma, St Louis, Mo, USA) is added to stop further action of trypsin.

The epidermis and the dermis are separated with the help of a pair of non-toothed forceps **(Fig. 11)**. Dermis is then transferred into a tube containing mealanocyte medium and the adherent cells are separated. Dermal tissue is then discarded. The medium used is Dulbecco's Modified Eagles Medium (DMEM) with F-12 nutrient mixture,1:1 v/v and a 15 mmole/L HEPES Buffer system (Sigma, St Louis, Mo, USA). Simple Phosphate Buffer Saline can also be used in place of DMEM.

The epidermis is broken down into multiple small pieces and washed in the media and the basal cells were separated. The epidermal pieces are then discarded. The media along with the cells is centrifuged at 2000 rpm for 10 minutes. A cell pellet rich in melanocyte and basal keratinocytes is formed at the bottom of the tube **(Fig. 12)**. The supernatant is discarded and the pellet is re-suspended in a total volume of 0.8 mL of fresh medium in a 1 mL syringe.

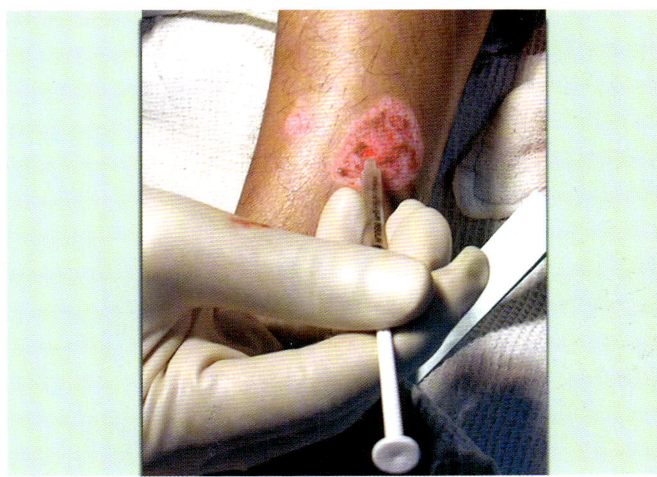

Fig. 13: Application of cell suspension over the dermabraded area

Transplantation: The recipient area is cleaned with povidone iodine and alcohol. Under local anesthesia, using a high speed diamond fraise dermabrader or carbon dioxide laser, the recipient area is abraded down to the dermoepidermal junction. The cell suspension is evenly applied with the syringe and spread out with its tip over the recipient area **(Fig. 13)**. Cells are covered with a thin transparent collagen film. This is then covered with a sterile pad and finally with Tegaderm (3M) dressing. The patient is sent home under antibiotic coverage and the dressings are removed after a week. The various stages of the procedure is given in **Figures 14A to H**.

Surgical outcome: The onset of pigmentation usually occurs in 3-6 weeks and it is complete in 2 to 6 months time **(Figs 15 to 17)**. The pigmentation is uniform with good textural and cosmetic color match. The method preformed is much simpler than culture based techniques and less time consuming. It does not require expensive culturing conditions and high-

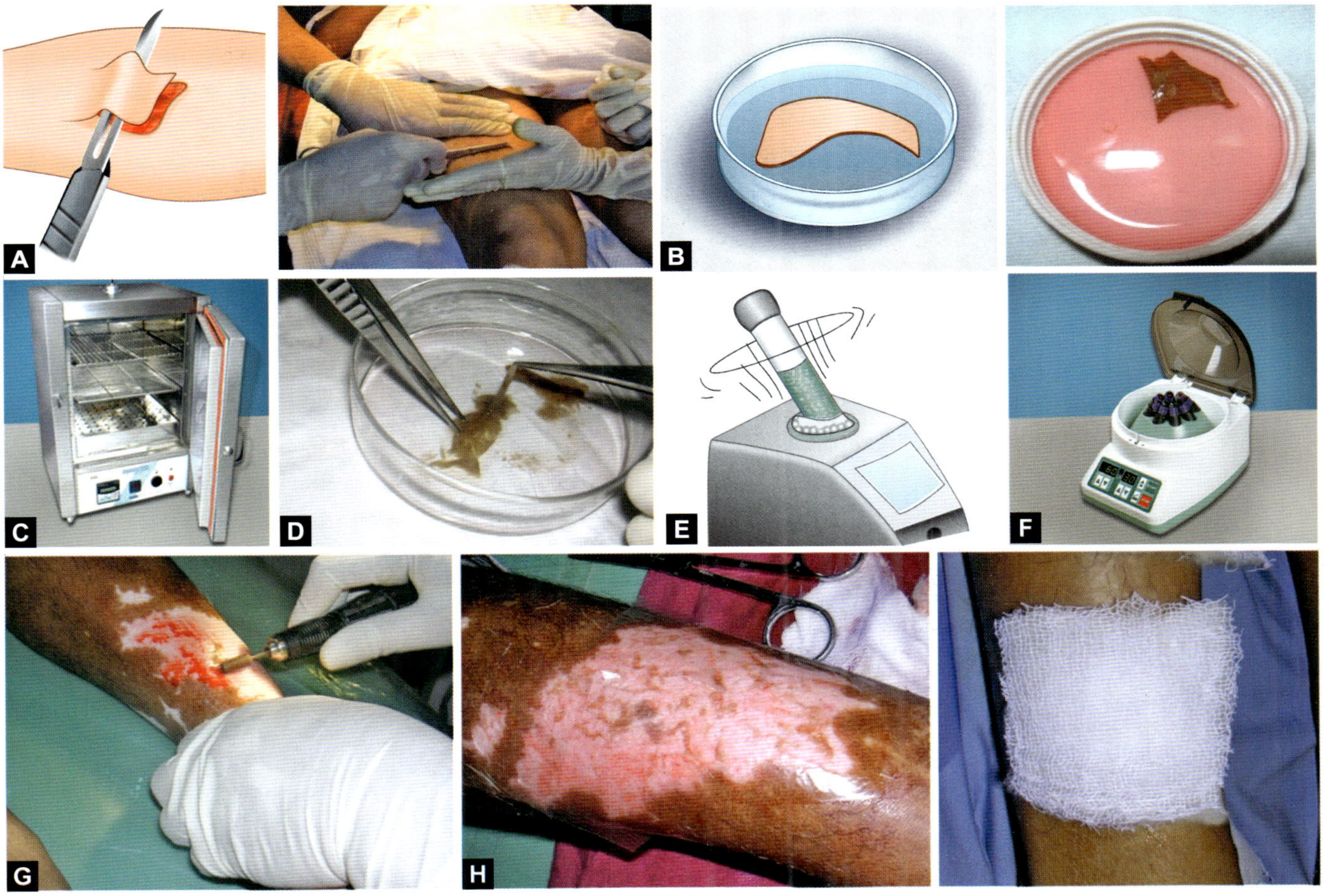

Figs 14A to H: Steps of noncultured epidermal cell suspension

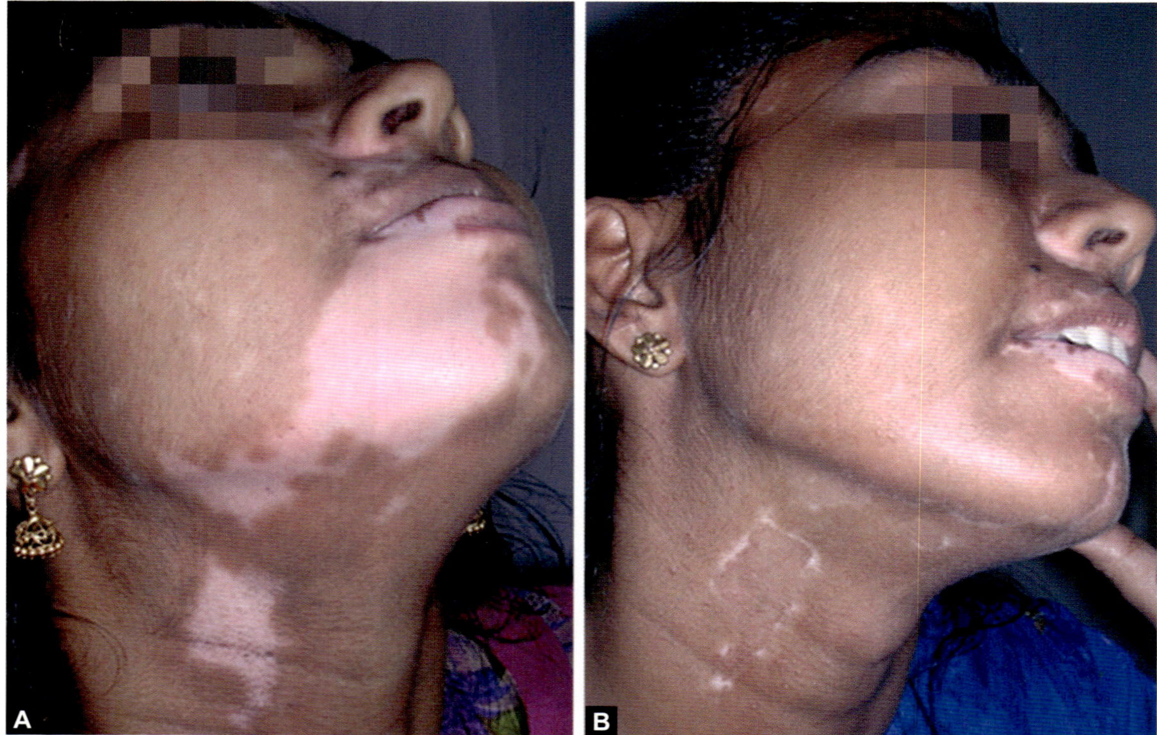

Figs 15A and B: (A) Segmental vitiligo before NECS; (B) Repigmentation after 2 months

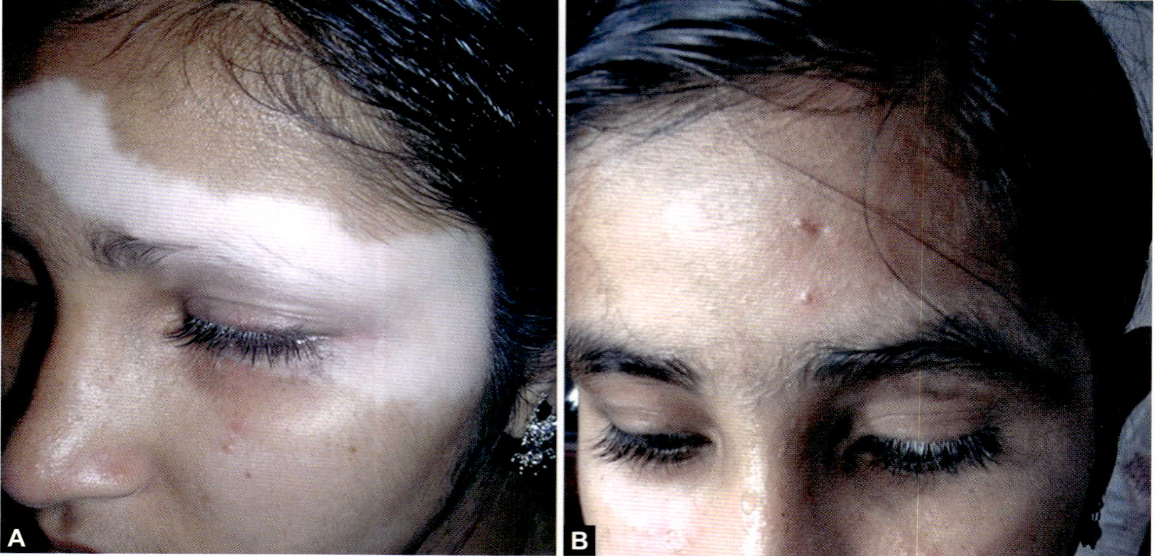

Figs 16A and B: (A) Segmental vitiligo with leukotrichea before NECS; (B) After 2 years. Note the improvement in leukotrichea

tech laboratories; but still requires trained personals familiar with cell separation to get an optimal survival rate of cells. Cell separation can be done under sterile conditions in the operating room itself. Key features of NECS are given in **Table 6**.

Hair Follicle Cell Suspension (HFCS)

This is an emerging area of noncultured cellular grafting technique in vitiligo. Cui J et al.[38] has proved the role of hair follicle in the pigmentation of the vitiliginous lesion. Inactive

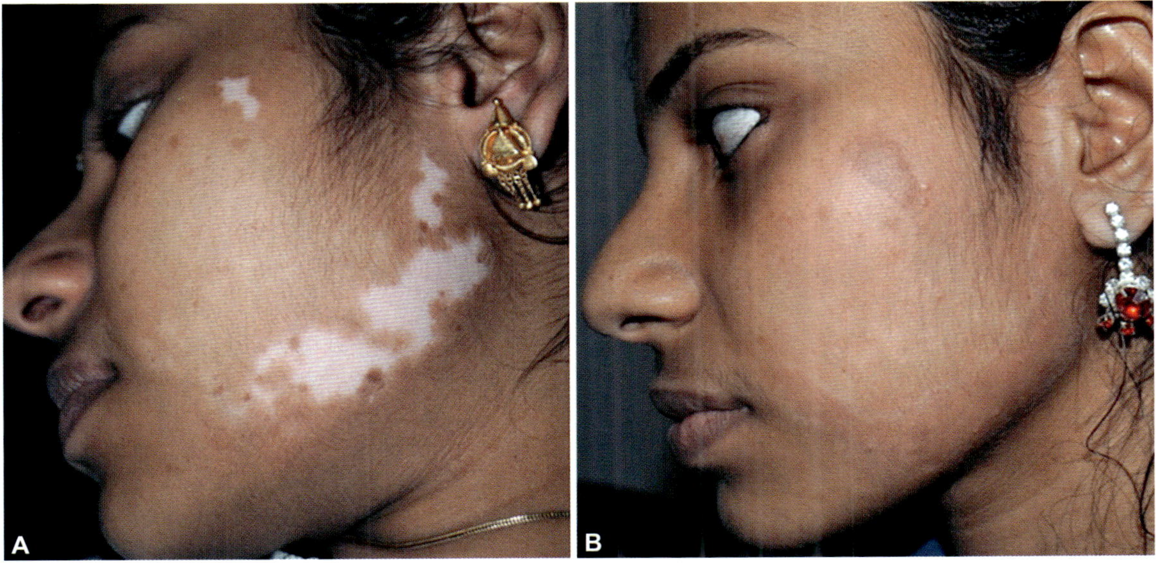

Figs 17A and B: (A) Segmental vitiligo before follicular cell transplantation; (B) 3 months after the surgery

Table 6: Advantages and disadvantages of noncultured epidermal cell suspension

Advantages
• Large area can be treated using a small skin sample. Donor recipient ratio 1:10 • Can be used in difficult areas like joints, pressure sites, mucosa, etc. • Faster, uniform pigmentation matching with adjoining skin • Does not need laboratory as the cell separation can be done in operating room itself • Day care procedure • Donor site pigments with minimal scaring
Disadvantages
• Requires specific cell culture grade biochemicals and media • The operating room has to be equipped with incubator, centrifuge and equipment for preparation of cell suspension • Surgical skill required to harvest adequate sized, thin grafts • Perilesional Halo seen in few cases

melanocytes or melanocyte stem cells are found to reside in the outer root sheath (ORS) and bulge areas of the hair follicle. These melanocytes did not produce melanin under normal conditions but became active to produce melanin when stimulated either by ultraviolet radiation or dermabrasion.[39] It was these melanocytes that were proposed to lead to repigmentation in vitiligo by dividing and migrating upward along the surface of hair follicle to the nearby epidermis where they continued to move radially and lead to repigmentation of surrounding skin as observed by Cui et al.[38]

Vaenscheidt et al.[40] in a small case series have used single cell suspension of 'plucked' hair follicles in the treatment of vitiligo. They found almost complete (>90%) repigmentation in 3 of 5 patients with vitiligo, around 50% repigmentation in one patient and less than 10% repigmentation in one patient. Mohanthy et al.[11] used follicular unit extraction followed by separation of melanocytes from ORS and transplantation in vitiligo patients with promising results.

Technique: Follicular unit extraction is done from the scalp using follicular extraction device or 1mm and 1.5 mm punches attached to micromotor. About 15-25 hair follicles are extracted. These are then trimmed and transferred to a petridish containing 10 mL of 0.25% of Trypsin EDTA solution. Three different incubations of 30 minutes at each at 37°C is required for cell separation. After each incubation, the hair is transferred to another pertridish containing DMEM and the separated cell are scraped. The cells fall into the DMEM. It is again transferred to Trypsin and incubated.

The cells are then concentrated by centrifugation and the cell pellet formed is resuspended in fresh medium. The cell suspension is spread over dermabraded reciepient area and covered with collagen sheet as in case of epidermal cell suspension technique. Postoperative care is same as in NCES.

Surgical outcome: The results are uniform with good color match as in case of NCES. Donor scaring is not evident since follicular extraction is done. 15-25 follicular units provide 25000–50000 cells comprising of a large number of melanocytes and heavily melanized keratinocytes, which is sufficient to treat up to 25 cm^2 of recipient area.[11] This procedure is a novel technique with good yield of melanocytes, melanocyte stem cells, and other stem cells like keratinocyte stem cells, and mesenchymal stem cells in the surrounding dermis. A recent randomized study on comparison between autologus noncultured extracted hair follicle outer root sheath cell suspension and autologous noncultured epidermal cell

Table 7: Comparison of noncultured epidermal cell suspension and follicular epithelial cells

Noncultured epidermal cell suspension	*Hair-follicle cell suspension*
• Easy to perform • Single incubation required • Melanocyte keratinocyte ration 1:36 • Load of melanocyte is less in comparison with HFCS • Skin melanocytes less influenced by age	• Follicular unit extraction and cellular suspension preparation is time consuming • Three incubations required • Melanocyte keratinocyte ration 1:1 to 1:6. • Load of melanocyte is much higher than NECS. Few hairs can yield large quantity of melanocyte. • Hair melanocyte undergo aging (graying)

Abbreviations: NCES, noncultured epidermal cell suspension; HFCS, hair follicle cell suspension.

Table 8A: Choice of method of surgery according to the area of involvement

Area involved	*First line surgical therapy*	*Second line surgical therapy*
Very large area	NCES, HFCS, CM, CE	-
Moderate	NCES, HFCS, STSG	PG
Small area	SBEG, STSG	PG
Site		
Face	NCES, HFCS, SBEG	STSG
Lips, genitals, eye lids	NCES, HFCS, SBEG	STSG, PG
Fingers and toes	PG, SBEG	NCES
Nipples and areola	SBEG, NCES, HFCS	
Palms and soles	PG	
Other areas like abdomen, legs	NCES, HFCS, CM, CE	PG

Abbreviations: NCES, noncultured epidermal cell suspension; HFCS, hair follicle cell suspension; CM, cultured melanocytes; CE, cultured epidermis; STSG, split-thickness skin grafting, SBEG, suction blister epidermal grafting; PG, punch grafting.

suspension revealed that both techniques were comparable in efficacy and safety. But the patient in NCES group was significantly more satisfied than the patients in HFCS group.[41]

One concern about the follicular melanocyte transplantation is the influence of aging. Hair graying is noticed as an age related phenomena in melanocytes. The future of the transplanted hair melanocytes in the skin can be predicted only through long term studies. The comparison of NCES and FECS is given in **Table 7**.

Culture Techniques

Melanocyte culture techniques are slowly moving out of vitiligo surgical scenario with the advent of less time consuming nonculture techniques yielding freshly prepared melanocytes. Moreover, culture techniques employed for the expansion of the cell number are time consuming, requires trained personals, expensive tissue culture laboratory and is not cost effective. In addition, the xenobiotic properties of some of the additives in the culture medium raise safety concerns.[42]

Cultured melanocytes (CM): Melanocytes are cultured *in vitro* for 15–30 days by the addition of media and growth factors. Once sufficient numbers are present, melanocytes are detached from the culture plates and suspension is transplanted onto the denuded recipient area in a density of 1000-2000 melanocytes/mm^2. The vitiliginous patch is dermabraded or laser abraded and cells suspension is applied.[32,42]

Cultured Epidermis (CE)

Basal cells separated by trypsinisation are seeded in a medium that allows co-cultivation of keratinocytes and melanocytes. A few weeks later, a cultured epidermal sheet is obtained, released by dispase and attached to petrolatum gauze. This is applied on a dermabraded recipient site.

Both the culture techniques are being replaced by nonculture techniques. The recent advances in cellular methods and their relatively easier availability have indeed brightened the outlook for vitiligo patients.

APPROACH TO SURGICAL MANAGEMENT OF VITILIGO

The choice of surgical intervention should be individualized according to the type of vitiligo, stability, localization of lesions, patient's attitude and requirements, facilities available, expertise of the surgeon and cost-effectiveness of the procedure. SBEG can yield outstanding results but has limitation of limited yield of graft. Cellular methods give the best cosmetically appealing results in treating larger area, but need more training and specific infrastructure. **Table 8A** summarizes the choice of method of surgery according to the area of involvement and **Table 8B** according to the surgical technique.[20]

In segmental vitiligo, especially associated with leucotrichea; surgical therapy can be the first line manage-ment. These cases rarely repigment with conventional medical treatments. Focal vitiligo can also be treated primarily by surgical methods with long lasting results. Surgical manage ment of acrofacial vitiligo and vitiligo vulgaris is complementary to the existing medical and physical modalities of treatments.

Table 8B: Choice of method of surgery according to the surgical technique

Technique	*Indications*
Punch grafting	Acral areas, palms and soles
Suction blister epidermal grafting	Mucosa, small area
Split-thickness skin grafting	Moderate area on skin
Noncultured epidermal cell suspension	All area can be treated
Hair follicle cell suspension	All area can be treated
Cultured melanocytes, cultured epidermis	All area can be treated

CONCLUSION

Vitiligo surgery have made major advances in techniques. Noncultured cellular grafting techniques, evolved from the culture techniques have outgrown from the cell culture laboratories. It is now possible to treat very large areas of vitiliginos patches with excellent cosmetic results in operating theatre settings. The improved techniques are able to encompass larger areas with better results at a substantially lower cost thus enabling us to reach a wider spectrum of the population.

ACKNOWLEDGMENT

The author sincerely thanks Dr S Prasannakumar (Calicut) for providing useful inputs.

REFERENCES

1. Spencer GA, Tolmach JA.Exchange grafts in vitiligo. J Invest Dermatol. 1952;19:1-5.
2. Olsson MJ, Juhlin L. Leukoderma treated by transplantation of basal cell layer enriched suspension. Br J Dermatol. 1998;138:644-8.
3. Falabella R. epidermal grafting: An original technique and its application in achromic and granulating areas. Arch Dermatol. 1971;104:592-600.
4. Behl PN. Homologous thin thiersch grafts in treatment of vitiligo. Curr Med Pract. 1964;8:218-21.
5. Orentriech N, Selmanwitz VJ. Autograft repigmentation of leucoderma. Arch Dermatol. 1972;105:734-6
6. Falabella R. Repigmentation of segmental vitiligo by autologus minigrafting. J Am Acad Dermatol. 1983;9:514-21.
7. Lerner AB, Halaban R, Leffell D. Melanocyte culture in patients with disorders of hypopigmentation. In: Programme abstracts of 14th International Pigment Cell Conference. Japan: The International Pigment Cell Soc; 1990. p. 100.
8. Olsson MJ, Juhlin L. Repigmentation of vitiligo by transplantation of cultured autologous melanocytes. Acta Derm Venereal (Stockholm). 1993;73:49-51.
9. Gauthier Y, Surleve-Brazeille JE. Autologous grafting with noncultured melanocytes: a simplified method for treatment of depigmentary lesions. J Am Acad Dermatol. 1992;26:191-4.
10. Olsson MJ, Juhlin L. Leukoderma treated by transplantation of basal cell layer enriched suspension. Br J Dermatol 1998;138:644-8.
11. Mohanty S, Kumar A, Dhawan J, Sreenivas V, Gupta, S. Non-cultured extracted hair follicle outer root sheath cell suspension for transplantation in vitiligo. Br J Dermatol 2011; DOI: 10.1111/j.1365-2133.2011.10234.x.
12. Falabella R, Arrunategui A, Barona MI, Alzate A. The minigrafting test for vitiligo: Detection of stable lesions for melanocyte transplantation. J Am Acad Dermatol. 1995;32:228-32.
13. Das SS, Pasricha JS. Punch grafting as a treatment of residual lesions of vitiligo. Indian J Dermatol Venereol Leprol 1992;58:315-9.
14. Falabella R, Escobar C, Borrero I. Treatment of refractory and stable vitiligo by transplantation of in vitro cultured epidermal autografts bearing melanocytes. J Am Acad Dermatol. 1992;26:230-6.
15. Savant SS. Autologous miniature punch grafting in vitiligo. Indian J Dermatol Venereol Leprol. 1992;58:310-4.
16. Jha AK, Pandey SS, Shukla VK. Punch grafting in vitiligo. Ind J Dermatol Venerol Leprol. 1992;58:328-30.
17. Boersma BR, Westerhof W, Bos JD. Repigmentation in vitiligo vulgaris by autologous minigrafting: Results in nineteen patients. J Am Acad Dermatol. 1995;33:990-5.
18. Falabella R. Grafting and transplantation of melanocytes for repigmenting vitiligo and other types of leukoderma. Int J Dermatol. 1989;28:363-9.
19. Falabella R. Surgical treatment of vitiligo: Why, when and how. J Eur Acad Dermatol Venereol. 2003;17:518-20.
20. Parsad D, Gupta S. Standard guidelines of care for vitiligo surgery. Indian J Dermatol Venereol Leprol. 2008;74:37-45.
21. Njoo MD, Das PK, Bos JD, Westerhof W. Association of the Kobner phenomenon with disease activity and therapeutic responsiveness in vitiligo vulgaris. Arch Dermatol 1999; 135:407-13.
22. Gupta S, Kumar B. Epidermal grafting in vitiligo: Influence of age, site of lesion, and type of disease on outcome. J Am Acad Dermatol. 2003;49:99-104.
23. Savant SS. Surgical therapy of vitiligo: Current status. Indian J Dermatol Venereol Leprol. 2005;71:307-10.
24. Savant SS. Miniature punch grafting. In: Savant SS (Ed). Association of scientific cosmetologists and dermatosurgeons textbook of dermatosurgery and cosmetology, 2nd edn. Mumbai: ASCAD; 2005. pp. 359-69.
25. Burm JS. Simple suction device for autologous epidermal grafting. Plast Reconstr Surg. 2000;106:1225-6.

26. Gupta S, Shroff S. Modified technique of suction blistering for epidermal grafting in vitiligo. Int J Dermatol. 1999;38: 306-9.
27. Albert S, Srinivas CR, Shenoi SD, Pai Sathish, Sabitha L. Phototoxic blister induction in vitiligo surgery. British Journal Dermatol. 1999;141:30-31.
28. Hann SK, Im S, Bong HW, Park YK. Treatment of stable vitiligo with autologous epidermal grafting and PUVA. J Am Acad Dermatol. 1995;32:943-8.
29. Khunger N. Thin split-thickness skin grafts for vitiligo. In: Gupta S, et al. editors. In surgical management of vitiligo. Blackwell Publishing Ltd; 2007. pp. 108-14.
30. Kahn AM, Cohen MJ. Repigmentation in vitiligo patients. Melanocyte transfer via ultra thin grafts. Dermatol Surg. 1998;24:365-7.
31. Njoo MD, Westerhof W, Bos JD, Bossuyt PMM. A systematic review of autologous transplantation methods in vitiligo. Arch Dermatol. 1998;134:1543-9.
32. Mysore V, Salim T. Cellular grafts in management of leucoderma. Indian J Dermatol. 2009;54:142-9.
33. Bahadoran P OJ-P. Classification of surgical therapies for vitiligo. In: Gupta S, Olsson M, Kanwar A, Ortonne JP, (Eds) Surgical Management of Vitiligo. Oxford: Blackwell Publishing; 2007. pp. 59-68.
34. Lontz W, Olsson MJ, Moellmann G, et al. Pigment cell transplantation for treatment of vitiligo: a progress report. J Am Acad Dermatol. 1994;30:591-7.
35. Falabella R. Surgical approaches for stable vitiligo. Dermatol Surg. 2005;31:1277-84.
36. Ongenae K, van Geel N, Naeyaert JM. Autologous cellular suspensions and sheets in the treatment of achromic disorders: the need for future controlled studies. Dermatology. 2001;202:158-61.
37. Olsson MJ, Juhlin L. Leucoderma treated by transplantation of a basal cell layer enriched suspension. Br J Dermatol. 1998;138:644-8.
38. Cui J, Shen LY, Wang GC. Role of hair follicles in the repigmentation of vitiligo. J Invest Dermatol. 1991;97:410-6.
39. Staricco RG, Miller-Milinska A. Activation of the amelanotic melanocytes in the outer root sheath of the hair follicle following ultraviolet rays exposure. J Invest Dermatol. 1962; 39:163-4.
40. Geel NV. A Review of Non-cultured Epidermal Cellular Grafting in Vitiligo. Journal of Cutaneous and Aesthetic Surgery. 2011;4:17-22.
41. Singh. C, Parsad. D*, Kanwar, AJ, Dogra S, Kumar R, Br J Dermatol. 2013 Mar 21. doi: 10.1111/bjd.12325. Comparison between autologus noncultured extracted hair follicle outer root sheath cell suspension and autologous non cultured epidermal cell suspension in the treatment of stable vitiligo: a randomized study. [Epub ahead of print]
42. Czajkowski R, Placek W, Drewa T, Kowaliszyn B, Sir J, Weiss W. Autologous cultured melanocytes in vitiligo treatment. Dermatol Surg. 2007;33:1027-36.

28

Autologous Mini Punch Grafting in Vitiligo

Koushik Lahiri

Key Features

- Minigrafting in vitiligo remains the easiest, fastest and cheapest of all surgical options in vitiligo.
- If deployed properly, it can produce excellent result.
- Stability must be assured before opting for surgical options in vitiligo.
- Optimal punch sizes are 1 mm, 1.2 mm and 1.5 mm. Punch sizes more than 1.5 mm are to be avoided.
- Cobblestoning and polka dotting remain the main complication if larger punches are used.
- Phototherapy, after minigrafting evokes encouraging results.

HISTORICAL PERSPECTIVE

Vitiligo is the most significant form of cutaneous achromia which is an illusive, if not enigmatic problem down the ages. In all the ancient civilizations and religions, there is some reference to vitiligo. In the *Rigveda,* it was referred to as '*Kilas*' meaning a white spotted deer. It is interesting to note that as per a Vedic myth the anthropomorphic adoration of the sun, Bhagavantam, developed vitiligo after being gazed upon by his illegitimate son.[1] The disease was mentioned in '*Tarkh-e-Tibbl-e-Iran*' in the period of the *Aushooriyan*, as early as 2200 BC. In 1550 BC, information regarding vitiligo was noted in the Ebers Papyrus.[2] Unfortunately in some of the prominent ancient texts, the disease was confused with leprosy and also other skin diseases like psoriasis. This was referred to as *Swethakushtha* (white leprosy) in the *Atharba Veda* (1400 BC).[3] An accurate description also exists in a collection of Japanese Shinto prayers, Amarakosa, dating from 1200 BC.[4] In the Old Testament, the white spots were also described in Verse 2 of Chapter 13 of Leviticus under the Hebrew word *Zora at* or *Tzaraat/Tzoraath. Tsoraath* was translated using the Greek word "Lepros," which means a scale or scales. Along with this the phonetic resemblance of the word *Tsoraath* (which in Ashkenazi pronunciation would read *tsoraas*) led to the belief that 'leprosy' was psoriasis. In truth, in all likelihood, most cases of biblical 'leprosy' were achromic or hypochromic disorders that would include vitiligo, some cases of psoriasis, cases of pityriasis alba, probably albinism, and also leprosy. The word got translated as 'lepra' in the Greek and English translations of the Bible. Also the theory of vitiligo as a dirty/polluted/contaminated disease was initiated, as the word *Tzaraat* refers to a group of skin diseases, which according to the Old Testament, renders one ritually unclean.[5] The exact word 'Vitiligo' may have been derived from the Latin word *vitium* meaning 'blemish,' or possibly *vitulum* meaning 'small blemish.[5] Another theory is that the Latin derivation is from the white, glistening flesh of calves (vitelius). Others believe that the actual word was first used by Celsus in his tome De Medicina in the first century AD.[4,6,7] References to this disease can also be found in the ancient Koran and Buddhist scripts.[7] The treatment has undergone an enormous evolutionary change from the Vedic days of *Vasuchika* to the most modern transplantation techniques. However, the ultimate goal remains the same, which is, replenishment of lost pigment. Among all the techniques described for surgical management of vitiligo, mini punch grafting (MPG) is the easiest, fastest, least aggressive and minimal expensive technique. Since the dermatologist is familiar with the punch, this technique is easily learnt and is usually the first technique performed by a beginner.[8-22]

PUNCH INSTRUMENT

The skin punch or surgical punch is an instrument which is used almost exclusively by dermatologists. It is interesting to note that originally, it was used as a trephine to cut through the skull bone. Its use was documented in abscess removal from tibia as early as in 1852.[23] In 1878, Watson described its use in the correction of accidental gunpowder disfigurement.[24]

But it was EL Keyes in 1887, who first established the importance of punch instrument in dermatology.[25]

The Keyes punch **(Fig. 1)** has been used in dermatology since then for diagnostic purpose. Its rounded sharp cutting end and thick handle make it very much appropriate for small skin biopsies. Because of the thick walls with angled sides above the cutting edge, tissue tends to be pushed away as the punch is made, causing less dermis (in diameter) to be cut through than overlying epidermis. This is also a function of the bevel, which is outside the barrel of the Keyes punch.[26]

To overcome these difficulties, other punches have been developed.[27]

The walls of the Loo trephine **(Fig. 2)** are thinner and less slanted than those of the Keyes punch, making it advantageous to use on depressed scars or minor autotransplants (where a straight vertical incision is needed). This is difficult to do with Keyes punch.

The newer disposable punches **(Fig. 3)** are excellent for punch biopsies or excisional work on cysts. The razor-sharp edge is a great benefit. The punch is available in different dimensions.

For vitiligo surgery, now the consensus favors using miniature punches with smaller diameter of the cutting edge.

EVOLUTION OF MINI PUNCH GRAFTING

In the history of skin grafting, few observations can be mentioned as a preamble to further discussion on punch grafting (PG).

The first documented successful result of experimental skin grafting was described in sheep by Baronio in 1804.[28]

But it took almost another one and half century for the first autograft response of dark-skinned autografts transplanted to fair skin in spotted guinea pigs to be published by Lewin and Peck in 1941.[29]

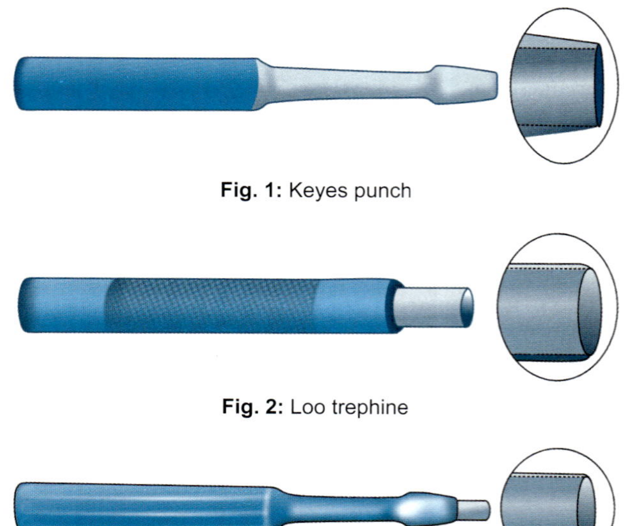

Fig. 1: Keyes punch

Fig. 2: Loo trephine

Fig. 3: Disposable punch

In 1972, Norman Orentriech first reported autograft repigmentation in humans. He treated a black woman with long-standing leukoderma that occurred after a chemical burn resulting from application of a home remedy, which included a copper penny dipped in vinegar for presumptive tinea infection on her cheek. Orentriech deployed nine 1 mm and 2 mm diameter normal skin autografts and observed the "pigment spread phenomenon". He reported a maximum of 1 mm pigment spread from both 1 mm and 2 mm grafts.[11]

In 1976, Labuono and Shatin made a similar observation after transplanting hair bulbs with hair PG within the leukodermic scars of discoid lupus erythematosus (DLE).[30]

Falabella in 1978 reported a novel method of repigmenting leukoderma. With the help of a power driven dermabrasion unit, he used dental burs to create abrasion 2–3 mm in diameter and less than 1 mm in depth and 5 mm apart. In the donor area, skin was raised by means of a curved needle and was sniffed off just below it to harvest 1–2 mm size minigrafts. He reported about 3 mm perigraft pigment spread by this technique. Three patients, one with piebaldism, another with chemical leukoderma and a third with postburn depigmentation were treated by this method.[12] He observed that this superficial split thickness grafts evoked a much better outcome than the full thickness hair PG by Labuono.

In the same article, interestingly, it was concluded that "true vitiligo is not treatable by transplantation of grafts of normally pigmented, autologous skin".[12]

Miniature punches on 1.5 mm diameter was used by Falabella while repigmenting three cases of segmental vitiligo in 1983.[13]

Behl (1995) expressed some reservation while commenting on Falabella's work on minigrafting and claimed better results with thin Thiersch grafting. In a rejoinder Falabella reiterated his faith on miniature PG and countered with his sets of reasons and logics in favor of PG.[31,32]

In the following years Falabella reported success with MPG in chemical leukoderma, postdermabrasion leukoderma, and focal and segmental vitiligo.[33-35]

While repigmenting stable leukoderma with autologous minigrafting, Falabella made an important observation regarding the relationship between the donor graft area and the area of surgical repigmentation and found that a 1 mm donor graft can originate a pigmented spot 25 times larger than its size.[33]

In 1995, it was Falabella again who combined epidermal grafting and minigrafting in treating vitiligo and piebaldism.[36]

Westerhof in 1994 reported success with PG in stable vitiligo and observed a maximum of 5 mm of pigment spread.[37] In the subsequent year (1995), Boersma stressed on the importance of proper selection of cases before minigrafting.[38]

Various studies point toward the high effectiveness of the procedure.[39-42] An assortment of different evaluation parameters of MPG has also evolved over the years.[43-45]

It has now been documented that MPG can be combined with narrowband ultraviolet B (NB-UVB) (311 nm) with encouraging results.[22]

TEST GRAFTING

Punch grafting is also used for determining stability.[46] The objectives of this test are:

- Establishing the stability of the depigmenting process
- Identifying patients who may respond to pigment cell transplantation.

In the original suggested procedure,[46] a few grafts (1.0–1.2 mm) were placed in the center of the depigmented lesion to be tested. Dressing was done by Micropore® adhesive tape and kept for a couple of weeks. After removal of the tape, the area was exposed to sunlight for 15 minutes daily for a period of 3 months. No treatment was permitted during this test period. All test sites are visualized under Wood's light. The test was considered positive if unequivocal repigmentation takes place beyond 1 mm from the border of the implanted grafts. On the other hand, if less than 1 mm or no repigmentation was observed, the test was considered as negative.

Test grafting (TG) has been found to be a more reliable exercise than the unreliable dependence on period of stability alone.[22,42,47]

PROCEDURE OF MINIGRAFTING[13,40-42] (FIG. 4)

After proper assessment of the stability status, routine physical examination and investigations, an informed consent is taken

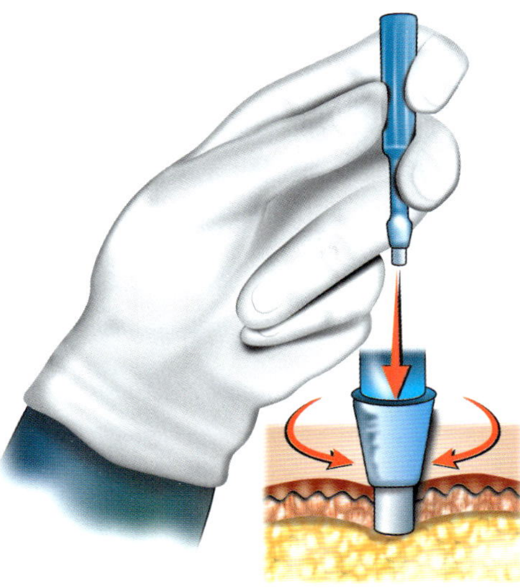

Fig. 4: Correct positioning of the hand while taking grafts with a miniature punch

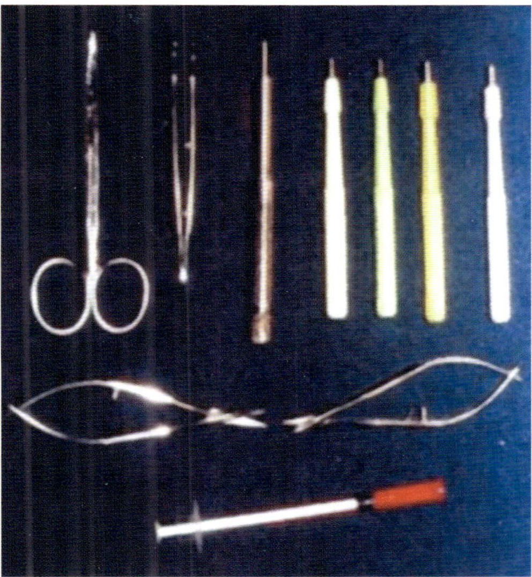

Fig. 5: Instrument required for minigrafting

from the patient. The donor and recipient areas are surgically prepared.

1. The instruments required are 1.5 mm or 1.2 mm punches, small jeweler's or graft holding forceps and small curved tip scissors **(Fig. 5)**.
2. Recipient area is prepared first. Two percent lignocaine with or without adrenaline is infiltrated as local anesthetic.
3. To minimize the chance of developing any perigraft halo, the initial recipient chambers are made on or very close to the border of the lesion. The punched out chambers are spaced according to the result of TG or at a gap of 5–10 mm from each other.
4. The donor area is either upper lateral portion of thigh or gluteal area. Punch impressions are made very close to each other so that from a small area maximum number of grafts can be taken.
5. Same sized punches are used for both donor and recipient area.
6. The grafts were placed directly from donor (buttock or upper thigh) to the recipient areas. This speeds up the procedure and lessens the chance of infection. Care is taken so that the graft edges are not folded, the tissue is not crushed or placed upside down. The needle of the syringe or the tip of the scissors is used for proper placement of grafts in the recipient chambers.
7. Hemostasis is achieved by pressing a saline soaked gauze piece over the area.
8. For the recipient area three layers of dressing from inside out: paraffin-embedded nonadherent sterile gauze (Jelonet®), sterile Surgipad® and bio-occlusive Micropore® **(Figs 6A to E)**.
9. For the donor area only Surgipad® and Micropore® are used.

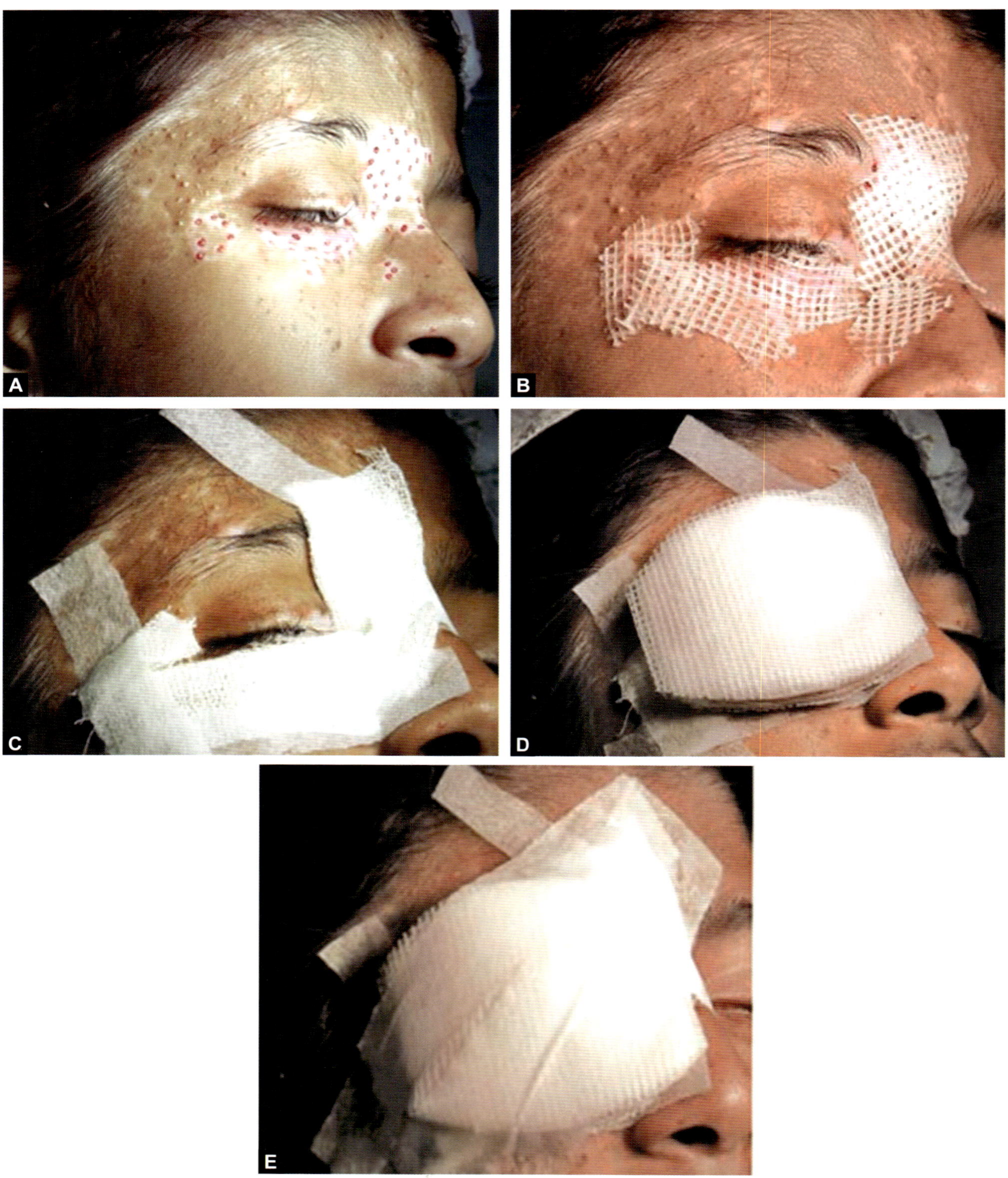

Figs 6A to E: Three layers of dressing from inside out: Paraffin-embedded nonadherent sterile gauze (Jelonet®), sterile Surgipad® and bio-occlusive Micropore®

10. The recipient area may be immobilized if necessary. Proper instructions for special areas like lips are necessary. To secure the recipient area, these patients are advised to take liquid diet for first 24 hours, preferably with a straw. Patients are allowed normal diet after this period.
11. Sometimes dressings are opened after 24 hours to look for any dislodgment of grafts, if found any, they are replaced.
12. Finally, after 4–7 days the dressings are removed.

FOLLOW-UP AND COURSE OF EVENTS

Postsurgically the patients are exposed to psoralen plus ultraviolet A (PUVA)[17,18] or psoralen plus ultraviolet A from solar radiation (PUVASOL)[41,42] or NB-UVB[22] or even kept as such in some studies.[42] The patients are followed up fortnightly for initial 2 months and then monthly up to complete repigmentation is achieved.

In the donor site, after healing with secondary intention, minimal superficial scarring is expected and acceptable.

Scabs may fall off from the recipient site within 7–14 days. Though in many instances there may not be any scab formation. Perigraft repigmentation is expected to start around 3–4 weeks.[22,41-43]

The entire depigmented and grafted area is expected to be completely repigmented within 3–6 months, based on the area of grafting and body part involved.

Minigrafting can be deployed on any parts of the body **(Figs 7 to 11)**.

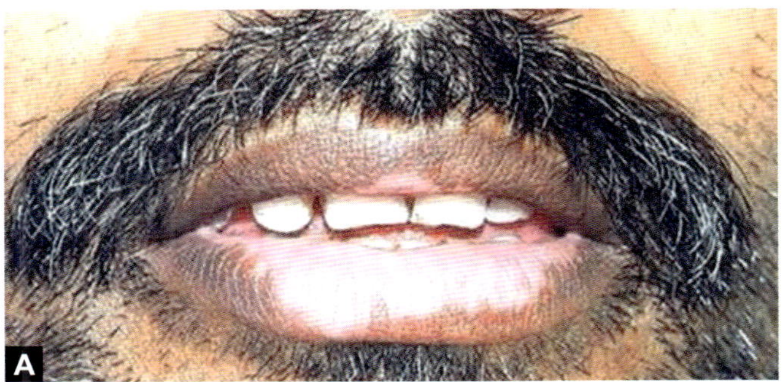

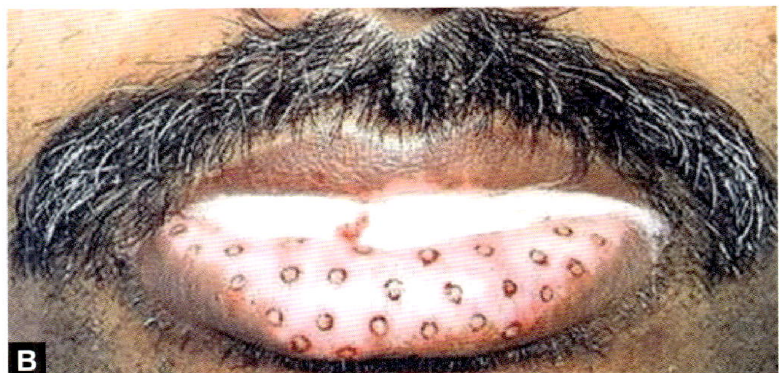

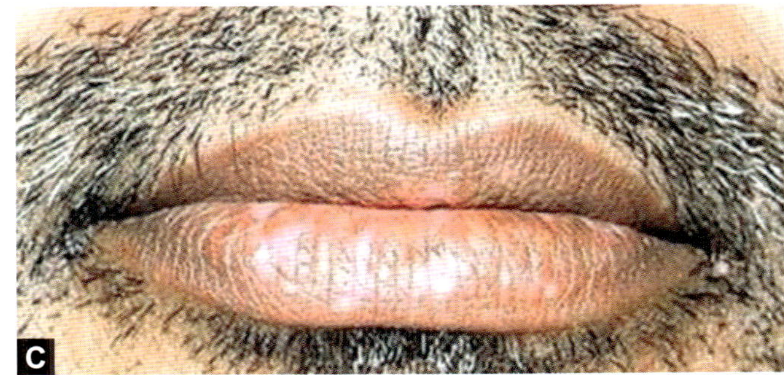

Figs 7A to C: (A) Lip vitiligo; (B) Correct positioning of graft; (C) Excellent repigmentation after 9 months

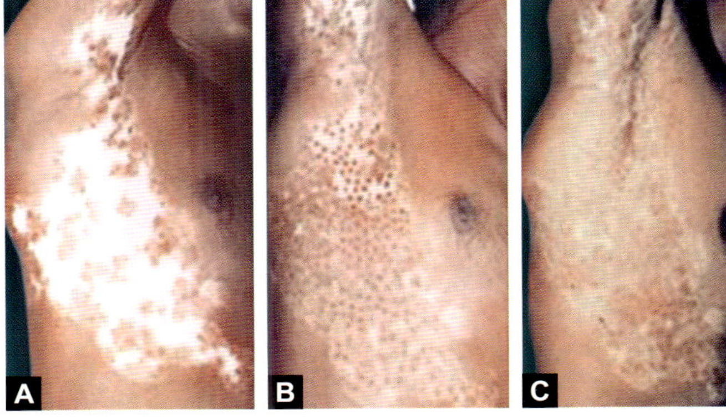

Figs 8A to C: (A) Large segmental vitiligo; (B) After second session of minigrafting; (C) Complete repigmentation after 6 months

COMPLICATIONS[22,40-42]

Complications are seen in PG frequently and are enumerated in **Table 1**. By proper selection of cases and with proper technique, most of these complications are entirely avoidable. Cobblestoning is regarded as the most common of them all.[22,41,42,47] It was observed that with time it got corrected in most of the cases.[41] In resistant cases, corrective electrofulguration may be needed.[48]

It can be avoided by avoiding punches more than 1.5 mm in diameter. On face and lips, it should be even smaller (1.2 or 1 mm).[22]

Rejection of grafts is another complication, particularly seen in herpes labialis-induced lip leukoderma.[49-52]

ANALYSIS OF SPECIAL FEATURES

Among all surgical methods, autologous miniature PG has established its place as the easiest means of vitiligo surgery. When the graft is taken off, the piece of tissue is completely detached from the donor site and then it is placed on the

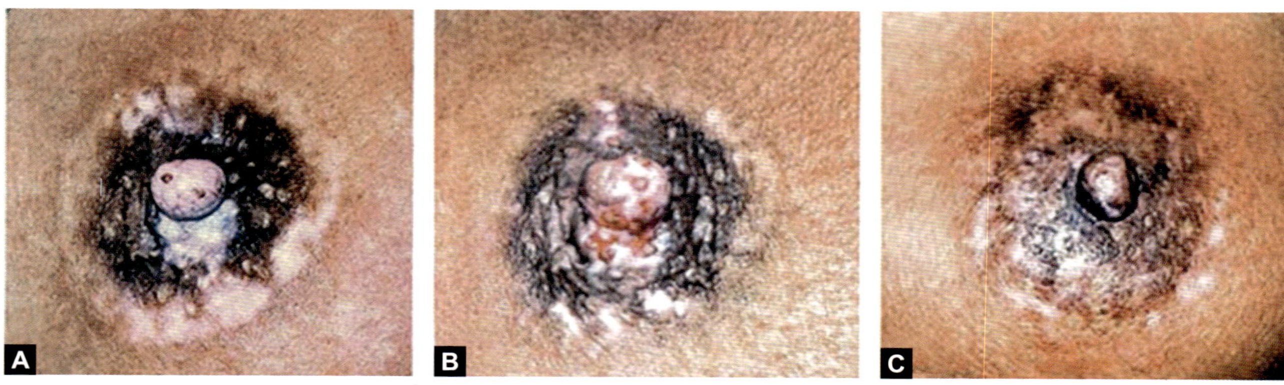

Figs 9A to C: (A) Depigmented right nipple and areola with two test grafts on nipple; (B) More grafts are placed on areola and nipple; (C) Almost complete repigmentation

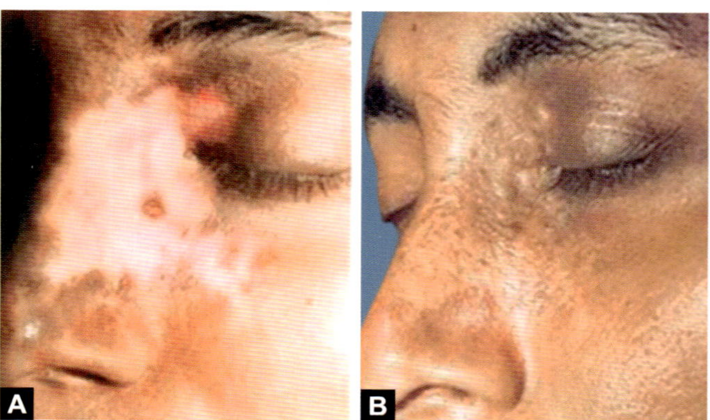

Figs 10A and B: (A) Segmental vitiligo on side of the nose; (B) Complete repigmentation after 5 months

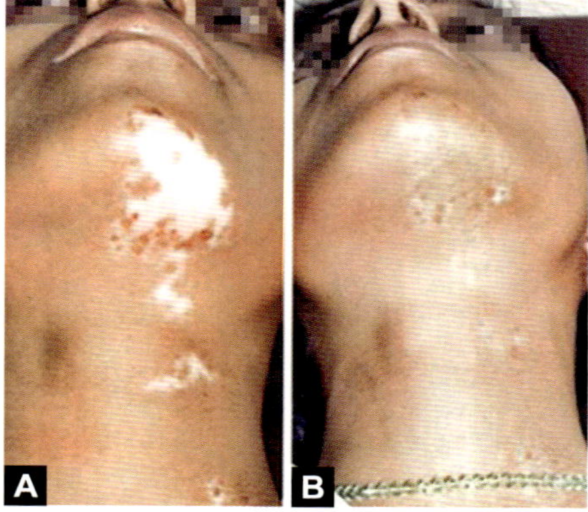

Figs 11A and B: (A) Segmental vitiligo on neck; (B) Complete repigmentation after 7 months

vascular bed in the recipient holes. From this vascular bed it derives its blood supply. Initially the graft adheres to its new bed by fibrin. There is diffusion of nutrients through this fibrinous layer which keeps the graft alive initially. Within 2–3 days, capillary linkage occurs with vascularization of the graft. The thinner the graft the denser the capillary network in the superficial dermis and thus earlier is the process of vascularization.[53] Several aspects of PG need special consideration:

- *Mechanism of pigmentation of grafting procedures*: The mechanism of pigmentation of grafting procedures has been studied in several studies. Melanocytes have been shown to spread centrifugally from the infundibulum of hair follicle to the basal cell layer and recolonize the epidermis with active and functional melanocytes.[54,55] The presence of pilosebaceous apparatus within the grafts is not at all necessary for the repigmentation process; suction blister grafts possess only epithelial cells and still achieve repigmentation.[56] Billingham and Silvers demonstrated the phenomenon of melanocytes migration from graft's edge within the achromic skin to recolonize and replenish the area with functional and active melanocytes.[57]
- *Relapse after grafting*: The major limitation of all grafting techniques is lack of specific criteria for defining

Table 1: Complications of minigrafting

Recipient site	*Donor site*
• Cobblestoning **(Fig. 12)** • Polka dot • Variegated appearance and color mismatch • Static graft (no pigment spread) • Depigmentation of graft **(Fig. 12)** • Perigraft halo • Graft dislodgment/rejection • Hypertrophic scar and keloid formation	• Keloid • Hypertrophic scar • Superficial scar **(Fig. 13)** • Depigmentation/spread/ activation of disease • Contact dermatitis to adhesive tapes

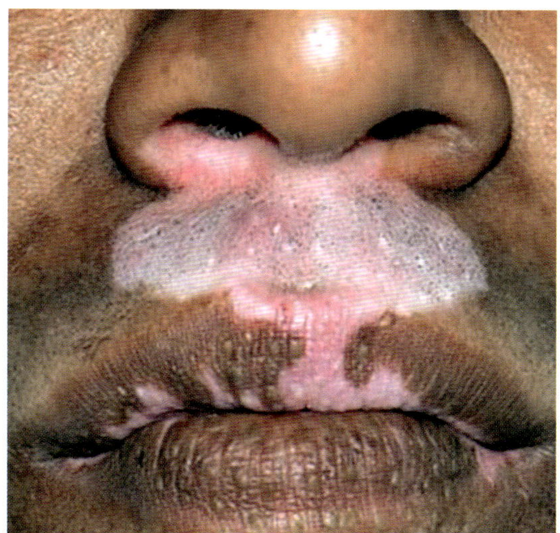

Fig. 12: Cobblestoning on lips and depigmentation of grafts on moustache area

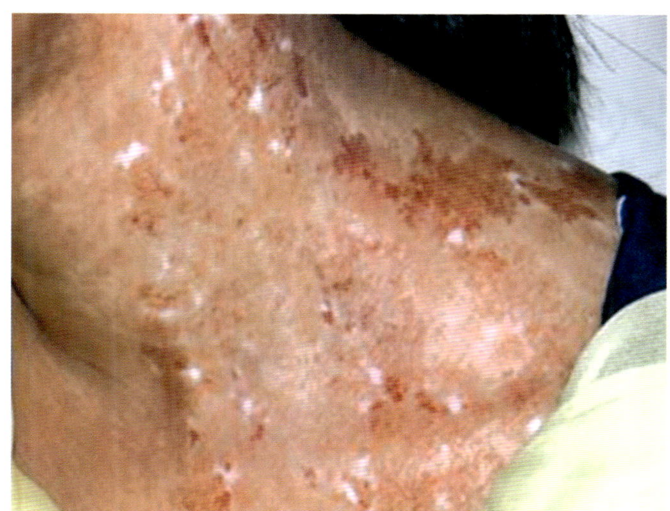

Fig. 13: Variegated appearance

Table 2: Maximum grafted area in different studies

Author (Reference)	*Year*	*Maximum grafted area (cm²)*
Jha AK, et al.[59]	1992	15
Das SS, et al.[58]	1992	80
Boersma BR, et al.[38]	1995	96
Malakar S, et al.[42]	1999	>100
Falabella R[35]	1988	110
Lahiri K, et al.[41]	1997	144

Figs 14A and B: (A) Segmental vitiligo with leukotrichia; (B) Complete repigmentation with resolving cobblestoning and repigmentation of leukotrichia

Table 3: Size of graft in different studies

Author (Reference)	*Year*	*Size of punch (diameter in mm)*
Das SS, et al.[58]	1992	4
Jha AK, et al.[59]	1992	3 and 4
Boersma BR, et al.[38]	1995	2
Lahiri K, et al.[41]	1997	2
Malakar S, et al.[42]	1999	2
Malakar S, et al.[47]	2004	1.5
Falabella R[35]	1988	1.2
Orentriech N, et al.[11]	1972	1 and 2

Table 4: Appearance of repigmentation (AOR) time in different studies

Author (Reference)	*Year*	*Earliest AOR (in days)*
Lahiri K, et al.[22]	2006	14
Lahiri K, et al.[41]	1997	14
Malakar S, et al.[42]	1999	16
Savant SS[39]	1992	30

stability.[58-60] It is often hard to predict how long the disease will remain stable. Similarly, it is difficult to envisage when it will start to become unstable.[61,62] This fact has made assessment of results difficult. Treatment of relapsed cases is considered difficult. However, repigmentation has been successfully induced in previous graft failure cases under NB-UVB (311 nm) phototherapy.[63]

- The author has reported curious phenomenon reverse Koebner's phenomenon after PG; spontaneous repigmentation of distant non-grafted vitiligo patches after PG.[64-66] It was attributed to possible release of cytokines from grafts.
- Size of the grafted lesion varied between 15 cm^2 and 144 cm^2 in different studies **(Table 2)**. Likewise the size of the punch instrument differed in different studies **(Table 3)**. But now the consensus is toward using smaller punches like 1.2 mm or 1.5 mm. Falabella even recommends 1 mm grafts for facial region and 1.2 mm for other body parts.[67,51]
- Treatment of leukotrichia is difficult and is not generally corrected by grafting. However, recently repigmentation of leukotrichia with PG and NB-UVB[22] and PUVASOL[68] was reported **(Figs 14A and B)**.[68]
- *Appearance of repigmentation time*: Another important parameter is the postgraft appearance of repigmentation (AOR) time. It was found to be between 2 weeks and 6 weeks in different studies **(Table 4)**. After PG and PUVASOL, AOR time in different regions varied between 14 days and 39 days, with an overall average being approximately 21.6 days as shown in one study.[41] With the deployment of NB-UVB along with PG AOR time in different regions varied between 14 days and 32 days, with an overall average being approximately 20.6 days.[22] Falabella found that a 1 mm donor graft can repigment an area 25 times larger than the graft itself.[33] In a recent study with 1.5 mm grafts and NB-UVB in type IV and V skin type subjects, this value was found to be more than double of that (56.21 times).[22] Previously in one study with PUVASOL, this relationship was found to be 42 times.[45]

CONCLUSION

Considering all the indicators and parameters, it can be concluded that minigrafting is an easy, inexpensive, effective method of treating stable and recalcitrant vitiligo.[69] The advantages and disadvantages are summarized in **Box 1**.

Box 1

Advantages and disadvantages of minigrafting

Advantages
- Easiest, fastest and least expensive method
- Can be performed any where on any site (except angle of the mouth)
- Particularly suitable for areola
- It is perhaps the only suitable method for palm, though results may not be fully satisfactory

Disadvantages
- Side effects are common, particularly cobblestoning
- Phototherapy is always necessary after grafting
- Perfect match does not occur

ACKNOWLEDGMENTS

Some Figures and Tables used in this chapter have also been used in the following chapter and chapters by me and my coauthors. With the permission of the concerned editors and publisher, I would like to properly acknowledge the original source:

- Lahiri K, Malakar S, Sarma N, et al. Repigmentation of vitiligo with punch grafting and narrow-band UV-B (311 nm)—a prospective study. Int J Dermatol. 2006;45(6):649-55.
- Malakar S, Lahiri K. Spontaneous repigmentation in vitiligo: why it is important? Int J Dermatol. 2006;45(4): 478-9.
- Malakar S, Lahiri K. Mini grafting for vitiligo. In: Gupta S, Olsson MJ, Kanwar AJ, Ortonne JP (Eds). Surgical Management of Vitiligo, 1st edn. Oxford: Blackwell Publishing; 2007. pp. 87-95.
- Lahiri K. Evolution and evaluation of autologous mini punch grafting in vitiligo. Indian J Dermatol. 2009; 54(2):159-67.
- Lahiri K. Autologous Mini Punch Grafting in Vitiligo. In: M Venkatram (Ed): ACSI Textbook of Vitiligo Surgery, 1st edn. New Delhi: Jaypee Brothers Medical Publishers, 2012.

REFERENCES

1. Millington GW, Levell NJ. Vitiligo: the historical curse of depigmentation. Int J Dermatol. 2007;46(9):900-5.
2. Ebbel B. The Papyrus Ebers. Copenhagen. Levin and Muntisgaard; 1937.
3. Whitney MD. Atharvaveda Samhita (Translation and notes). Harvard Oriental series, volume 7, Lannman, Cambridge: Harvard University Press; 1905.
4. Nair BK. Vitiligo—a retrospect. Int J Dermatol. 1978;17(9): 755-7.
5. Freilich AR. Tzaraat—biblical leprosy. J Am Acad Dermatol. 1982;6(1):131-4.
6. Mercurialis H. De morbidis cutaneis et omnibus corporis humani excrementis tractatus. Venezia. Paulus et Antonium Meietos; 1572.
7. Sutton RL. On definition of vitiligo. Arch Dermatol. 1965;91:288.
8. Ortonne JP, Mosher DB, Fitzpatrick TB. Vitiligo and Other Hypomelanoses of Hair and Skin. New York: Plenum Medical; 1983.
9. Behl PN. Homologous thin Thiersch's grafts in treatment of Vitiligo. Curr Med Pract. 1964;8:218-21.
10. Falabella R. Epidermal grafting: an original technique and its application in achromic and granulating areas. Arch Dermatol. 1971;104(6):592-600.
11. Orentriech N, Selmanwitz VJ. Autograft repigmentation of leucoderma. Arch Dermatol. 1972;105(5):734-6.

12. Falabella R. Repigmentation of leukoderma by minigrafts of normally pigmented, autologous skin. J Dermatol Surg Oncol. 1978:4:916-9.
13. Falabella R. Repigmentation of segmental vitiligo by autologous minigrafting. J Am Acad Dermatol. 1983;9:514-21.
14. Lerner AB, Halaban R, Klaus SN, et al. Transplantation of human melanocytes. J Invest Dermatol. 1987;89:219-24.
15. Lerner AB. Repopulation of pigmented cells in patients with vitiligo. Arch Dermatol. 1988;124(11):1701-2.
16. Falabella R, Escobar C, Borrero I. Treatment of refractory and stable vitiligo by transplantation of *in vitro* cultured epidermal autografts bearing melanocytes. J Am Acad Dermatol. 1992;26(2 Pt 1):230-6.
17. Skouge JW, Morison WL, Diwan RV, et al. Autografting and PUVA. A combination therapy for vitiligo. Dermatol Surg Oncol. 1992;18(5):357-60.
18. Hann SK, Im S, Bong HW, et al. Treatment of stable vitiligo with autologous epidermal grafting and PUVA. J Am Acad Dermatol. 1995;32(6):943-8.
19. Olsson MJ, Juhlin L. Repigmentation of vitiligo by transplantation of cultured autologous melanocytes. Acta Derm Venereol (Stockh). 1993;73:49-51.
20. Malakar S, Dhar S. Repigmentation of vitiligo patches by transplantation of hair follicles. Int J Dermatol. 1999;38(3):237-8.
21. Olsson MJ, Juhlin L. Long-term follow-up of leucoderma patients treated with transplants of autologous cultured melanocytes, ultrathin epidermal sheets and basal cell layer suspension. Br J Dermatol. 2002;147(5):893-904.
22. Lahiri K, Malakar S, Sarma N, et al. Repigmentation of vitiligo with punch grafting and narrow-band UV-B (311 nm)—a prospective study. Int J Dermatol. 2006;45(6):649-55.
23. Thompson CJ. The evolution and development of surgical instruments, IV: the trepan. Br J Surg. 1937;25:726.
24. Watson BA. Gunpowder disfigurements. St. Louis Med Surg J. 1878;35:145.
25. Keyes EL. The cutaneous punch by Edward L. Keyes (J Cutan Genitourin Dis, 1887). Arch Dermatol. 1982;118(11):940-2.
26. Hagerman D, Wilson H. The skin biopsy punch: evolution and modification. Cutis. 1970;6:1139.
27. Stegman SJ. Commentary: the cutaneous punch. Arch Dermatol. 1982;118(11):943-4.
28. Baronio G. Degli innesti animali, Stamperia e Fonderia del Genio. Milano, 1804.
29. Lewin ML, Peck SM. Pigment studies in skin grafts on experimental animals. J Invest Dermatol. 1941;4:504.
30. Labuono P, Shatin H. Transplantation of hair bulbs and melanocytes into leucodermic scars. J Dermatol Surg Oncol. 1976;2(1):53-5.
31. Behl PN. Repigmentation of segmental vitiligo by autologous minigrafting. J Am Acad Dermatol. 1985;12 (1 Pt 1):118-9.
32. Falabella R. Reply. J Am Acad Dermatol. 1985;12:119.
33. Falabella R. Repeigmentation of stable leucoderma by autologous minigrafting. J Dermatol Surg Oncol. 1986;12: 172-9.
34. Falabella R. Postdermabrasion leukoderma. J Dermatol Surg Oncol. 1987;13(1):44-8.
35. Falabella R. Treatment of localized vitiligo by autologous minigrafting. Arch Dermatol. 1988;124:1649-55.
36. Falabella R, Barona M, Escobar C, et al. Surgical combination therapy for vitiligo and piebaldism. Dermatol Surg. 1995; 21(10):852-7.
37. Westerhof W, Boersma B. Grafting techniques in leucoderma. Book of Abstract. 7th International Congress of Dermatology New Delhi, India; 1994.
38. Boersma BR, Westerhof W, Bos JD. Repigmentation in vitiligo vulgaris by autologous minigrafting: results in nineteen patients. J Am Acad Dermatol. 1995;33 (6):990-5.
39. Savant SS. Autologous miniatures punch grafting in vitiligo. Indian J Dermatol Venereol Leprol. 1992;58:310-4.
40. Malakar S. Punch grafting. An Approach to Dermatosurgery, 1st edn. Calcutta: A Paul; 1996. pp. 44-6.
41. Lahiri K, Sengupta SR. Treatment of stable and recalcitrant depigmented skin conditions by autologous punch grafting. Indian J Dermatol Venereol Leprol. 1997;63(1):11-4.
42. Malakar S, Dhar S. Treatment of stable and recalcitrant vitiligo by autologous miniature punch grafting: a prospective study of 1,000 patients. Dermatology. 1999;198(2):133-9.
43. Lahiri K, Sengupta SR. A regionwise comparative study of the extent of post punch graft surgical repigmentation in cutaneous achromia. Indian J Dermatol Venereol Leprol. 1998;64:173-5.
44. Lahiri K, Sengupta SR. A clinico-microscopic corroboration of surgical repigmentation—a study of 30 cases. Indian J Dermatol. 1998;43(3):99-101.
45. Lahiri K, Sengupta SR. Relationship between donor graft area and area of surgical repigmentation. Indian J Dermatol. 1999;44(1)11-4.
46. Falabella R, Arrunategui A, Barona MI, et al. The minigrafting test for vitiligo: detection of stable lesions for melanocyte transplantation. J Am Acad Dermatol. 1995;32:228-32.
47. Malakar S, Lahiri K. Punch grafting for lip leucoderma. Dermatol. 2004;208(2):125-8.
48. Malakar S, Lahiri K. Electrosurgery in cobblestoning. Indian J Dermatol. 2000;45(1):46-7.
49. Malakar S, Dhar S. Rejection of punch grafts in three cases of herpes-simplex-induced lip leucoderma, caution and precaution. Dermatology. 1997;195(4):414.
50. Malakar S, Dhar S. Acyclovir can abort rejection of punch grafts in herpes-simplex-induced lip leucoderma. Dermatology. 1999;199(1):75.
51. Malakar S, Lahri K. Successful repigmentation of six cases of herpes labialis-induced lip leucoderma by micropigmentation. Dermatology. 2001;203(2):194.
52. Lahiri K, Malakar S, Sarma N. Herpes-simplex-induced lip leucoderma revisited. Dermatology. 2004;208(2):182.
53. Burge S, Rayment R. Free skin grafts. In: Simple Skin Surgery, Ist edn. Bombay. Blackwell Scientific Publications; 1986. pp. 71-84.

54. Parrish JA, Fitzpatrick TB, Shea C, et al. Photochemotherapy of vitiligo: use of orally administered psoralen and a high intensity long-wave ultraviolet light system. Arch Dermatol. 1976;112(11):1531-4.
55. Ortonne JP, Schmnitt D, Thivolet J, et al. PUVA-induced repigmentation of vitiligo, scanning electron microscopy of hair follicles. J Invest Dermatol. 1980;74(1):40-2.
56. Suvanprakorn P, Dee-Analap S, Pongsomboon CH, et al. Melanocyte autologous grafting for treatment of leukoderma. J Am Acad Dermatol. 1985;13(6):968-74.
57. Billingham RE, Silvers WK. Studies on the migratory behaviour of melanocytes in guinea pig skin. J Exp Med. 1970;131(1):101-17.
58. Das SS, Pasricha JS. Punch grafting as a treatment for residual lesions in vitiligo. Indian J Dermatol Venereol Leprol. 1992;58:315-9.
59. Jha AK, Pandey SS, Shukla VK. Punch grafting in vitiligo. Indian J Dermatol Venereol Leprol. 1992;58:328-30.
60. Singh KG, Bajaj AK. Autologous miniature skin punch grafting in vitiligo. Indian J Dermatol Venereol Leprol. 1995;61:77-80.
61. Malakar S, Lahiri K. How unstable is the concept of stability in surgical repigmentation of vitiligo? Dermatol. 2000;201: 182-3.
62. Lahiri K, Malakar S, Banerjee U, et al. Clinico-cellular stability of vitiligo in surgical repigmentation: an unexplored frontier. Dermatology. 2004;209:170-1.
63. Lahiri K, Malakar S. Inducing repigmentation by regrafting and phototherapy (311 nm) in punch failure cases of lip vitiligo—a pilot study. Indian J Dermatol Venereol Leprol. 2004;70:156-8.
64. Malakar S. Spontaneous repigmentation of vitiligo patches other than the grafted site. Indian J Dermatol. 1997;47(2):68-70.
65. Malakar S, Dhar S. Spontaneous repigmentation of vitiligo patches distant from the autologous skin graft sites: a remote reverse Koebner's phenomenon? Dermatology. 1998;197(3):274.
66. Malakar S, Lahiri K. Spontaneous repigmentation in vitiligo: why it is important. Int J Dermatol. 2006;45(4):478-9.
67. Falabella R. Surgical treatment of vitiligo: why, when and how. J Eur Acad Dermatol Venereol. 2003;17(5):518-20.
68. Malakar S, Dhar S. Repigmentation of leukotrichia over vitiligo patches after punch grafting. Indian J Dermatol Venereol Leprol. 1998;64(5):252-3.
69. Malakar S, Lahiri K. Mini grafting for vitiligo. In: Gupta S, Olsson MJ, Kanwar AJ, Ortonne JP (Eds). Surgical Management of Vitiligo, 1st edn. Oxford: Blackwell Publishing; 2007. pp. 87-95.

29

Meshed Split Skin Graft for Extensive Vitiligo

CR Srinivas, Reena Rai

Key Features

- Useful when the pigmented donor skin is limited.
- Meshing increases size of graft by 4 times.
- Meshing releases cytokines which enhance wound healing.

INTRODUCTION

Surgical treatment is indicated when vitiligo is stable. It is difficult to treat large depigmented areas surgically when it fails to respond to medical treatment. So, when the donor area is limited; donor skin has to be enlarged by meshing to cover a larger body surface area.

The skin is passed through a machine that makes small slits, which allows expansion similar to that in fish netting. In a meshed skin graft, the skin from the donor site is stretched to allow it to cover an area larger than itself. The size of the mesh varies in ratios from 1:1 to 1:6. Following mesh grafting, pigmentation occurs at the spaces between the mesh, which fill in with new epithelial skin growth. This technique enables large areas to be grafted when the pigmented donor skin is limited.[1]

TECHNIQUE

Instruments

Padgett dermatome: Electrically operated dermatome for harvesting. The thickness is adjustable in thousandths of an inch by setting pointer on calibrated scale.

Ampligreffe (Collin, France): Machine with a slightly inclined metal plate with spiral barrels which rotate and help to mesh the graft by rotating the handle.

Dermabrader: Kurtin wire planning brushes (Robbins).

Preoperative Workup

The patient's consent is obtained. The preoperative workup includes complete blood count, bleeding time, clotting time, prothrombin time, platelet count, blood sugar and screening for hepatitis B, venereal disease research laboratory (VDRL), human immunodeficiency virus (HIV), and fitness for general anesthesia.

Treatment of the Recipient and Donor Area before Surgery

On the vitiliginous areas 0.075% of 8-methoxy psoralen is applied and after 10 minutes the affected part is exposed to ultraviolet A (UVA) in full body phototherapy unit for two consecutive days before surgery. The dosage of UVA would depend on the type and thickness of skin; 10–14 J/cm^2 usually induces blisters over the vitiliginous skin; which facilitates easy removal of epidermis before grafting.[2]

Preoperative Preparation

Both donor and recipient sites are shaved and pre-medication as required for general anesthesia administered.

PROCEDURE

Harvesting

Povidone iodine is used to sterilize the donor and recipient sites at the beginning of the procedure. It is useful to lubricate the skin at the donor site with sterilized white petrolatum to facilitate easy gliding of the dermatome over the skin.

Under general anesthesia 0.0252 inch split thickness graft is harvested using electrically operated Padgett or Duvals dermatome. A Humby knife can also be used. The dermatome is held in the dominant hand of the operator at the 30–45° angle from the donor skin surface. Greater angulation of the dermatome leads to gouging or trenching of the donor site skin. With the non-operating hand providing traction behind the dermatome and the assistant providing traction in front of the dermatome, the dermatome is activated and advanced in a smooth, continuous motion over the skin and the graft is harvested, removed and gently washed to remove the lubricant and wrapped in a moistened saline sponge until it is ready to be used.

The donor site typically has numerous small punctuate bleeding spots with thin-to-intermediate thickness grafts; thicker grafts have fewer, larger bleeding points that bleed more briskly. Any exposure of fat indicates that excision of the graft was performed too deeply, probably because of incorrect assembly of the dermatome or error in technique.

Meshing

The graft is transferred to an Ampligreffe for meshing. The Ampligreffe contains a slightly inclined metal plate over which the graft is placed with the dermis facing upwards. One end of the graft is gently inserted between the spiral barrels of the Ampligreffe. The handle of the Ampligreffe is then rotated. This results in the graft passing between the two barrels which forms diamond shaped sieves or mesh in the graft. This increases the size to two or four times depending on the size of the sieve. Different Ampligreffe is used to obtain different size. We recommend 1:4 ratio expansions for vitiligo. This meshed skin with the dermal surface facing upward is spread on a non-adherent paraffin and framycetin gauze.

The vitiliginous skin with phototoxic erythema and blister is rubbed with saline-soaked gauze held between thumb and index finger to remove the epidermis. Areas of epidermis not removed by this procedure are dermabraded using Kurtins stainless steel wire planning brush (Robbin). Hemostasis is easily obtained if the phototoxic blister is well formed. If in the event a dermabrader is used, the bleeding is easily controlled by saline-soaked gauze piece within 4–5 minutes. The Sofratulle® with meshed skin is placed on the dermabraded area. Once the graft has been placed, the recipient site should be re-inspected for hemostasis. The grafts are kept in position by bandaging using saline-soaked gauze. Movement of muscles and joints may lead to displacement of the graft. So when large areas are to be grafted it is better to cut the graft into smaller sizes by cutting the Sofratulle® on which the graft has been placed. Since the graft is already meshed there is no risk of lifting up of the graft due to bleeding or oozing. Attention must be paid to placing the dermal side down, as the dermis and epidermis can appear very similar without close inspection in lighter-skinned individuals. Care should also be taken to prevent wrinkling or excessive stretching of the graft. The graft must then be secured in place to provide stability during initial adherence and healing. After grafting, Sofratulle® followed by saline-soaked gauze is placed to prevent drying. We have observed that chances of drying are greater when the humidity is less and this can be prevented by placing saline-soaked gauze over the Sofratulle®.

The dressing is placed to provide uniform pressure over the entire grafted area. These dressings are intended to immobilize the graft. Grafts placed on the extremities may be managed with elevation and compression dressing for the entire extremity distal to the graft to prevent edema. A plaster of Paris cast can be used over joints to immobilize the graft.

Donor Site Dressing

Donor site dressing in an aseptic way is crucial for a successful re-epithelialization of the donor site avoiding any morbidity secondary to infection or poor wound healing. A generous layer of absorbent gauze and soakage pads are put on top of this and bandaged in place with Crepe bandage securely. The donor site is inspected in 10–14 days, by which time the donor site usually re-epithelializes.

Postoperative Care

Adequate rest to the grafted area with antibiotics and anti-inflammatory drugs is given. Rapid re-epithelialization occurs and the dressing becomes loose after a week and it can easily be removed. The patient is advised to undergo phototherapy after 7–10 days.

CONCLUSION

Mesh grafts is useful in extensive vitiligo or in a convoluted surface where a graft might not adhere well. Meshing of the skin graft, also releases maximal amounts of cytokines favoring wound healing. There is a minimal risk of scarring at the donor site as very thin grafts are taken. The irregularity of pigmentation which is noticed following all surgical procedures is likely to improve in due course. This procedure is recommended when large areas have to be grafted and pigmented donor skin is limited.

REFERENCES

1. Albert S, Srinivas CR, Shenoi SD, et al. Phototoxic blister induction in vitiligo surgery. Br J Dermatol. 1998;138:644-8.
2. Srinivas CR, Rai R, Kumar PU. Meshed split skin graft for extensive vitiligo. Indian J Dermatol Venereol Leprol. 2004;70:165-7.

30

Therapeutic Guidelines in Vitiligo

Shyamanta Barua

Key Features

- Topical corticosteroids (TCS) can be advised for children and adults with limited, extrafacial involvement.
- Facial lesions can be treated as effectively and more safely by topical calcineurin inhibitors (TCIs).
- Oral minipulse (OMP) is a safe, cheap and convenient option for fast-spreading vitiligo.
- Narrowband ultraviolet B (NB-UVB) is indicated for generalized nonsegmental vitiligo (NSV) and is more efficacious and safe than psoralen plus ultraviolet A (PUVA).
- Targeted phototherapy is best indicated for localized and childhood vitiligo.
- Surgical treatments are best reserved for cosmetically sensitive sites in patients in whom there have been no new lesions, no Koebner phenomenon and no extension of the lesion in the previous 12 months.
- In light colored skin, the policy of no active treatment other than use of camouflage cosmetics and sunscreens may be the initial approach.
- Psychological interventions should be offered as a way of improving coping mechanisms in patients with vitiligo.

INTRODUCTION

Vitiligo is a commonly acquired cutaneous achromia characterized by amelanotic macules and patches that affects approximately 0.5–2% of the global population without predilection for age, sex, skin type or ethnicity.[1] Its pathogenesis is multifactorial and not clearly elucidated, and may include mechanisms involving autoimmunity, intrinsic defects of melanocytes, and oxidative stress.[2]

Although vitiligo is physically asymptomatic in most patients, the cosmetic disfigurement evokes profound psychosocial distress in skin of color. Vitiligo can, therefore, be a psychologically devastating disease which has a significant impact on quality of life (QoL) and self-esteem.[3,4] The contrast in color between healthy pigmented skin and the depigmented vitiligo patches may cause social isolation, stigmatization and significant depression.[5-7] Further, it may lead to difficulties in sexual relationships, and affect perceived suitability for marriage.[8,9]

A wide array of therapeutic modalities, both medical and surgical, are used in the management of vitiligo but none is clearly a definitive cure or leads to predictably good results in all cases. Treatment for vitiligo is, therefore, arduous and prolonged. Commonly used treatments include, but are not limited to, topical corticosteroids (TCS), topical calcineurin inhibitors (TCIs), systemic immunomodulators, phototherapy, laser therapy, and repigmentation surgical therapies.[10]

TOPICAL THERAPY

Topical Corticosteroids

Topical corticosteroids have been used as first-line treatment for limited forms of vitiligo since the 1950s for their anti-inflammatory and immunomodulating effects.[11] TCS have the best results on sun-exposed areas such as the face and neck.[12,13] TCS are effective in repigmenting vitiligo patches in skin of color[14] and those of recent onset[15] whereas acral lesions show a poor response.

A meta-analysis of nonsurgical therapies for vitiligo showed significant effectiveness of TCS with a success rate of 33% compared to no response in the placebo groups.[12] No differences in efficacy were found between clobetasol and tacrolimus,[16] and between clobetasol[17] or mometasone[18] and pimecrolimus. TCS, however, might be more effective than the TCIs for extrafacial lesions. TCS appear to be safe and effective for both children and adults when used over a short term.[11]

Steroid-induced repigmentation occurs within 1–4 months of treatment in a perifollicular pattern and from the margins of the lesions. Local side effects include dermal atrophy, telangiectasia, hypertrichosis, acneiform eruptions and striae and are seen with potent or very potent TCS. Suppression of the hypothalamic-pituitary-adrenal axis may occur after prolonged applications over large areas. Currently, there are no studies available on optimal duration and mode of TCS therapy that could improve the therapeutic index.[11]

Recommendations[19]

- Continuous once-daily application of potent TCS can be advised for children and adults with limited, extrafacial involvement for a period no longer than 3 months.
- Facial lesions can be treated as effectively and with lesser side effects by TCI.
- Potent TCS should score over very potent TCS as the first and safest choice as they appear to be at least as effective as the latter.
- Systemic absorption is a concern when large areas of skin, regions with thin skin and children are treated for a prolonged time with potent steroids.

Topical Calcineurin Inhibitors

The TCIs are used in a variety of inflammatory dermatoses and have been tried successfully in vitiligo since 2002. The beneficial effects of TCIs have been reported for patients with vitiligo, particularly in areas where prolonged use of potent corticosteroids is contraindicated. Tacrolimus and pimecrolimus are ascomycin-derived topical immuno-modulating macrolactams (TIMs) and act as calcineurin inhibitors affecting the activation or maturation of T cells and subsequently inhibiting the production of various cytokines, such as tumor necrosis factor (TNF)α. In addition to its immunosuppressive effects, TCIs have been shown to increase melanin biosynthesis and melanocyte migration *in vitro*.[20,21] Its ability to reduce inflammation and thus counter the autoimmune destruction of melanocytes in addition to its ability to induce melanin production and/or melanocyte migration led investigators to explore its use in the treatment of vitiligo.

Tacrolimus

Clinical application of topical tacrolimus for the treatment of localized and generalized vitiligo has been met with mixed results and most of the early studies were not controlled. In her initial report, Grimes reported moderate to excellent repigmentation of vitiligo areas in five out of six study participants.[22] Later on, she reported repigmentation in 17 of 19 (89%) patients treated with topical tacrolimus in an open trial, but with statistically significant repigmentation only on head/neck areas.[23] Similarly, Tanghetti reported partial repigmentation in 13 of 15 (87%) patients, but only patients with limited facial lesions achieved greater than 75% repigmentation.[24] In a later study of 22 children, topical tacrolimus resulted in repigmentation in 19 (86.4%) patients, but the authors state that the best repigmentation was noted on facial areas.[25] Other studies have also resulted in similar conclusion regarding the more substantial effect of topical tacrolimus in the repigmentation of facial areas.[26,27] All these reports suggested that topical tacrolimus is most effective in head and neck areas and that this effect was likely due to increased ultraviolet (UV) exposure in these areas.

When clobetasol was compared with tacrolimus 0.1% ointment in children, clinical evaluation showed both to be effective with no significant difference between them. The lack of atrophy and surrounding hypopigmentation with the use of tacrolimus make it a better option than TCS in children or in areas of sensitive skin such as the eyelids.[16,28] In addition to the previous reports of the effectiveness of topical tacrolimus on facial areas, this report helped to establish topical tacrolimus as a corticosteroid-alternative treatment featuring similar results, an important consideration when treating facial skin that may be easily subjected to corticosteroid side effects. Hartmann et al.[29] confirmed the efficacy of tacrolimus and showed that occlusive dressings may augment its effects, as well as shorten time of onset.[30] However, majority of these early reports did not feature a control group, which is an integral aspect of evidence-based medicine. Radakovic et al.[31] observed that twice-daily application of tacrolimus was superior to once daily and was found to be most effective for facial vitiligo.

Combination Therapy

Several studies have been performed to evaluate the synergism of tacrolimus with other therapeutic modalities. Passeron et al. reported a synergistic effect with a combination treatment of 308 nm excimer laser and topical tacrolimus twice daily versus the excimer laser alone.[32] Studies specifically regarding tacrolimus plus a UV source versus tacrolimus alone have not been supportive for using topical tacrolimus alone and suggest that most of the repigmentation is due to UV exposure. In a comparative right/left trial with nine patients, Ostavari et al.[33] showed poor repigmentation response in areas treated with topical tacrolimus while areas treated with a combination of topical tacrolimus and excimer laser showed good to excellent repigmentation. In a pilot study of nine patients, Mehrabi and Pandya also reported no significant difference in areas treated with petrolatum and narrowband ultraviolet B (NB-UVB) versus topical tacrolimus and NB-UVB over 12 weeks.[34] These latter two studies would support that UV radiation is the primary cause of repigmentation, and that the addition of topical tacrolimus has no additional benefit. More reproducible studies are needed to substantiate whether the addition of topical tacrolimus to UV exposure has any benefit. Another study compared topical pimecrolimus with topical tacrolimus and NB-UVB light, showing modest repigmentation in all three groups without statistical significance between them. The best results were seen in the face with pimecrolimus followed by tacrolimus, and photoexposed areas showed more improvement compared with non-exposed areas.[35]

Pimecrolimus

The use of topical pimecrolimus in the treatment of generalized and localized vitiligo has been less studied than topical tacrolimus, and the results have been mixed. Coskun and colleagues compared topical pimecrolimus with topical clobetasol in a left versus right comparison over an 8-week period in 10 adults.[17] They found topical pimecrolimus resulted in 50–100% repigmentation in 8 of 10 patients, most noticeable for lesions on the trunk or extremities, compared with an equivalent degree of repigmentation in 7 of 10 patients treated with clobetasol. No skin atrophy was noted but burning was a side effect with pimecrolimus. The number of subjects in this study is small, making a reliable conclusion difficult. However, in another study directly comparing immunomodulator therapy with TCS, Eryilmaz et al.[36] showed that the mean percentage of repigmentation was significantly higher with clobetasol than pimecrolimus.

In an open proof-of-concept study of 26 children aged over 6 years and adults with generalized symmetrical forms of vitiligo, treated for head and neck lesions with topical 1% pimecrolimus twice daily, total repigmentation of a target lesion was found in 50% of patients after 6 months of therapy.[37] However, Dawid et al.[38] were unable to show efficacy and recreate previously shown results with pimecrolimus 1% cream twice daily for 6 months in a placebo-controlled study. A few recent studies have again demonstrated the efficacy of pimecrolimus in vitiligo, especially in children.[18,39,40]

Tacrolimus versus Pimecrolimus

In an open randomized study comparing topical pimecrolimus and tacrolimus, Stinco et al. have not shown significant differences in efficacy.[35] In another open study, Lotti et al. have shown slightly higher response rate in patients treated with tacrolimus alone (61%) than in those treated with pimecrolimus alone (54.6%).[41] Finally, in a case report describing a head-to-head comparison between topical tacrolimus and pimecrolimus, both agents induced repigmentation of pretibial lesions when used under occlusion overnight. Tacrolimus was slightly more effective (88% repigmentation) than pimecrolimus (73% repigmentation).[31]

Tolerance

The most common reported side effects for TIMs within the first days of treatment are local application reactions such as burning sensation, pruritus and erythema.[25,28,33,42] Although rare, transient skin hyperpigmentation has also been reported.[43] The association between TIM and UV or sun exposure is not recommended, according to "black box" Food and Drug Administration (FDA) warning for atopic dermatitis, even if the possible side effects are limited. In any case, long-term studies, although reassuring for atopic dermatitis, are still lacking for vitiligo which is an off-label prescription in most countries.

Recommendations[19]

- Topical calcineurin inhibitors can be considered as an alternative to topical steroids for new, actively spreading, vitiliginous lesions on thin skin in both adults and children. The topical safety profile of TCI is better compared with potent TCS, especially concerning risks of skin atrophy.
- The current data does not seem to support using TCI as a first-line treatment of vitiligo below the neck, especially if this is done without occlusion.
- Topical calcineurin inhibitors can be used in combination with excimer laser or NB-UVB to enhance the degree of repigmentation over UV-sensitive sites but not for areas over bony prominences.
- Topical calcineurin inhibitors can be used in combination with topical steroids to enhance their efficacy and for early repigmentation. Topical steroids can be used in the morning and TCIs at night.

SYSTEMIC THERAPY

Oral Steroids

Systemic steroids have been used in the management of vitiligo as high-dose pulsed therapy or minipulsed regimen or daily low-dose therapy to rapidly arrest spreading disease and attempt to induce repigmentation. The efficacy of low-dose oral corticosteroids in the treatment of vitiligo patients was observed by Kim et al.[44] and Banerjee et al.[45] Systemic steroids could arrest the activity of the disease,[46] but were not effective in repigmenting stable vitiligo. Moreover, there were side effects associated with long-term use of daily systemic corticosteroids. This led to the concept of pulsed regimens.

Pulse therapy refers to the intermittent administration of large (suprapharmacological) doses of a drug to enhance the therapeutic effect and reduce the side effects attendant with daily administration. Oral minipulse (OMP) of moderate doses of betamethasone has been pioneered in India by Pasricha et al.[47] They studied 40 patients having extensive and/or actively spreading vitiligo with 5 mg betamethasone tablets given as a single dose after breakfast on 2 consecutive days and noted that disease was arrested in 89% patients with 80% of the treated patients experiencing spontaneous repigmentation of the existing lesions within 2–4 months. Radakovic-Fijan et al.[48] used dexamethasone minipulses of 10 mg daily on 2 consecutive days per week up to 24 weeks. Disease activity was arrested in 88% of patients with progressive disease after 18.2 weeks of treatment. Overall, OMP with either betamethasone or dexamethasone can arrest, without inducing repigmentation, the progression of vitiligo.[49]

The efficacy of high dose methylprednisolone pulse therapy was studied by Sieter et al.[50] Methylprednisolone bolus dose of 8 mg/kg was administered on 3 consecutive days in six patients with generalized spreading vitiligo. It was observed that 85% of the patients presenting with progressive disease showed cessation of disease progression after the infusion therapy. Repigmentation was observed in 71% of patients with progressive vitiligo.

Other Immunosuppressants

Immunosuppressants other than oral steroids have been evaluated in a limited number of studies. There are anecdotal reports on the off-label use of biologic agents too in vitiligo.

Azathioprine

Azathioprine has been tried in adults with symmetrical types of vitiligo in combination with psoralen plus ultraviolet A (PUVA).[51] The dose used was 0.75 mg/kg daily. An earlier and a significant degree of repigmentation was noted compared with PUVA alone and there were no serious side effects.

Cyclophosphamide

Cyclophosphamide was assessed in a small case study of 33 patients at a dose of 50 mg twice a day. In 29 patients, some repigmentation was seen including over acral sites.[52] Side effects included hair loss, cytopenia and nausea.

Cyclosporine

Systemic cyclosporine was tried in six patients at a daily dose of 6 mg/kg.[53] Little or no repigmentation was seen in five out of six patients after several months of therapy. The most prominent side effects were renal dysfunction and hypertension.

Biologics

The therapeutic potential of etanercept was evaluated in a pilot study of four patients with progressive non-segmental vitiligo (NSV).[54] Etanercept 50 mg was given weekly for 12 weeks, followed by 25 mg weekly for a further 4 weeks. Although tolerability was good, none of the patients had a repigmentation response. In another case report,[55] a patient with ankylosing spondylitis and progressive NSV was treated with infliximab. After 6 months, spreading of vitiligo stopped and partial or complete repigmentation occurred on several spots. However, there is an instance of NSV itself being induced by anti-TNFα agents.[56]

Recommendations[19]

- Oral minipulse is a safe, cheap and convenient choice in Indian patients, despite it having only level B evidence.
- Weekend OMP is not useful for repigmenting stable vitiligo but can be considered for fast-spreading vitiligo.
- The benefit of adding OMP to phototherapy at the onset of treatment in progressive vitiligo is not proven and needs further assessment.
- The optimal duration of OMP therapy needed to stop vitiligo progression is between 3 months and 6 months.
- Other immunosuppressants need to be used with caution, in selected cases, after proper assessment of risk, and in those patients in whom steroids are contraindicated and/or not effective.

PHOTOTHERAPY

Phototherapy is considered one of the most effective therapeutic modalities in the management of vitiligo.[57] The various strategies used are based on immunomodulatory effects and include ultraviolet A (UVA) phototherapy, photochemotherapy such as PUVA, khellin plus ultraviolet A (KUVA), psoralen plus sunlight (PUVAsol), broadband ultraviolet B and narrowband ultraviolet B (BB-UVB and NB-UVB respectively) phototherapy, targeted phototherapy and combination phototherapy.

Ultraviolet A Phototherapy

Oral Psoralen Plus Ultraviolet A

Oral PUVA involves the oral intake of psoralens and subsequent exposure to UVA (320–400 nm) radiation.[58] It has been in vogue for vitiligo management since more than 2,500 years when topical application and ingestion of extract of plants *Psoralea corylifolia* in India and *Ammi majus linnaeus* in Egypt were used.[59] It was the first treatment to be established as efficacious in vitiligo. The first clinical studies were performed by El Mofty[60] in 1948 and later by Lerner et al.[61] The principle behind therapy is the phototoxic reactions which occur after psoralens are activated by UVA.

Psoralen plus ultraviolet A stimulate melanogenesis after photoconjugation of psoralens to DNA leading to proliferation of melanocytes, increased synthesis of tyrosinase, formation and melanization of melanosomes, and increased transfer of melanosomes to keratinocytes. PUVA additionally downregulates certain lymphocytic and antigen presenting cell functions, influences adhesion molecule expression and decreases number of Langerhans cells in epidermis.[62-64]

Psoralens are naturally occurring tricyclic furocoumarins present in plants.[60] Most widely used psoralens for oral PUVA are 8-methoxypsoralen (8-MOP; 0.6–0.8 mg/kg), 5-methoxypsoralen (5-MOP; 1.2–1.8 mg/kg) and 4,5,8 trimethylpsoralen (TMP; 0.6 mg/kg). These are given orally 1–3 hours before exposure to UVA. The initial dose is based on the skin type and can vary from approximately 0.5 J/cm^2 and 1 J/cm^2, with increments of 0.5 J/cm^2 given for each subsequent treatment or every other treatment until asymptomatic mild erythema is observed in the vitiliginous patches.[65,66] Alternatively, the initial dose can also be based on the minimum phototoxic dose (MPD), which is defined as the UVA dose that produces barely perceptible erythema with well-defined borders at 48–72 hours in a patient who has ingested the requisite dose of psoralen at the appropriate time interval before exposure.[67] The initial dose often given is 70% of the MPD and treatments are typically administered twice per week.

Patients should be motivated to continue PUVA therapy for at least 6 months before being considered nonresponsive, and 12–24 months of continuous therapy may be necessary to acquire maximal repigmentation.[68-70] Repigmentation is noted in 70–80% of patients with PUVA, but complete repigmentation is obtained in only 20% of patients. Relapse can occur in 75% of patients after 1 or 2 years.

Oral PUVA is not recommended in children aged less than 10–12 years because of the risk of retinal toxicity. Other contraindications include photosensitivity disorders, pregnancy and lactation, a history of skin cancer, arsenic exposure or cutaneous radiation therapy, cataract and retinal disease.[12]

Risk of squamous cell carcinoma is significantly increased with long-term high dose exposure to PUVA.[71] There is higher risk of genital cancer than other skin cancers in men on increasing the dose.[72] Hence genital protection with opaque clothing is mandatory. Proposed maximal cumulative PUVA dose is 1,000–1,500 J/cm^2 and a maximum of 150–200 sessions is recommended.[73]

Topical Psoralen Plus Ultraviolet A

Topical PUVA refers to application of a thin coat of 8-MOP cream or ointment or lotion at very low concentration (0.001%) followed by UVA exposure after half an hour. The initial dose should not exceed 0.25 J/cm^2. This treatment is performed once or twice a week on non-consecutive days with increments of 0.12–0.25 J/cm^2/week, until mild erythema is achieved at the treated sites. Following treatment, the area is washed, a broad-spectrum sunscreen is applied, and excessive sun exposure is avoided for at least 24 hours. The mean clinical response is about 60% repigmentation and is dependent on the anatomic site.[74] Topical PUVA is indicated when the body surface area involved is less than 20% and in children more than 5 years of age with local patches.[75] The advantage of topical therapy is the considerably smaller cumulative UVA doses, as well as lower plasma levels and consequently less systemic and ocular phototoxicity.[76] The main disadvantages are severe blistering reactions, perilesional hyperpigmentation, tedious method of application and lack of effectiveness in limiting the progression of actively spreading vitiligo.

Psoralen with Solar Ultraviolet Light

Psoralen with solar ultraviolet light (PUVAsol) is commonly used in countries where sunlight is in abundance and where the facilities for artificial sources of light are often lacking. It works on the same principle as PUVA, except that natural sunlight is used instead of UVA. PUVAsol can be systemic or topical and the same oral and topical preparations are used as for PUVA. The short initial exposure is gradually prolonged at subsequent sittings until satisfactory erythema is achieved. TMP is usually used at a dose of 0.3 mg/kg, administered 2–4 hours before the sun exposure.[30] Fairly good results have been reported in the past.[77,78] The combination of PUVAsol and calcipotriol has been reported to be highly effective and works faster than PUVA alone.[79] Nevertheless, when artificial sources for PUVA and NB-UVB are readily available, this rather empiric procedure should be discouraged due to its potentially dangerous and frequent side effects.

Khellin Plus Ultraviolet A

This is another photochemotherapy regimen that consists of khellin as the photosensitizer, a furanochrome extract of the plant, *Amni visnaga* (5,8-dimethoxy-2 methyl-4,5-furo-6,7 chromone) and UVA.[80] Khellin is less phototoxic and mutagenic than psoralens and it promotes less darkening of normal skin. Khellin is given orally at a dose of 100 mg, 2 hours before UVA exposure. Systemic KUVA, however, has nowadays been largely abandoned due to concern about hepatic toxicity. Khellin can also be applied topically in a moisturizing cream or carbopol gel at a concentration of 3–5%.[81]

Ultraviolet B Phototherapy

Broadband Ultraviolet B

Wavelengths from 290 nm to 320 nm (BB-UVB) were once widely used in the treatment of a variety of skin disorders. UVB spectrum possesses greater energy than UVA and has a more superficial depth of penetration in the skin. As such, it primarily affects the function of keratinocytes and Langerhans cells in epidermis.[58] There is a solitary report of its efficacy in vitiligo.[82] Fourteen patients were treated and eight (57.1%) of them achieved 75% repigmentation in 12 months. In this series, the best results were seen in patients with facial lesions and skin types V and VI. These results have been negated by a subsequent comparative study which showed significantly better repigmentation with NB-UVB than with BB-UVB.[83] As such, NB-UVB has largely replaced BB-UVB phototherapy in management of vitiligo.

Narrowband Ultraviolet B

Narrowband fluorescent tubes (Philips TL01/Waldman) with an emission spectrum of 311 nm are used for this form of phototherapy. The use of NB-UVB phototherapy for vitiligo was first reported in 1997 by Westerhof and Nieuweboer-Krobotova.[84] The mechanism of action of NB-UVB in vitiligo has not been completely understood. It may exert its effect by stabilization of depigmentation process by local and systemic immunomodulation and simultaneous stimulation of residual follicular melanocytes. NB-UVB causes induction of various cytokines like interleukin-1, TNFα, endothelin-1, leukotriene-C4 and basic fibroblast growth factor that lead to melanocyte mitogenesis, melanogenesis and melanocyte migration.[85]

A meta-analysis of the literature concluded that NB-UVB therapy is the most effective and safe therapy for generalized vitiligo.[12] The starting dose varies from 150 mJ/cm^2 to 250 mJ/cm^2, with increments of 10–40% at each subsequent exposure till development of perceptible erythema.[84] Treatment sessions are administered twice or thrice weekly on non-consecutive days. Several studies have demonstrated the effectiveness of NB-UVB as monotherapy.[86-93] Greater than 75% repigmentation is noted in about 60% of patients. Usually, maximal repigmentation occurs in children with vitiligo. Njoo et al.[94] recommended that responsive patient can be given therapy for 24 months maximum and a resting period of 3 months after 1 year to minimize annual cumulative dose. In children the period recommended was 12 months. If there was no response at 6 months further therapy was discouraged.

The acute side effects of NB-UVB include erythema, pruritus, xerosis, reactivation of herpes simplex and exposure-related conjunctivitis or keratitis.[95] The long-term risks of NB-UVB remain unclear and the question as to the carcinogenicity of UVB still remains unanswered. The only available human data has a mean follow-up of 5 years.[96] The carcinogenic potential of NB-UVB as seen in animal studies is negligible and far less than BB-UVB or PUVA.[97] In Indian patients, in whom prevalence of skin cancer is very low and even PUVA has not been shown to be of any risk, NB-UVB is thought to be a relatively safe option.

The advantages of NB-UVB over oral PUVA include shorter treatment times with obviation of post-exposure photoprotection, no requirement for oral medications, less carcinogenicity, better efficacy and color matching between repigmented and normal skin, and suitability for use in children, pregnant or lactating women, and in individuals with hepatic and renal dysfunction.[86,87,98] NB-UVB is, hence, considered the treatment of choice for generalized vitiligo. Factors that contribute to a good response in vitiligo patients are higher initial doses, more frequent exposure, darker skin type and shorter duration of disease.[86] Potential limitations of NB-UVB are scheduling difficulties and time commitment. Lesions localized on hands and feet, segmental lesions and lesions resistant to systemic PUVA show poorer response.[87] NB-UVB is absolutely contraindicated in patients of xeroderma pigmentosum and lupus erythematosus.

Targeted Phototherapy

Targeted phototherapy is a new form of phototherapy, which seeks to overcome some of the disadvantages with conventional phototherapy.[99-102] This modality involves application of light energy directly focused on, or targeted at, the lesion through special delivery mechanisms such as fiberoptic cables. It has proved effective for localized vitiligo. Different technologies can deliver targeted phototherapy and these include excimer laser (a xenon chloride laser), excimer light (a non-coherent monochromatic light source) and several non-chromatic broadband or narrowband light sources.[103] The advantages of the light sources over excimer laser include smaller size, less maintenance problems, lesser cost. An added advantage of some of these machines over the excimer light or laser is that both UVA and UVB (narrowband) spectra are available.

The following advantages have been claimed for targeted phototherapy: (1) Exposure of involved areas only and sparing of uninvolved areas minimizes acute side effects such as erythema and long-term risk of skin cancer over unaffected skin, (2) Quick delivery of energy ensures shortened duration of treatment, (3) Delivery of higher doses (super-erythemogenic doses) of energy selectively to the lesions enhances efficacy and achieves faster response, (4) Shortened duration of treatment leads to less frequent visits to clinic, and thereby lessens the inconvenience for the patient, (5) The maneuverable hand piece allows treatment of difficult areas such as scalp, nose, genitals, oral mucosa, ear, etc., (6) Ease of administration in children as delivery is hand-held and (7) Targeted phototherapy machines occupy less space.[101,103] However, at the same time, targeted phototherapy devices have certain disadvantages. They are more expensive. Also, they are not adequate to treat extensive areas in view of the cost of treatment and time involved in treatment. They are not recommended for use if lesions occur over more than 10% of the body area.

Excimer Laser

A pilot study in 2002[102] showed significant benefits in twenty-nine patches of vitiligo from 18 patients that were treated three times a week for a maximum of twelve times. The parameters used for the excimer laser were 120 nanosecond, 20 Hz pulse with a 10 × 10 mm spot size and a power output of 60 mW of laser light. The study concluded that the degree of repigmentation in a short period of 2–4 weeks is much higher than that achieved with any other present therapy for vitiligo. These results were confirmed by other studies, which showed benefit with excimer laser in patients of localized vitiligo that had been unsuccessfully treated with other modalities of treatment.[104] A large study of 140 patients with vitiligo treated by excimer laser showed excellent results in UV-sensitive areas, while UV-resistant areas such as acral lesions and lesions in joint areas responded poorly.[105] However these and other studies[106] were small studies conducted in small number of patients, and uncontrolled.

Excimer Light

Several studies have been published which demonstrate their efficacy. In a pilot study of excimer light in 37 patients of vitiligo, Leone et al.[107] obtained initial repigmentation in the first eight treatments and excellent repigmentation in 50% of patients at 6 months. Some patients who had not previously responded to NB-UVB therapy were also found to respond. The results were comparable to excimer laser and superior to narrowband phototherapy. Studies have suggested that combination with topical immunomodulators[108] and fluticasone[109] could enhance the clinical response in vitiligo, especially in more resistant anatomical sites and in segmental vitiligo (SV).[110]

Non-coherent Targeted UVB Phototherapy Devices

Several non-coherent light sources have been shown to be effective in vitiligo.[111,112] A study by Akar et al.[113] demonstrated that therapeutic effectiveness is limited and depends on the locations of vitiligo lesions. Out of a total of 32 patients, only four (12.5%) showed visible repigmentation. All the lesions responsive to treatment were facial lesions. Welsh et al.[114] too demonstrated that extremities did not respond satisfactorily.

Recommendations[19]

- Oral PUVA is currently used in adult patients with generalized vitiligo as a second-line therapy. Compared with NB-UVB it has the disadvantage of lower efficacy and higher short- and long-term risks. Oral KUVA has been largely abandoned due to significant liver toxicity.
- For topical PUVA, psoralens should be formulated in creams at very low concentration. Topical khellin might be combined with artificial UVA irradiation or exposure to natural sunlight.
- Narrowband ultraviolet B is indicated for generalized NSV. Total body treatment is suggested for lesions involving more than 15–20% of the body area.
- Targeted phototherapies are indicated for localized vitiligo and in particular for small lesions of recent onset and childhood vitiligo, to avoid side effects due to total body irradiation with UVB, and in all cases where contraindications exist for total body irradiation with conventional NB-UVB.
- There is as yet no consensus as to the optimum treatment duration of NB-UVB or targeted phototherapy. Phototherapy is usually continued as long as there is ongoing repigmentation or over a maximum period of 1 or 2 years. Maintenance irradiation is not recommended, but regular follow-up examinations are suggested for detecting relapse.
- Although prospective studies are still lacking, the combination of TCS and UVB sources (NB-UVB and 308 nm excimer lasers or lamps) may be promising for difficult-to-treat areas, e.g. over bony prominences.
- There is good evidence that the combination of TCI and UV radiation is effective and provides better results than the two treatments used alone.
- There is now a good level of evidence that phototherapy (NB-UVB or PUVA) should be used for 3 or 4 weeks after surgical procedures to enhance repigmentation.

SURGERY

The concept of surgically treating vitiligo was first proposed in the mid-20th century and specific techniques were developed in the 1970s and early 1980s. The aim of surgical induction of repigmentation is to replenish melanocytes in the depigmented lesions of vitiligo which either have no reservoir or fail to activate melanocytes with medical therapy.

Surgical procedures aim to replace the melanocytes with ones from a normally pigmented autologous donor site. Several melanocyte transplantation techniques can be performed under local anesthesia in an outpatient facility.[115-121]

Tissue Grafts

Punch Grafts

In this procedure, punch grafts (1.2–2.0 mm diameter) are taken from donor areas over the thighs, buttocks, postauricular areas/posterior earlobe or the medial aspect of the upper arm. These are grafted into recipient sites, 5–10 mm apart, in stable vitiligo lesions. Dressings are postoperatively placed to ensure immobilization. Grafts are taken up in 7–10 days after which phototherapy or topical therapy is started to ensure even spread of perigraft pigment.

Advantages: This is the easiest and least expensive method and may be used satisfactorily in all areas other than the nipples and the angle of the mouth, where involuntary muscle contraction may interfere with graft uptake. It is even suitable for "difficult-to-treat" locations such as the fingers, toes, palms and soles.

Disadvantages and complications: This method is not suitable for large lesions as uniform pigmentation may not always be achieved. Other important complications include scar formation at the donor site, cobblestoning and a polka dot appearance.

Suction Blister Epidermal Grafts

A physiological split is made at the dermoepidermal junction by the application of prolonged suction at a negative pressure of –200 to –500 mm Hg to the donor site. The recipient site is dermabraded and thin grafts are placed over it. Alternatively, the recipient site may be denuded by an erbium-doped yttrium aluminum garnet (Erbium:YAG) or carbon dioxide laser.

Advantages: It yields excellent cosmetic results as the graft is very thin. Chances of scarring at the donor or recipient sites are minimal as the graft is purely epidermal.

Disadvantages: The major disadvantage of this procedure is that it is time-consuming as donor site blistering requires a few hours. Large areas cannot be treated by this method.

Split-thickness Grafts

Split-thickness skin grafting involves the free transfer of the epidermis along with a portion of the dermis from one site to another. It consists of obtaining very thin, split-thickness skin grafts, consisting of the epidermis and a part of the upper papillary dermis, and grafting them on the dermabraded or laser-abraded recipient site. The grafts are further secured with pressure and immobilization.

Advantages: This method has the advantage of treating a relatively large area (up to 200 cm^2) in a short period of time.

Disadvantages: Taking split-thickness grafts of uniform thickness requires skill and experience. Other disadvantages include "stuck-on" or "tire patch" appearance, curling of the border with beaded appearance, color mismatch, milia, perigraft halo of depigmentation, and donor site scarring.

Cellular Grafts

Cellular grafts consist of a basal cell layer autologous suspension containing melanocytes and keratinocytes. A given area can be treated with a good donor to recipient ratio. Initially, this procedure required a laboratory facility for cell processing, but single-use kits for enzymatic separation of thin shave biopsies from the graft area have been developed, allowing the generation of cell suspension in the operating room within an hour. Transplants of pure cultured melanocytes expanded *in vitro* can treat lesions up to 500 cm^2. This method is more expensive, time-consuming and requires specialized staff.

Indications

Surgery is indicated for stable vitiligo that does not respond to medical treatment. The best indications are stabilized segmental or focal vitiligo, especially when characterized by leukotrichia and large lesional areas. While there is no consensus on definitive parameters for stability, the Indian Association of Dermatologists, Venereologists and Leprologists (IADVL) Dermatosurgery Task Force[121] suggests the absence of progression of disease for the past 1 year as a definition of stability. Test grafting may be performed in doubtful cases to detect stability. In 1999, Njoo et al.[122] suggested a set of objective criteria—the Vitiligo Disease Activity (VIDA) score—to follow the progress of the patient. It is a 6-point scale on which the activity of the disease is evaluated by the appearance of new vitiligo lesions or the enlargement of pre-existing lesions gauged during a period ranging from less than 6 weeks to 1 year **(Table 1)**. The IADVL Dermatosurgery Task Force recommends that surgery for vitiligo should be performed only in patients with VIDA scores of –1 or 0 (Level D).[121] Although no uniformly accepted opinion exists concerning the minimal age for surgery, vitiligo surgery is generally not attempted in children as all the melanocyte transplantation techniques are performed under local anesthesia.[115,123]

Adverse Events

The highest incidence of adverse events occurs with punch grafting followed by ultrathin epidermal grafting and suction blister epidermal grafting.[118] Cellular grafting was associated with the lowest number of adverse events. Follow-up studies have documented long-term stability and safety.[117]

The choice of the procedure is dependent upon the site, area, availability of infrastructure (applicable especially for cellular grafts), expertise of the dermatological surgeon, cost of the procedure and the patient's preference **(Table 2)**.[121]

It has to be stressed that surgery does not change the overall prognosis of the disease in the case of NSV. When a surgical treatment is conducted in NSV it should be combined with other medical and or UV-light treatment for best outcome and long-term stability.

Recommendations[19]

- The surgical option should be reserved for patients with SV and other localized forms of vitiligo, after the documented failure of medical interventions.
- For NSV, patients with stable disease and a negative history of Koebner phenomenon are eligible, but the risk of relapse must be explained thoroughly to the patient.

Table 1: Vitiligo disease activity (VIDA) 6-point score

Disease activity	*VIDA score*
Active in past 6 weeks	+4
Active in past 3 months	+3
Active in past 6 months	+2
Active in past 1 year	+1
Stable for at least 1 year	0
Stable for at least 1 year and spontaneous repigmentation	-1

Table 2: Choice of surgical method according to area size and site

	Preferred	*Alternative*
Area		
Small area	SBEG, STG	PG
Moderate	NCES, STG	PG
Relatively large area	CM, CE, NCES, STG	
Site		
Fingers and toes	PG, SBEG	NCES
Palm and soles	PG	
Lips	SBEG	PG
Eyelids	SBEG, NCES, STG	MPG
Nipple and areola	SBEG, NCES	
Genitals	NCES, SBEG, CM	

Abbreviations: SBEG, suction blister epidermal grafting; STG, split-thickness grafting; PG, punch grafting; NCES, noncultured epidermal suspension; CM, cultured melanocytes; CE, cultured epidermis

MISCELLANEOUS THERAPY

Calcipotriol

Calcipotriol, a vitamin D_3 analog has been shown to repigment vitiliginous lesions either as monotherapy or in combination with phototherapy. The exact mode by which calcipotriol brings about repigmentation in vitiligo is debatable but the possible mechanism is through 1,25 dihydro vitamin D3 receptors or by modifying the calcium homeostasis in melanocytes.[124] Topical calcipotriol is available in ointment and lotion form and is applied twice daily.

Many randomized controlled studies have been undertaken with calcipotriol as monotherapy or in combination with phototherapy. A preliminary study to see the effect of calcipotriol in vitiligo was done by Parsad et al.[125] Twenty-one children aged between 5 years and 17 years were enrolled in this study. They were asked to apply calcipotriol 50 µg/g in the evening and take sunlight exposure the next day. As many as 10 patients had marked to complete repigmentation and 4 had moderate improvement.

Yalcin et al.[126] studied the effect of combination topical calcipotriol and PUVA in patients who were refractory to 70 sittings of PUVA alone and observed cosmetically acceptable overall repigmentation in 29% of patients. Repigmentation was maximal on the truncal lesions and nil in the acral areas.

Randomized controlled studies by Ermis et al.,[127] clinical trials by Parsad et al.,[79] Kullavanijaya et al.[128] and Goktas et al.[129] have shown combination of phototherapy and calcipotriol brings about faster repigmentation, reduces the number of phototherapy cycles and decreases the side effects of phototherapy. On the other hand, a few other randomized placebo-controlled studies by Baysal et al.,[130] Hartman et al.[131] and Ada et al.[132] have shown contradictory results.

Pseudocatalase

Researchers have demonstrated low catalase levels and defective calcium uptake in the epidermis of vitiligo skin and suggested both as a cause of depigmentation.[133-135] Topical pseudocatalase formulation is an inorganic low molecular weight complex which shows catalase activity in combination with calcium chloride. It is recommended to be applied twice daily.

Schallreuter et al. first studied the efficacy of topical pseudocatalase combined with BB-UVB phototherapy in 33 vitiligo patients and reported a complete repigmentation of vitiliginous lesions over face and hands in 90% of the patients.[136] In another study, the combined effect of topical pseudocatalase and Dead Sea climatotherapy was studied in 59 patients with vitiligo. A faster repigmentation and significant decrease in the hydrogen peroxide levels was observed in the combination treatment group.[137]

In a recent uncontrolled retrospective study, 71 children treated with topical pseudocatalase along with NB-UVB were analyzed and it was observed that greater than 75% repigmentation was seen in 66 children and the disease attained stability in 70 of them.[138] However consecutive studies that followed showed contradictory results. Patel et al. studied effect of pseudocatalase and NB-UVB in 26 vitiligo patients and concluded that no significant repigmentation was achieved at the end of the study and in fact there was worsening of the disease in many patients.[139] A randomized double-blind, placebo-controlled study by Bakis-Petsoglou found that topical pseudocatalase and NB-UVB combination was no better than placebo and NB-UVB combination.[140] Two more recent studies did not find a statistically significant role for pseudocatalase as a treatment modality in vitiligo.[141,142]

Prostaglandins

Prostaglandins (PGs) are active biological derivatives of polyunsaturated essential fatty acids which are released from cell membrane phospholipids. PGE2, synthesized in skin, affects keratinocytes, Langerhans cells and melanocytes and regulates melanocyte proliferation.[143] PGE2 is available commercially as sterile translucent gel containing dinoprostone 0.25 mg/g in a prefilled syringe and catheter, in blister packing. It is applied twice daily.

Parsad et al.[143] studied the effect of topical PGE2 analog in 27 patients with limited vitiligo for 6 months. At the completion of study period, 15 patients showed marked to complete repigmentation and three patients showed moderate repigmentation. The remaining patients showed none to minimal repigmentation. The application was well tolerated except for complaint of burning sensation in two patients.

In another open label study by Kapoor et al.[144] topical PGE2 therapy was given in 56 patients for 6 months. Excellent response was seen in 22 of 40 patients who had demonstrated repigmentation. The incidence of side effects was 18% and mainly involved a transient burning sensation, especially on the lips.

Other Antioxidants

The occurrence of cellular oxidative stress during the progression of vitiligo is the rationale for the topical or systemic administration of antioxidants.[145] Vitamins E and C, ubiquinone, lipoic acid, *Polypodium leucotomos*, catalase/superoxide dismutase combination, and *Ginkgo biloba* are antioxidants that have been used alone or, more frequently, in combination with phototherapy. The administration of antioxidants during or before phototherapy aims to counteract the oxidative stress induced by UV radiation itself, increasing its effectiveness.

Open trials suggested that oral or topical administration of single or multiple antioxidants stopped the progression of the disease and promoted repigmentation.[146] Randomized controlled trials (RCTs) reported to date suggest that vitamin E is effective for the recovery of skin lipid peroxidation induced by PUVA treatment.[147] A mixture of alpha lipoic acid, and vitamins E and C, administered in a double-blind, placebo-controlled trial, promoted a reduction of UV dosage together with improvement of the repigmentation.[148] *Polypodium leucotomos*, an antioxidant photosensitizing and immunomodulator agent, was effective when used in association with PUVA or UVB.[149] *Ginkgo biloba*, a polyphenol compound with anti-inflammatory, immunomodulatory and antioxidant activities, also showed promising results.[150] No side effects have been reported but long-term administration has raised concerns.[151]

Recommendations[19]

- There are no randomized double-blind, placebo-controlled studies which can authenticate the significance of these miscellaneous therapies in the management of vitiligo.
- Antioxidant supplementation could be useful during UV therapy, and during the reactivation phase of vitiligo. However, further evidence is needed before recommending their prescription in vitiligo.

OTHER INTERVENTIONS

Camouflage

Considering the negative impact of the disease on the patient's self-body image, camouflage techniques play a significant role in the global management of vitiligo.[152-155] It is usually suitable for extensive lesions over the face and the dorsa of hands and feet, areas that are generally recalcitrant to conventional treatment modalities.

Ongenae et al.[9] clearly demonstrated that cosmetic camouflage improves QoL in patients with vitiligo. Corrective cosmetics are available in various shades and formulations and allow a perfect match to normal skin color in most patients.[156] Products developed to disguise esthetic skin disfigurement require specialized application techniques.[152,153] Permanent camouflage, micropigmentation and tattoos should be considered with particular caution due to the unpredictable course of the vitiligo.[155]

Suga et al.[157] introduced the use of dihydroxyacetone (DHA) to camouflage the depigmented lesions of patients with vitiligo vulgaris and SV. DHA preparations color the stratum corneum brown owing to its oxidative properties and provide temporary pigmentation resembling a UV-induced tan. Dark-skin subjects need a higher concentration of DHA cream than lighter-skin subjects.[158]

Depigmentation

In patients with extensive and refractory vitiligo, depigmenting the remaining islands of normally pigmented skin on the face or other exposed areas through chemical or physical methods may be cosmetically acceptable. The most common agent used for depigmentation is monobenzyl ether of hydroquinone (MBEH) which almost always causes nearly irreversible depigmentation.[159,160]

Monobenzyl ether of hydroquinone 20% cream is applied twice a day. Prolonged exposure to sunlight should be avoided during treatment, or a sunscreen should be used, as exposure to sunlight reduces the depigmenting effect. Depigmentation is usually noted after 1–4 months of treatment.[160] Mild transient skin irritation or sensitization causing eczema may occur. Ocular side effects have been rarely reported. Sometimes areas of normal skin distant to the site of application have become depigmented.[161]

The Q-switched 755 nm ruby laser has been proposed as a physical depigmenting agent.[162] It can be used alone or in combination with methoxyphenol.[163,164] It destroys melanin and melanin-bearing cells. Cryotherapy has been reported as an inexpensive depigmentation therapy, but due to the risk of scarring, it should be used only by experienced dermatologists.[165-167]

Psychological Interventions

Vitiliginous loss of pigment exerts a negative impact on the patient's appearance and self-esteem.[168] Most patients with vitiligo find their disfigurement moderately or severely intolerable, and suffer from poor body image, low self-esteem and social isolation in both personal and professional relationships. The levels of disability vary according to extension and site of the disease, phototype, ethnicity and cultural background.[169,170]

The prevalence of psychiatric morbidity ranges from 25–30% in Western Europe, with a predominance of fair-skinned subjects, and from 56–75% in India, with a predominance of dark-skinned patients.[171] Perceived severity of the disease is more influenced by the patient's personality than by objective traits of the vitiligo.[171] Additional discomforting aspects are the chronic, unpredictable nature of the disease and the lack of a universally effective treatment.[172] All patients appreciate the opportunity to express difficulties related to their disease and to be listened to and understood.

Recommendations[19]

- Camouflage may be useful in vitiliginous areas resistant to medical and surgical treatments such as the extremities of hands and feet. Cosmetic tattoo may be suitable for depigmented lips and nipples.
- Depigmentation should be reserved for patients with extensive disfiguring vitiligo and only after exploring other possible therapies.
- Psychosocial assessment should be included as part of the evaluation of disease severity. In many instances, community interventions may be necessary besides individual psychosocial therapeutic interventions.

CONCLUSION

Vitiligo patients are in need of a global therapeutic approach. The disease and its course are to be fully explained to the patients and all therapeutic options discussed. Considering the growing menace of charlatanism in the management of vitiligo, especially in a country as India, counseling patients to avoid some therapies of dubious efficacy is of great significance. The Cochrane review on vitiligo[3] describes the various limitations in deriving a valuable algorithm of treatment for all patients with vitiligo based on RCTs. In spite of such constraints, the European Dermatology Forum Consensus,[19] drawing from an earlier consensus report of the Vitiligo European Task Force,[173] has outlined a stepwise treatment approach based on the type and extent of vitiligo. This has been adapted into modified treatment algorithms for both SV **(Flow chart 1)** and NSV **(Flow chart 2)** that might be useful for use of clinicians and researchers alike.

Flow chart 1: Treatment algorithm for segmental vitiligo (SV)

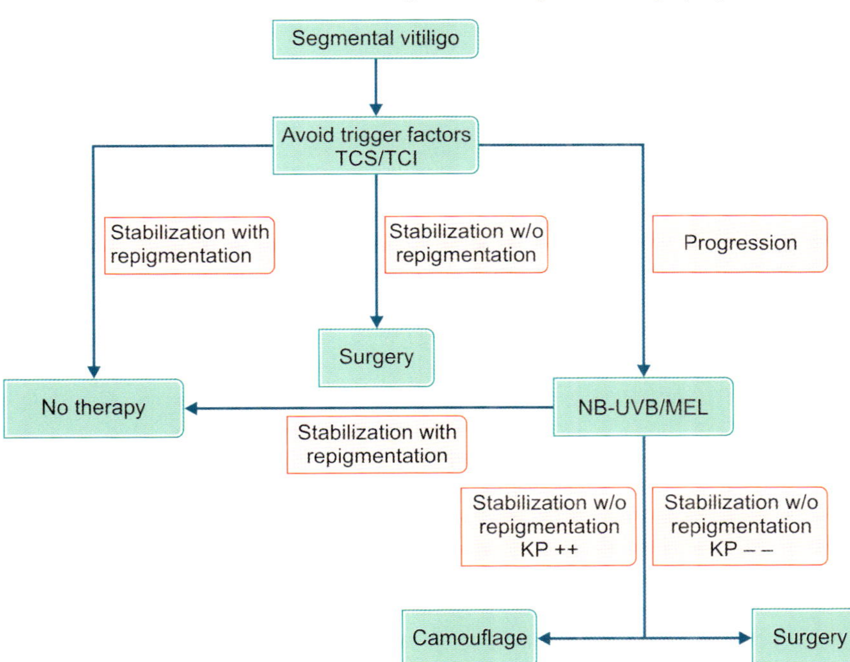

Abbreviations: TCS, topical corticosteroid; TCI, topical calcineurin inhibitor; w/o, without; NB-UVB, narrowband ultraviolet B; MEL, monochromatic excimer lamp; KP, Koebner phenomenon

Flow chart 2: Treatment algorithm for non-segmental vitiligo (NSV)

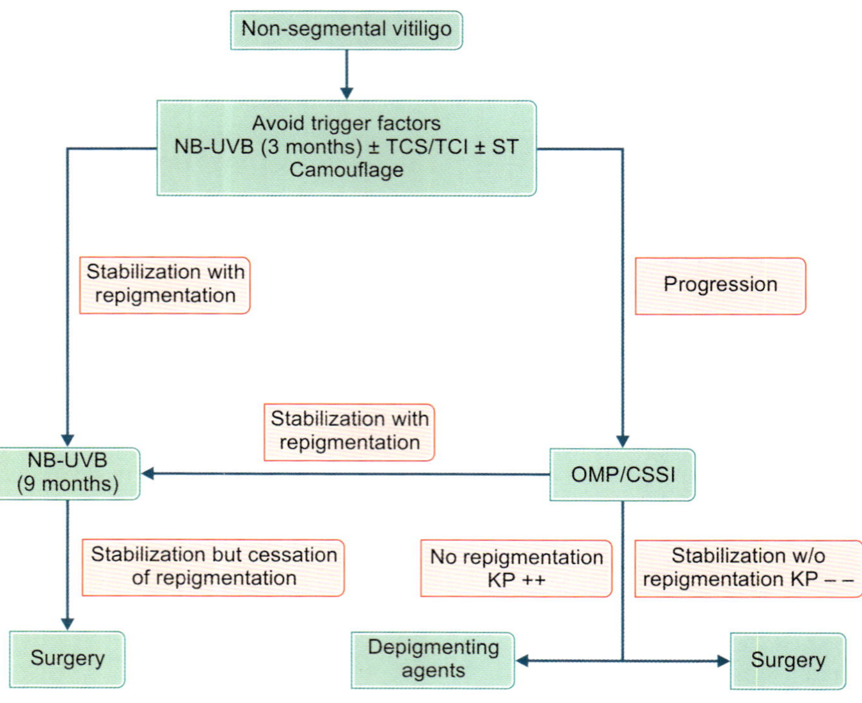

Abbreviations: NB-UVB, narrowband ultraviolet B; TCS, topical corticosteroid; TCI, topical calcineurin inhibitor; ST, systemic therapy; OMP, oral minipulse (steroids); CSSI, corticosteroid sparing immunosuppressive; w/o, without; KP, Koebner phenomenon

REFERENCES

1. Hann SK, Nordlund JJ. Vitiligo: a monograph on basic and clinical science. Oxford: Blackwell Science; 2000.
2. Taieb A, Picardo M. Clinical practice: vitiligo. N Engl J Med. 2009;360:160-9.
3. Whitton ME, Ashcroft DM, Barrett CW, et al. Interventions for vitiligo. Cochrane Database Syst Rev. 2006;1:CD003263.
4. Firooz A, Bouzari N, Fallah N, et al. What patients with vitiligo believe about their condition? Int J Dermatol. 2004;43: 811-14.
5. McMichael AJ, Shaw K, Cayce K. Facial blemishes and QoL. J Cosmet Dermatol. 2004;17:107-13.
6. Mattoo SK, Handa S, Kaur I, et al. Psychiatric morbidity in vitiligo: prevalence and correlates in India. J Eur Acad Dermatol Venereol. 2002;16:573-8.
7. Papadopoulos L, Bor R, Legg C. Coping with the disfiguring effects of vitiligo: a preliminary investigation into the effects of cognitive-behavioural therapy. Br J Med Psychol. 1999; 72:385-96.
8. Parsad D, Pandhi R, Dogra S, et al. DLQI score in vitiligo and its impact on treatment outcome. Br J Dermatol. 2003;148:373-4.
9. Ongenae K, Dierckxsens L, Brochez L, et al. Quality of life and stigmatization profile in a cohort of vitiligo patients and effect of the use of camouflage. Dermatology. 2005;210:279-85.
10. Falabella R. Treatment of localized vitiligo by autologous minigrafting. Arch Dermatol. 1988;124:1649-55.
11. Gawkrodger DJ, Ormerod AD, Shaw L, et al. Guideline for the diagnosis and management of vitiligo. Br J Dermatol. 2008;159:1051-76.
12. Njoo MD, Spuls PI, Bos JD, et al. Nonsurgical repigmentation therapies in vitiligo: meta-analysis of the literature. Arch Dermatol. 1998;134:1532-40.
13. Westerhof W, Nieuweboer-Krobotova L, Mulder PG, et al. Left-right comparison study of the combination of fluticasone propionate and UV-A vs. either fluticasone propionate or UV-A alone for the long-term treatment of vitiligo. Arch Dermatol. 1999;135:1061-6.
14. Kumari J. Vitiligo treated with topical clobetasol propionate. Arch Dermatol. 1984;120:631-5.
15. Schaffer JV, Bolognia JL. The treatment of hypopigmentation in children. Clin Dermatol. 2003;21:296-310.
16. Lepe V, Moncada B, Castanedo-Cazares JP, et al. A double-blind randomized trial of 0.1% tacrolimus vs. 0.05% clobetasol for the treatment of childhood vitiligo. Arch Dermatol. 2003;139:581-5.

17. Coskun B, Saral Y, Turgut D. Topical 0.05% clobetasol propionate versus 1% pimecrolimus ointment in vitiligo. Eur J Dermatol. 2005;15:88-91.
18. Kose O, Arca E, Kurumlu Z. Mometasone cream versus pimecrolimus cream for the treatment of childhood vitiligo. J Dermatolog Treat. 2010;21:133-9.
19. Taieb A, Alomar A, Bohm M, et al. Guidelines for the management of vitiligo: the European Dermatology Forum consensus. Br J Dermatol. 2013;168:5-19.
20. Lan CC, Chen GS, Chiou MH, et al. FK506 promotes melanocyte and melanoblast growth and creates a favourable milieu for cell migration via keratinocytes: possible mechanisms of how tacrolimus ointment induces repigmentation in patients with vitiligo. Br J Dermatol. 2005;153:498-505.
21. Kang HY, Choi YM. FK506 increases pigmentation and migration of human melanocytes. Br J Dermatol. 2006;155:1037-40.
22. Grimes PE, Soriano T, Dytoc MT. Topical tacrolimus for repigmentation of vitiligo. J Am Acad Dermatol. 2002;47: 789-91.
23. Grimes PE, Morris R, Avaniss-Aghajani E, et al. Topical tacrolimus therapy for vitiligo: therapeutic responses and skin messenger RNA expression of proinflammatory cytokines. J Am Acad Dermatol. 2004;51:52-61.
24. Tanghetti EA. Tacrolimus ointment 0.1% produces repigmentation in patients with vitiligo: results of a prospective patient series. Cutis. 2003;71:158-62.
25. Kanwar AJ, Dogra S, Parsad D. Topical tacrolimus for treatment of childhood vitiligo in Asians. Clin Exp Dermatol. 2004;29:589-92.
26. Silverberg NB, Lin P, Travis L, et al. Tacrolimus ointment promotes repigmentation of vitiligo in children: a review of 57 cases. J Am Acad Dermatol. 2004;51:760-6.
27. Almeida P, Borrego L, Rodriguez-Lopez J, et al. Vitiligo. Treatment of 12 cases with topical tacrolimus. Actas Dermosifiliogr. 2005;96:159-63.
28. Ho N, Pope E, Weinstein M, et al. A double-blind randomized placebo-controlled trial of topical tacrolimus 0.1% versus clobetasol propionate 0.05% in childhood vitiligo. Br J Dermatol. 2011;165:626-32.
29. Hartmann A, Brocker EB, Hamm H. Occlusive treatment enhances efficacy of tacrolimus 0.1% ointment in adult patients with vitiligo: results of a placebo controlled 12-month prospective study. Act Derm Venereol. 2008; 88:272-9.
30. Hartmann A, Brocker EB, Hamm H. Repigmentation of pretibial vitiligo with calcineurin inhibitors under occlusion. J Dtsch Dermatol Ges. 2008;6:383-5.
31. Radakovic S, Breier-Maly J, Konschitzky R, et al. Response of vitiligo to once vs. twice-daily topical tacrolimus: a controlled prospective, randomized, observer-blinded trial. J Eur Acad Dermatol Venereol. 2009;23:951-3.
32. Passeron T, Ostovari N, Zakaria W, et al. Topical tacrolimus and the 308-nm excimer laser: a synergistic combination for the treatment of vitiligo. Arch Dermatol. 2004;140:1065-9.
33. Ostovari N, Passeron T, Lacour JP, et al. Lack of efficacy of tacrolimus in the treatment of vitiligo in the absence of UV-B exposure. Arch Dermatol. 2006;142:252-3.
34. Mehrabi D, Pandya AG. A randomized, placebo-controlled, double-blind trial comparing narrowband UV-B Plus 0.1% tacrolimus ointment with narrowband UV-B plus placebo in the treatment of generalized vitiligo. Arch Dermatol. 2006;142:927-9.
35. Stinco G, Piccirillo F, Forcione M, et al. An open randomized study to compare narrow band UVB, topical pimecrolimus and topical tacrolimus in the treatment of vitiligo. Eur J Dermatol. 2009;19;588-93.
36. Eryilmaz A, Seckin D, Baba M. Pimecrolimus: a new choice in the treatment of vitiligo? J Eur Acad Dermatol Venereol. 2009;23:1327-49.
37. Boone B, Ongenae K, Van Geel N, et al. Topical pimecrolimus in the treatment of vitiligo. Eur J Dermatol. 2007;17:55-61.
38. Dawid M, Veensalu M, Grassberger M, et al. Efficacy and safety of pimecrolimus cream 1% in adult patients with vitiligo: results of a randomized, double-blind, vehicle-controlled study. J Dtsch Dermatol Ges. 2006;4;942-6.
39. Souza Leite RM, Craveiro Leite AA. Two therapeutic challenges: periocular and genital vitiligo in children successfully treated with pimecrolimus cream. Int J Dermatol. 2007;46:986-9.
40. Esfandiarpour I, Ekhlasi A, Farajzadeh S, et al. The efficacy of pimecrolimus 1% cream plus narrow-band ultraviolet B in the treatment of vitiligo: a double-blind, placebo-controlled clinical trial. J Dermatolog Treat. 2009;20:14-8.
41. Lotti T, Buggiani G, Troiano M, et al. Targeted and combination treatments for vitiligo. Comparative evaluation of different current modalities in 458 subjects. Dermatol Ther. 2008;21:S20-6.
42. Kawalek AZ, Spencer JM, Phelps RG. Combined excimer laser and topical tacrolimus for the treatment of vitiligo: a pilot study. Dermatol Surg. 2004;30:130-5.
43. De D, Kanwar AJ. Tacrolimus-induced hyperpigmentation in a patch of vitiligo. Skinmed. 2008;7;93-4.
44. Kim SM, Lee HS, Hann SK. The efficacy of low-dose oral corticosteroids in the treatment of vitiligo patients. Int J Dermatol. 1999;38:546-50.
45. Banerjee K, Barbhuiya JN, Ghosh AP, et al. The efficacy of low-dose oral corticosteroids in the treatment of vitiligo patient. Indian J Dermatol Venereol Leprol. 2003;69:135-7.
46. Pasricha JS, Seetharam KA, Dashore A. Evaluation of five different regimes for the treatment of vitiligo. Indian J Dermatol Venereol Leprol. 1989;55:18-21.
47. Pasricha JS, Khaitan BK. Oral mini-pulse therapy with betamethasone in vitiligo patients having extensive or fast-spreading disease. Int J Dermatol. 1993;32:753-7.

48. Radakovic-Fijan S, Furnsinn-Fridl AM, Honigsmann H, et al. Oral dexamethasone pulse treatment for vitiligo. J Am Acad Dermatol. 2001;44:814-7.
49. Rath N, Kar HK, Sabhnani S. An open labeled, comparative clinical study on efficacy and tolerability of oral minipulse of steroid (OMP) alone, OMP with PUVA and broad/narrow band UVB phototherapy in progressive vitiligo. Indian J Dermatol Venereol Leprol. 2008;74:357-60.
50. Seiter S, Ugurel S, Tilgen W, et al. Use of high-dose methylprednisolone pulse therapy in patients with progressive and stable vitiligo. Int J Dermatol. 2000;39:624-7.
51. Radmanesh M, Saedi K. The efficacy of combined PUVA and low dose azathioprine for early and enhanced repigmentation in vitiligo patients. J Dermatolog Treat. 2006; 17:151-3.
52. Gokhale BB. Cyclophosphamide and vitiligo. Int J Dermatol. 1979;18:92.
53. Gupta AK, Ellis CN, Nickoloff BJ, et al. Oral cyclosporine in the treatment of inflammatory and noninflammatory dermatoses. A clinical and immunopathologic analysis. Arch Dermatol. 1990;126:339-50.
54. Rigopoulos D, Gregoriou S, Larios G, et al. Etanercept in the treatment of vitiligo. Dermatology. 2007;215:84-5.
55. Smith DI, Heffernan MP. Vitiligo after the resolution of psoriatic plaques during treatment with adalimumab. J Am Acad Dermatol. 2008;58:S50-1.
56. Ramirez-Hernández M, Marras C, Martinez-Escribano JA. Infliximab-induced vitiligo. Dermatology. 2005;210:79-80.
57. Passeron T. UVB therapy for pigmentary disorders. In: Nordlund JJ, Boissy RE, Hearing VJ, King RA, Ortonne JP (Eds). The Pigmentary System, 2nd edn. New York: Oxford University Press; 2006. pp. 1183-7.
58. Mosher DB, Fitzpatrick PB, Ortonne PJ, et al. Hypomelanosis and Hypermelanosis. In: Freedberg IM, Eisen AZ, Wolff K, Austen KJ, Goldsmith LA, Katz SI (Eds). Dermatology in General Medicine, 6th edn. New York; McGraw-Hill; 2003. pp. 839-47.
59. Morrison WL, Hann SK, Nordlund JJ. PUVA therapy in Vitiligo. Bangalore: Panther Publishers Ltd.; 2000. pp. 168-72.
60. El Mofty AM. A preliminary clinical report on the treatment of leucoderma with Ammi Majjus Linn. J Eygpt Med Assoc. 1948;31:651-65.
61. Lerner AB, Deuton CR, Fitzpatrick TB. Clinical and experimental studies with 8 methoxypsoralen in vitiligo. J Invest Dermatol. 1953;20:299-314.
62. Pathak MA, Fitzpatrick TB. The evolution of photochemotherapy with psoralens and UVA (PUVA): 2000 BC to 1992. J Photochem Photobiol B. 1992;14:3-22.
63. Carrascosa JM, Gardeazabal J, Perez-Ferriols A, et al. Consensus document on phototherapy: PUVA therapy and narrow-band UVB therapy. Actas Dermosifiliogr. 2005;96:635-58.
64. Wu CS, Lan CC, Wang LF, et al. Effects of psoralen plus ultraviolet A irradiation on cultured epidermal cells in vitro and patients with vitiligo *in vivo*. Br J Dermatol. 2007;156:122-9.
65. Gupta AK, Anderson TF. Psoralen photochemotherapy. J Am Acad Dermatol. 1987;17:703-34.
66. Ibbotson SH, Dawe RS, Farr PM. The effect of methoxsalen dose on ultraviolet-A-induced erythema. J Invest Dermatol. 2001;116:813-5.
67. Ibbotson SH, Farr PM. The time-course of psoralen ultraviolet A (PUVA) erythema. J Invest Dermatol. 1999;113:346-50.
68. Bhatnagar A, Kanwar AJ, Parsad D. Comparison of systemic PUVA and NB-UVB in the treatment of vitiligo: an open prospective study. J Eur Acad Dermatol Venereol. 2007;21:638-42.
69. Pathak MA, Mosher DB, Fitzpatrick TB. Safety and therapeutic effectiveness of 8-methoxypsoralen, 4,5,8-trimethylpsoralen, and psoralen in vitiligo. Natl Cancer Inst Monogr. 1984;66:165-73.
70. Yones SS, Palmer RA, Garibaldinos TM, et al. Randomized double-blind trial of treatment of vitiligo: efficacy psoralen UVA therapy versus narrowband UVB therapy. Arch Dermatol. 2007;143:578-84.
71. Stern R, Lunder EJ. Risk of squamous cell carcinoma and methoxsalen and UVA radiation. Arch Dermatol. 1998; 134:1582-5.
72. Stern RS. Genital tumors among men with psoriasis exposed to psoralens with ultraviolet A radiation (PUVA) and ultraviolet B radiation. N Engl J Med. 1990;322:1093-7.
73. British Photodermatology Group. Appraisal guidelines for PUVA. Br J Dermatol. 1994;130:246-55.
74. Grimes PE. Psoralen photochemotherapy for vitiligo. Clin Dermatol. 1997;15:921-6.
75. Drake LA, Dinehart SM, Farmer ER, et al. Guidelines of care for vitiligo. J Am Acad Dermatol. 1996;35:620-6.
76. Morrison WL, Marwaha S, Beck L. PUVA-induced phototoxicity: incidence and causes. J Am Acad Dermatol. 1997;36:183-6.
77. Theodoridis A, Tsambaos D, Sivenas C, et al. Oral trimethylpsoralen in the treatment of vitiligo. Acta Derm Venereol. 1976;56:253-6.
78. Handa S, Pandhi R, Kaur I. Vitiligo: a retrospective comparative analysis of treatment modalities in 500 patients. J Dermatol. 2001;28:461-6.
79. Parsad D, Saini R, Verma N. Combination of PUVAsol and topical calcipotriol in vitiligo. Dermatology. 1998;197: 167-70.
80. Ortel B, Tanew A, Honigsmann H. Treatment of vitiligo with khellin and ultraviolet A. J Am Acad Dermatol. 1988;18:693-701.
81. Orecchia G, Perfetti L. Photochemotherapy with topical khellin and sunlight in vitiligo. Dermatology. 1992;184: 120-3.

82. Koster W, Wiskemann A. Phototherapy with UV-B in vitiligo. Z Hautkr. 1990;65:1022-4.
83. Hartmann A, Lurz C, Hamm H, et al. Narrow-band UVB 311 nm vs. broad-band UVB therapy in combination with topical calcipotriol vs. placebo in vitiligo. Int J Dermatol. 2005;44:736-42.
84. Westerhof W, Nieuweboer-Krobotova L. Treatment of vitiligo with UV-B radiation vs topical psoralen plus UV-A. Arch Dermatol. 1997;133:1525-8.
85. Imokawa G, Miyagishi M, Yada Y. Endothelin 1 as a new melanogen: coordinated exposure of its gene and the tyrosinase gene in UVB exposed human epidermis. J Invest Dermatol. 1995;105:32-7.
86. Natta R, Somsak T, Wisuttida T. Narrow band UVB radiation therapy for recalcitrant vitiligo in Asians. J Am Acad Dermatol. 2003;49:473-6.
87. Scherschun L, Kim JJ, Lim HW. Narrow band ultraviolet B is a useful and well-tolerated treatment for vitiligo. J Am Acad Dermatol. 2001;44:999-1003.
88. Njoo MD, Bos JD, Westerhof W. Treatment of generalized vitiligo in children with narrow-band (TL-01) UVB radiation therapy. J Am Acad Dermatol. 2000;42:245-53.
89. Hamzavi I, Jain H, McLean D, et al. Parametric modeling of narrowband UV-B phototherapy for vitiligo using a novel quantitative tool-the vitiligo area scoring system. Arch Dermatol. 2004;140:677-83.
90. Kanwar AJ, Dogra S, Parsad D, et al. Narrow-band UVB for the treatment of vitiligo: an emerging effective and well-tolerated therapy. Int J Dermatol. 2005;44:57-60.
91. Kanwar AJ, Dogra S. Narrow-band UVB for the treatment of generalized vitiligo in children. Clin Exp Dermatol. 2005;30:332-6.
92. Brazzelli V, Antoninetti M, Palazzini S, et al. Critical evaluation of the variants influencing the clinical response of vitiligo: study of 60 cases treated with ultraviolet B narrow-band phototherapy. J Eur Acad Dermatol Venereol. 2007;21:1369-74.
93. Kishan Kumar YH, Rao GR, Gopal KV, et al. Evaluation of narrow-band UVB phototherapy in 150 patients with vitiligo. Indian J Dermatol Venereol Leprol. 2009;75:162-6.
94. Njoo MD, Westerhof W, Bos JD. The development of guidelines for treatment of vitiligo. Arch Dermatol. 1999;135:1514-21.
95. Perna JJ, Mannix ML, Rooney JF, et al. Reactivation of latent herpes simplex virus by ultraviolet light - a human model. J Am Acad Dermatol. 1987;17:473-8.
96. Man I, Crombie IK, Dawe RS. The photocarcinogenic risk of narrow band TL-01 ultraviolet B therapy: early follow up data. Br J Dermatol. 2003;149:12.
97. Young AR. Carcinogenicity of UVB phototherapy assessed. Lancet. 1995;345:1431-2.
98. Parsad D, Kanwar AJ, Kumar B. Psoralen-ultraviolet A vs. narrow-band ultraviolet B phototherapy for the treatment of vitiligo. J Eur Acad Dermatol Venereol. 2006;20:175-7.
99. Hamzavi I, Lui H. Using light in dermatology: an update on lasers, ultraviolet phototherapy, and photodynamic therapy. Dermatol Clin. 2005;23:199-207.
100. Spencer JM, Hadi SM. The excimer lasers. J Drugs Dermatol. 2004;3:522-5.
101. Grimes PE. Advances in the treatment of vitiligo: targeted phototherapy. Cosm Dermatol. 2003;16:18-22.
102. Spencer JM, Nossa R, Ajmeri J. Treatment of vitiligo with the 308-nm excimer laser: a pilot study. J Am Acad Dermatol. 2002;46:727-31.
103. Mysore V. Targeted phototherapy. Indian J Dermatol Venereol Leprol. 2009;75:119-25.
104. Taneja A, Trehan M, Taylor CR. 308-nm excimer laser for the treatment of localized vitiligo. Int J Dermatol. 2003;42:658-62.
105. Choi KH, Park JH, Ro YS. Treatment of Vitiligo with 308-nm xenon-chloride excimer laser: therapeutic efficacy of different initial doses according to treatment areas. J Dermatol. 2004;31:284-92.
106. Hadi S, Tinio P, Al-Ghaithi K, et al Treatment of vitiligo using the 308-nm excimer laser. Photomed Laser Surg. 2006;24:354-7.
107. Leone G, Iacovelli P, Paro Vidolin A, et al. Monochromatic excimer light 308 nm in the treatment of vitiligo: a pilot study. J Eur Acad Dermatol Venereol. 2003;17:531-7.
108. Nisticò S, Chiricozzi A, Saraceno R, et al. Vitiligo treatment with monochromatic excimer light and tacrolimus: results of an open randomized controlled study. Photodermatol Photoimmunol Photomed. 2011;27:108-10.
109. Coelho JD, Ferreira A. Letter: Association of targeted intense pulse light system UVA1-UVB and fluticasone in the treatment of vitiligo: prospective study of 10 patients. Photodermatol Photoimmunol Photomed. 2009;25:161-3.
110. Lee DY, Kim CR, Lee JH. Targeted phototherapy in combination with drug therapy for segmental vitiligo. Photodermatol Photoimmunol Photomed. 2011;27:108-10.
111. Lotti TM, Menchini G, Andreassi L. UV-B radiation microphototherapy: An elective treatment for segmental vitiligo. J Eur Acad Dermatol Venereol. 1999;13:102-8.
112. Menchini G, Tsoureli-Nikita E, Hercogova J. Narrow-band UV-B micro-phototherapy: a new treatment for vitiligo. J Eur Acad Dermatol Venereol. 2003;17:171-7.
113. Akar A, Tunca M, Koc E, et al. Broadband targeted UVB phototherapy for localized vitiligo: a retrospective study. Int J Dermatol. 2009;48:529-34.
114. Welsh O, Herz-Ruelas ME, Gómez M, et al. Therapeutic evaluation of UVB-targeted phototherapy in vitiligo that affects less than 10% of the body surface area. Int J Dermatol. 2009;48:529-34.
115. Njoo MD, Bos JD, Westerhof W, et al. A systematic review of autologous transplantation methods in vitiligo. Arch Dermatol. 1998;134:1543-9.
116. Gauthier Y. Complications and limitations of melanocyte transplantation. In: Gupta S, Olsson M, Kanwar AJ, Ortonne

JP (Eds). Surgical Management of Vitiligo. Oxford: Blackwell Publishing; 2007. pp. 144-7.
117. Olsson MJ, Juhlin L. Long-term follow-up of leucoderma patients treated with transplants of autologous cultured melanocytes, ultrathin epidermal sheets and basal cell layer suspension. Br J Dermatol. 2002;147:893-904.
118. Falabella R. Surgical treatment of vitiligo. Why, when and how? J Eur Acad Dermatol Venereol. 2003;17:518-20.
119. Olsson MJ. What are the needs for transplantation treatment in vitiligo, and how good is it? Arch Dermatol. 2004; 104:1273-4.
120. Gupta S, Narang T, Olsson MJ, et al. Surgical management of vitiligo and other leukodermas: evidence-based practice guidelines. In: Gupta S, Olsson M, Kanwar AJ, Ortonne JP (Eds). Surgical Management of Vitiligo. Oxford: Blackwell Publishing; 2007. pp. 69-79.
121. Parsad D, Gupta S. Standard guidelines of care for vitiligo surgery. Indian J Dermatol Venereol Leprol. 2008;74: 37-45.
122. Njoo MD, Das PK, Bos JD, et al. Association of the Kobner phenomenon with disease activity and therapeutic responsiveness in vitiligo vulgaris. Arch Dermatol. 1999;135: 407-13.
123. Gupta S, Kumar B. Epidermal grafting in vitiligo: influence of age, site of lesion, and type of disease on outcome. J Am Acad Dermatol. 2003;49:99-104.
124. Ameen M, Exarchou V, Chu AC. Topical calcipotriol as monotherapy and in combination with psoralen plus ultraviolet A in the treatment of vitiligo. Br J Dermatol. 2001;145:476-9.
125. Parsad D, Saini R, Nagpal R. Calcipotriol in vitiligo: a preliminary study. Pediatr Dermatol. 1999;16:317-20
126. Yalçin B, Sahin S, Bükülmez G, et al. Experience with calcipotriol as adjunctive treatment for vitiligo in patients who do not respond to PUVA alone: a preliminary study. J Am Acad Dermatol. 2001;4:634-7.
127. Ermis O, Alpsoy E, Cetin L, et al. Is the efficacy of psoralen plus ultraviolet A therapy for vitiligo enhanced by concurrent topical calcipotriol? A placebo-controlled double-blind study. Br J Dermatol. 2001;3:472-5.
128. Kullavanijaya P, Lim HW. Topical calcipotriene and narrowband ultraviolet B in the treatment of vitiligo. Photodermatol Photoimmunol Photomed. 2004;20:248.
129. Goktas EO, Aydin F, Senturk N, et al. Combination of narrow band UVB and topical calcipotriol for the treatment of vitiligo. J Eur Acad Dermatol Venereol. 2006;20:553-7.
130. Baysal V, Yildirim M, Erel A, et al. Is the combination of calcipotriol and PUVA effective in vitiligo? J Eur Acad Dermatol Venereol. 2003;17:299-302.
131. Hartmann A, Lurz C, Hamm H, et al. Narrow-band UVB 311 nm vs. broadband UVB therapy in combination with topical calcipotriol vs. placebo in vitiligo. Int J Dermatol. 2004;44:736-42.
132. Ada S, Sahin S, Boztepe G, et al. No additional effect of topical calcipotriol on narrow-band UVB phototherapy in patients with generalized vitiligo. Photodermatol Photoimmunol Photomed. 2004;21:79-83
133. Schallreuter KU, Wood JM, Berger J. Low catalase levels in the epidermis of patients with vitiligo. J Invest Dermatol. 1991;97:1081-5.
134. Schallreuter KU, Pittelkow MR. Defective calcium uptake system in vitiligo. Arch Dermatol Res. 1988;280:137-9.
135. Westerhof W. Vitiligo—a window in the darkness. Dermatology. 1995;190:181-2.
136. Schallreuter KU, Wood JM, Lemke KR, et al. Treatment of vitiligo with a topical application of pseudocatalase and calcium in combination with short-term UVB exposure. Case study on 33 patients. Dermatology. 1995;190:223-9.
137. Schallreuter KU, Moore J, Behrens-Williams S, et al. Rapid initiation of repigmentation in vitiligo with Dead Sea climatotherapy in combination with pseudocatalase (PC-KUS). Int J Dermatol. 2002;41:482-7.
138. Schallreuter KU, Krüger C, Würfel BA, et al. From basic research to the bedside: efficacy of topical treatment with pseudocatalase PC-KUS in 71 children with vitiligo. Int J Dermatol. 2008;47:743-53.
139. Patel DC, Evans AV, Hawk JL. Topical pseudocatalase mousse and narrowband UVB phototherapy is not effective for vitiligo: an open, single centre study. Clin Exp Dermatol. 2002;27:641-4.
140. Bakis-Petsoglou S, Le Guay J, Wittal R. A randomized, double blinded, placebo-controlled trial of pseudocatalase cream and narrow band UVB in the treatment of vitiligo. Br J Dermatol. 2009;161:910-7.
141. Sanclemente G, Garcia JJ, Zuleta JJ, et al. A double-blind, randomized trial of 0.05% betamethasone vs. topical catalase/dismutase superoxide in vitiligo. J Eur Acad Dermatol Venereol. 2008;22:1359-64.
142. Yuksel EP, Aydin F, Senturk N, et al. Comparison of the efficacy of narrow band ultraviolet B and narrow band ultraviolet B plus topical catalase superoxide dismutase treatment in vitiligo patients. Eur J Dermatol. 2009;19:341-4.
143. Parsad D, Pandhi R, Dogra S, et al. Topical prostaglandin analog (PGE2) in vitiligo—a preliminary study. Int J Dermatol. 2002;41:942-5.
144. Kapoor R, Phiske MM, Jerajani HR. Evaluation of safety and efficacy of topical prostaglandin E2 in treatment of vitiligo. Br J Dermatol. 2009;160:861-3.
145. Dell'Anna ML, Picardo M. A review and a new hypothesis for non-immunological pathogenetic mechanisms in vitiligo. Pigment Cell Res. 2006;19:406-11.
146. Picardo M, Dell'Anna ML. Vitamins and antioxidants: topical and systemic. In: Picardo M, Taieb A (Eds). Vitiligo. Berlin: Springer; 2010. pp. 369-74.
147. Akyol M, Celik VK, Ozcelik S, et al. The effects of vitamin E on the skin lipid peroxidation and the clinical improvement in vitiligo patients treated with PUVA. Eur J Dermatol. 2002;12:24-6.
148. Dell'Anna ML, Mastrofrancesco A, Sala R, et al. Antioxidants and narrow band-UVB in the treatment of vitiligo: a

double-blind placebo controlled trial. Clin Exp Dermatol. 2007;32:631-6.
149. Middelkamp-Hup MA, Bos JD, Rius-Diaz F, et al. Treatment of vitiligo vulgaris with narrow band UVB and oral Polypodium leucotomos extract: a randomized double-blind placebo controlled study. J Eur Acad Dermatol Venereol. 2007;21:942-50.
150. Parsad D, Pandhi R, Juneja A. Effectiveness of oral Ginkgo biloba in treating limited, slowly spreading vitiligo. Clin Exp Dermatol. 2002;28:285-7.
151. Hercberg S, Ezzedine K, Guinot C, et al. Antioxidant supplementation increases the risk of skin cancers in women but not in men. J Nutr. 2007;137:2098-105.
152. Tanioka M, Yamamoto Y, Kato M, et al. Camouflage for patients with vitiligo vulgaris improved their quality of life. J Cosmet Dermatol. 2010;9:72-5.
153. DePase A. 'La Voce dei Pazienti'. Evidence Based Dermatology. Milan: Masson Publisher; 2003.
154. Savin J. The hidden face of dermatology. Clin Exp Dermatol. 1993;18:393-5.
155. De Cuyper C. Permanent makeup: indications and complications. Clin Dermatol. 2008;26:30-4.
156. Levy SB. Tanning prepaprations. Dermatol Clin. 2000;18: 591-6.
157. Suga Y, Ikejima A, Matsuba S, et al. Medical pearl: DHA application for camouflaging segmental vitiligo and piebald lesions. J Am Acad Dermatol. 2002;47:436-8.
158. Rajatanavin N, Suwanachote S, Kulkollakarn S. Dihydroxyacetone: a safe camouflaging option in vitiligo. Int J Dermatol. 2008;47:402-6.
159. Njoo MD, Vodegel RM, Westerhof W. Depigmentation therapy in vitiligo universalis with topical 4-methoxyphenol and the Q-switched ruby laser. J Am Acad Dermatol. 2000;42:760-9.
160. Rao J, Fitzpatrick RE. Use of the Q-switched 755-nm alexandrite laser to treat recalcitrant pigment after depigmentation therapy for vitiligo. Dermatol Surg. 2004; 30:1043-5.
161. Kasraee B, Fallahi MR, Ardekani GS, et al. Retinoic acid synergistically enhances the melanocytotoxic and depigmenting effects of monobenzylether of hydroquinone in black guinea pig skin. Exp Dermatol. 2006;15:509-14.
162. Kim YJ, Chung BS, Choi KC. Depigmentation therapy with Q-switched ruby laser after tanning in vitiligo universalis. Dermatol Surg. 2001;27:969-70.
163. Nordlund JJ. Depigmentation for the treatment of extensive vitiligo. In: Hann SK, Nordlund JJ (Eds). Vitiligo. Oxford: Blackwell Science; 2000. pp. 207-13.
164. Solano F, Briganti S, Picardo M, et al. Hypopigmenting agents: an updated review on biological, chemical and clinical aspects. Pigment Cell Res. 2006;19:550-71.
165. Alghamdi K, Kumar A. Depigmentation therapies for normal skin in vitiligo universalis. J Eur Acad Dermatol Venerol. 2011;25:749-57.
166. Radmanesh M. Depigmentation of the normally pigmented patches in universal vitiligo patients with cryotherapy. J Eur Acad Dermatol Venereol. 2000;14:149-52.
167. Di Nuzzo S, Masotti A. Depigmentation therapy in vitiligo universalis with cryotherapy and 4-hydroxyanisole. Clin Exp Dermatol. 2010;35:215-6.
168. Linthorst Homan MW, Spuls PI, de Korte J, et al. The burden of vitiligo: patient characteristics associated with quality of life. J Am Acad Dermatol. 2009;61:411-20.
169. Thompson AR, Clarke SA, Newell RJ, et al Vitiligo linked to stigmatization in British South Asian women: a qualitative study of the experiences of living with vitiligo. Br J Dermatol. 2010;163:481-6.
170. Kostoupolou P, Taieb A. Psychological interventions. In: Picardo M, Taieb A (Eds). Vitiligo. Berlin: Springer; 2009. pp. 433-5.
171. Kostopoulou P, Jouary T, Quintard B, et al. Objective vs. subjective factors in the psychological impact of vitiligo: the experience from a French referral centre. Br J Dermatol. 2009;161:128-33.
172. Talsania N, Lamb B, Bewley A. Vitiligo is more than skin deep: a survey of members of the Vitiligo Society. Clin Exp Dermatol. 2009;35:736-9.
173. Taieb A, Picardo M; VETF members. The definition and assessment of vitiligo: a consensus report of the Vitiligo European Task Force. Pigment Cell Res. 2007;20:27-35.

31

Pigmentary Changes in Pregnancy

M Sendhil Kumaran, Amrinder Jit Kanwar

Key Features

- Pigmentary changes are the most common physiological change occurring during pregnancy.
- Most of the pigmentary changes are due to changes in hormonal milieu occurring during pregnancy.
- No specific treatment is required as most of them return back to near normal postdelivery.

INTRODUCTION

Pregnant women experience a myriad of physiological changes throughout their gestational period, affecting different organs in the body. The cutaneous and appendageal variance manifest commonly early during the course of pregnancy and are by in large modulated by complex interplay of hormonal, immunological and metabolic factors. They occur so regularly during pregnancy that they are considered normal, but may become pathological when the presentation is severe and extensive.

Many changes are reversed postpartum, while some persist in less severe form. It is important for dermatologists to be familiar with various normal physiological changes occurring during pregnancy and to understand their genesis, in order to recognize and study the pathogenesis of abnormal changes.

Physiological alterations in pregnancy can be broadly considered under:

- Pigmentary
- Vascular
- Structural
- Appendageal
- Miscellaneous changes.

In this chapter, we will be discussing the pigmentary changes only.

PATHOGENESIS

There is an overall hyperpigmentation of the skin in pregnancy. Its exact etiology remains obscure, but it is probably due to increased levels of pituitary, placental and ovarian hormones. Rise in levels of melanocyte stimulating hormone (MSH), estrogen and progesterone have been implicated as causative factors for hyperpigmentation in pregnancy. However, the role of MSH in causing hyperpigmentation has been disputed because hyperpigmentation in pregnancy begins during the first trimester of pregnancy and regresses during the postpartum period, whereas the levels of alpha-MSH are high only during later stages in pregnancy. Additionally, there is no difference noted in the plasma levels of beta-MSH during late pregnancy and postpartum.

Some investigators consider the cause of hyperpigmentation to be related to an elevated level of estrogen and progesterone. Blood levels of progesterone increase throughout pregnancy and estrogen production increases from the 8th week onwards and begins to fall only after the 30th week of pregnancy. This pattern of estrogen and progesterone levels coincides with the progression of hyperpigmentation. Additional factors responsible for hyperpigmentation could be a greater population of melanocytes at the affected sites or a greater estrogen or progesterone receptor sensitivity.[1] It is well known that folic acid reduces the risk of neural tube defects in babies, and reports have also shown a relation between folic acid deficiency and hyperpigmentation.

Various types of pigmentary changes during pregnancy can be broadly classified into facial and nonfacial. These are enumerated in **Table 1**.

Table 1: Pigmentary changes in pregnancy

Nonfacial	*Facial*
• Diffuse hyperpigmentation	Melasma
• Selective hyperpigmentation	
• Secondary areola	
• Linea nigra	
• Prominent pigmentary demarcation lines	
• Nevi and melanoma	
• Halo nevi	
• Striae	
• Melanonychia	
• Reactivation of dormant dermal melanocytes	

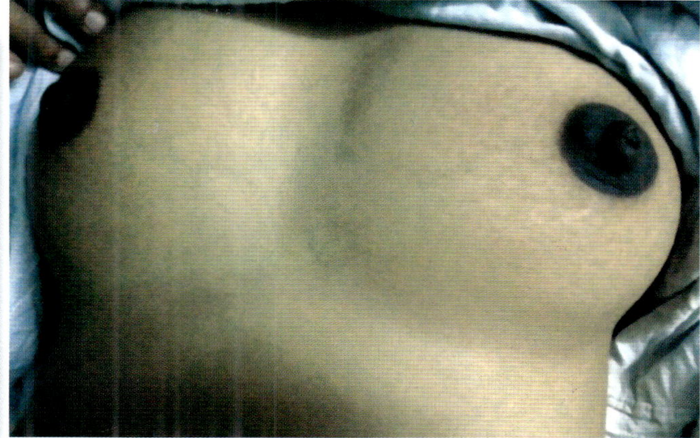

Fig. 1: Darkened areolar and nipple skin

Hyperpigmentation

Hyperpigmentation is one of the earliest signs and is the most frequently encountered physiological change in pregnancy. It occurs in majority (90%) of pregnant women and is usually more accentuated in women of a darker complexion. It takes place during the first trimester and progresses until delivery. Most of it reverses after delivery, but the skin does not always return back to its original color.

Areas normally displaying hyperpigmentation become darker during pregnancy. However, this change is often more localized, targeting areola, **Figure 1**, nipples, which are the most commonly affected site (40%), anogenital, axillae, inner thighs, periumbilical region, melanocytic nevi, scars and freckles.[2] In a study of 140 pregnant women of skin types III and IV, hyperpigmentation of the areolar region was observed in all the cases.[3]

Secondary areola refers to hyperpigmentation of the region in between the two areolae. Areolar pigmentation must be differentiated from nevoid hyperkeratosis of the nipple and areola, a rare condition that has been reported to develop during pregnancy or even at puberty with histology showing rete ridge elongation, papillomatosis and hyperkeratosis with greatly dilated keratin filled spaces.[4] Hyperpigmentation of recent scars occasionally manifests.[5]

Nevi

The change, which is of concern, is the alteration of clinical appearance in pre-existing freckles and nevi. Pigmented nevi can increase in number, size, and pigmentation. Darkening may be attributed to the upregulation of estrogen and progesterone receptors on the surface of nevoid cells. Growth and increase in number of nevi have been reported and may be alarming at times. Changes in the clinical appearance of benign dermal nevi during pregnancy may be a concern for malignant change. Mild cellular atypia may be encountered on histology, but the rate of dysplastic changes is undetermined. The occurrence of any significant change in nevi is debatable and so far there is no concrete evidence for the risk of malignant transformation because the hormonal milieu of pregnancy has not been proven to alter their banal behavior. Histological characterization is needed to prevent over-diagnosis and unnecessary treatment.

Linea Nigra

Linea nigra (Latin for black line) is a dark vertical line that appears on the abdomen in 75% of pregnant females **(Fig. 2)**. It occurs due to darkening of the line alba which is a blended aponeurosis that extends from the symphysis pubis to the xiphisternum, with the umbilicus at or below its center. The brownish streak is about a centimeter in width. The line runs vertically along the midline of the abdomen from the pubis to the umbilicus, but can also run from the pubis to the top of the abdomen. Fair-skinned women show this phenomenon less often than women with darker pigmentation. The reason for the distinctive pigmentary change in the linea nigra is again thought to be due to a local increase in the number of melanocytes. Linea nigra is often accompanied by the displacement of umbilicus at term, to the right side of the patient (ligamentum teres sign). This shift persists during the postpartum period until the abdominal muscles regain their tone.[6]

Melanonychia

Few women notice transient longitudinal melanonychia, which usually fades spontaneously after delivery, only to recur during subsequent pregnancies.[5]

Furthermore, accentuation of patches of dermal melanocytosis also becomes evident, and *de novo* lesions have been reported as early as the first trimester.[7] Reactivation of pre-existing dormant dermal melanocytes by a variety of

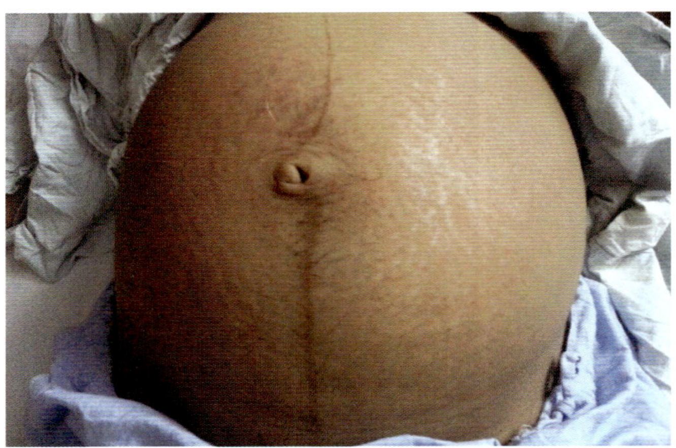

Fig. 2: Linear pigmented line over abdomen in pregnancy

hormonal factors is thought to occur. Elevations in levels of progesterone and estrogen, keratinocyte derived endothelin-1 and MSH have been implicated as its etiology.

Pigmentary Demarcation Lines

Pigmentary demarcation lines (PDL), also known as Futcher's or Voigt's lines, are physiological, abrupt flux from deeper pigmented skin to a lighter pigmented skin. Five naturally manifesting PDLs, labeled A–E **(Table 2)**, have been described in text.

- Increase of the pigmentation in the demarcation lines is consistently observed in pregnant women of darker complexion, but seldom in white subjects.[8] Type B pigmentary demarcation lines have been reported over the legs during pregnancy that regresses after delivery.[9] Recently, three more lines F, G, H have been delineated for the Asian population.
- After delivery, the hyperpigmentation usually resolves spontaneously even though the outcome may widely vary among patients.

Table 2: Pigmentary demarcation lines

A	On the lateral aspect of the upper arm extending over the pectoral area
B	On the posteromedial portion of the lower limb
C	Midsternal line, a vertical hypopigmented line in the pre and parasternal area
D	On the posteromedial area of the spine
E	Bilateral hypopigmented streaks, bands or lanceolate areas over the chest in the zone between the mid-third of the clavicle and the periareolar skin

Table 3: Stages in the onset of a halo nevus

Stage 1	A rim of pale skin surrounds a mole
Stage 2	The mole may become pinker or less pigmented, and fades away
Stage 3	A circular or oval area of depigmentation persists
Stage 4	The affected skin gradually returns to its normal color

Striae Gravidarum

Striae gravidarum is a physiological skin change occurring commonly over the abdomen, buttocks and thighs of pregnant women. They appear in up to 90% of fair-skinned individuals, usually in the 6th and 7th months.[10] It is a scar formation of the skin opposite to the skin tension lines due to sudden weight gain amidst pregnancy, caused by the tearing of the dermis, resulting in atrophy and loss of rete pegs.[11] The striae are often accompanied by a reddish purple color hue during pregnancy (striae rubra), and then pigmentation decreases to become atrophic in the long-term after pregnancy (striae alba). It is a common condition that does not cause any significant medical problems but can be of cosmetic concern. Proposed hypotheses include increased lateral stress on connective tissue and increased glucocorticoid levels due to elevated adrenocortical activity, relaxin and estrogens.[12]

Halo Nevi

The halo nevus (also known as leukoderma acquisitum centrifugum, or Perinevoid vitiligo or Sutton nevus)[13] is a mole that is surrounded by a depigmented ring or "halo", occurs infrequently, usually in young individuals. Appearance of halo corresponds with the regression of the nevus, and depigmentation is usually followed by complete repigmentation. Its underlying etiology is elusive. Vitiligo, is often associated with halo nevi. Halo nevi can occur as an isolated event, in association with vitiligo, in association with prominent and/or atypical nevi, or rarely represent a new primary melanoma.[14] The development of a halo may also coincide with the onset of puberty or pregnancy.[15] The halo is due to the loss of pigment, which corresponds to the body's attempt to launch an immune response against the mole. There are four stages in the onset of a halo nevus **(Table 3)**. It may take several years to complete the cycle.

MELASMA

Melasma, or chloasma or "mask of pregnancy" may affect close to 75% of pregnant women.[16] It displays various symmetrical distributions. The most common is centrofacial type of melasma developing on the forehead, cheeks, upper lip, and chin. Maxillary and mandibular patterns are less frequent. Pigmentation consists of gray-brown, poorly demarcated plaques. The diagnosis is very easy. Wood's light examination helps to differentiate epidermal-type (enhanced pigmentation) from dermal-type (unchanged pigmentation). Mixed-type is less common.

Melasma usually begins after 3rd month of gestation and is responsible for asthetical aversion in many women. Pigmentation usually regresses in postpartum but may persist in less than 10% of the cases[5] and/or worsen again after sun exposure. Recurrence in future pregnancies or with oral contraception is common.

Histopathology, although not required, would show melanin deposits within the epidermis and/or dermal macrophages. There is also an increase in melanogenesis without modification in the number of melanocytes.[17] Of note, estrogen receptor expression is enhanced in melasma-affected skin.[18]

The use of sunscreens is advised. Topical demelanizing agents can be given, if melasma persists after delivery. Treatment in some cases can be annoying and discouraging, and the extent of dermal melanization often influences success rates.

CONCLUSION

The chapter focuses attention on the various pigmentary changes during pregnancy as they are a frequent and polymorphous feature. Dermatologists' expertise in distinguishing between physiological skin changes and specific dermatoses of pregnancy is of vital importance for better patient care of pregnant women.

This chapter focuses on the various pigmentary changes in pregnancy which can be subtle and missed. A through knowledge of the same will help us in identifying these changes.

REFERENCES

1. Huber J, Gruber C. Immunological and dermatological impact of progesterone. Gynecol Endocrinol. 2001;15(S6):18-21.
2. Estève E, Saudeau L, Pierre F, et al. Signes cutanés lors des grossesses normales. Étude de 60 cas. Ann Dermatol Vénéréol. 2004;121:227-31.
3. Muzaffar F, Hussein I, Haroon TS. Physiologic skin changes during pregnancy: a study of 140 cases. Int J Dermatol. 1998;37:429-31.
4. Aytekin S, Tarlan N, Alp S, et al. Naevoid hyperkeratosis of the nipple and areola. J Eur Acad Dermatol Venereol. 2003;17:232-3.
5. Barankin B, Silver SG, Carruthers A. The skin in pregnancy. J Cutan Med Surg. 2002;6:236-40.
6. Beisher NA, Wein P. Linea alba pigmentation and umbilical deviation in nulliparous pregnancy: the ligamentum teres sign. Obstet Gynecol. 1996;87:254-6.
7. Rubin A, Van Laborde S, Stiller MJ. Acquired dermal melanocytosis: appearance during pregnancy. J Am Acad Dermatol. 2001;45:609-13.
8. Somani VK, Razvi F, Sita VN. Pigmentary demarcation lines over the face. Indian J Dermatol Venereol Leprol. 2004;70:336-41.
9. James WD, Meltza MS, Giml MA, et al. Pigmentary demarcation lines associated with pregnancy. J Am Acad Dermatol. 1984;11:438-40.
10. Demis DJ, Dobson RL, McGuire J. In: Clinical dermatology. Vol 2:New York: Harper & Row; 1975. pp. 1–9 Unit 12-25.
11. Kroumpouzos G, Cohen LM. Specific dermatoses of pregnancy: an evidenced-based systematic review. Am J Obstet Gynecol. 2003;188:1083-92.
12. Nigman PK. Striae cutis distensae. Int J Dermatol. 1989; 28:426-8.
13. James WD, Timothy B, E Dirk. Andrews' diseases of the skin. Clinical Dermatology. Saunders Elsevier; 2006.
14. Milton GW, McCarthy WH, Carlton A. Malignant melanoma and vitiligo. Aust J Dermatol. 1971;12:131-42.
15. Kliegman RM, Stanton BF, Geme JW, Schor NF, Behrman RE. Cutaneous Nevi. In: Morelli JG. Nelson Textbook of Pediatrics, 19th edn. Elsevier Saunders; 2011.
16. Smith AG, Shuster S, Thody AJ, et al. Chloasma, oral contraceptives, and plasma immunoreactive beta melanocyte stimulating hormone. J Invest Dermatol. 1976; 68: 367-76.
17. Grimes PE, Yamada N, Bhawan L. Light microscopic, immunohistochemical and ultrastructural alterations in patients with melasma. Am J Dermatopathol. 2005;27: 96-101.
18. Lieberman R, Moy L. Estrogen receptor expression in melasma: results from facial skin of affected patients. J Drugs Dermatol. 2007;7:463-5.

32

Quality of Life in Pigmentary Disorders

Sudhir Nayak UK, Smitha Prabhu, Shrutakirthi D Shenoi

Key Features

- Disorders of pigmentation have negligible physical, but considerable psychological morbidity.
- Quality of life indices are patient reported outcome measures which are carefully designed and validated questionnaires which measure the psychosocial distress faced by sufferers of various chronic illnesses.
- In pigmentary disorders, measurement of quality of life do not show concordance between physician and the patient, as there is psychological debility rather than measurable physical defects.

INTRODUCTION

Quality of life (QoL) is a universal concept that has different political, philosophical and health related definitions. Health-related QoL (HRQoL) includes physical, functional, social and emotional well-being of an individual and is a patient-reported outcome measure based on carefully designed and validated instruments such as questionnaires or semi structured interview schedules.[1] The World Health Organization (WHO) has defined QoL as "individual's perceptions of their position in life in the context of the culture and value systems in which they live and in relation to their goals, expectations, standards and concerns".[2] Thus QoL encompasses physical, psychological, social and environmental health, thus including all factors which tend to influence an individual.

The necessity to evaluate QoL in dermatological diseases stems from the fact that even though generally not life threatening, there is considerable emotional trauma as skin is cosmetologically important. QoL questionnaires are nowadays being used in regular dermatological practice and not just for clinical studies as this can help in evaluating the patient's perception of the dermatological concerns. QoL scales also evaluate the therapeutic efficacy of intervention. QoL questionnaire needs to be adapted to the local populace in view of the cultural variations and language usage and it is also important to validate this QoL questionnaire.[2]

Quality of life has been studied in various chronic skin diseases such as atopic dermatitis, psoriasis, alopecia areata, chronic urticaria, vitiligo, acne, etc. using various questionnaires among which dermatology life quality index (DLQI),[3] the first dermatology specific QoL questionnaire by Finlay and Khan which is universally accepted and used for numerous dermatoses and Skindex[4] are frequently used.

Beauty is considered skin deep. The impairment or alteration of normal cutaneous pigmentation often has a deep impact on psychological well-being and QoL of patients. This is especially so when exposed areas are involved. Indians tend to have a darker complexion than their western counterparts and further hyperpigmentation or depigmentation can negatively affect their psyche. Often, the QoL of close family members is also affected, especially of parents with marriageable children.

Leading causes for hypermelanoses include lentigines, melasma, pigmented contact dermatitis, post-inflammatory hyperpigmentation secondary to lichen planus and macular amyloidosis whilst causes for hypomelanoses include vitiligo, albinism and post-inflammatory hypopigmentation secondary to tinea versicolor, etc.

QUALITY OF LIFE IN DISORDERS OF HYPERPIGMENTATION

India is a large country with varied populace with skin types ranging from FitzPatrick skin types II to VI. Indian obsession with fair skin, which is erroneously equated with beauty and superiority, especially in the "fairer" gender has its roots in Hindu mythology.[5] The importance given to fair skin in India is best highlighted by Indian movie songs which often fixate on lighter skin tone, by innumerable advertisements for lightening agents and by the numerous matrimonial advertisements requesting a "fair" bride. The use of skin lightening agents is universal irrespective of skin type, tone, gender and socioeconomic strata. The need for skin lightening creams ranges from treatment of hyperpigmentation to just lightening the skin "tone".[6] QoL thus tends to be important in such a wide population with hyperpigmentation being a concern in the people with "fair" skin. In a person with an already dark complexion, further hyperpigmentation may be a source of great concern. Moreover, facial pigmentation is notoriously chronic and relatively resistant to treatment with only 50–60% improvement noticed following treatment with various bleaching creams and chemical peels. It may recur on discontinuation of treatment and re-exposure to sunlight.

Hyperpigmentation involving exposed areas is associated with greater morbidity to the patient with a greater negative impact on QoL. The psychosocial impact is often severe with patients complaints ranging from being self-conscious, feeling others focus on their skin, feeling unattractive, taking measures to cover pigmentary aberration and restriction of activities.[7] Pigmentary alteration can lead to embarrassment, frustration, interpersonal relationship disturbances, difficulty in showing affection, reduced sense of importance and productivity, restricted freedom,[1] depression, desocialization, avoidance of sexual contact, anxiety and sometimes even suicide. Over a period of time, people tend to be indifferent to their cosmetic concern.

Dermatology life quality index for pigmentary diseases is equal to that of leg ulcers and drug eruption. However, is significantly less than that for atopic dermatitis, psoriasis, pruritus, urticaria, scabies and even birth marks.[8] The psychosocial scale for pigmentary disorders is comparable to psoriasis on using dermatology QoL scales.[9] Many a time, measurement of QoL in pigmentary disorders do not show concordance between physicians and patients.[10]

Melasma is the prototype of facial pigmentation and has considerable impact on the patients. Men with melasma also reported a higher DLQI scores.[11] Melasma quality of life (MelasQoL) instrument was developed and validated by Dr Balkrishnan in 2003.[12] It is a 10-item QoL scale, with each question rated from 0 to 7 specific for melasma that determines the effect on three domains viz. social life, recreational and leisure life, and emotional well-being. This is found to be superior with higher discriminatory power and consistency.[12,13] MelasQoL has been developed by modifying Skindex-16 and skin discoloration index.[14]

Higher MelasQoL scores indicating greater negative QoL is seen in melasma of longer duration, older age group and patients undergoing treatment: this has been attributed to patients seeking treatment at the time of greater distress/impairment in QoL.[13] Social life, emotional, well-being and recreation/leisure are more affected in MelasQoL.[14] No correlation is seen between severity of melasma and MelasQoL and even a small area of pigmentation can affect QoL.[14] Worldwide, several studies have determined QoL in melasma.[12-14] Pre-treatment DLQI in patients with melasma is high and tends to become less post-treatment.[15] QoL of patients tends to improve significantly subsequent to treatment of the hyperpigmentation and this correlates with objective scales of measurement which measure the improvement in hyperpigmentation.[1]

Post-inflammatory hyperpigmentation tends to affect the QoL significantly, and may even be more disturbing than the primary dermatosis.

Patients with facial blemishes who use facial foundations reported a poorer HRQoL than those not using foundations[16] though DLQI of patients with pigmentary disorders after attending a cosmetic camouflage clinic statistically improves in comparison with pre-clinic DLQI.[17]

OTHER RELATED QoL INDICES

Beauty QoL is an internationally covalidated and reliable instrument that measures physical appearance QoL due to cosmetic products, techniques and/or agents.[18] Another similar scale which has been used is the cosmeti-QoL.[19]

Cutaneous diseases also impact the QoL of families and this has been assessed by questionnaires like family DLQI[20] and family dermatitis impact questionnaire.[21] QoL in children is often measured by children's CDLQI.[21] Pigmentary disorders in children rate on a lower scale both among children and parents of affected children in comparison to other dermatoses.[22]

QUALITY OF LIFE IN DISORDERS OF DEPIGMENTATION

Disorders of depigmentation rarely cause physical discomfort, but the associated social stigma and isolation is severe enough to cause depression, anxiety and a negative self-image, especially in adolescents and young adults, who have an active social and sexual life. The patients are more concerned when the depigmented area is large or when there is depigmentation on cosmetically important and exposed sites, like face, genitals and dorsae of hands.

Vitiligo is the prototype of depigmenting disorder and has been the focus of almost all studies and research on QoL. There are barely any studies on other disorders of depigmentation or hypopigmentation, like albinism or post-inflammatory hypopigmentation. It an acquired, usually progressive autoimmune disease appearing usually in childhood or in young adulthood, a period of life in which the individual is most concerned about his or her appearance.

Prevalence of vitiligo is higher in India (0.46–8.8%)[23] and is of particular concern as the condition is more visible in dark skinned and stigma is more, especially in Asian culture, where there is perceived unsuitability for marriage.[24] There are various modalities of treatment for vitiligo, but none are fully effective with the best treatment rates not more than 70%.[25] Patients feel they are disfigured for life and naturally QoL is impaired.

STIGMATIZATION IN VITILIGO[24,26,27]

Vitiligo is a disease known to ancient civilizations and patients with generalized lesions and disease affecting exposed parts are subjected to social discrimination and stigmatization, which is unrelated to age or gender, though females of marriageable age and even afflicted parents and relatives suffer the most as vitiligo is perceived to be a hereditary condition. So people, especially in certain cultures, like Indian and Asian, tend to conceal the disease.

PSYCHOLOGICAL AND PSYCHIATRIC CO-MORBIDITY[28-31]

Vitiligo can be "psychologically devastating"[32] and patients suffer from anxiety,[24,33] depression,[26,29,31] adjustment disorders,[28] social and sexual phobias and various obsessions. Increased prevalence of alexithymia and avoidance behaviors have been noted.[34] Patients are often embarrassed, suffer from depression and are stigmatized; interestingly, the psychological impact of vitiligo does not correlate with the extent of the lesions, and patient satisfaction with treatment does not correlate with the clinical response.[35] Furthermore patients' beliefs about the onset of their disease may positively or negatively affect their psyche. Indian studies show a high prevalence of psychiatric morbidity in vitiligo (56–75%)[24,28,36,37] as compared to UK and Italy.[38,39] Studies from Iran,[40] Saudi Arabia[41] and Tunisia have found that 21–84% of people believe that their disease was pre-ordained by fate, the "evil eye" or other agents like envious people and evil spirits (28–46%) or stress (33–63%). Vitiligo has a major impact on the life and self-esteem in 42–50% of patients.[35,40]

STRESS PRECIPITATING VITILIGO

A study based on illness perception questionnaire found that 62.5% believed that stress was a major factor in onset or worsening, 49% believed that their illness had a major effect on their lives and about 58% had a low self-esteem. There was no variation between the sexes. As the duration of disease increased, there was increasing hopelessness and a belief that the disease would be permanent.[42] In an Indian study, 2.19% of cases associated precipitation of their disease with emotional stress.[23]

PSYCHOSOCIAL ASSESSMENT SCALES

There are various scales and indices to assess the psychosocial and general impact of vitiligo in patients. General scales include Short Form-36,[43] Rosenberg's self-esteem scale,[44] WHOQoL-BREF,[45] etc. whereas specific ones include DLQI,[3] dermatological HRQoL instrument, Skindex-29,[4] etc. All these scales assess various aspects like psychosocial morbidity, disability, cognitive functioning, emotional components, etc. Many studies have correlated vitiligo to a higher DLQI score, i.e. more impact on QoL. Impairment in HRQoL usually is seen in areas like self-esteem,[38] body image, social,[28] and sexual[46,47] interactions.

VITILIGO SPECIFIC SCALES

As vitiligo is more of a cosmetic problem than a physical disease, "perceived severity" is more important than physician rated severity,[48,49] which are not usually satisfactorily addressed by the general health scales. So, specific scales have been developed to assess domains not covered by general scales.

The vitiligo impact scale (VIS) is a 27 point questionnaire specific for vitiligo patients and assesses aspects like attitude to the disease, anxiety and depression, self-confidence, interpersonal interactions and problems related to marriage, family, education, occupation and also treatment related issues.[35] VitiQoL is another 16-item scale exclusive for vitiligo.[50]

PREDICTORS OF INCREASED SEVERITY IN VARIOUS SCALES

Individual factors include young adulthood (ages 20–29),[51] patient's personality (traits like high anxiety, low self-esteem, negative body self-image) as well as the perceived severity,[49] unstable marital status,[47,52] darker skin,[28,30,52] female sex,[26,35,40,41,47,53,54] Asian and African cultures and unsatisfactory treatment in the past[30,49,55] whereas disease related factors include extensive lesions,[46,47,56,57] lesions on anatomically important parts[30] and on exposed parts,[55] prolonged duration and increase in progression. Vitiligo also has a negative impact on the sexual life.[58] Skindex-29 studies on vitiligo have revealed that patients suffer in functional and emotional aspects.[48]

Gender difference in QoL is worthy of special mention as females suffer more from the psychological effects of vitiligo, especially in patriarchal societies. An Indian study which assessed 180 patients with vitiligo using the VIS found that women had a higher distress rate[35] which is in accordance with many other studies.[26,40,41,47,53,54]

QUALITY OF LIFE IN CHILDREN AND ADOLESCENTS WITH VITILIGO

As compared to adults, there are few studies on the effect of psychosocial stress in children and adolescents with vitiligo. Some opine that childhood onset of vitiligo can lead to considerable psychological distress during the growing years[59,60] and stress may impact disease onset as well as exacerbation,[61] whereas others say that early onset can in fact act as a protective factor as children are not yet focused on their physical appearance and develop mechanisms to cope up and strengthen their self-esteem.[62,63] A study assessing depression, anxiety and QoL using various scales, like Child Depression Inventory, State-Trait Anxiety Inventories for Children and Pediatric Quality of Life Inventories (PedsQL-P and PedsQL-C) in 41 children found depression rather than anxiety in affected children but adolescents were spared.[64] This is slightly confounding as adolescence is more equated with development of self-consciousness and self-image. The score was worse in children with more number of affected body areas, female sex, involvement of face in males and legs and genitalia in females. The extent of disease could not be correlated to the increased scores. Prolonged duration correlated with a better physical health score of PedsQL-P which may be due to the enhanced compliance and coping skills in children. Children with vitiligo were found more prone to avoid strangers and respond more to unexpected changes in relatives and associates.[65]

EFFECTIVENESS OF THERAPEUTIC INTERVENTIONS IN QoL IN VITILIGO PATIENTS[66]

Treatment has shown considerable improvement in DLQI score, especially with modalities like topical tacrolimus, epidermal cell graft transplantation, narrowband ultraviolet B (NB-UVB) treatment, 308-excimer laser, psoralen + ultraviolet A with 8-methoxy psoralen. In two studies of phototherapy in vitiligo, the improvement was more with emotional and social functioning subscales of Skindex-29. Life style changing methods like cognitive behavior therapy and camouflaging also have improved QoL in vitiligo patients, but only if the initial score was very high.

ROUTINE PSYCHOLOGICAL ASSESSMENT IN VITILIGO

According to current recommendations, psychological assessment, especially in children with vitiligo has a level of evidence C/2++ (directly applicable to target population and showing overall consistency) and psychological intervention for helping to cope with the disease has a level of D/4 (based on non-analytical studies and expert opinion). It is also advised that parents of vitiligo children should be offered psychological counseling.[32]

OVERCOMING QUALITY OF LIFE ISSUES IN VITILIGO[37]

As a complete cure is often difficult to attain, focus should be upon improving the body image and self-esteem of the sufferers by helping them to confront their problem and improve their social skills, leading to social and psychological well-being. Assertiveness training and teaching relaxation techniques will help the patients to achieve a better QoL.

LIMITATIONS OF QoL STUDIES

- Scores range widely between various studies
- Different scales are used by different studies
- Patient's perception of the condition varies significantly from the physician's.

CONCLUSION

QoL in a disease tends to provide a clue to the extent to which a disease affects an individual as perception of a disease by a patient is quite different from that perceived by a doctor, and may vary from patient to patient as there are multiple factors that influence it like age, sex, community, upbringing and individual emotional fitness. In a society 'obsessed' with fairness and uniformity of skin color, pigmentary alterations (both hyper- and hypo- or depigmentation) tend to cause distress to the patient. Thus, QoL questionnaires provide a valuable tool for assessing the distress of a patient with pigmentary disorder and hence its incorporation in the evaluation of a patient with pigmentary disorders is essential.

REFERENCES

1. Cestari TF, Hexsel D, Viegas ML, et al. Validation of a melasma quality of life questionnaire for Brazilian Portuguese language: the MelasQoL-BP study and improvement of QoL of melasma patients after triple combination therapy. Br J Dermatol. 2006;156(Suppl 1):13-20.
2. WHOQoL Measuring Quality of Life. Division of mental health and substance abuse. World Health Organization. Report number:WHO/MSA/MNH/PSF/97.4, 1997.
3. Finlay AY, Khan GK. Dermatology Life Quality Index (DLQI)—a simple practical measure for routine clinical use. Clin Exp Dermatol. 1994;19(3):210-6.

4. Chren MM, Lasek RJ, Quinn LM, et al. Skindex, a quality-of-life measure for patients with skin disease: reliability, validity and responsiveness. J Invest Dermatol. 1996;107(5):707-13.
5. Chand P, Choudhary S. (2012) Advertising discourse: Studying creation and perception of meaning. [online] Available from http://www.academicjournals.org/IJEL. [Accessed October, 2013].
6. Hamed SH, Tayyem R, Nimer N, et al. Skin-lightening practice among women living in Jordan: prevalence, determinants, and user's awareness. Int J Dermatol. 2010;49(4):414-20.
7. Taylor A, Pawaskar M, Taylor SL, et al. Prevalence of pigmentary disorders and their impact on quality of life: a prospective cohort study. J Cosmet Dermatol. 2008;7(3):164-8.
8. Harlow D, Poyner T, Finlay AY, et al. Impaired quality of life of adults with skin disease in primary care. Br J Dermatol. 2000;143(5):979-82.
9. Morgan M, McCreedy R, Simpson J, et al. Dermatology quality of life scales—a measure of the impact of skin diseases. Br J Dermatol. 1997;136(2):202-6.
10. Sampogna F, Picardi A, Melchi CF, et al. The impact of skin diseases on patients: comparing dermatologists' opinions with research data collected on their patients. Br J Dermatol. 2003;148(5):989-95.
11. Pichardo R, Vallejos Q, Feldman SR, et al. The prevalence of melasma and its association with quality of life in adult male Latino migrant workers. Int J Dermatol. 2009;48(1):22-6.
12. Balkrishnan R, McMichael AJ, Camacho FT, et al. Development and validation of a health-related quality of life instrument for women with melasma. Br J Dermatol. 2003;149(3):572-7.
13. Misery L, Schmitt A, Boussetta S, et al. Melasma: measure of the impact on quality of life using the French version of MELASQoL after cross-cultural adaptation. Acta Derm Venereol. 2010;90(3):331-2.
14. Sheth VM, Pandya AG. Melasma: a comprehensive update. J Am Acad Dermatol. 2011;65(4):689-97.
15. Hexsel D, Arellano I, Rendon M. Ethnic considerations in the treatment of Hispanic and Latin-American patients with hyperpigmentation. Br J Dermatol. 2006;156(Suppl 1):7-12.
16. Pawaskar MD, Parikh P, Markowski T, et al. Melasma and its impact on health-related quality of life in Hispanic women. J Dermatolog Treat. 2007;18(1):5-9.
17. Holme SA, Beattie PE, Fleming CJ. Cosmetic camouflage advice improves quality of life. Br J Dermatol. 2002; 147(5):946-9.
18. Krueger G, Beresniak A, Walkiewicz-Cyranska B, et al. International covalidation of a new international quality of life instrument specific to physical appearance: BeautyQoL. J Am Acad Dermatol. 2011;64(2):AB70.
19. Taieb C, Sibaud V. Cosmeti-QoL: a tool for assessing quality of life in cosmetic dermatology. J Am Acad Dermatol. 2012;66(4):AB87.
20. Basra MKA, Finlay AY. The family impact of skin diseases: the Greater Patient concept. Br J Dermatol. 2007;156(5): 929-37.
21. Finlay AY. Quality of life indices. Indian J Dermatol Venereol Leprol. 2004;70(3):143-8.
22. Beattie PE, Lewis-Jones MS. A comparative study of impairment of quality of life in children with skin disease and children with other chronic childhood diseases. Br J Dermatol. 2006;155(1):145-51.
23. Shah H, Mehta A, Astik B. Clinical and sociodemographic study of vitiligo. Indian J Dermatol Venereol Leprol. 2008; 74(6):701.
24. Parsad D, Dogra S, Kanwar AJ. Quality of life in patients with vitiligo. Health Qual Life Outcomes. 2003;1:58.
25. Parsad D. Vitiligo: emerging paradigms. Indian J Dermatol Venereol Leprol. 2012;78(1):17-8.
26. Schmid-Ott G, Kunsebeck HW, Jecht E, et al. Stigmatization experience, coping and sense of coherence in vitiligo patients. J Eur Acad Dermatol Venereol. 2007;21(4): 456-61.
27. Kent G, Al'Abadie M. Psychologic effects of vitiligo: a critical incident analysis. J Am Acad Dermatol. 1996;35(6):895-8.
28. Mattoo SK, Handa S, Kaur I, et al. Psychiatric morbidity in vitiligo: prevalence and correlates in India. J Eur Acad Dermatol Venereol. 2002;16(6):573-8
29. Sampogna F, Raskovic D, Guerra L, et al. Identification of categories at risk for high quality of life impairment in patients with vitiligo. Br J Dermatol. 2008;159(2):351-9.
30. Linthorst Homan MW, Spuls PI, de Korte J, et al. The burden of vitiligo: patient characteristics associated with quality of life. J Am Acad Dermatol. 2009;61(3):411-20.
31. Agarwal G. Vitiligo: an under-estimated problem. Fam Pract. 1998;15 Suppl 1:S19-23.
32. Gawkrodger DJ, Ormerod AD, Shaw L, et al. Guideline for the diagnosis and management of vitiligo. Br J Dermatol. 2008;159(5):1051-76.
33. Gieler U, Brosig B, Schneider U, et al. Vitiligo-coping behavior. Dermatol Psychosom. 2000;1:6-10.
34. Picardi A, Pasquini P, Cattaruzza MS, et al. Stressful life events, social support, attachment security and alexithymia in vitiligo. A case-control study. Psychother Psychosom. 2003;72(3):150-8.
35. Krishna GS, Ramam M, Mehta M, et al. Vitiligo impact scale: an instrument to assess the psychosocial burden of vitiligo. Indian J Dermatol Venereol Leprol. 2013;79(2): 205-10.
36. Mattoo SK, Handa S, Kaur I, et al. Psychiatric morbidity in vitiligo and psoriasis: a comparative study from India. J Dermatol. 2001;28(8):424-32.
37. Parsad D, Pandhi R, Dogra S, et al. Dermatology life quality index score in vitiligo and its impact on treatment outcome. Br J Dermatol. 2003;148(2):373-4.
38. Kent G, Al'Abadie M. Factors affecting responses on Dermatology Life Quality Index items among vitiligo sufferers. Clin Exp Dermatol. 1996;21(5):330-3.
39. Picardi A, Abeni D, Melchi CF, et al. Psychiatric morbidity in dermatological outpatients: an issue to be recognized. Br J Dermatol. 2000;143(5):983-91.

40. Alghamdi KM. Beliefs and perceptions of Arab vitiligo patients regarding their condition. Int J Dermatol. 2010;49(10):1141-5.
41. Borimnejad L, Parsa Yekta Z, Nikbakht-Nasrabadi A, et al. Quality of life with vitiligo: comparison of male and female muslim patients in Iran. Gen Med. 2006;3(2):124-30.
42. Firooz A, Bouzari N, Fallah N, et al. What patients with vitiligo believe about their condition. Int J Dermatol. 2004;43(11):811-4.
43. Ware JE. SF-36 health survey update. [online] Available from: http://www.sf-36.org/tools/sf36.shtml. [Accessed March, 2013].
44. Robins RW, Hendin HM, Trzesniewski KH. Measuring global self-esteem: construct validation of a single-item measure and the Rosenberg self-esteem scale. Personality and Social Psychology Bulletin. 2001;27:151-61.
45. WHO. (2004). WHOQoL-BREF. [online] WHO website. Available from http://www.who.int/substance_abuse/research_tools/en/english_whoQoL.pdf. [Accessed March, 2013].
46. Porter JR, Beuf AH, Lerner AB, et al. The effect of vitiligo on sexual relationships. J Am Acad Dermatol. 1990;22(2 Pt 1):221-2.
47. Wang KY, Wang KH, Zhang ZP. Health-related quality of life and marital quality of vitiligo patients in China. J Eur Acad Dermatol Venereol. 2011;25(4):429-35.
48. Kim do Y, Lee JW, Whang SH, et al. Quality of life for Korean patients with vitiligo: Skindex-29 and its correlation with clinical profiles. J Dermatol. 2009;36(6):317-22.
49. Kostopoulou P, Jouary T, Quintard B, et al. Objective vs. subjective factors in the psychological impact of vitiligo: th experience from a French referral centre. Br J Dermatol. 2009;161(1):128-33.
50. Lilly E, Lu PD, Borovicka JH, et al. Development and validation of a vitiligo-specific quality-of-life instrument (VitiQoL). J Am Acad Dermatol. 2013;69(1):e11-8.
51. Radtke MA, Schäfer I, Gajur A, et al. Willingness-to-pay and quality of life in patients with vitiligo. Br J Dermatol. 2009;161(1):134-9.
52. Dolatshahi M, Ghazi P, Feizy V, et al. Life quality assessment among patients with vitiligo: comparison of married and single patients in Iran. Indian J Dermatol Venereol Leprol. 2008;74(6):700.
53. Belhadjali H, Amri M, Mecheri A, et al. Vitiligo and quality of life: a case control study. Article in French. Ann Dermatol Venerol. 2007;134(3 Pt 1):233-6.
54. Al Robaee AA. Assessment of quality of life in Saudi patients with vitiligo in a medical school in Qassim province, Saudi Arabia. Saudi Med J. 2007;28(9):1414-7.
55. Ongenae K, Dierckxsens L, Brochez L, et al. Quality of life and stigmatization profile in a cohort of vitiligo patients and effect of the use of camouflage. Dermatology. 2005;210(4):279-85.
56. Ongenae K, van Geel N, De Schepper S, et al. Effect of vitiligo on self-reported health-related quality of life. Br J Dermatol. 2005;152(6):1165-72.
57. Linthorst Homan MW, Sprangers MA, de Korte J, et al. Characteristics of patients with universal vitiligo and health-related quality of life. Arch Dermatol. 2008;144(8):1062-4.
58. Sukan M, Maner F. The problems in sexual functions of vitiligo and chronic urticaria patients. J Sex Marital Ther. 2007;33(1):55-64.
59. Silverberg NB. Update on childhood vitiligo. Curr Opin Pediatr. 2010;22(4):445-52.
60. Barisic-Drusko V, Rucevic I. Trigger factors in childhood psoriasis and vitiligo. Coll Antropol. 2004;28(1):277-85.
61. Manolache L, Petrescu-Seceleanu D, Benea V. Correlation of stressful events with onset of vitiligo in children. J Eur Acad Dermatol Venereol. 2009;23(2):187-8.
62. Prcic S, Durovic D, Duran V, et al. Some psychological characteristics of children and adolescents with vitiligo—our results. Med Pregl. 2006;59(5-6):265-9.
63. Hill-Beuf A, Porter JD. Children coping with impaired appearance: social and psychological influences. Gen Hosp Psychiatry. 1984;6(4):294-301.
64. Bilgiç O, Bilgiç A, Akiş HK, et al. Depression, anxiety and health-related quality of life in children and adolescents with Vitiligo. Clin Exp Dermatol. 2010;36(4):360-5.
65. Schwartz R, Sepulveda JE, Quintana T. Possible role of psychological and environmental factors in the genesis of childhood vitiligo. Rev Med Chil. 2009;137(1):53-62.
66. Lert CT, Fai CM. A systematic review of the effectiveness of therapeutic interventions on quality of life for adult vitiligo patients. JBI Library of Systematic Reviews. 2010;8: 1169-201.

33

Epidemiology of Melasma

Sanjay K Rathi, Paschal D'Souza

Key Features

- No randomized studies for prevalence of melasma.
- Commonly seen in women, but in Indian scenario, around 19–26% of men can develop melasma.
- UV exposure and genetic influence considered important reasons; further studies needed worldwide.

INTRODUCTION

Melasma is a common hypermelanosis that happens to develop on sun exposed area of face. Despite being a very common skin condition, the exact prevalence of melasma is unknown in most of the countries.[1,2]

There have been various studies to ascertain prevalence of melasma in general population, but all lack randomization. It accounts for 2.5–4% of the patients seen in the dermatology clinic in Southeast Asia and is the most common pigmentary disorder among Indians.[3,4]

Worldwide, melasma is a frequent disorder that affects over 5 million people in the United States.[5] In Southeast Asia, the prevalence of melasma is very high (40% in women and 20% in men),[4] while studies done in India reported approximately 19–26% of males having melasma.[6,7] It represents the fifth common cutaneous disorder with a prevalence of 14.5% in case of Arab-American individuals living in the United States.[8]

The disease affects all racial groups, but is more common in individuals of Hispanic, Asian and African origin. This reflects that people with dark skin and Fitzpatrick phototypes IV, V and VI are more frequently affected.[9,10]

A multicentric study on melasma was carried out in nine countries. It showed that familial cases of melasma are more commonly seen in Afro-Americans. Melasma appearing after pregnancy but before menopause is seen in 41% of women. Spontaneous remission may occur in only 8% of cases. Twenty-five percent of patients taking oral contraceptives developed melasma after having started taking the contraception.[11]

In an Indian study of 312 patients, the women to men ratio were approximately 4:1.[6] The average age of onset of melasma was 30 years. In 55% of patients, the melasma was exacerbated by sun exposure. Amongst the 250 women, 56 had precipitation of melasma during pregnancy and 46 were on contraceptive pills which could have been the causative factor in their cases. Only 34 patients reported an exacerbation of melasma during pregnancy. Family history of melasma was reported in 104 patients (33.3%).[6]

The disorder is more common in women of child bearing age indicating hormonal activity. However, since males are also involved it could not hold as the only causative reason for melasma.[7] Even though genetic influence and UV radiation are considered to be important reasons, melasma represents chronic disorder that may last for decades and still much more is to be learnt about the epidemiology of it worldwide.[1]

REFERENCES

1. Sheth VM, Pandya AG. Melasma: a comprehensive update: part I. J Am Acad Dermatol. 2011;65(4):689-97.
2. Tamega Ade A, Miot LD, Bonfietti C, et al. Clinical patterns and epidemiological characteristics of facial melasma in Brazilian women. J Eur Acad Dermatol Venereol. 2013;27(2):151-6.
3. Pasricha JS, Khaitan BK, Dash S. Pigmentary disorders in India. Dermatol Clin. 2007;25(3):343-522.
4. Sivayathorn A. Melasma in orientals. Clin Drug Invest. 1995;10(Suppl 2):34-40.

5. Grimes PE. Melasma: etiologic and therapeutic considerations. Arch Dermatol. 1995;131(12):1453-7.
6. Achar A, Rathi SK. Melasma: a clinico-epidemiological study of 312 cases. Indian J Dermatol. 2011;56(4):380-2.
7. Sarkar R, Puri P, Jain RK, et al. Melasma in men: a clinical, aetiological and histological study. J Eur Acad Dermatol Venereol. 2010;24(7):768-72.
8. El-Assawi D, Musial JL, Hammad A, et al. A survey of skin disease and skin-related issues in Arab-Americans. J Am Acad Dermatol. 2007;56(6):933-8.
9. Lapeere H, Boon B, Scheffer SD, et al. Hypomelanoses and hypermelanoses. In: Wolff K, Goldsmith LA, Katz SI, Gilchrist BA, Patter AS, Leffell DT (Eds). Dermatology in General Medicine, 5th edition. New York: McGraw-Hill; 2008. pp. 622-40.
10. Bandyopadhyay D. Topical treatment of melasma. Indian J Dermatol. 2009;54(4):303-9.
11. Ortonne JP, Arellano I, Berneburg M, et al. A global survey of the role of ultraviolet radiation and hormonal influences in the development of melasma. J Eur Acad Dermatol Venereol. 2009;23(11):1254-62.

34

Etiopathogenesis of Melasma

Hee Young Kang

Key Features

- Combined factors such as family history and sun exposure are likely associated with the development of melasma.
- Melasma pigmentation occurs in the epidermis; however, factors related to the dermis are thought to be the major causes of why this disorder is persistent and difficult to treat.
- How cutaneous blood vessels influence the pathogenesis of melasma is a recommended theme for subsequent work.

INTRODUCTION

Melasma is a common acquired hyperpigmentary disorder of the face and the treatment is still challenging.[1] Classical etiological factors typically include genetic effects, female sex hormones and instances of ultraviolet (UV) radiation exposure. A recent major survey of 324 patients internationally suffering from melasma was conducted in an effort to deepen our knowledge of the causes of melasma.[2] In the present study, family history was found to be crucial in terms of its effect on the development of melasma, and almost half of the patients here had a familial history of melasma. The hormonal influence, although playing some role at least in some of the patients appeared to be weaker than previous thought. Melasma was not always associated with pregnancy, and only 20% of melasma occurred in the peripregnancy period. This study concluded that combined factors such as family history and UV exposure are likely associated with the development of this disorder.

The pathogenesis of melasma is not fully understood, but the current studies suggest that endogenous or exogenous stimuli cause the microenvironment to become stimulated, initiating the release of various mediators that activate melanocytes as melasma develops. In melasma skin, not only melanocytes but also other factors most likely play a key role in the development and in relapses of melasma.

SUN EXPOSURE AND MELASMA

Melasma arises in areas exposed to strong sunlight. Patients report that melasma can become more pronounced upon exposure to the sun. The use of solely a sunscreen as a means of treating melasma has not been investigated, though the usage of this type of protection is recommended based on clinical experience. The regular use of a broad-spectrum sunscreen is effective both in preventing melasma and in enhancing the effectiveness of other topical therapies after the development of melasma.[3,4] Immunohistochemical studies have shown that melasma skin shows features of prominent solar damaged skin.[5,6] An enhanced degree of lesional skin showing solar elastosis has been noted, leading to the suggestion that the solar damage process affects the development of hyperpigmentation in the melasma skin.

During exposure to the sun's rays, UV irradiation has been considered as the main triggering or exacerbating factor in the development of melasma. It is well known that UV radiation causes melanogenesis and melanocyte proliferation as well as cell migration. Moreover, the creation of multiple cytokines, including α-melanocyte-stimulating hormone (MSH) and adrenocorticotropic hormone (ACTH) derived from proopiomelanocortin, is known to be increased by UV irradiation in keratinocytes, thus upregulating melanocyte proliferation while also increasing the synthesis of melanin by stimulating tyrosinase-related protein-1 (TRP-1) and tyrosinase activity.[7] In a comparison of perilesional and lesional normal skin biopsies in 10 melasma patients, a statistically significant increase in the expression of α-MSH was noted in lesional skin.[8] This implies that the persistent overexpression of α-MSH after lesional skin is exposed to UV light has an important effect during the development of melasma.

Interestingly, it has been recently suggested that visible light is also able to induce hyperpigmentation, at least on type IV–VI skin.[9] In dark types of skin, both UVA and visible light induce pigmentation, but the pigmentation was more intense and more stable after visible light exposure as compared with UVA. Therefore, it is emphasized that patients with melasma should use a broad-spectrum UVA- and UVB-protective sunscreen in conjunction with a physical block, for instance zinc oxide or titanium dioxide.

ROLE OF DERMAL FACTORS IN THE DEVELOPMENT OF MELASMA

Melasma pigmentation occurs in the epidermis; however, factors related to the dermis are thought to be the major causes of why this disorder is persistent and difficult to treat. Indeed, melasma dermal skin is different from perilesional normal skin and shows the features of prominently solar-damaged skin. When skin is exposed to the sun, combinations of cellular interactions between melanocytes and fibroblasts, keratinocytes and the vasculature system may play an important role in the occurrence of epidermal hyperpigmentation in melasma.

Role of Fibroblasts

The fibroblasts in the dermis may be linked to the occurrence of melasma. It is known that the protein expression of stem cell factor (SCF) from fibroblasts and c-Kit in melanocytes shows a significant increase in the lesional skin of melasma.[10] The messenger ribonucleic acid (mRNA) expressions of SCF or c-Kit also show increases in melasma. Cytokines derived from fibroblasts cause melanogenesis while also causing melanocytes to proliferate in cultures.[11] A clinical case also supported the role of dermal SCF in epidermal pigmentation.[12] The patient applied topical tacrolimus to treat lichen sclerosus et atrophicus and developed hyperpigmentation. Histological work showed an increased amount of epidermal pigmentation and an increase in the expression of fibroblast-derived SCF in the hyperpigmented skin. This case supported that fibroblast-derived SCF is strongly linked to how epidermal hyperpigmentation develops *in vivo*. Therefore, it is speculated that dermal inflammation caused by UV irradiation is related to fibroblast activation, in turn resulting in dermal SCF upregulation in patients with melasma and in fact enhancing melanogenesis.

Role of Blood Vessels

The presence of hyperpigmented patches is among the main clinical features of melasma, but patients with melasma have other distinguishing features such as pronounced telangiectatic erythema, which is commonly found only on the lesional skin of melasma patients **(Figs 1A and B)**. Vascularization has been found to be greater in melasma lesions relative to the amount in perilesional normal skin.[13,14] The erythema index was also noted as being significantly higher in lesional skin as compared to in perilesional normal skin. A positive correlation was also found in the melanin and erythema index. It was suggested that "erythema" in melasma reflects the severity of the disease and that deeper erythema and less pigmentation in melasma are associated with a poorer response to laser treatments.[15] The immunohistochemistry for vascular markers revealed that the upper dermis contained relatively more vessels.[13] This number was correlated positively with epidermal pigmentation in the lesional skin of melasma. Chronic sun exposure stimulates vascular endothelial growth factor (VEGF) secretion from keratinocytes. The increased expression of VEGF in keratinocytes has been proposed as the main angiogenic cause of the different vessels in melasma.[13]

Whereas how cutaneous blood vessels act in the pathogenesis of melasma has not been studied to a great extent, recent studies suggested that targeting both melanin pigment and blood vessels would be beneficial for the treatment of melasma.[16,17] A controlled, prospective and comparative split-face study was performed to evaluate the effects of pulsed dye laser (PDL) therapy when used in conjunction with a triple combination cream to treat melasma.[16] Triluma cream® combined with PDL decreased pigmentation considerably as compared to the cream alone. Moreover, the progress caused by PDL when combined with the cream continued to be remarkably significant after a summer had passed. In contrast, relapses were noted in a group given only the cream. This implies that targeting vascularization in melasma lesions can lessen melanocyte stimulation. Another study showed that the treatment of melasma with tranexamic acid, an antifibrinolytic used to prevent and to treat some hemorrhagic events, caused epidermal pigmentation linked with melasma to decrease while reversing dermal changes related to melasma, i.e. the number of vessels.[17] Considering that tranexamic acid suppresses angiogenesis, the decline in the number of vessels and the reduction of erythema may have resulted from the antiangiogenic action.

REFERENCES

1. Kang HY, Ortonne JP. What should be considered in the treatment of melasma. Ann Dermatol. 2010;22:373-8.
2. Ortonne JP, Arellano I, Berneburg M, et al. A global survey of the role of ultraviolet radiation and hormonal influences in the development of melasma. J Eur Acad Dermatol Venereol. 2009;23:1254-62.
3. Lakhdar H, Zouhair K, Khadir K, et al. Evaluation of the effectiveness of broad-spectrum sunscreen in the prevention of chloasma in pregnant women. J Eur Acad Dermatol Venereol. 2007;21:738-42.
4. Vazquez M, Sanchez JL. The efficacy of a broad-spectrum sunscreen in the treatment of melasma. Cutis. 1983;32:95-6.
5. Kang WH, Yoon KH, Lee ES, et al. Melasma: histopathological characteristics in 56 Korean patients. Br J Dermatol. 2002;146:228-37.
6. Hernández-Barrera R, Torres-Alvarez B, Castanedo-Cazares JP, et al. Solar elastosis and presence of mast cells as key features in the pathogenesis of melasma. Clin Exp Dermatol. 2008;33:305-8.
7. Suzuki I, Kato T, Motokawa T, et al. Increase of pro-opiomelanocortin mRNA prior to tyrosinase, tyrosinase-related protein 1, dopachrome tautomerase, Pmel-17/gp100, and P-protein mRNA in human skin after ultraviolet B irradiation. J Invest Dermatol. 2002;118:73-8.
8. Im S, Kim J, On WY, et al. Increased expression of alpha-melanocyte-stimulating hormone in the lesional skin of melasma. Br J Dermatol. 2002;146:165-7.
9. Mahmoud BH, Ruvolo E, Hexsel CL, et al. Impact of long-wavelength UVA and visible light on melanocompetent skin. J Invest Dermatol. 2010;130:2092-7.
10. Kang HY, Hwang JS, Lee JY, et al. The dermal stem cell factor and c-kit are overexpressed in melasma. Br J Dermatol. 2006;154:1094-9.
11. Imokawa G. Autocrine and paracrine regulation of melanocytes in human skin and in pigmentary disorders. Pigment Cell Res. 2004;17:96-110.
12. Kim YJ, Kang HY. Pigmentation after using topical tacrolimus to treat lichen sclerosus: possible role of stem cell factor. J Am Acad Dermatol. 2007;57:S125-7.
13. Kim EH, Kim YC, Lee ES, et al. The vascular characteristics of melasma. J Dermatol Sci. 2007;46:111-6.
14. Kang HY, Bahadoran P, Suzuki I, et al. *In vivo* reflectance confocal microscopy detects pigmentary changes in melasma at a cellular level resolution. Exp Dermatol. 2010;19:e228-33.
15. Choi JR, Won CH, Oh ES, et al. The degree of erythema in melasma lesion is associated with the severity of disease and the response to the low-fluence Q-switched 1064-nm Nd:YAG laser treatment. J Dermatol Treat. 2013;24(4):297-9.
16. Passeron T, Fontas E, Kang HY, et al. Melasma treatment with pulsed-dye laser and triple combination cream: a prospective, randomized, single-blind, split-face study. Arch Dermatol. 2011;147:1106-8.
17. Na JI, Choi SY, Yang SH, et al. Effect of tranexamic acid on melasma: a clinical trial with histological evaluation. J Eur Acad Dermatol Venereol. 2013;27(8):1035-9.
18. Lee DJ, Park KC, Ortonne JP, et al. Pendulous melanocytes: a characteristic feature of melasma and how it may occur. Br J Dermatol. 2012;166:684-6.
19. Torres-Álvarez B, Mesa-Garza IG, Castanedo-Cázares JP, et al. Histochemical and immunohistochemical study in melasma: evidence of damage in the basal membrane. Am J Dermatopathol. 2011;33:291-5.
20. Iriyama S, Ono T, Aoki H, et al. Hyperpigmentation in human solar lentigo is promoted by heparanase-induced loss of heparan sulfate chains at the dermal–epidermal junction. J Dermatol Sci. 2011;64:223-8.
21. Park GH, Lee JH, Choi JR, et al. Does altered basement membrane of melasma lesion affect treatment outcome in Asian skin? Am J Dermatopathol. 2013;35:137-8.
22. Kang HY, Suzuki I, Lee DJ, et al. Transcriptional profiling shows altered expression of the Wnt pathway and lipid metabolism-related genes as well as melanogenesis-related genes in melasma. J Invest Dermatol. 2011;131:1692-700.
23. Lee DJ, Lee J, Ha J, et al. Defective barrier function in melasma skin. J Eur Acad Dermatol Venereol. 2012;26:1533-7.
24. Rhodes LE, Gledhill K, Masoodi M, et al. The sunburn response in human skin is characterized by sequential eicosanoid profiles that may mediate its early and late phases. FASEB J. 2009;23:3947-56.
25. Kapoor R, Phiske MM, Jerajani HR. Evaluation of safety and efficacy of topical prostaglandin E2 in treatment of vitiligo. Br J Dermatol. 2009;160:861-3.

35

Histopathological Evaluation of Melasma and Other Facial Hyperchromias

Asha Kubba, Meenakshi Batrani

Key Features

- Facial hyperchromia is a broad category comprising of entities with diverse etiologies; melasma being the most common.
- Melasma is clinically characteristic but requires distinction from melasma mimickers.
- Histopathological evaluation is valuable to establish a specific diagnosis.

DEFINITION OF TERMS

The terms "hyperchromia", "hyperpigmentation", "melanosis" and "melanocytosis" are being used inaccurately and interchangeably. Each of these terms is distinctive and signifies a unique pathophysiology[1,2] **(Flow chart 1)**.

HYPERCHROMIA AND HYPERPIGMENTATION

Hyperchromia implies macular skin darkening due to any cause. Based on the underlying etiology, hyperchromia is broadly classified into melanotic type and non-melanotic type. Melanotic type is related to increase in melanin or melanocytes. Pigmentary disorder academy proposes that the term "hyperpigmentation" should be restricted to melanotic type of hyperchromia. Non melanotic hyperchromia is caused by deposition of non melanin endogenous substances (collagen, hemoglobin and its derivatives, porphyrin, ochronosis) or exogenous chemicals (drugs, metals).[1] In some situations as exemplified by drugs both melanotic and non melanotic pathogenetic mechanisms are responsible. Epidermal and stratum corneum thickening is another mechanism of hyperchromia.[2]

Flow chart 1: Classification of hyperchromia

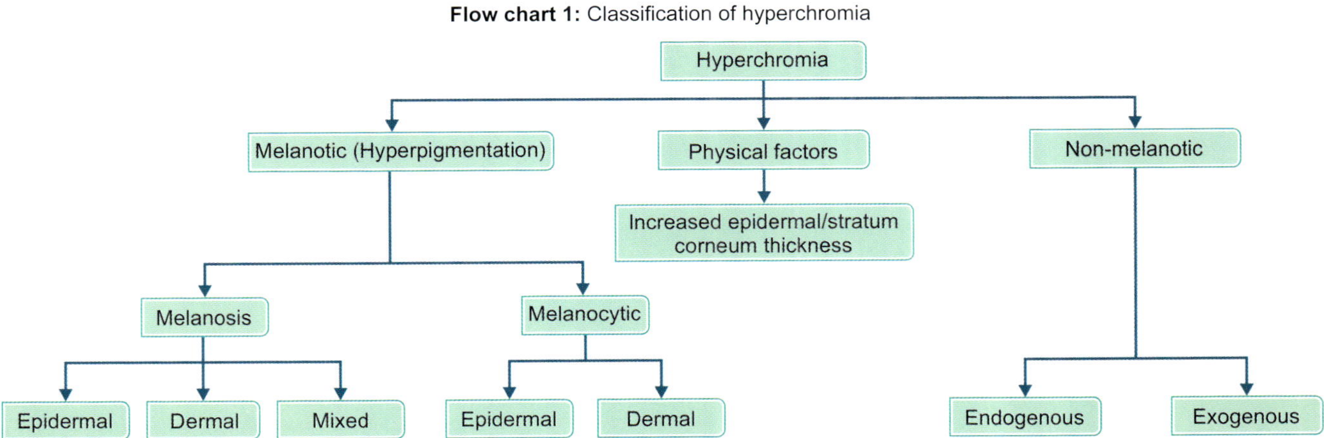

Melanosis

It is a form of hyperpigmentation caused by an increase in melanin pigment which can be epidermal and/or dermal. There may be an associated mild proliferation of melanocytes along the basal layer, but the cause of pigmentation is increase in pigment and not the number of melanocytes *per se*.

Melanocytosis

Literally, this term would imply an increase in number of melanocytes. However, from a pathological perspective, the melanocytic nevi (which also represent increase in melanocytes albeit nevoid melanocytes) are not included. The term melanocytosis is mainly used in the context of dermal melanocytosis which is the umbrella category representing a group of disorders characterized by ectopic presence of dendritic melanocytes in the dermis.[3] Epidermal increase in melanocytes other than melanocytic nevi is seen in lentigines, characterized by elongated rete ridges with increase in single melanocytes along the basal layer, which theoretically can be labelled as epidermal melanocytosis, a term which is not often used.

FACIAL HYPERCHROMIA

Hyperchromias involving the face form a distinct subset of disorder of color. This group is clinically important for the psychosocial implications related to facial involvement and due to diverse underlying etiological conditions **(Box 1)** which need to be distinguished for the prognosis and therapeutic purposes.

Histopathological evaluation is important in facial hyperchromias for diagnostic purpose as well as a useful tool for accurate determination of location and extent of pigment which aids to patient management **(Box 2)**.

This chapter deals with histopathological aspects of various causes of facial hyperchromias.

Box 1

Causes of facial hyperchromias

1. Melanotic hyperchromias (Hyperpigmentation)
   A. Hypermelanosis
   - Melasma
   - Lichen planus pigmentosus
   - Riehl's melanosis
   - Poikiloderma of Civatte
   - Berloque's dermatitis
   - Erythrosis pigmentosa peribuccalis of Brocq
   - Macular amyloidosis
   - Freckles (Ephelids)
   - Erythromelanosis follicularis faciei et colli
   - Periorbital melanosis and pigment demarcation line
   - Post-inflammatory hyperpigmentation
   - Post-Chikungunya melanosis
   - Pigmented discoid lupus erythematosus
   - Facial melanosis of systemic diseases
     - Addison's disease
     - Porphyria cutanea tarda

   B. Hypermelanocytosis
   - Epidermal melanocytic hyperplasia
     - Lentigines
   - Dermal melanocytic hyperplasia (Melanocytosis)
     - Nevus of Ota
     - Hori's nevus (ABNOM)
2. Non-melanotic hyperchromia
   - Endogenous deposits
     - Alkaptonuric ochronosis
   - Exogenous deposits
     - Exogenous ochronosis
     - Drugs
     - Heavy metals (Silver, Gold)
3. Mixed melanotic and non-melanotic hyperchromia
   - Hemochromatosis
   - Drugs
4. Epidermal and stratum corneum alterations
   - Acanthosis nigricans

Box 2

Keys to histopathological evaluation

Lesional and perilesional skin: Essential for evaluation
- Histochemical stains
  - Melanin: Masson-Fontana
  - Elastic fibers: Verhoeff-Van Gieson
  - Hemosiderin: Perl's
- Immunohistochemistry
  - Melanocyte: Melan-A (Mart-1), SOX 10, NKI/beteb, S-100, Microphthalmia-associated transcription factor (MITF)

Diagnosis: Based on clinicopathological correlation

MELASMA

Melasma is the most common cause of facial melanosis, therefore, often used synonymously.

Histopathology

Traditionally, Wood's light examination divides melasma into epidermal, dermal and mixed types.[4] Except an odd past study,[5] most of the recent histopathology based studies on melasma have found an increased epidermal melanin in almost all cases of melasma with or without an increase in dermal pigment. Thus, refuting the existence of pure dermal melasma.[6-8] Reflectance confocal microscopy (RCM) has also substantiated the histopathological findings.[7,9-11] RCM has also demonstrated a heterogeneous topographic distribution of melanophages.[10] This may be the reason for pure dermal melasma being reported in rare past studies based on single biopsies.[7] A better classification which can be achieved using

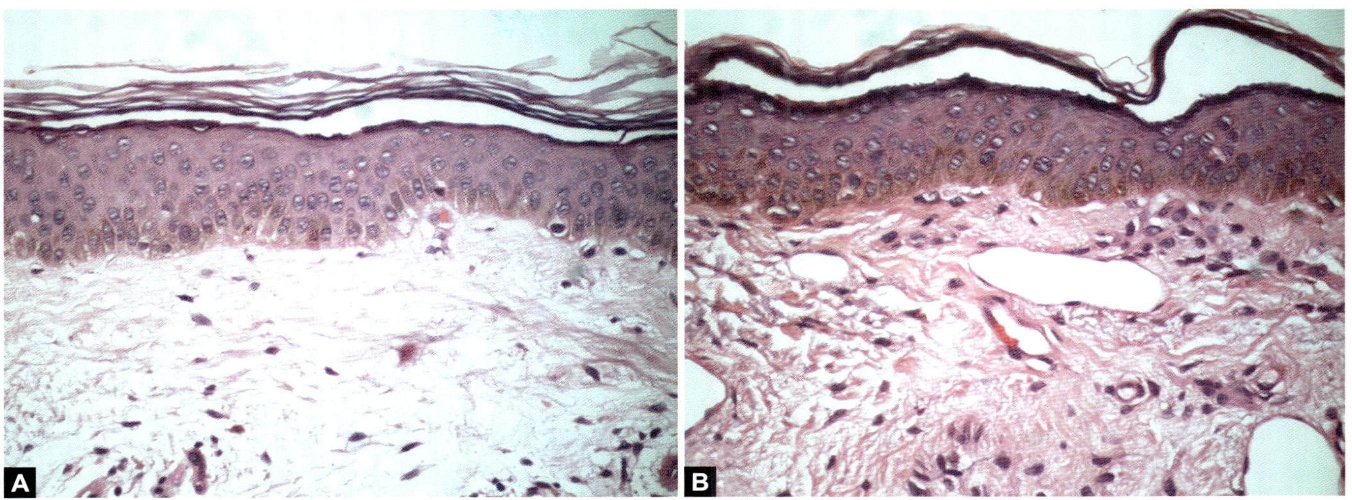

Figs 1A and B: Melasma: (A) Peri-lesional skin as normal control; (B) Lesional skin showing epidermal hypermelanosis, and telangiectatic vessels, no dermal inflammation, (H&E, x400)

RCM would be based on epidermal/dermal melanin ratio covering the entire involved skin.[7]

Histopathology shows increase in epidermal melanin at all levels including stratum corneum but is more pronounced in basal layers **(Figs 1A and B)**.[5,6,8,12-16] Melanin granules are often seen as caps over the keratinocytic nuclei.[6] The dermal melanin is variably present in melanophages, as well as free form, in perivascular area in upper dermis.[6,8,13-15] Increase in melanin is better appreciated by comparing lesional skin to patient's control skin using Masson-Fontana stain to highlight the pigment **(Figs 2A and B)**. Epidermis shows mildly flattened rete ridges which may be either more prominent or comparable to normal control skin.[6,10,15] Mild perivascular lymphohistiocytic inflammation may be present in superficial dermis.[5,6,8,13,14] Solar elastosis better appreciated by Verhoeff-Van Gieson (VVG) is increased with thicker, curled and fragmented elastic fibers in lesional skin as compared to normal skin **(Figs 3A and B)**.[6,10,15] However, in two studies, the difference in degree of solar elastosis between lesional and control skin was not significant.[8,12] Increase in number and size of the blood vessels of the lesional skin as compared to control may be apparent on hematoxylin and eosin (H&E) stain **(Fig. 1)**.

Melanocyte immunostaining with markers, like Mel-5/MART-1, NKI/beteb and microphthalmia-associated transcription factor (MITF) shows enlarged intensely stained melanocytes exhibiting prominent dendrites.[6,8] The melanocytes are variable in number either increased, similar, or decreased in comparison to control skin.[6-8,16]

A feature observed on immunohistochemistry (IHC) and Masson-Fontana stain is melanocytes protruding into the dermis labelled as "pendulous melanocytes" which are related to hyperactivity.[10,17] However, pendulous melanocytes are also observed in other hyperpigmentary disorders, thus, are not pathognomonic for melasma.[17] Torres-Álvarez et al. have demonstrated that protrusion of melanocytes at dermoepidermal junction is associated with disruption to total absence of basement membrane using periodic acid schiff (PAS) stain and collagen IV immunostaining.[18] However, in a previous study by Kang et al. no basement membrane alteration was observed on PAS staining.[6]

Melasma skin shows increased expression of melanogenesis related proteins including tyrosinase, tyrosinase-related proteins TRP-1 and TRP-2.[7,19] The paracrine linkage between keratinocytes, melanocytes and fibroblasts has been demonstrated using immunohistochemical expression for various cytokines, growth factors, hormones and their receptors in melasma skin. Epidermis in melasma shows an increased expression of α-MSH, c-kit, vessel endothelial growth factor, nerve growth factor (NGF), NGF receptor and progesterone receptor.[12,16,18-22] Dermis of the lesional skin shows increase in the size and number of blood vessels with either factor VIII-related antigen or CD31 immunostaining,[7,10,12,22] and increased number of fibroblasts immunostained with vimentn.[21] Increase in mast cells localized to elastotic area in melasma skin has been documented using metachromatic staining with Giemsa and with anti mast cell tryptase imunostaining.[15,17] An increased expression of stem cell growth factor and estrogen receptor β (ERβ) has been documented around dermal fibroblasts and blood vessels.[12,16,18,19,21]

Ultrastructurally, there is an increase in the number of melanosomes which are more widely dispersed through keratinocytes. However, there are no alterations in maturation status and morphology of melanosomes in melasma skin in comparison to control skin. Melanocytes exhibit an increase in mitochondria, Golgi apparatus, rough endoplasmic reticulum and ribosomes.[6,8]

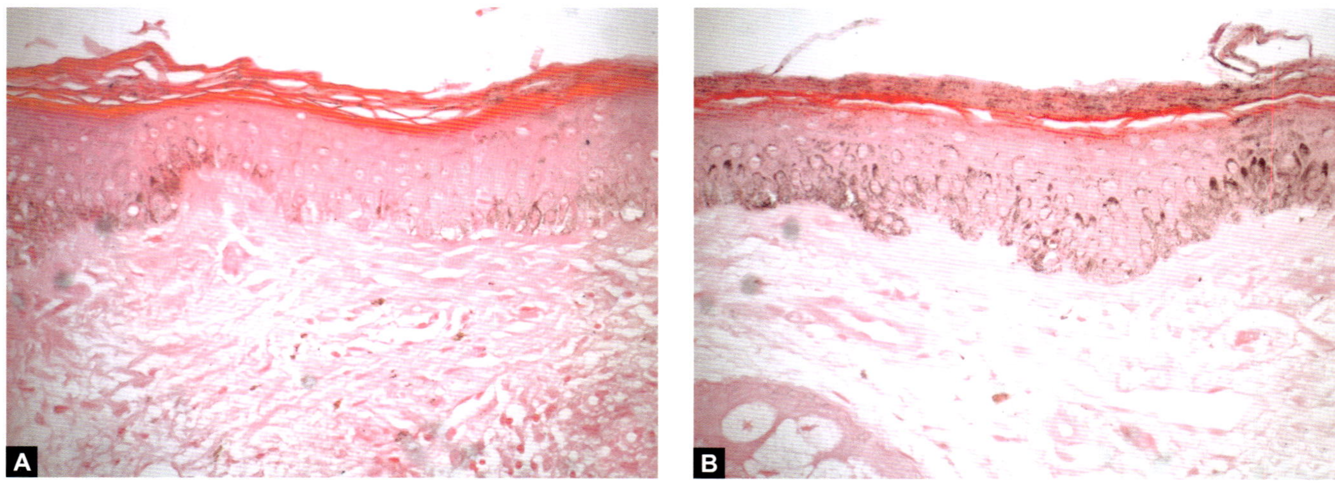

Figs 2A and B: Melasma. (A) Peri-lesional skin as normal control; (B) Hypermelanosis in lesional skin, (Masson-Fontana, x400)

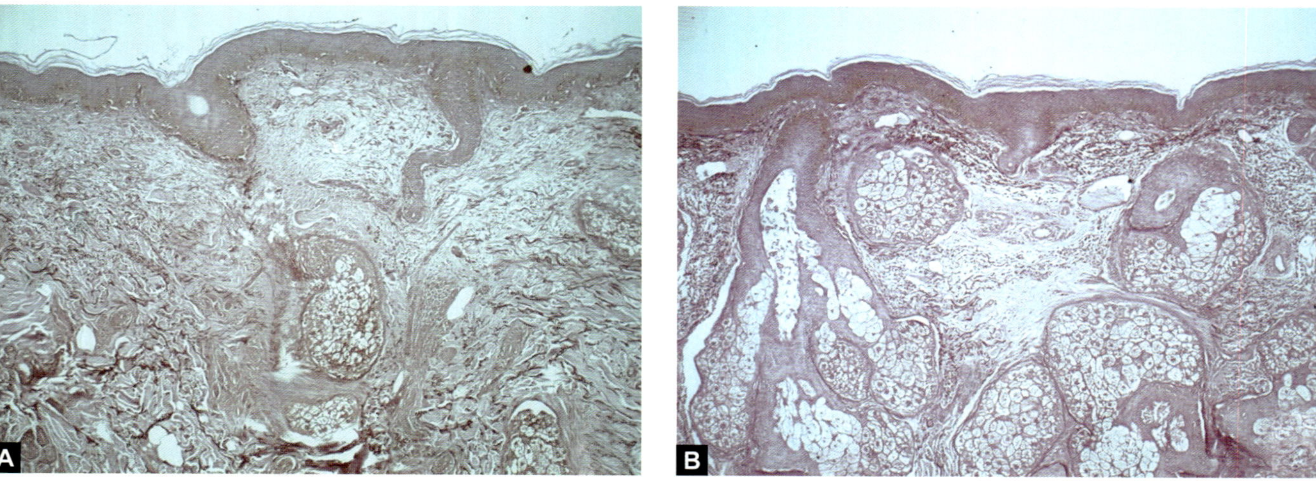

Figs 3A and B: Melasma: (A) Peri-lesional skin as normal control; (B) Increased solar elastosis in lesional skin (Verhoeff-Van Gieson, x100)

DIFFERENTIAL DIAGNOSIS OF MELASMA

Melasma is diagnosed clinically in most cases. However, other causes of facial hyperchromias as listed in **Box 1** require clinical distinction from melasma, lichen planus pigmentosus (LPP), actinic lichen planus, Riehl's melanosis, pigmented discoid lupus erythematosus, bilateral acquired nevus of Ota, exogenous ochronosis, postinflammatory hyperpigmentation, drug/heavy metal induced hyperchromias, systemic diseases (Addison's disease and porphyria cutanea tarda), poikiloderma of Civatte, macular amyloidosis and acanthosis nigricans, can closely mimic melasma in some cases. Rarely, unusual presentation of melasma as exemplified by a case mimicking morphea poses a diagnostic difficulty.[23] Histopathological evaluation as discussed below is valuable in distinguishing these entities.

Lichen Planus Pigmentosus and Actinic Lichen Planus

Both entities are considered as clinically distinctive variants of lichen planus. LPP is particularly significant in the differential diagnosis of facial melanosis in Indian context because of its high prevalence rate.[24] LPP may present in melasma-like pattern in some patients.[25] Lichen planus actinicus (LPA) has four clinical forms and it is the pigmented form which closely resembles melasma.[26-28]

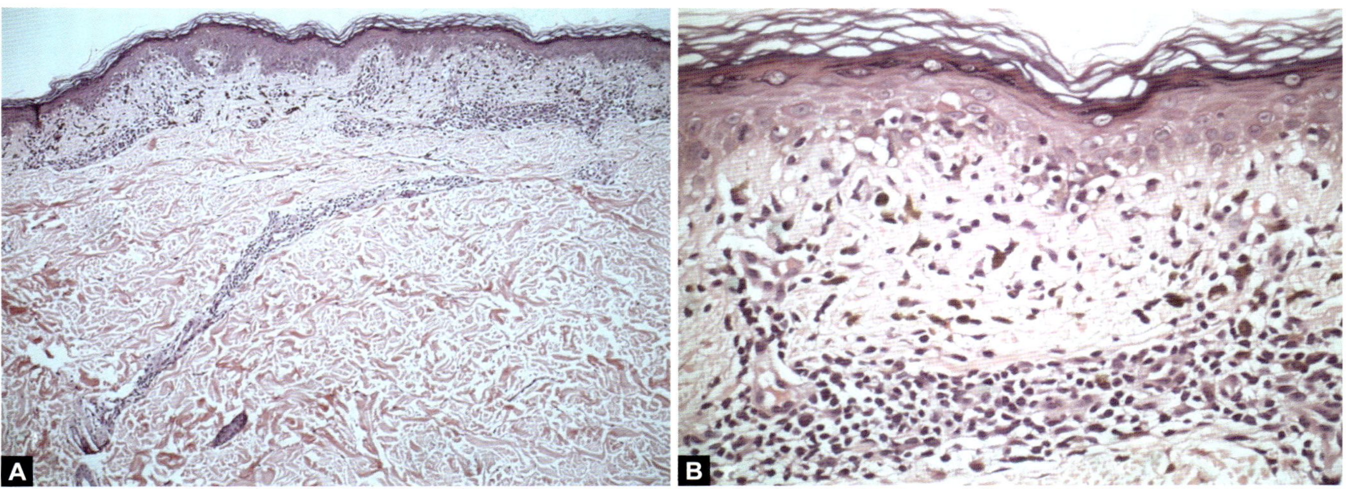

Figs 4A and B: Fully evolved lesion of lichen planus pigmentosus: (A) Mild basket weave hyperkeratosis and preserved rete ridges (H&E, x100); (B) Vacuolar damage to basal layer, lichenoid inflammation and melanophages in papillary dermis (H&E, x400)

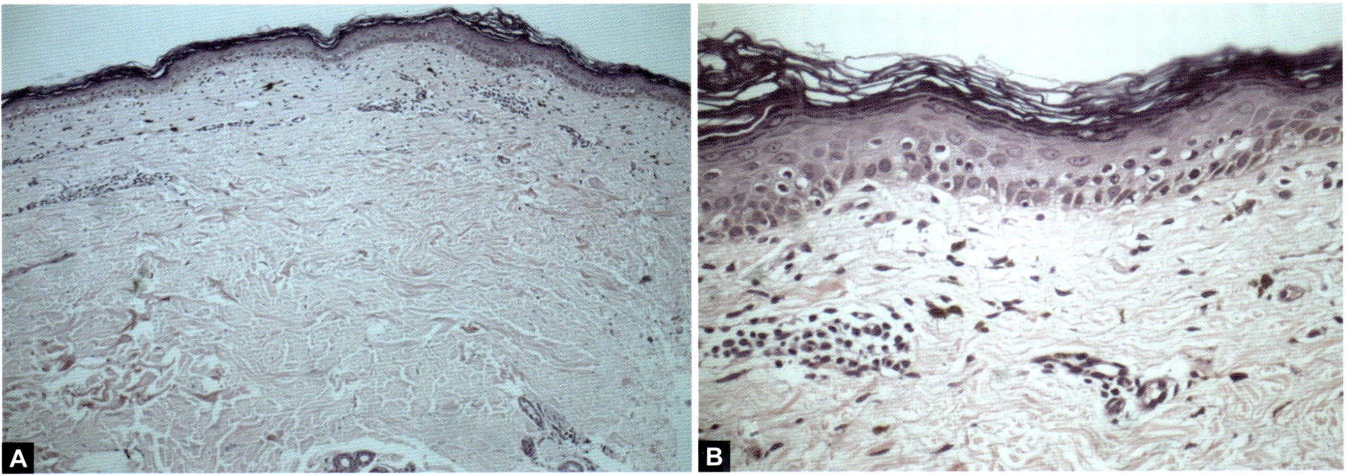

Figs 5A and B: Late lesion of lichen planus pigmentosus: (A) Compact orthokeratosis and flattened epidermis, (H&E, x100); (B) Subtle vacuolar damage, occasional colloid body, sparse inflammation and melanophages, (H&E, x400)

The spectrum of pathologic changes in LPP is explained by the life of the lesion that spans from early to fully evolved to late/resolving lesion. Fully developed lesion shows basal layer vacuolization, and few necrotic keratinocytes with perivascular lymphocytic and variable band like lichenoid lymphocytic inflammation abutting the basal epidermis. Epidermis is normal in thickness and may show mild basket weave hyperkeratosis **(Figs 4A and B)**. A late lesion, on the other hand, shows squamatized basal layer and an occasional colloid body indicating previous damage and sparse perivascular inflammation with little or no lichenoid inflammation. Epidermis is flat or atrophic and shows compact orthokeratotic hyperkeratosis **(Figs 5A and B)**. Melanophages and free melanin in the dermis are more prominent in late lesions.[24,25,29] In contrast to classic lichen planus, acanthosis is not seen in LPP and associated features of hyperkeratosis, hypergranulosis and dermal inflammation are mild in LPP.

In pigmented LPA, the pathology resembles lichen planus to some degree in most cases. The epidermis shows mild to moderate acanthosis with jagged saw toothed elongation of rete ridges and focal wedge shaped hypergranulosis. Less commonly epidermal thinning is present. Moderately dense band like lichenoid infiltrate abutting the basal layer with variable perivascular lymphocytic inflammation and melanophages are seen. Focal parakeratosis and solar elastosis have been described in some cases.[26-28]

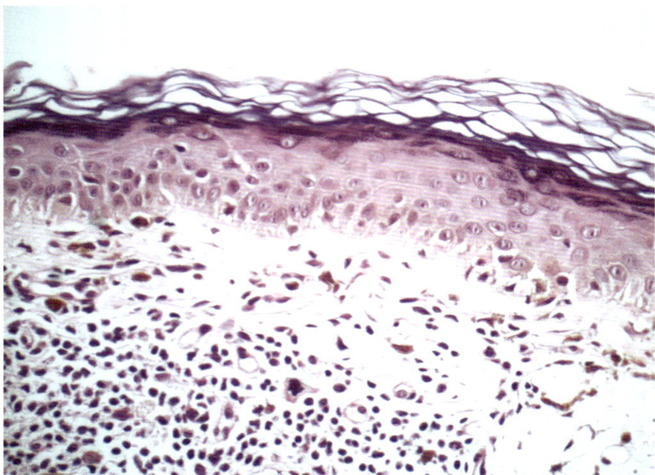

Fig. 6: Riehl's melanosis: Epidermis shows vacuolar basal cell damage, necrotic keratinocyte, dermal inflammation and melanophages, (H&E, x400)

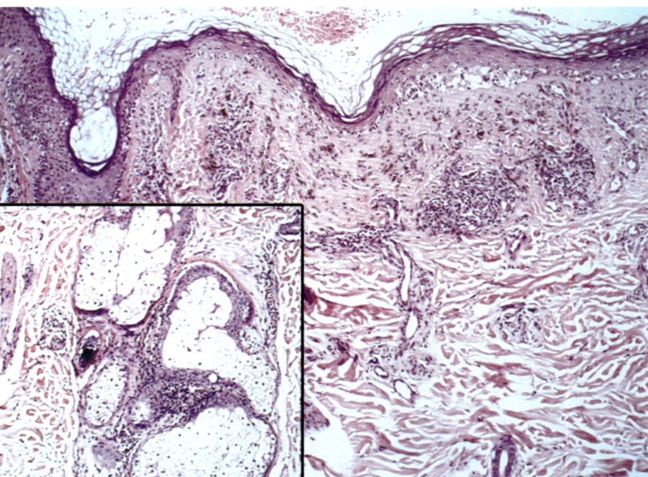

Fig. 7: Pigmented discoid lupus erythematosus: Vacuolar damage, necrotic keratinocyte, dermal inflammation and melanophages, (H&E, x100); inset shows deep dermal, perifollicular inflammation (H&E, x100)

Riehl's Melanosis

The other name for Riehl's melanosis is pigmented contact dermatitis. In India "Kumkum" is the most common allergen implicated in its pathogenesis.[4,30] The disease presents primarily as facial melanosis and contrary to the expected (being a contact dermatitis) the eczematous changes of contact dermatitis are usually not seen.[30]

Unlike the spongiotic features seen in contact dermatitis, the predominant pathology in Riehl's melanosis is basal cell damage in the form of vacuolization. The papillary dermis shows perivascular and/or lichenoid lymphocytic infiltrate with numerous melanophages.[4,31] Epidermis may be atrophic **(Fig. 6)**. PAS stain demonstrates thickening of basal lamina. Increase in basal epidermal melanin in comparison to control skin is seen on Masson-Fontana stain.[31]

Pigmented Discoid Lupus Erythematosus

Discoid lupus erythematosus (DLE) may present as hyperpigmented macules on the face and neck in a focal distribution without attendant erythema, telangiectasia, induration, adherent scaling, atrophy or scarring.[32,33] This presentation of DLE is rarely reported in the literature.[33] In a clinical study on Indian patients by George et al. pigmented DLE constituted 25% of all DLE patients.[32] Author's have also observed few (unpublished) cases of this variant. Therefore, this form of DLE might be more common in Indian population than reported in literature.

Histopathology, reveals a relatively thin epidermis with basal cell vacuolization, necrotic keratinocytes, pigment incontinence along with perivascular and lichenoid infiltrate of lymphocytes and plasma cells in both superficial and deep dermis **(Fig. 7)**.[32,33] Variable dermal changes of telangiectasia and mucin deposition are seen. In our cases, deep dermal infiltrate was less dense than seen in classic DLE. Direct immunofluorescence study demonstrating multiple deposits of immunoglobulin IgG, IgM and C3 is confirmatory.

Hori's Nevus [Synonym: Acquired Bilateral Nevus of Ota like Macules (ABNOM)]

Hori's nevus is an acquired dermal melanocytosis presenting as bilateral nevus of Ota-like macules. Because of its symmetrical bilateral involvement of malar areas it simulates melasma.

Histopathology is distinctive. Features are similar but not identical to nevus of Ota. Bipolar or dendritic melanocytes are seen in the upper and mid dermis predominantly in perivascular location **(Fig. 8)**. The depth of dermis to which melanocytes extend is less than that in nevus of Ota.[34] There may be increase in solar elastosis. No epidermal alterations are seen. Because of clinical similarity with melasma, the possibility of shared pathogenesis between the two entities was investigated with regard to vascularity and paracrine factors. There was an increased expression of stem cell factor in the dermis and increased mast cells similar to melasma. Higher c-kit expression in the dermis and lack of increased vascularity were unlike that seen in melasma.[35]

Exogenous Ochronosis

The term ochronosis refers to deposition of yellow-brown (ocher) color pigment in the dermis. Exogenous ochronosis particularly that caused by hydroquinone closely mimics melasma.[36,37]

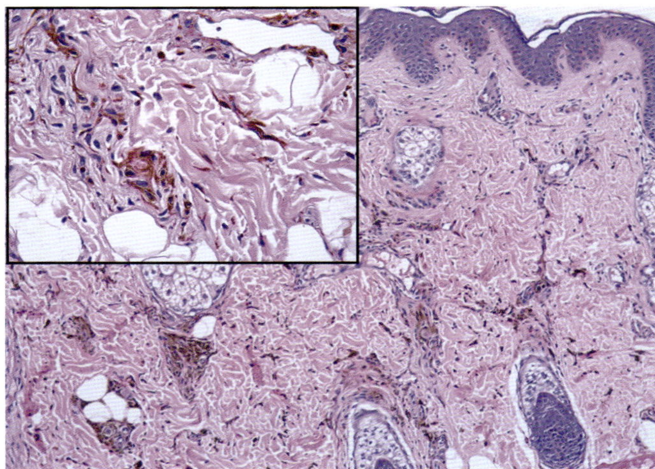

Fig. 8: Hori's nevus: Heavily pigmented melanocytes in dermis particularly in perivascular location, (H&E, x100); inset shows dendritic bipolar melanocytes, (H&E, x400)

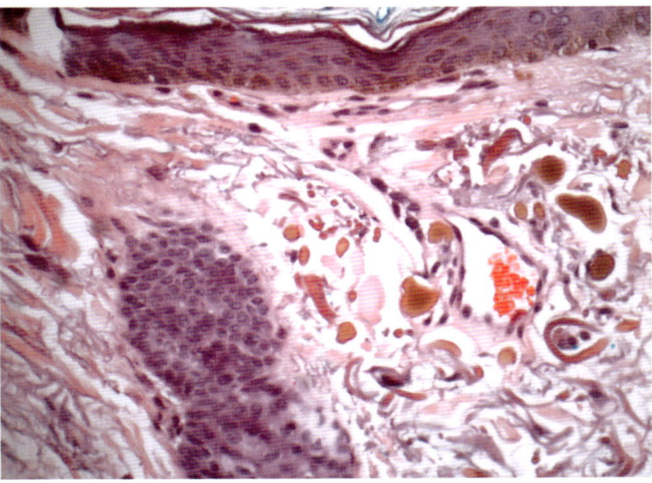

Fig. 9: Ochronosis: Banana shaped ochre colored collagen fibers, (H&E, x400)

The most characteristic feature is deposition of yellow brown (ochre) color pigment within the damaged collagen bundles which appear rigid, sharp, fractured with jagged borders, irregularly shaped often crescentic famously called as banana bodies **(Fig. 9)**.[38] In the early stages, the fibers appear swollen and basophilic and subsequently develop into the characteristic morphology in a fully evolved lesion.[39] There may be associated solar elastosis. In addition fine yellow-brown (ochre) colored pigment is also seen lying free in the dermis as well as in macrophages. Pigment may also be seen in endothelial cells of blood vessels, in sweat glands and in the elastic fibers. The pigment is autofluorescent, stains black with methylene blue and crystal violet. It is negative for elastic stain (VVG), iron stain (Perl's) and melanin stain (Masson-Fontana) except in antimalarial induced ochronosis where pigment is positive for iron and melanin.[38] Late in the disease amorphous eosinophilic deposits resembling colloid milium develop. Other features described in exogenous ochronosis include foreign body granulomatous response resembling sarcoidosis, transepidermal and transfollicular elimination of ochronotic fibers with lichenoid infiltrate, pseudoepitheliomatous hyperplasia and actinic granuloma, like morphology.[38,40]

Electron microscopy demonstrates electron dense deposit within the damaged scalloped collagen fibers with loss of fibrillar structure.[39]

Post-inflammatory Hyperpigmentation

Post-inflammatory hyperpigmentation is an acquired melanosis which develops secondary to preceding inflammatory dermatosis.[41] Histopathologically, both epidermal type with increased basal keratinocyte melanin pigment or dermal type with upper dermal melanophages can be seen.[41] The features of underlying dermatosis are usually not evident. The diagnosis is based on clinical correlation.

Post Chikungunya Melanosis

Chikungunya is an acute viral fever. Maculopapular rash is the most common skin manifestation.[4] Reports of different patterns of hyperpigmentation including melasma like malar involvement have emerged mostly from India.[4,42] The exact cause is not known, however, it is considered to be post-inflammatory response. It has been proposed that epidermal melanin dispersion and retention may be triggered by the virus.[4] Histopathology described, is, of increased epidermal melanin, focal basal layer vacuolization and perivascular dermal mononuclear infiltrate with melanophages.[4,42]

Poikiloderma of Civatte

The reticulate pigmentation involving the face and "V" of neck with features of telangiectasia and erythema are distinctive for specific clinical diagnosis. Associated erythema and telangiectasia are not present in 20% of the patients,[43,44] also, these features may not be evident in dark skin individuals. These cases require distinction from other causes of facial melanosis.

Epidermis is flattened and atrophic with hyperkeratosis. The melanin granules are irregularly distributed in lower epidermis. There may be mild or patchy vacuolar change in some cases. Dermal changes include mild perivascular lymphocytic infiltrate with numerous melanophages, dermal fibrosis, invariable presence of solar damage and telangiectatic vessels **(Fig. 10)**.[44] In author's experience the degree of solar elastosis seen in Indian patients is less prominent unlike Caucasians. Occasionally, increased number of perivascular mast cells are observed.[44]

Electron microscopy demonstrates significant alteration in dermal connective tissue in the form of degeneration and disruption of collagen fibers with foci of degenerated

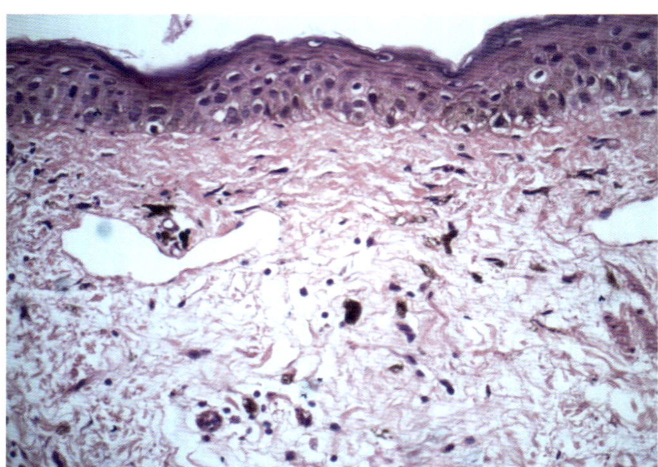

Fig. 10: Poikiloderma of Civatte: Atrophy, subtle fibrosis, elastosis, melanophages and telangiectasia, (H&E, x400)

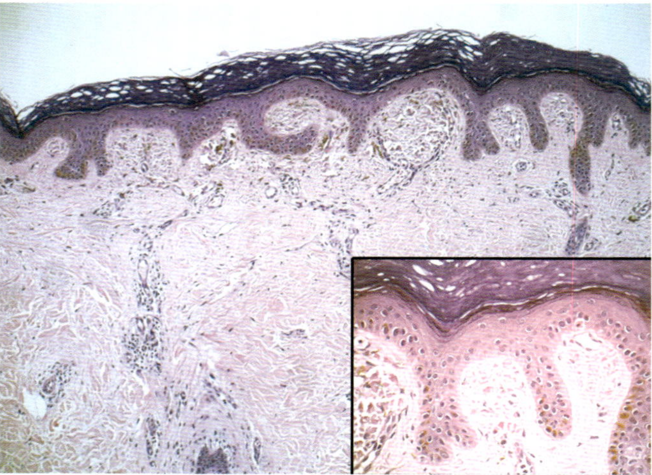

Fig. 11: Amyloid deposit and melanophages within distended dermal papilla (H&E, x100); inset shows apoptotic keratinocytes (H&E, x400)

organelles. Inactive fibroblasts are seen in between the collagen bundles. Dermoepidermal junction remains intact.[44]

Macular Amyloidosis

Macular amyloidosis classically presents as reticulate pigmentation involving chest and upper back. Less frequently, face is involved.[45] A diffuse dark brown homogeneous photodistributed facial pigmentation without rippled pattern mimicking melasma has been documented.[46]

Small, sometimes subtle, globular deposits of eosinophilic amyloid are focally present within mildly distended dermal papillae **(Fig. 11)**. Upper dermis exhibits sparse perivascular lymphocytic infiltrate and melanophages. Additional findings which may be seen are focal basal layer vacuolar damage, Civatte bodies and apoptotic keratinocytes. Mild hyperkeratosis is usually present.[46,47] Special stains such as Congo red **(Fig. 12)**, and Crystal violet which metachromatically stain amyloid are helpful to detect and confirm the deposits. The apple green birefringence of amyloid with Congo red stain under polarizing light is characteristic but not always appreciated.[47] At times, the deposits are very subtle and serial sections and IHC are required to demonstrate the deposits.

Immunohistochemically, cutaneous amyloid stains with cytokeratin antibodies. CK5 being the major constituent of cutaneous amyloid, the deposits stain with cocktail of AE1/AE3 and with anti-CK5/6 antibodies. Cutaneous amyloid also stains with various other cytokeratin antibodies including EAB-903 (which recognizes 66K and 57K dalton keratin), 34betaE12, MNF116, and LP34.[47]

Ultrastructurally, amyloid is a fibrillar protein composed of nonbranching fibrils between 60 Å and 130 Å. In primary cutaneous amyloidosis filamentous degeneration of keratinocytes, tonofilaments coexisting with amyloid filaments and continuation of epidermal filaments with

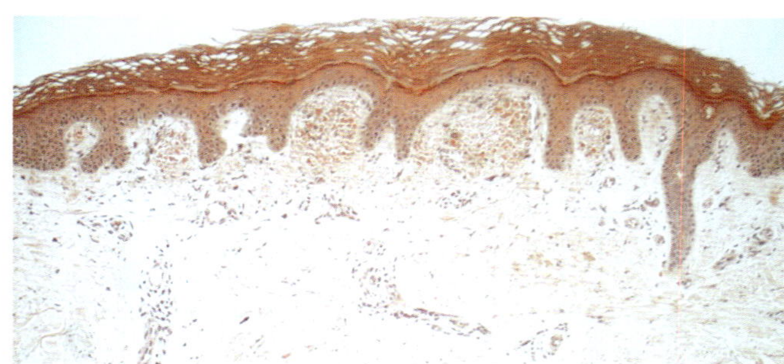

Fig. 12: Orange-pink amyloid deposit (Congo red, x100)

dermal deposits have been demonstrated supporting the epidermal origin of primary cutaneous amyloidosis.[47]

Systemic Diseases

Porphyria cutanea tarda (PCT) is a disorder of heme biosynthesis. Many patients have facial pigmentation resembling melasma.[48,49] The histopathology of the pigmented lesions shows increased epidermal melanin without the typical changes of PCT in most cases. In some patients, separation of dermoepidermal junction suggestive of an early blister may be seen.[49]

Addison's disease is the result of primary adrenocortical insufficiency. Cutaneous hyperpigmentation on sun exposed areas including face, flexures and mucous membranes is one of the most common presenting symptom of the disease.[50,51] There may be few melanophages in the dermis.[50]

Drugs

Apart from causing fixed drug eruption and ochronosis which are distinct entities, a variety of drugs have been implicated in diffuse cutaneous hyperchromia. Face is commonly involved in drug induced hyperchromias.[52]

The histopathological findings vary depending on the offending drug. Various patterns described are lichenoid reaction pattern (diltiazem and amlodipine);[53,54] complexes of iron (Perl's stain)–melanin (Masson-Fontana stain) with or without calcium (Von-Kossa stain) deposited in melanophages, myoepithelial cells of eccrine units, along the elastic fibers and lying free in the dermis reaching up to subcutis (tetracycline, minocycline, doxycycline and antimalarials);[52,55,56] deposits of drug-melanin complexes which are refractile as well as stain with Masson-Fontana (phenothiazines);[52,57] deposits of lipofuscin which is autofluorescent and stains pink with Mallory lipofuscin, PAS and acid fast stains (amiodarone and clofazimine)[52,58] and deposition of drug crystal itself (amiodarone and clofazimine).[52,58]

Hemochromatosis

Hemochromatosis is a disorder of iron metabolism. Hyperpigmentation is an early sign of the disease and is seen in more than 90% of patients. Cutaneous hyperpigmentation involves sun exposed area including face.[59] The major contribution to the skin pigmentation is increased melanin with some degree of pigmentation due to hemosiderin deposition. It is hypothesized that hemosiderin deposition enhances the melanin synthesis by melanocytes.[60]

There is an increase in basal epidermal melanin. Golden brown hemosiderin pigment is seen in the dermis concentrated around the blood vessels and sweat glands.[48,59] Hemosiderin deposit in the epidermis and epithelium of sweat glands have been demonstrated with Perl's stain for hemosiderin.[61]

Heavy Metals

Silver and gold are characteristically associated with pigmentation of sun exposed area particularly face.

Argyria refers to the cutaneous pigmentation due to deposition of silver. Histologically, it is characterized by the deposition of fine, brown-black granules along the elastic fibers of the papillary dermis **(Fig. 13A)**, in the basal lamina of the secretory portion of eccrine glands **(Fig. 13B)**, blood vessel walls and connective tissues sheath surrounding pilosebaceous units. Granules are refractile under dark field microscopy and do not stain with melanin or iron stains.[62]

The term chrysiasis refers to cutaneous pigmentation resulting from deposition of gold salts. Gold granules are larger than silver and are deposited in the macrophages around blood vessels in the upper and mid reticular dermis.[62] The granules are refractile under dark field microscopy and exhibit orange-red birefringence under polaroscopic examination.[63]

Acanthosis Nigricans

Acanthosis nigricans is characterized by occurrence of velvety, brownish-black plaques typically located on intertriginous areas and neck. Face is uncommonly affected.[64] Facial lesions involve cheeks, forehead or sulcus nasi and sulcus mentolabialis akin to other intertriginous area.[65]

Stratum corneum is hyperkeratotic. Papillomatosis is seen in the form of finger like dermal projections covered by thin epidermis whereas the epidermis in the valleys in between the papillae is mildly acanthotic **(Fig. 14)**. Occasionally, pseudohorn cyst reminiscent of seborrheic keratosis are seen. Sparse upper dermal perivascular lymphocytic infiltrate may be seen. There may be some increase in basal layer melanin

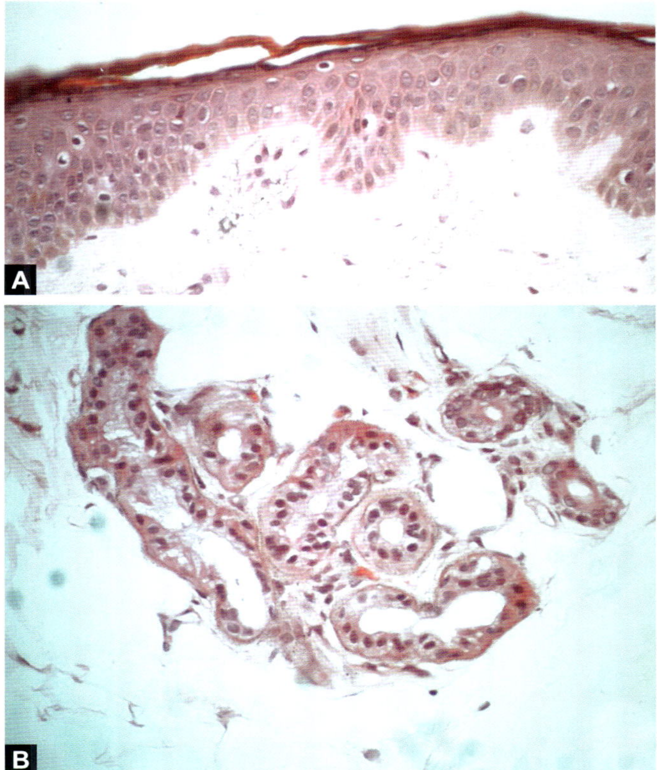

Figs 13A and B: Argyria: (A) Fine black silver granules coating elastic fibers, (H&E, x400); (B) Silver granules deposited in basement membrane of sweat units, (H&E, x400)

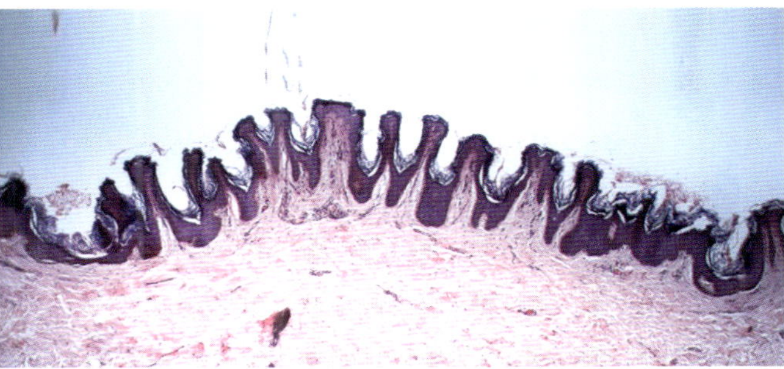

Fig. 14: Acanthosis nigricans: Papillomatosis, with peaks and valleys, (H&E, x40)

Flow chart 2: Algorithm for the diagnosis of facial hyperchromia

Facial hyperchromia

- Epidermal melanosis with or without dermal melanosis → Melasma, PIH, Drugs, PCT → CPC
- Dermal melanosis → Interface pathology
  - +ve → Deep PV/PA infiltrate
    - +ve → DLE, Drugs → CPC
    - –ve → LPP/LPA, Riehl's melanosis, Drugs → CPC
  - –ve → Dermal features
    - Solar elastosis and telangiectasia → POC
    - Metachromatic Congo red +ve deposit → Macular amyloidosis
- Dermal melanocytosis → NOO, Hori's nevus → CPC
- Epidermal thickening → AN
- Non-melanin/Melanin+ non-melanin deposit
  - Refractile granules –ve with Perl's and Masson-Fontana → Drugs, Argyria, Chrysiasis
  - Crystal violet +ve → Ochronosis
  - +ve with Masson-Fontana and/or Perl's and/or Von Kossa → Hemochromatosis, Drugs

Abbreviations: AN, acanthosis nigricans; CPC, clinicopathological correlation; DLE, discoid lupus erythematosus; LPA, lichen planus actinicus; LPP, lichen planus pigmentosus; NOO, nevus of Ota; PA, periadnexal; PV, perivasular; POC, poikiloderma of Civatte; PCT, porphyria cutanea tarda; PIH, postinflammatory hyperpigmentation

pigment, but it should be noted that the basis of pigmentation is hyperkeratosis and not increased melanin.[64]

PRACTICAL APPROACH IN DIAGNOSING FACIAL HYPERCHROMIA

The diagnosis of facial hyperchromia relies on clinico-pathological correlation. The algorithm summarizes the various differential diagnosis based on histopathological patterns/findings **(Flow chart 2)**.

Hypermelanosis in melasma is best assessed comparing lesional skin with patient's normal skin on H&E and Masson-Fontana stains for routine diagnosis. Stains for melanocytic markers such as Melan-A, NKI/beteb and S-100 are useful in distinguishing melanocytosis from melanosis. Many of the immunostains mentioned in the text are more of academic and research interest to elucidate the pathogenesis.

REFERENCES

1. Nordlund JJ, Ortonne JP, Cestari T, et al. Confusions about color: formulating a more precise lexicon for pigmentation, pigmentary disorders, and abnormalities of "chromatics". J Am Acad Dermatol. 2006;54:S291-7.
2. Hori, Yoshiaki, Yasuo Kubota. Acquired, circumscribed hypermelanotic disorders. Dermatol Sinica. 1993;11:1-19.
3. Zembowicz A, Mihm MC. Dermal dendritic melanocytic proliferations: an update. Histopathology. 2004;45:433-51.
4. Khanna N, Rasool S. Facial melanoses: Indian perspective. Indian J Dermatol Venereol Leprol. 2011;77(5):552-63.
5. Sanchez NP, Pathak MA, Sato S, et al. Melasma: a clinical, light microscopic, ultrastructural, and immunofluorescence study. J Am Acad Dermatol. 1981;4:698-710.
6. Kang WH, Yoon KH, Lee ES, et al. Melasma: histopathological characteristics in 56 Korean patients. Br J Dermatol. 2002;146:228-37.
7. Young Kang H, Ortonne JP. Melasma update. Actas Dermosifiliogr. 2009;100(Suppl 2):110-3.
8. Grimes PE, Yamada N, Bhawan J. Light microscopic, immunohistochemical, and ultrastructural alterations in patients with melasma. Am J Dermatopathol. 2005;27(2):96-101.
9. Ardigo M, Cameli N, Berardesca E, et al. Characterization and evaluation of pigment distribution and response to therapy in melasma using in vivo reflectance confocal microscopy: a preliminary study. J Eur Acad Dermatol Venereol. 2010;24:1296-303.
10. Kang HY, Bahadoran P, Suzuki I, et al. In vivo reflectance confocal microscopy detects pigmentary changes in

melasma at a cellular level resolution. Exp Dermatol. 2010;19:e228-33.

11. Liu H, Lin Y, Nie X, et al. Histological classification of melasma with reflectance confocal microscopy: a pilot study in Chinese patients. Skin Res Technol. 2011;17:398-403.
12. Jang YH, Sim JH, Kang HY, et al. The histopathological characteristics of male melasma: comparison with female melasma and lentigo. J Am Acad Dermatol. 2012;66:642-9.
13. Sarkar R, Puri P, Jain RK, et al. Melasma in men: a clinical, aetiological and histological study. J Eur Acad Dermatol Venereol. 2010;24(7):768-72.
14. Sarvjot V, Sharma S, Mishra S, et al. Melasma: a clinicopathological study of 43 cases. Indian J Pathol Microbiol. 2009;52(3):357-9.
15. Hernández-Barrera R, Torres-Alvarez B, Castanedo-Cazares JP, et al. Solar elastosis and presence of mast cells as key features in the pathogenesis of melasma. Clin Exp Dermatol. 2008;33:305-8.
16. Jang YH, Lee JY, Kang HY, et al. Oestrogen and progesterone receptor expression in melasma: an immunohistochemical analysis. J Eur Acad Dermatol Venereol. 2010;24(11):1312-6.
17. Lee DJ, Park KC, Ortonne JP, et al. Pendulous melanocytes: a characteristic feature of melasma and how it may occur. Br J Dermatol. 2012;166:684-6.
18. Torres-Álvarez B, Mesa-Garza IG, Castanedo-Cázares JP, et al. Histochemical and immunohistochemical study in melasma: evidence of damage in the basal membrane. Am J Dermatopathol. 2011;33(3):291-5.
19. Kim JE, Chang SE, Yeo UC, et al. Histopathological study of the treatment of melasma lesions using a low-fluence Q-switched 1064-nm neodymium:yttrium-aluminium-garnet laser. Clin Exp Dermatol. 2013;38(2):167-71.
20. Im S, Kim J, On WY, et al. Increased expression of alpha-melanocyte-stimulating hormone in the lesional skin of melasma. Br J Dermatol. 2002;146:165-7.
21. Kang HY, Hwang JS, Lee JY, et al. The dermal stem cell factor and c-kit are overexpressed in melasma. Br J Dermatol. 2006;154:1094-9.
22. Kim EH, Kim YC, Lee ES, et al. The vascular characteristics of melasma. J Dermatol Sci. 2007;46:111-6.
23. Tabata H, Yamakage A, Yamazaki S. Bandlike melasma mimicking linear morphea ("en coup de sabre" type). Cutis. 1998;61(4):225-6.
24. Kanwar AJ, Dogra S, Handa S, et al. A study of 124 Indian patients with lichen planus pigmentosus. Clin Exp Dermatol. 2003;28:481-5.
25. Al-Mutairi N, El-Khalawany M. Clinicopathological characteristics of lichen planus pigmentosus and its response to tacrolimus ointment: an open label, non-randomized, prospective study. J Eur Acad Dermatol Venereol. 2010;24:535-40.
26. Salman SM, Khallouf R, Zaynoun S. Actinic lichen planus mimicking melasma. A clinical and histopathologic study of three cases. J Am Acad Dermatol. 1988;18:275-8.
27. al-Fouzan AS, Hassab-el-Naby HM. Melasma-like (pigmented) actinic lichen planus. Int J Dermatol. 1992; 31(6):413-5.
28. Aloi F, Solaroli C, Giovannini E. Actinic lichen planus simulating melasma. Dermatology. 1997;195(1):69-70.
29. Vega ME, Waxtein L, Arenas R, et al. Ashy dermatosis and lichen planus pigmentosus: a clinicopathologic study of 31 cases. Int J Dermatol. 1992;31(2):90-4.
30. Shenoi SD, Rao R. Pigmented contact dermatitis. Indian J Dermatol Venereol Leprol. 2007;73:285-7.
31. Serrano G, Pujol C, Cuadra J, et al. Riehl's melanosis: pigmented contact dermatitis caused by fragrances. J Am Acad Dermatol. 1989;21:1057-60.
32. George R, Mathai R, Kurian S. Cutaneous lupus erythematosus in India: immunofluorescence profile. Int J Dermatol. 1992;31:265-9.
33. Boyd AS. Localized chronic cutaneous lupus erythematosus masquerading as pigmented lesions: a new clinical subset? Lupus. 2006;15:292-5.
34. Lee B, Kim YC, Kang WH, et al. Comparison of characteristics of acquired bilateral nevus of Ota-like macules and nevus of Ota according to therapeutic outcome. J Korean Med Sci. 2004;19:554-9.
35. Lee JY, Kim EH, Kim KH, et al. Acquired bilateral naevus of Ota-like macules: an immunohistological analysis of dermal melanogenic paracrine cytokine networks. Br J Dermatol. 2011;164:580-5.
36. Ribas J, Schettini AP, Cavalcante Mde S. Exogenous ochronosis hydroquinone induced: a report of four cases. An Bras Dermatol. 2010;85(5):699-703.
37. Tan SK. Exogenous ochronosis in ethnic Chinese Asians: a clinicopathological study, diagnosis and treatment. J Eur Acad Dermatol Venereol. 2011;25:842-50.
38. Touart DM, Sau P. Cutaneous deposition diseases. Part II. J Am Acad Dermatol. 1998;39:527-44.
39. Phillips JI, Isaacson C, Carman H. Ochronosis in black South Africans who used skin lighteners. Am J Dermatopathol. 1986;8:14-21.
40. Jordaan HF, Mulligan RP. Actinic granuloma-like change in exogenous ochronosis: case report. J Cutan Pathol. 1990;17:236-40.
41. Davis EC, Callender VD. Postinflammatory hyperpigmentation: a review of the epidemiology, clinical features, and treatment options in skin of color. J Clin Aesthet Dermatol. 2010;3(7):20-31.
42. Shivakumar V, Okade R, Rajkumar V, et al. Unusual facial melanosis in viral fever. Indian J Dermatol. 2007;52:116-7.
43. Katoulis AC, Stavrianeas NG, Georgala S, et al. Poikiloderma of Civatte: a clinical and epidemiological study. J Eur Acad Dermatol Venereol. 2005;19(4):444-8.
44. Katoulis AC, Stavrianeas NG, Panayiotides JG, et al. Poikiloderma of Civatte: a histopathological and ultrastructural study. Dermatology. 2007;214(2):177-82.

45. Bandhlish A, Aggarwal A, Koranne RV. A clinico-epidemiological study of macular amyloidosis from north India. Indian J Dermatol. 2012;57:269-74.
46. Ranu H, Lee J, Sen P. Photodistributed macular amyloidosis presenting as diffuse facial pigmentation mimicking melasma: the surprising reveal. Hong Kong J Dermatol Venereol. 2010;18:209-13.
47. Fernandez-Flores A. Cutaneous amyloidosis: a concept review. Am J Dermatopathol. 2012;34(1):1-14.
48. Nicolaidou E, Antoniou C, Katsambas AD. Origin, clinical presentation, and diagnosis of facial hypermelanoses. Dermatol Clin. 2007;25(3):321-6.
49. Tsega E, Damtew B, Landells JW, et al. Hyperpigmentation of the face and hands without blisters: porphyria cutanea tarda. Br J Dermatol. 1980;103(2):187-90.
50 Ross IL, Levitt NS. Addison's disease symptoms—a cross sectional study in urban South Africa. PLoS One. 2013;8(1): e53526.
51. Vega Gutiérrez J, Miranda Romero A, Martínez G, et al. Hyperpigmentation mimicking Laugier syndrome, levodopa therapy and Addison's disease. J Eur Acad Dermatol Venereol. 2003;17:324-7.
52. Dereure O. Drug-induced skin pigmentation. Epidemiology, diagnosis and treatment. Am J Clin Dermatol. 2001;2(4):253-62.
53. Erbagci Z. Amlodipine associated hyperpigmentation. Saudi Med J. 2004;25(1):103-5.
54. Saladi RN, Cohen SR, Phelps RG, et al. Diltiazem induces severe photodistributed hyperpigmentation: case series, histoimmunopathology, management, and review of the literature. Arch Dermatol. 2006;142(2):206-10.
55. Böhm M, Schmidt PF, Lödding B, et al. Cutaneous hyperpigmentation induced by doxycycline: histochemical and ultrastructural examination, laser microprobe mass analysis, and cathodoluminescence. Am J Dermatopathol. 2002;24:345-50.
56. Bowen AR, McCalmont TH. The histopathology of subcutaneous minocycline pigmentation. J Am Acad Dermatol. 2007;57:836-9.
57. Ming ME, Bhawan J, Stefanato CM, et al. Imipramine-induced hyperpigmentation: four cases and a review of the literature. J Am Acad Dermatol. 1999;40(2 Pt 1):159-66.
58. Job CK, Yoder L, Jacobson RR, et al. Skin pigmentation from clofazimine therapy in leprosy patients: a reappraisal. J Am Acad Dermatol. 1990;23:236-41.
59. Chevrant-Breton J, Simon M, Bourel M, et al. Cutaneous manifestations of idiopathic hemochromatosis. Study of 100 cases. Arch Dermatol. 1977;113(2):161-5.
60. Tsuji T. Experimental hemosiderosis: relationship between skin pigmentation and hemosiderin. Acta Derm Venereol. 1980;60(2):109-14.
61. Weintraub LR, Demis DJ, Conrad ME, et al. Iron excretion by the skin. Selective localization of Iron-59 in epithelial cells. Am J Pathol. 1965;46:121-7.
62. Granstein RD, Sober AJ. Drug- and heavy metal—induced hyperpigmentation. J Am Acad Dermatol. 1981;5(1):1-18.
63. al-Talib RK, Wright DH, Theaker JM. Orange-red birefringence of gold particles in paraffin wax embedded sections: an aid to the diagnosis of chrysiasis. Histopathology. 1994;24(2):176-8.
64. Puri N. A study of pathogenesis of acanthosis nigricans and its clinical implications. Indian J Dermatol. 2011;56(6):678-83.
65. Barabash-Neila R, Freire LR, Zulueta-Dorado T, et al. Thickening of the skin on the forehead: a quiz. Acanthosis nigricans with forehead location. Acta Derm Venereol. 2011;91(1):108, 110.

36

Update Scoring Methods and Non-invasive Measurement Methods in Melasma

(Reliability Assessment and Validation of the Melasma Area and Severity Index and a New Modified MASI Scoring Method)

Jean-Paul Ortonne

Key Features

- The MASI is the most commonly used scoring system for melasma and has good reliability and validity.
- Modified MASI is easy to learn and perform.
- MelasQoL is helpful to evaluate objectively the effect of melasma on a patient's HRQoL, can help guide treatment methods as well as track the improvement of patient's HRQoL.
- MelasQoL-BP can be used to evaluate the QoL and response to melasma treatment.
- Applications of RCM for melasma diagnosis and treatment.

MELASMA AREA AND SEVERITY INDEX

The melasma area and severity index (MASI), an outcome measure developed to provide a more accurate quantification of the severity of melasma and changes during therapy, was developed by Kimbrough-Green et al. who based it on a similar scoring system devised for psoriasis. The MASI score is calculated by subjective assessment of three factors: area (A) of involvement, darkness (D), and homogeneity (H), with the forehead (f), right malar region (rm), left malar region (lm), and chin (c), corresponding to 30%, 30%, 30% and 10% of the total face, respectively. The area of involvement in each of these four areas is given **(Fig. 1)** a numeric value of 0 to 6 (0 = no involvement; 1 = < 10%; 2 = 10–29%; 3 = 30–49%, 4 = 50–69%; 5 = 70–89%, and 6 = 90–100%). Darkness and homogeneity are rated on a scale from 0 to 4 (0 = absent; 1 = slight; 2 = mild; 3 = marked; and 4 = maximum). The MASI score is calculated by adding the sum of the severity ratings for darkness and homogeneity, multiplied by the value of the area of involvement, for each of the four facial areas.

$$\begin{aligned}\text{MASI total score} = {} & 0.3\,(f)\,[D(f) + H(f)] \\ & + 0.3A(lm)\,[D(lm) + H(lm)] \\ & + 0.3A(rm)\,[D(rm) + H(rm)] \\ & + 0.1A(c)\,[D(c) + H(c)]\end{aligned}$$

The total score range is 0–48. The MASI is the most commonly used outcome measure for melasma trials but has never been validated. The purpose of this prospectively designed study was to determine the reliability and validity of the MASI score.

The modified MASI we propose is easy to learn and perform and is scored as follows:

$$\begin{aligned}\text{Modified MASI total score} = {} & 0.3A(f)\,D(f) \\ & + 0.3A(lm)\,D(lm) \\ & + 0.3A(rm)\,D(rm) \\ & + 0.1A(c)\,D(c)\end{aligned}$$

The range of the total score is 0–24. Area and darkness are scored as follows: area of involvement: 0 = absent; 1 = less than 10%; 2 = 10–29%; 3 = 30–49%; 4 = 50–69%; 5 = 70–89%;

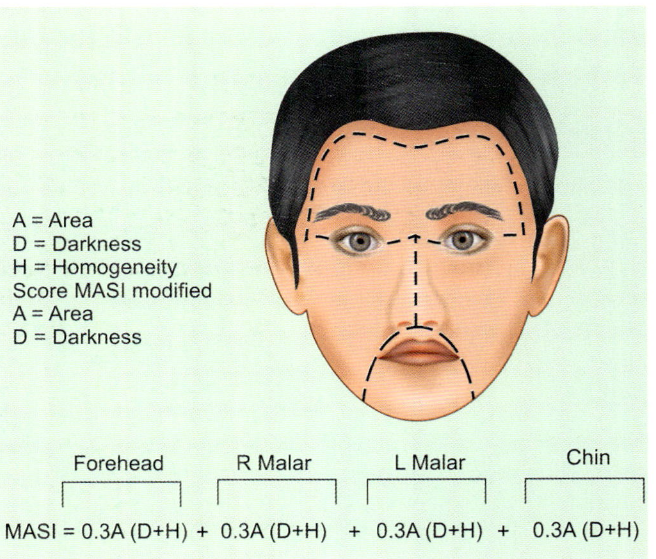

Fig. 1: MASI score calculated by subjective assessment 3 factors. (*Source:* Pandya AG, et al. J Am Acad Dermatol. 2011;64:78-83.)

and 6 = 90–100%; darkness: 0 = absent; 1 = slight; 2 = mild; 3 = marked; and 4 = severe.

Validity testing showed that the MASI scale being a continuous scale is able to provide more precise numeric estimates of the melasma severity than the categorical scale of melasma severity score (MSS). Importantly, the mean MASI scores presented may be useful as threshold scores for entry of patients with moderate and severe melasma in future studies, as there is currently no consensus on threshold levels for entry into a melasma study. For the modified MASI proposed in the current study, the values should be reduced by half.

In summary, the MASI score shows good reliability within and between raters and good validity when compared with the MSS, mexameter readings, and computer-assisted area measurements. Removing chin and homogeneity measurements does not improve intraclass correlation coefficient reliability but because kappa statistics were poor for homogeneity and because it is a difficult assessment to reach and perform, we recommend removal of homogeneity from the MASI score. We also recommend that chin assessments are preserved in the MASI as it is an important part of facial assessment and because it only represents 10% of the whole index. Practice of raters is important, as more agreement was noted on day 2 versus day 1. The validation and reliability testing of the modified MASI score required a training module, including practice images, before initiating patient assessments, therefore, this training should be given to raters to ensure reliability in future studies. If desired, readers may contact the corresponding author for access to this training module. Future studies assessing the modified MASI over time in individual patients should be performed to determine the sensitivity to change this outcome measure.

MEASURING THE IMPACT OF MELASMA

Validation of a Melasma Quality of Life for the Turkish Language: The MelasQoL-Tr Study

Methods

The study included 114 melasma patients. The MASI, MelasQoL-Tr and the Turkish short version of the quality of life (QoL) assessment instrument from the World Health Organization (WHOQoL-BREF) were used to assess melasma severity and QoL at baseline. The reliability and validity of MelasQoL-Tr were computed.

Results

The mean age of the patients in the study was 31.8 ± 7.3 years. The internal consistency of the scale (Cronbach's alpha coefficient) was 0.88. The melasQoLTr score was 29.9 ± 14.6 (range 10–66). The total WHOQoL-BREF score was 54.8 ± 9.8. The comparison of MelasQoL-Tr and WHOQoL-BREF questionnaires showed an inverse significant correlation on total scores, which indicated a sufficient convergent validity. According to the subscale of WHOQoL-BREF, the inverse correlation was most significant between the MelasQoL-Tr score and psychological domain and less significant between the MelasQoL-Tr score and environmental domain.

Conclusion

The Turkish version of the Melasma Quality of Life (MelasQoL) was valid and reliable for evaluating the QoL of Turkish melasma patients.

Development and Validation of a Health-related Quality of Life Instrument for Women with Melasma

Patient and Methods

A random sample of 102 women identified by an investigator as having melasma was evaluated by the investigator using the MASI. The patients were then anonymously surveyed with the Skindex-16, the fear of negative evaluation scale, the dermatology life quality index (DLQI), a skin discoloration evaluation questionnaire, and a measure of perceived life quality difference without melasma. The 10-item MelasQoL scale was devised from the comprehensive health-related quality of life (HRQoL) assessment battery.

Results

The psychometric properties of the MelasQoL were comparable with the properties of the DLQI and the Skindex-16. The MelasQoL scores were highly correlated with the other HRQoL measures. The discriminatory ability of the MelasQoL is superior to the Skindex-16 and the DLQI for melasma. The three life domains most adversely affected by melasma (social life, recreation/leisure and emotional well-being) were highlighted by this instrument. These were the same three areas of life that patients believed would improve the most if they no longer were affected by the disease.

Conclusion

The MelasQoL can be used to evaluate objectively the effect of melasma on a patient's HRQoL. The high correlation with the DLQI, the Skindex-16 and the skin discoloration questionnaire suggests that the new scale is a valid instrument, which can be used to monitor the level of impairment individuals suffer due to their melasma. The MelasQoL scores can help guide treatment methods as well as track the improvement of patient's HRQoL.

Validation of a Melasma Quality of Life Questionnaire for Brazilian Portuguese Language: The MelasQoL-BP Study and of QoL of Melasma-Patients after Triple Combination Therapy

Background

Pigmentation disorders, such as melasma, greatly influence the QoL of affected individuals who usually consider the disorder to be more severe than the objective clinical scores. Several instruments have been successfully developed to evaluate QoL. However, they must be adapted to the target population in terms of language and cultural diversity. The first, specific QoL questionnaire for melasma (MelasQoL) was developed for english speaking patients.

Objectives

To validate the Brazilian Portuguese version of the MelasQoL evaluation questionnaire for patients with melasma (MelasQoL-BP) and to assess the impact of treatment with a triple combination cream (hydroquinone, fluocinolone acetonide and tretinoin) on the QoL of patients with moderate-to-severe melasma.

Methods and Results

Three hundred individuals from the five Brazilian geographic regions took part in this multicenter study. Their mean age was 42 years and skin phototype distribution was: type II 7–10% of patients, III 23.7%; IV 42.7% and V 22.7%. MASI, MelasQoL-BP and the short version of the QoL assessment instrument from the World Health Organization (WHOQoL-BREF) were used to assess melasma severity and QoL at baseline. MelasQoL-BP was previously translated and culturally adapted from the English version, with participation of the authors and according to the standards of the World Health Organization (WHO). From the original sample, we randomized 150 volunteers to treat melasma and repeated the evaluation after 8 weeks. The analysis of the MelasQoL-BP baseline answers demonstrated an important impact of the disease on skin appearance (65% of patients were bothered all the time or most of the time), frustration (55%), embarrassment (57%) and influence of the disease on interpersonal relationships (42%). Forty-three percent of patients felt not attractive or even dirty due to their skin condition. MelasQoL-BP results showed significant internal consistency (Cronbach's alpha coefficient 0.919; $p < 0.001$) and good correlation with MASI scores. After treatment, the global assessment showed good or excellent results in 91.4% of the patients. The clinical outcome was not associated with the initial MASI score ($p = 0.814$; chi-square), skin color ($p = 0.449$; probability ratio) or skin pigmentation ($p = 0.814$; chi-square). There was also a significant reduction on MelasQoL-BP scores (Wilcoxon test; $p < 0.001$) after treatment, with the mean ± SD results shifting from 44.4 ± 14.9 at baseline to 24.3 ± 15.5 after treatment. The analysis of the MelasQoL-BP before and after treatment showed an important effect of the impact of treatment on a number of QoL measures. Of note, skin appearance (69.8% vs 10.1% of patients were bothered all the time or most of the time, respectively), frustration (59.7% vs 12.2%, respectively), embarrassment (56% vs 9.3%, respectively), and influence of the disease on interpersonal relationships (35.3% vs 5.8%, respectively) were greatly improved.

Conclusion

This study demonstrates that MelasQoL-BP is a valid instrument and can be used to evaluate the QoL and response to melasma treatment in Brazilian patients. The triple combination treatment produced significant results, regarding both clinical severity and QoL.

Melasma in Latina Patients: Cross Cultural Adaptation and Validation of a Quality of Life Questionnaire in Spanish Language

Background

Melasma has been shown to have a significant emotional and psychological effect on affected patients. Although this pigmentary disorder is thought to be more prevalent among Latinos, the effect of melasma on QoL in this population is unknown.

Objectives

The goals of this study were to translate and culturally adapt the previously validated MelasQoL scale into Spanish language, to confirm the new scale's reliability and validity, and to administer the scale to characterize melasma's effect on the health-related QoL of Spanish language-speaking Latino patients.

Methods

Cross-cultural adaptation of the original questionnaire was performed using previously established guidelines. After pretesting the questionnaire in a group of 30 patients, it was tested in a group of 112 patients recruited from a community outpatient clinic. A Spanish-language health-related QoL assessment battery was also administered for validation purposes. The degree of melasma was determined on clinical examination by the investigator using the MASI.

Results

Cross-cultural adaptation of the questionnaire was successful in producing a working and understandable Spanish-language version of the MelasQoL. The Spanish-language MelasQoL scale was internally reliable and demonstrated construct and content validity. The Spanish-language MelasQoL scores of patients with little to no formal education were significantly higher than those with at least a seventh-grade education. Scores were proportional to the length of time, a patient had lived with melasma and were higher in patients who had previously sought treatment. Spanish-language MelasQoL score and MASI were shown to be moderately correlated, but no differences were seen according to patient age, marital status, employment, or coexisting medical or psychiatric conditions.

Limitations

Limitations are a lack of data regarding socioeconomic status and limitation to Mexican and Central American female patients.

Conclusion

We have developed a semantically equivalent translation of MelasQoL in the Spanish language and have begun to characterize the effects of melasma on the QoL in a population that has not been previously studied. Further studies in larger populations of Spanish language-speaking patients from various geographic and socioeconomic groups are warranted.

Measure of the Impact on Quality of Life Using the French Version of MelasQoL after Cross-cultural Adaptation

Melasma has significant emotional and psychological effects. These repercussions can be measured using general measures of skin disease. Skindex-16 was used in a pilot study to show a significant impact on HRQoL and a correlation with disease severity measured by MASI.

A melasma-specific scale, the MelasQoL is highly correlated with the discoloration questionnaire. The discriminatory abilities of MelasQoL were found to be superior to those of Skindex-16 and DLQI for melasma (social life, recreation/leisure, and emotional well-being) has been highlighted by MelasQoL. We constructed a French version of MelasQoL (MelasQoL-F) following thorough cross-cultural adaptation, and then used it to evaluate the impact of melasma in French outpatients with melasma.

Twenty-eight women participated in the study. The proportion of women under the age of 45 years was 60.7% and over 45 years 39.3%. Almost one-half (48.2%) had melasma for 5 years or less and 29.6% for 10 years.

Melasma Quality of Life has been shown to have discriminatory power and high consistency; social life, recreation and leisure, and emotional well-being are the most affected domains of QoL. MelasQoL was constructed in English, and cross-cultural adaptations were then made in Spanish, Brazilian Portuguese and Turkish. We used the same methodology to construct the French version.

The absence of modification of MelasQoL-F score in association with high body mass index or an associated disease is a supplementary argument in favor of the specificity of MelasQoL-F. The correlations with alterations of mental QoL (assessed by MCS-12), general dermatological QoL (assessed by DLQI) and self-perceived stress (assessed by PCV-Metra) show that MelasQoL-F is as reliable as other scales. Our cross-cultural adaptation allowed correlation when melasma is more severe or when QoL is more altered. It is also possible that melasma experienced for a longer period of time is more severe, as shown by Dominguez et al. but the MASI score does not coincide with alterations in MelasQoL.

REFLECTANCE CONFOCAL MICROSCOPY FOR PIGMENTARY DISORDERS

In vivo reflectance confocal microscopy (RCM) is a noninvasive, repetitive imaging tool that provides real-time images at nearly cellular histological resolution. Application of RCM to skin imaging during the last decade has been a great advance in dermatology. RCM has been used mainly for the differentiation between benign and malignant skin lesions showing great potential for melanoma and melanocytic assessment. RCM also showed potential for diagnosis in inflammatory skin conditions including psoriasis, contact dermatitis and bacterial and fungal infections. Furthermore, as RCM provides the opportunity to determine *in vivo* kinetics of the skin after the application of therapeutics such as antiageing agent, RCM may be a useful tool in developing cosmetics.

As melanin is the strongest endogenous contrast in human skin, pigmentary disorders caused by abnormal amounts of melanin in the skin could be the most suitable candidates for RCM examination. This chapter reviews the RCM applications in the characterization and management of hyper- and hypopigmentary disorders as well as pigmented skin tumors.

The basic concept of confocal microscopy is the selective collection of light from the focused spot of the skin. A confocal microscope consists of a light source, condenser and objective lenses, and a detector. The light source, near-infrared wavelength laser beam **(Figs 2A and B)**, illuminates a specific point within a skin and reflected light is collected through a pinhole of the detector. The present commercially available confocal laser microscope (Vivascope 1500; Lucid Inc, Rochester, NY, USA) that we use, is equipped with an 830

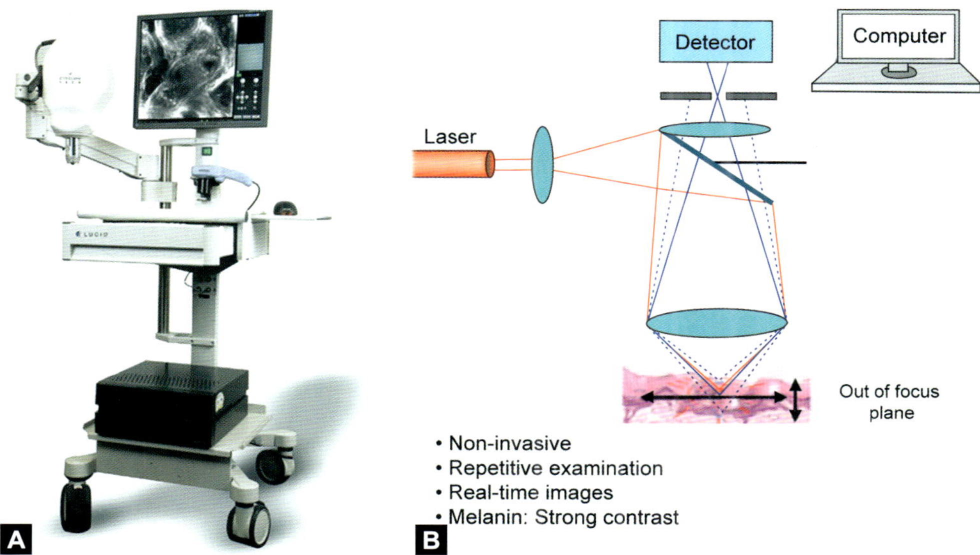

Figs 2A and B: *In vivo* reflectance confocal microscopy

nm diode laser with a low power of 5–10 mW, which causes no tissue damage. The light source, the illuminated spot, and the pinhole are in optically conjugated focal planes, leading to the name "confocal". The illuminated spot is then scanned horizontally, producing black and white images depth of up to 250–300 μm. To visualize a larger area, a two-dimensional sequence of images are captured and stitched in software to create a mosaic that displays up to 8 × 8 mm of tissue. Highly reflective skin components including melanin, collagen and keratin appear bright (white) in RCM images.

VISUALIZATION OF MELANIN AND MELANOCYTES BY REFLECTANCE CONFOCAL MICROSCOPY

Normal Skin

When examining the skin, the corneal layer is the first image seen as a highly refractile layer because of back scattering of light at the immersion medium-tissue junction. The granular layer appears next consisting of cells with bright grainy cytoplasm surrounding an oval dark nucleus. The spinous layer presents as a honeycombed pattern of smaller cells. The basal cell layer, is seen as a cobblestone pattern created by bright clusters of cells at the dermoepidermal junction (DEJ) of 40–130 μm depth. The brightness is stronger in the basal layer than in the spinous layer, because of the abundant supranuclear melanin caps in the basal cells. When imaging a little deeper, the supra-papillary epidermis at the DEJ appears as bright rings of basal cells surrounding a dark dermal papillae, which show a papillary dermal vasculature. Below DEJ, a network of collagen fibers and bundles can be observed in the papillary dermis and superficial reticular dermis.

Different brightness's correspond to endogenous variation among skin phototypes and the anatomic location. For examples, the brightness is stronger on the dorsal than on the volar forearm and particularly pronounced in heavily pigmented individuals. In skin phototype I, the basal keratinocytes have low refractivity and dermal papillary rings are difficult to elucidate.

Typical dendritic melanocytes were hardly observed in the normal human skin, although supranuclear melanin caps were easily visible. It was suggested that this might be because melanocytes rapidly transfer the produced melanin to keratinocytes and do not accumulate it. On the contrary, the melanocytes are observed in the pigmented animal skin such as Weiser-Maples guinea pig and during the pigmentation process of human skin (e.g. UV exposure). As activated Langerhans cells appear as highly refractile dendritic cells in suprabasal epidermal layer, it should be differentiated from the dendritic melanocytes.

Melanophages can be distinguished in the superficial dermis of pigmented skin as large, fuzzy, bright cells with illdefined cytoplasmic borders.

Ultraviolet-exposed Skin

Reflectance confocal microscopy has been used to show dynamic pigmentary changes in human or animal skin over time in response to UV irradiation. In the human skin after single UVA exposure, the brightness in the basal layer temporarily decreased and gradually increased from day 4.

Activated melanocytes were clearly visualized 8 days after UV exposure. The melanocytes then gradually disappeared and could no longer be observed in the RCM images. Instead, the supranuclear melanin caps became clear from day 29. Melanin appeared to be distributed more scattered than before UVA exposure. However, changes in the melanin immediately after the exposure, i.e. in immediate pigment darkening were hardly detectable, and RCM images only showed accelerated capillary flow patterns. There was also report showing a reduction of dermal reflectivity (dermal edema) and an increase in vessel diameter as well as increased brightness of the basal layer 72 hours after ultraviolet band irradiation.

Melasma

Melasma is characterized by epidermal hyperpigmentation, possibly because of an increased melanin and to an increased number or activity of melanocytes. We investigated the relevant *in vivo* RCM features of melasma in our preliminary study. Twenty-five patients with melasma, who gave informed consent, were enrolled in the study with approval of the ethic committee. Multiple mosaic and stack RCM images were acquired from the lesional skin and perilesional normal skin. Skin biopsy was obtained from seven patients. RCM images of melasma showed characteristic significantly increased hyper-refractile cobblestone pattern at the level of basal cell layer in lesional skin compared with perilesional normal skin (Kang HY et al. unpublished observations) **(Figs 3A to C)**. Dendritic cells and plump bright dermal cells corresponding to activated melanocytes and melanophages, respectively, were also observed in some patients. Most melasma skin showed an abrupt transition from stratum spinosum to papillary dermis and moderately refractile lacy structures (solar elastosis) in the dermis, suggesting the existence of chronic solar damage in the melasma. These findings suggested the possibility of future clinical applications of RCM for melasma diagnosis and treatment.

IN VIVO REFLECTANCE CONFOCAL MICROSCOPY DETECTS PIGMENTARY CHANGES IN MELASMA AT A CELLULAR LEVEL RESOLUTION

Epidermal Reflectance Confocal Microscopy Features Melasma

Reflectance confocal microscopy images of all melasma patients showed a characteristic hyper-refractile cobblestone pattern in the basal cell layer and sometimes lower stratum spinosum. Cobblestoning was significantly more pronounced in the lesion compared with perilesional normal skin (2.0 ± 0.7 versus 0.7 ± 0.8, $P \leq 0.001$). Histological studies confirmed that this pattern corresponded to epidermal hyperpigmentation. The dermal papillary rings were usually invisible in lesional and perilesional normal skin. Instead an abrupt transition from stratum spinosum to papillary dermis, corresponding to flattened rete ridges was seen in most RCM images. In five cases of melasma with preserved rete ridges (one check, three forehead and one supralip area), brighter papillary rings appeared in the lesion compared with perilesional normal skin (data not shown) **(Figs 4 to 7)**. In 6 of 26 patients, RCM images showed bright dendritic cells at the level of the DEJ in melasma but not in control skin. Immunohistochemical studies confirmed that these cells corresponded to activated melanocytes, and Langerhans cells.

Dermal Reflectance Confocal Microscopy Features of Melasma

In 9 of 26 patients, RCM images showed plump bright cells in the papillary dermis. Histological studies involved a 39-year-old woman with a 3-year history of melasma on the cheek

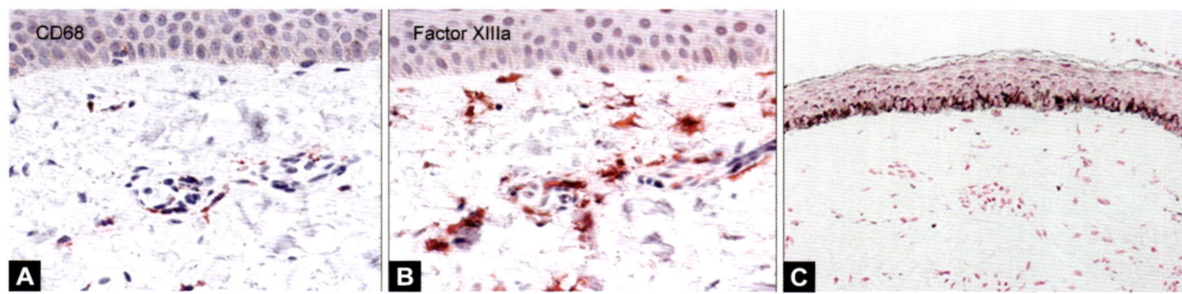

Figs 3A to C: Melasma and melanophages in the dermis.
(*Source:* Hee-Young Kang)

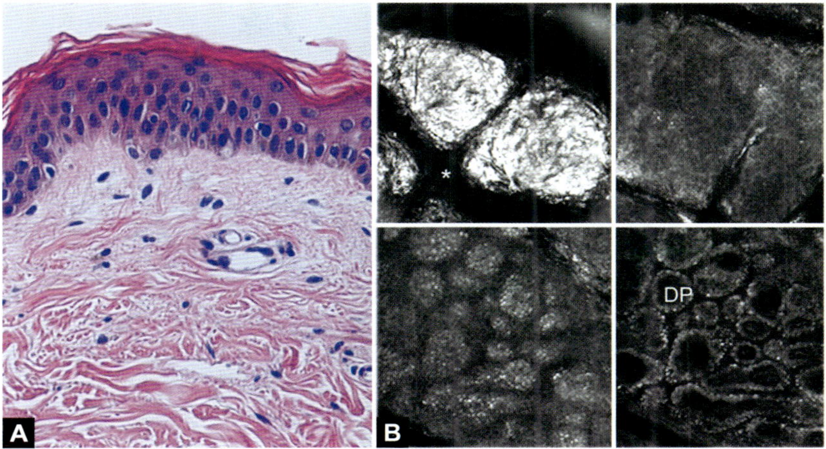

Figs 4A and B: Normal skin

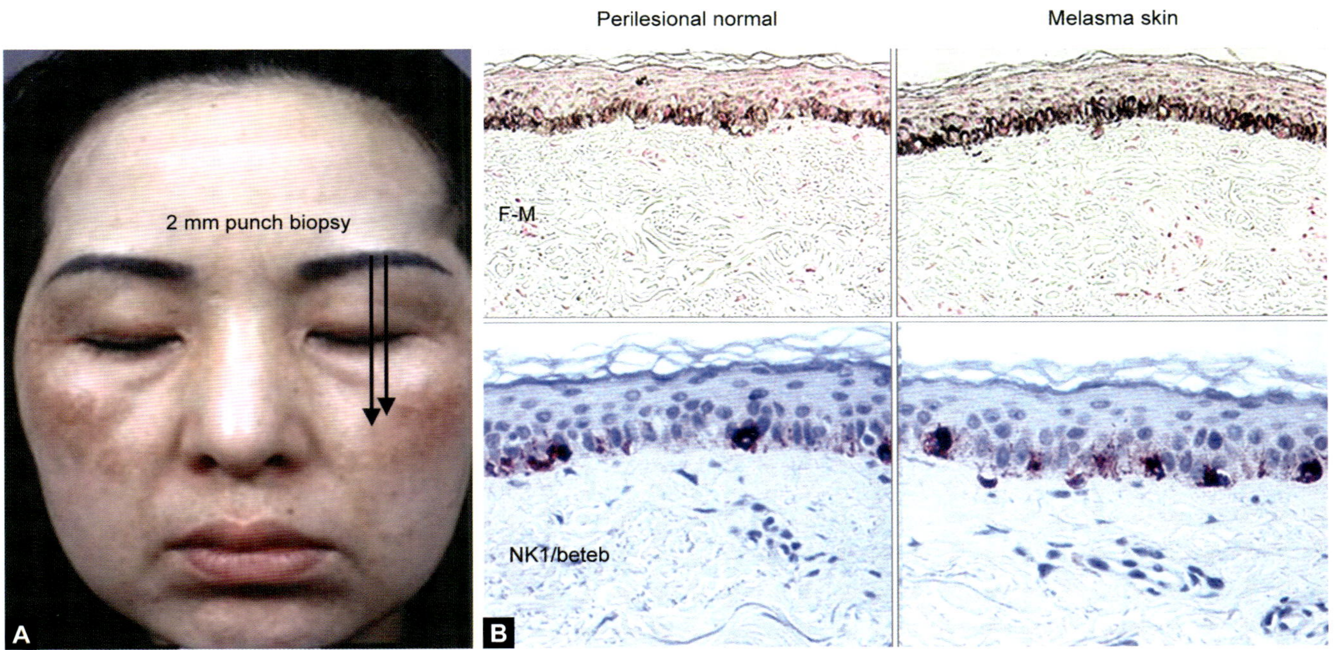

Figs 5A and B: Epidermal pigmentation in melasma

and supralip. The RCM images of right cheek demonstrated melanophages localized exclusively on the left lower corner of the RCM mosaic image. No melanophages were observed in the left cheek and supralip area **(Figs 8 and 9)**. These findings suggested the distribution of melanophages is very heterogeneous because it can vary from one melasma region to another and even inside a given melasma region **(Figs 10 to 16)**.

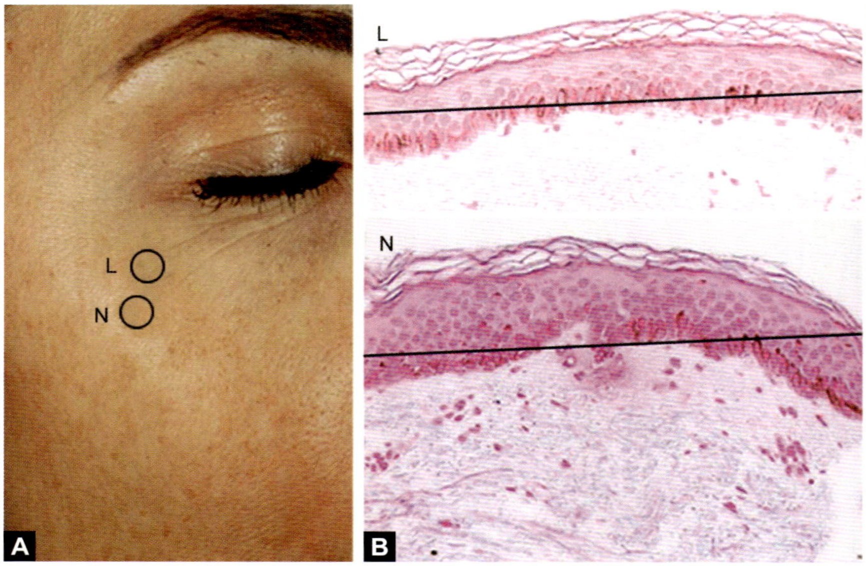

L	N	p value
2.0 ± 0.7	0.7 ± 0.8	0.00002

0, 0–25%; 1, 25–50%; 2, 50–75%; 3, 75–100%

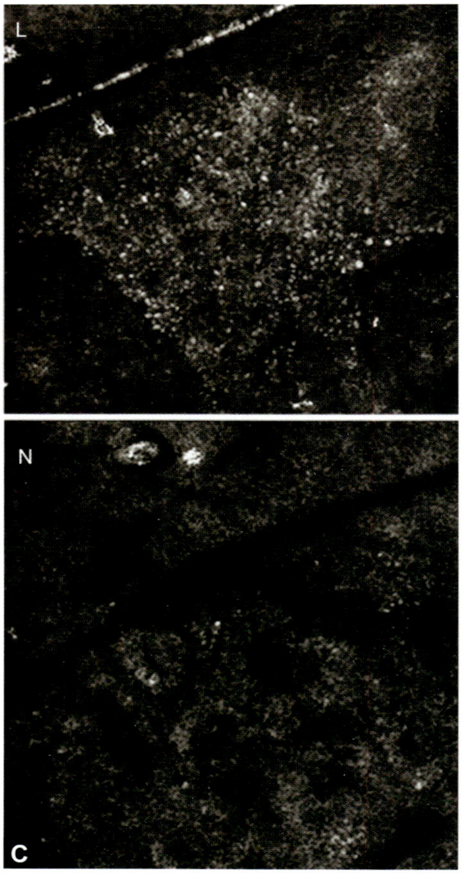

Figs 6A to C: Epidermal pigmentation (25/25)

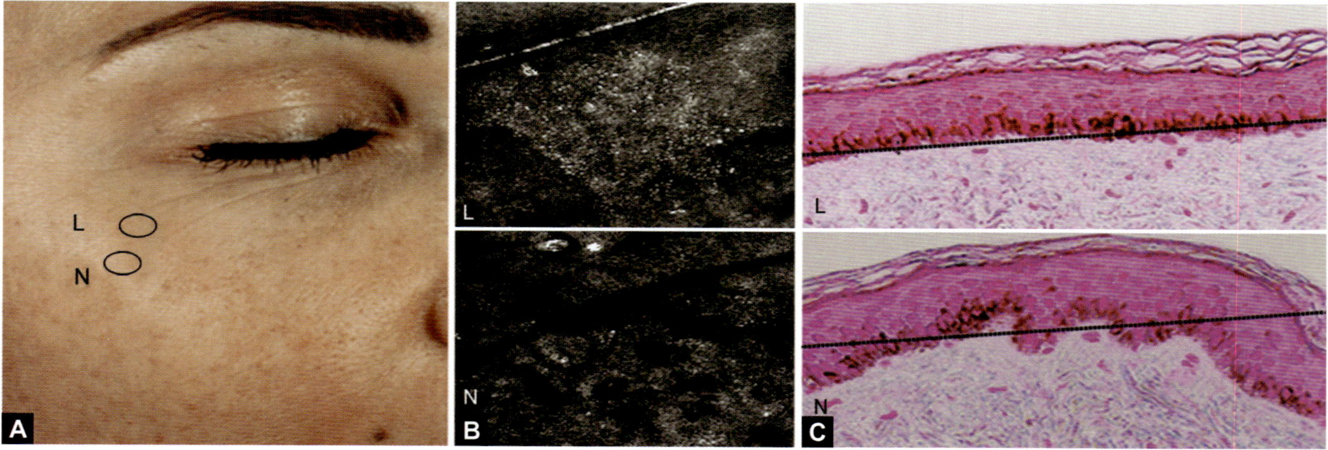

Figs 7A to C: Melasma with epidermal pigmentation. Melasma with epidermal pigmentation. (A) Clinical photograph of hyperpigmented macules (circled) on the cheek. The lesional (L) and perilesional normal skin (N) were evaluated; (B) Confocal images show increased cobblestonings and loss of dermal papillary rings at the basal layer in lesion (L) compared to perilesional normal skin (N). Scale bar: 50 μm (C) corresponding histopathology shows more pronounced epidermal hyperpigmentation and flattened rete ridges in lesion compared to perilesional normal skin (Fontana-Masson staining, x 200). Horizontal line indicates where reflectance confocal microscopy image is captured from. (*Source:* Kang HY, Bahadoran P, Ortonne JP. Exp Dermatol. 2010;19:233-9.)

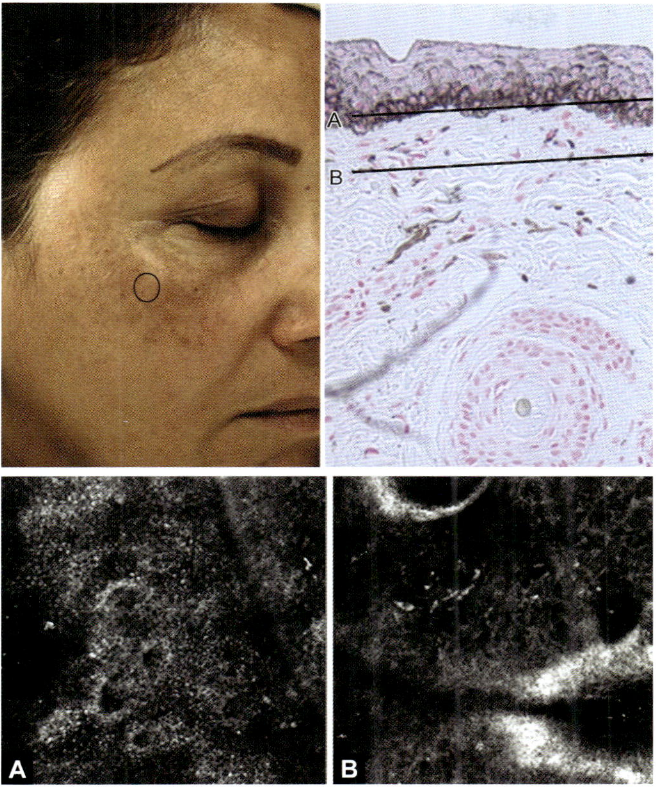

Figs 8A and B: Dermal pigmentation (8/25)

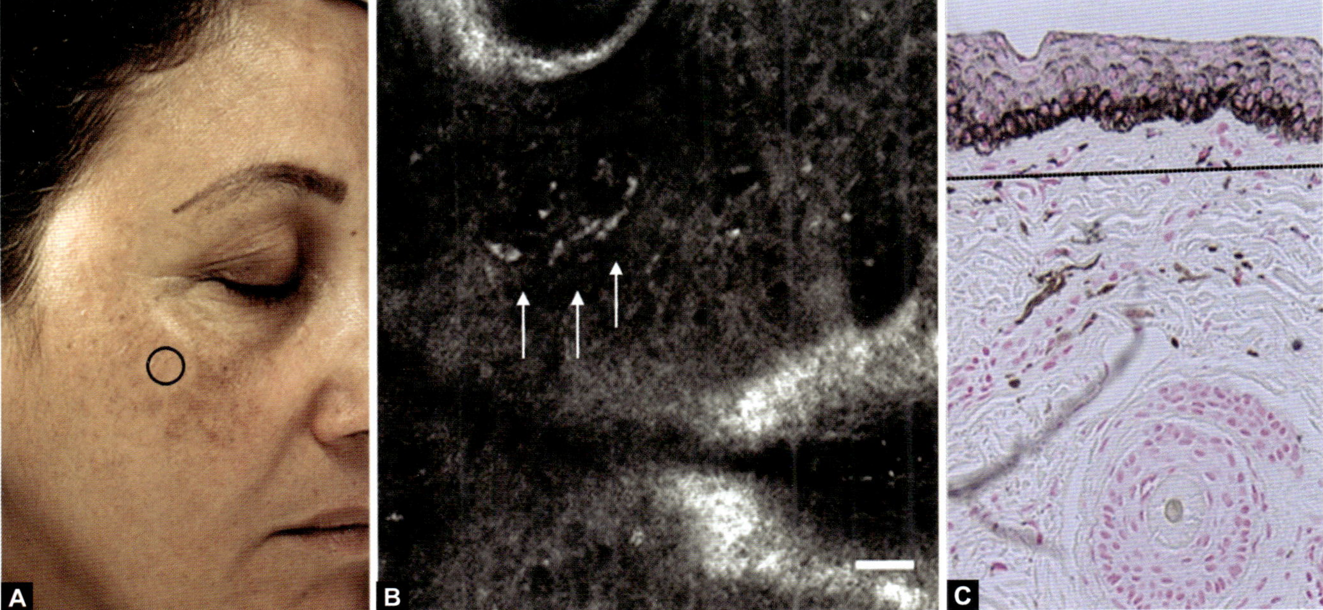

Figs 9A to C: Melasma with dermal pigmentation. (A) Clinical photograph of hyperpigmented macules; (B) Confocal photograph of melasma show plump brighter cells in the dermis; (C) Melanophages in the dermis. (*Source:* Kang HY, Bahadoran P, Ortonne JP. Exp Dermatol. 2010;19:233-9.)

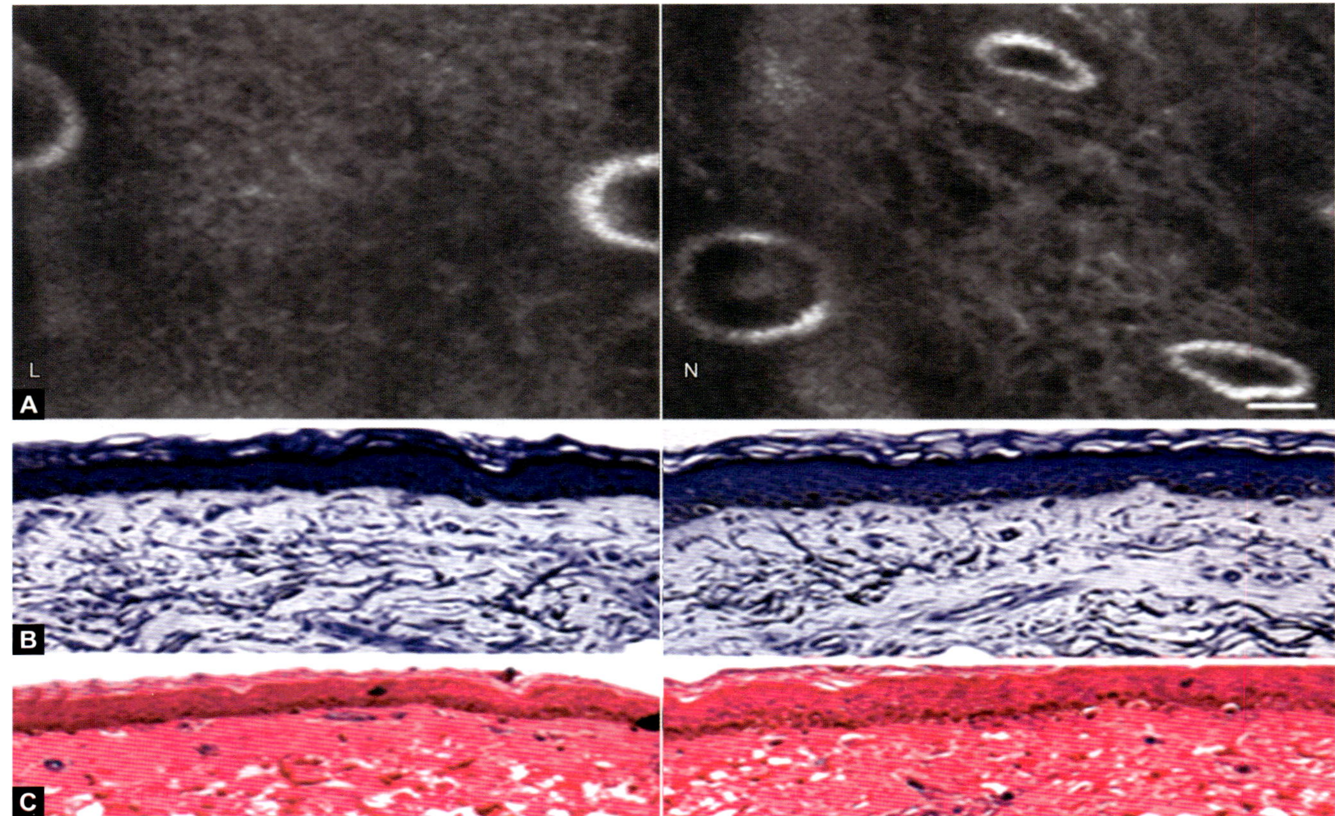

Figs 10A to C: *In vivo* reflectance confocal microscopy detects pigmentary changes in melasma at a cellular level resolution. Confocal and vasculature in melasma. (A) Confocal image at the level of upper dermis show ragged, less refractile, lacy structures corresponding to solar elastosis on histology. The degree of solar elatosis is more severe in the lesion (L) compared with perilesional normal skin (N). Blood vessels appeared as dark round to tubular structures; (B) Lesional skin demonstrates abundant elastotic material compared with perilesional normal skin in the upper dermis; (C) CD31 immunostaining shows increased number of blood vessels in the upper dermis compared with perilesional normal skin. (*Source:* Experimental Dermatology Volume 19, Issue 8, pages e228-e233.)

Comparison of Reflectance Confocal Microscopy Findings with Histology

For eight patients for whom a biopsy was available, RCM features were compared to histological findings. In all patients, the amount of melanin was increased in the epidermis of lesional skin. Image analysis showed significant increase in pigmented area per epidermal area in the lesional skin compared with perilesional normal skin (0.26 versus 0.09, $P \leq 0.01$), confirming RCM results. All specimens of lesional and perilesional normal skin also showed rete ridge flattening, as expected from RCM examination. In one patient, Fontana-Masson staining showed numerous melanized dropping cells in the lesion.

CD1a immunostaining ruled out the possibility that dendritic cells correspond to Langerhans cells and NKI/beteb immunostaining confirmed these cells were melanocytes. These cells were correctly identified as activated melanocytes by RCM. In four patients, scattered melanophages were detected in the upper dermis. These melanophages were correctly identified by RCM in three patients. The uneven distribution of melanophages in melasma lesions may explain why in one case biopsy-proven melanophages were not retrieved by RCM examination. Solar elastosis was significantly increased in lesional skin compared with perilesional normal skin (0.37 versus 0.21, $p \leq 0.01$). The number of vessels was significantly increased in lesional skin compared with perilesional normal skin (11 versus 7, $p \leq 0.05$). Sensitivity and specificity were determined for each individual RCM parameter. The sensitivity ranged from

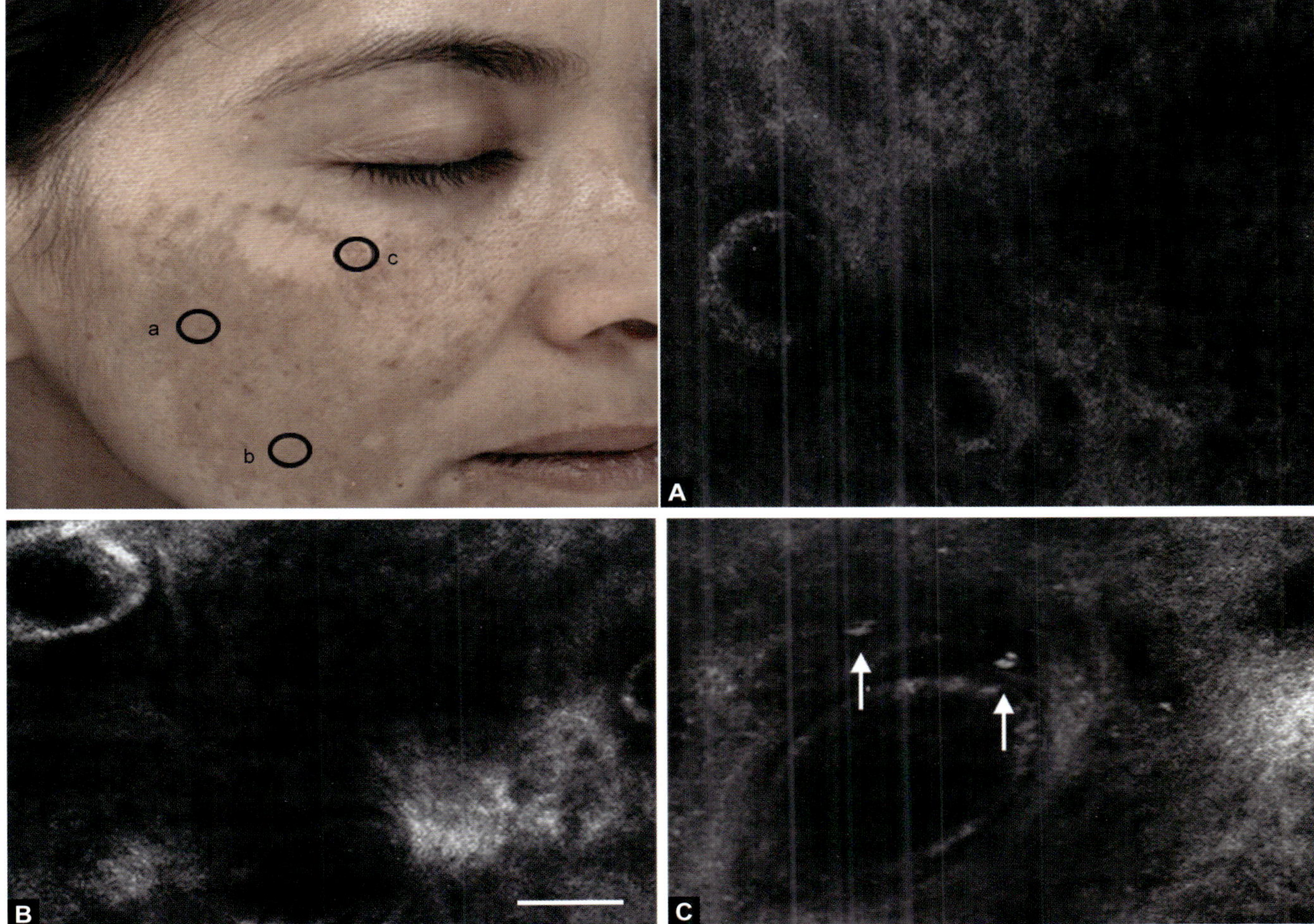

Figs 11A to C: Topographic variation of dermal melanin in melasma. (A) Uneven distribution of melanophages from one to another region in melasma; (B) The circles labelled a, b, c indique the area where confocal examination was performed; (C) Confocal taken from area c reveals melanophages in the papillary dermis. (*Source:* Kang HY, Bahadoran P, Ortonne JP. Exp Dermatol. 2010;19:233-9.)

50% to 100%, whereas the specificity was high. There was a good agreement between RCM images and histology except increased vascularity.

HISTOLOGICAL CLASSIFICATION OF MELASMA WITH REFLECTANCE CONFOCAL MICROSCOPY: A PILOT STUDY IN CHINESE PATIENTS

Objective

To investigate the histological classification of melasma with RCM *in vivo*.

Methods

Two hundred and ten cases with facial melasma lesions were enrolled. After informed consent, the target melasma lesion of 10 patients were imaged with RCM and then biopsied as well. Under the RCM scanning, the distribution of the melanin determined the histological types, and then, the results of RCM images were compared with those of the histopathology. The other 200 cases were tested only with RCM.

Results

For the 10 cases compared with that of the perilesional normal skin, the amount of melanin was significantly increased in the epidermis in all lesions under RCM, while three cases also found melanin in the dermis. Thus, imaged and biopsied

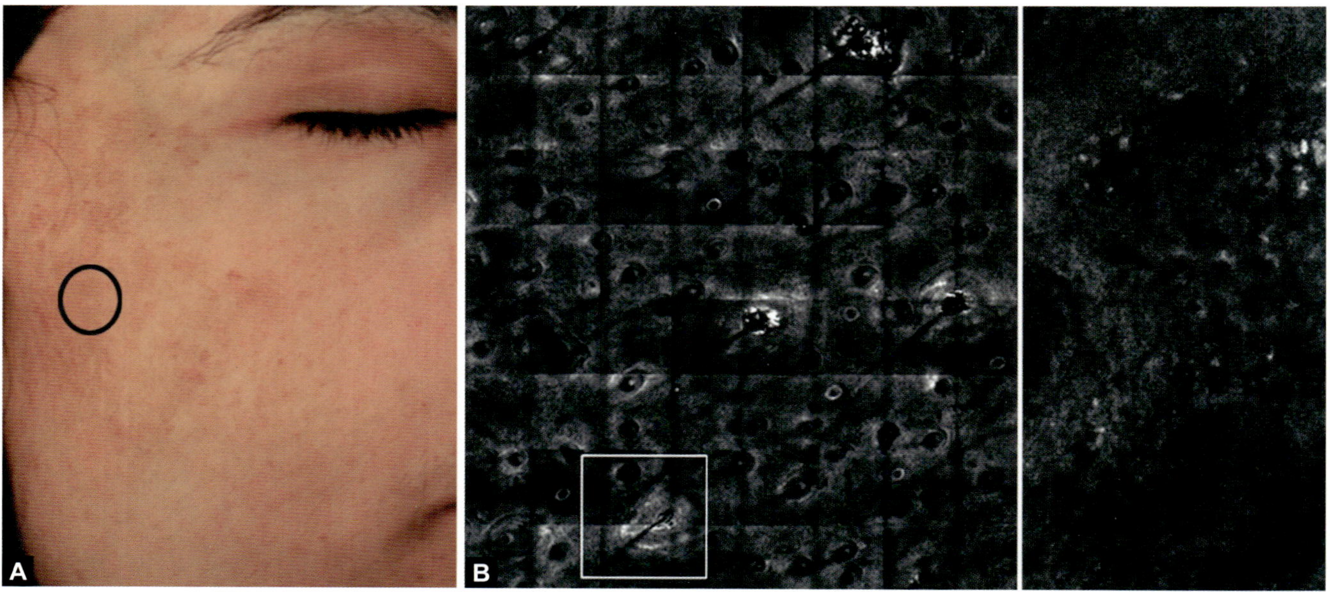

Figs 12A and B: Topographic variation of dermal melanin in melasma. (A) Uneven distribution of melanophages in the same melasma region; (B) Reflectance confocal microscopy mosaics suggest that melanophages are localized in the lower corner. (*Source:* Kang HY, Bahadoran P, Ortonne JP. Exp Dermatol. 2010;19:233-9.)

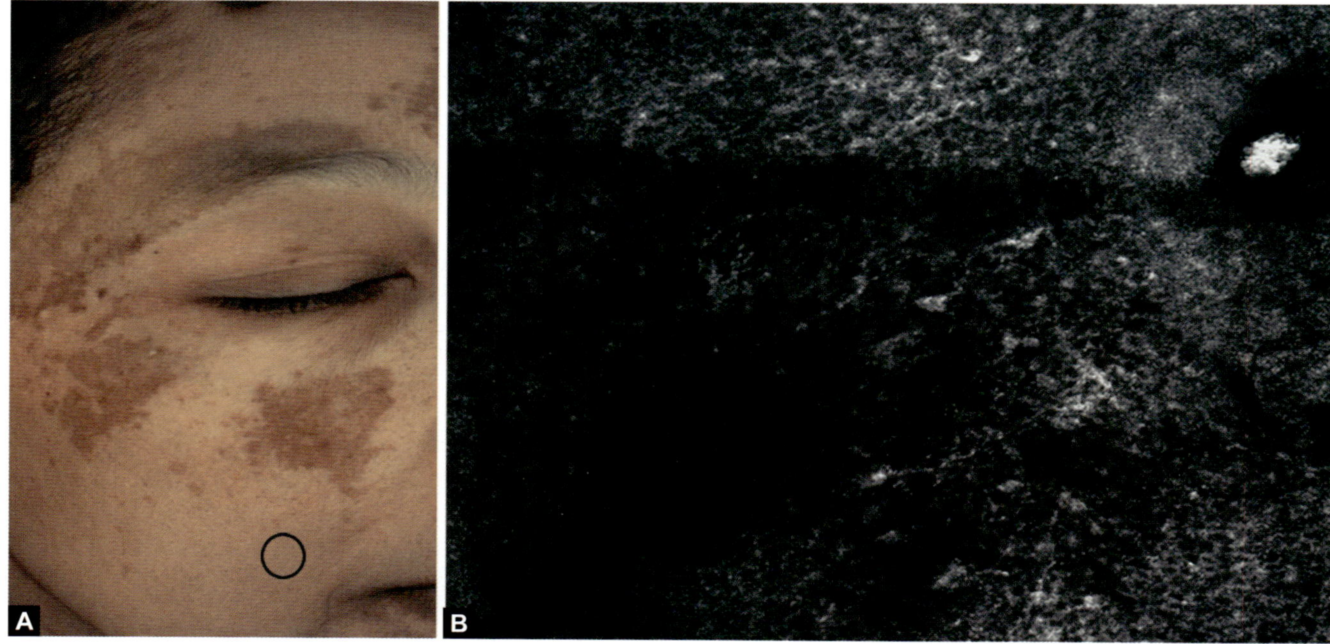

Figs 13A and B: Melasma with activated melanocytes. (A) Clinical photograph; (B) Reflectance confocal microscopy image shows dendritic cells at the level of dermoepidermal junction of the lesional skin (L)

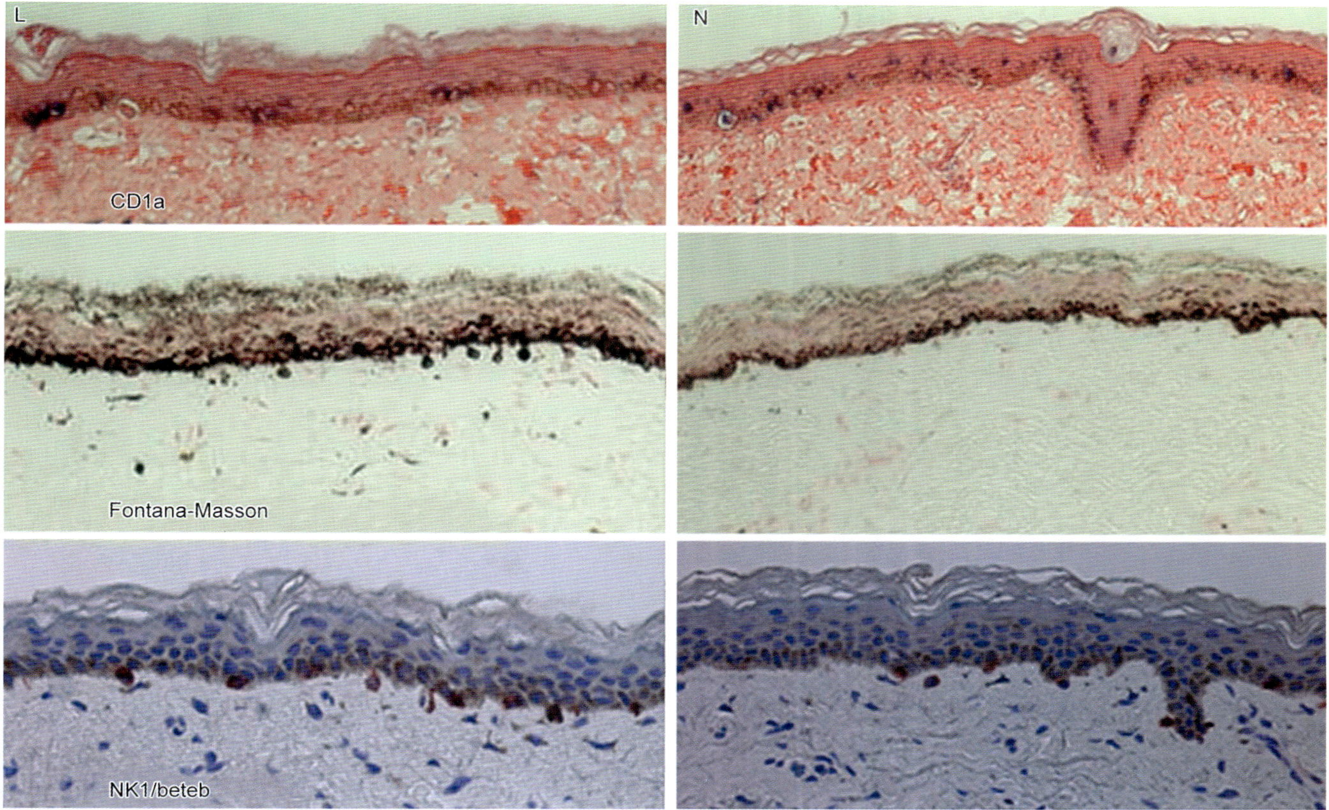

Fig. 14: Melasma with activated melanocytes. CD1a immunostaining shows reduced number of Langerhans in the lesion (L) compared to perilesional normal skin (N). FM staining shows numerous melanized dendritic dropping cells in lesion in comparison with the perilesional normal skin. NK1/beteb staining confirmed these cells are melanocytes

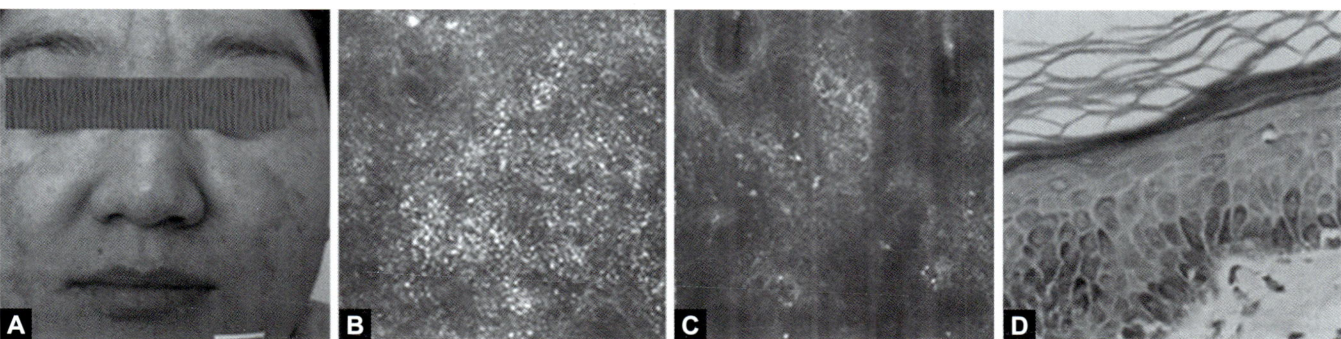

Figs 15A to D: Histological classification of melasma with reflectance confocal microscopy: a pilot study in Chinese patients. (A) Facial melasma lesion; (B) The increased melanin in the basal cell layer of the melasma lesion; (C) The increased melanin in the superficial dermis; (D) H-stain shows that the amount of melanin was significantly increased in the epidermal and dermal layers in melasma skin. (*Source:* Skin Research and Technology. Volume 17, Issue 4, pages 398-403, 21 FEB 2011 DOI: 10.1111/j.1600-0846.2011.00517.*xhttp://onlinelibrary.wiley.com/doi/10.1111/j.1600-0846.2011.00517.x/full#f1.*)

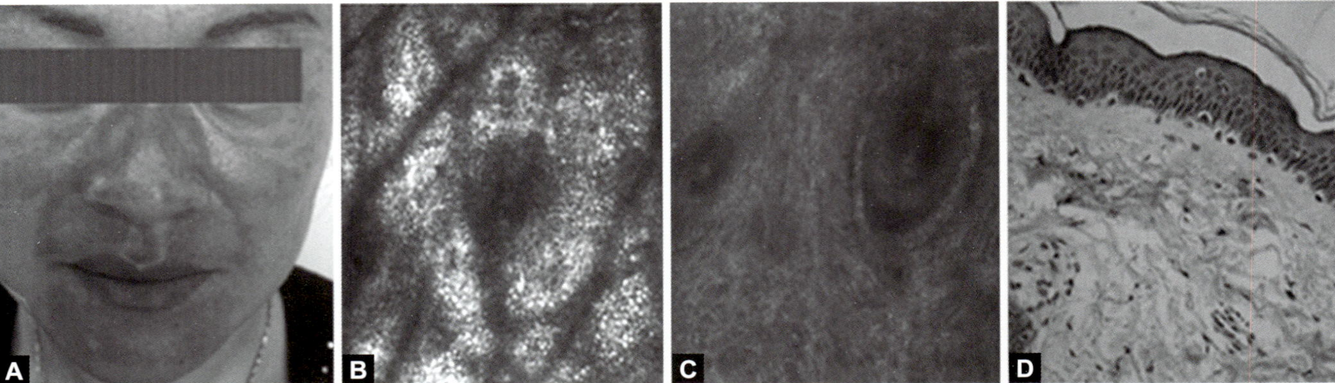

Figs 16A to D: Histological classification of melasma with reflectance confocal microscopy: a pilot study in Chinese patients. (A) Facial melasma lesion; (B) The increased melanin in the basal cell layer of the melasma lesion; (C) No melanin in the superficial dermis; (D) In HE section the amount of melanin was significantly increased in the epidermal layers in melasma skin, while there was no melanin in the dermis. (*Source:* Skin Research and Technology. Volume 17, Issue 4, pages 398-403, 21 FEB 2011 DOI: 10.1111/j.1600-0846.2011.00517.*xhttp://onlinelibrary.wiley.com/doi/10.1111/j.1600-0846.2011.00517.x/full#f1.*)

7 of the 10 patients were categorized as the epidermal type while the other three as mixed ones, and the results were well-correlated with those of the histopathology. Of the other 200 patients, 143 cases (71.5%) were categorized as the epidermal type while the other 57 (28.5%) cases as mixed ones.

Limitations

If more melasma cases are biopsied, the data will be more convincing.

Conclusion

Reflectance confocal microscopy *in vivo* analysis shows complete coherence with histopathology results, which could be an alternative for the classification of melasma, and based on the results of RCM imaging, melasma is classified into two major types: the epidermal type and mixed type.

The identification of the location and extent of the abnormal deposit of pigment in melasma lesions compared with that of the perilesional normal skin determines the types of melasma. Although quite a few studies attempted to use Wood's light to classify melasma as epidermal, dermal, mixed, and indeterminate types, a comparative study found discordance between Wood's light and histology. A new method, consistent with histology results, is needed for the classification of melasma.

Reflectance confocal microscopy is a noninvasive tool for in vivo imaging and microscopic analysis of the skin, at a high resolution and contrast without the requirement of physically dissecting the tissue. As melanin and melanosomes are strong sources of contrast for RCM images, pigmentary disorders are the most suitable candidates for RCM examination at a cellular-level resolution, but RCM features of melasma have seldom been reported.

In this study, we performed a two-stage investigation; first, we tested the feasibility of RCM in histological classification using histology as the gold standard and found a good concordance between the RCM and the histological analysis results, which proved that RCM was a good tool in the histological classification of melasma. Commonly, the distributions of melanin in the basal cell layer and spinous cell layer increase simultaneously in melasma lesions compared with that in controls. We found that all melasma lesions had increased melanin in the epidermis, and a few cases with melanin in the dermis based on the distribution of melanin, most cases were determined to be the epidermal type, while a few as the mixed type, and we found no dermal type. Then we performed the second stage, a large-scale study, in which 200 melasma cases were enrolled, to investigate whether a genuine dermal type does exist or not with *in vivo* RCM. Finally, we found no genuine dermal-type melasma in our two-stage study.

Reflectance confocal microscopy not only reflects histological changes in melasma but it provides a potential advantage over biopsies, as an entire lesion can be analyzed *in vivo*, despite its noninvasive nature. Moreover, compared with the perilesional normal skin, the semiqualitative scale of pigmentation could also be scored. We found that the distribution and amount of melanophages in melasma lesions differed in different cases. In some cases, the activated melanocytes with a dendritic or a polymorphic shape may respond to sun exposure or some extent of treatment. The degree of abnormal melanin deposition, the role of the active pigmentation, and influence of treatment still need further investigation.

In summary, our preliminary results highlight a different classification of melasma, which may provide a new view of the treatment modality selection.

BIBLIOGRAPHY

1. Balkrishanan R, McMichael AJ, Camacho FT, et al. Development and validation of a health-related quality of life instru ment for women with melasma. Br J Dermatol. 2003;149(3): 572-7.
2. Cestari TF, Hexsel D, Viegas ML, et al. Validation of a melasma quality of life questionnaire for Brazilian Portuguese language: the MelasQoL-BP study and improvement of QoL of melasma patients after triple combination therapy. Br J Dermatol. 2007;156(Suppl.1):13-20.
3. Dogramaci AC, Havlucu DY, Inandi T, et al. Validation of a melasma quality of life questionnaire for the Turkish language: The MelasQoL. J Dermatol Treat. 2009;20(2):95-9.
4. Dominguez AR, Balkrishnan R, Ellzev AR, et al. Melasma in Latina patients: cross cultural adaptation and validation of a quality of life questionnaire in Spanish language. J Am Acad Dermatol. 2006;55(1):59-66.
5. Kang HY, Bahadoran P, Ortonne JP. Reflectance confocal microscopy for pigmentary disorders. Exp Dermatol. 2009; 19(3):233-9.
6. Kang HY, Bahadoran P, Suzuki I, et al. In vivo reflectance confocal microscopy defects pigmentary changes in melasma at a cellular level resolution. Exp Dermatol. 2010; 19(8):228-33.
7. Liu H, Nie W, Chen X, et al. Histological classification of melasma with reflectance confocal microscopy: a pilot study in Chinese patients. Skin Res Technol. 2011;17(4): 398-403.
8. Misery L, Schmitt S, Boussetta N, et al. Letters; Acta Derm Venereol. 2010;90(3):331-2.
9. Pandya A, Hynan L, Bhore R, et al. Reliability assessment and validation of the melasma area and severity index (MASI) and a new modified MASI scoring method. J Am Acad Dermatol. 2011;64(1):78-83.

37

Cutaneous Biophysical Characteristics of Melasma

Jean-Paul Ortonne

Key Features

- Photodamaged skin has delayed barrier recovery with downregulation of lipid metabolism-associated genes.
- Melasma skin has normal hydration of stratum corneum and normal sebaceous gland activity.
- Melasma skin has reduced stratum corneum thickness with abnormal barrier function.
- Chronic UV exposure and increased epidermal pigmentation may cause the defective barrier function in melasma skin.
- Treatment of melasma should include improving the function of stratum corneum.

DEFECTIVE BARRIER FUNCTION IN MELASMA SKIN

Melanin is concentrated in the basal layer but also distributed throughout the epidermis. It has been thought that skin pigmentation is associated with multiple cutaneous functions. Stratum corneum (SC) in black skin contains more cell layers and greater electrical resistance and requires more tape strips to remove it than that of white skin, suggesting better intercellular cohesion in black skin. Moreover, epidermal barrier function is different between black and white skin, although the results are inconclusive. Darker skin has been shown to recover faster after barrier damage. Whereas, another scientist found significant higher transepidermal water loss (TEWL) after stripping blacks and Asian that in whites.

Photodamaged skin has been thought to have modified cutaneous functions. Barrier recovery is delayed in photoaged skin as compared to chronologically aged skin. Moreover, recently we found that most lipid metabolism-associated genes, such as peroxisome proliferator-activated receptor alpha (PPARA) and arachidonate 15-lipoxygenase, type B (ALOX15B), were downregulated accompanying a delayed barrier recovery rate in lesional skin. These findings suggest that cutaneous biophysical characteristics may have a significant impact on melasma patients. Therefore, in this study, scientist measured the cutaneous biophysical characteristics of melasma including SC hydration, sebum content, and TEWL and made comparisons between lesional and perilesional normal skin.[1]

MATERIAL AND METHODS

A total of 16 female Korean volunteers with melasma were recruited. The mean age was 44.2 ± 5.36 years old (31–55 years old), and the average of disease duration was 12.9 ± 7.2 years. All subjects have Fitzpatrick skin type III or IV. All subjects had a washout period of at least 1 month from a bleaching agent or steroid containing triple agents and a washout period of at least 1 year from lasers, dermabrasion and chemical peeling.

MELANIN INDEX AND ERYTHEMA INDEX

The melanin index was significantly higher in lesional skin compared to perilesional normal skin (221.4 ± 54.3 vs 150.4 ± 29.9, $p<0.001$). The erythema index was significantly increased in lesional skin that perilesional normal skin (323.2 ± 60.3 vs 272.3 ± 34.8, $p<0.012$). The melanin and erythema index showed a positive correlation (Correlation coefficient 0.703, $p<0.01$).

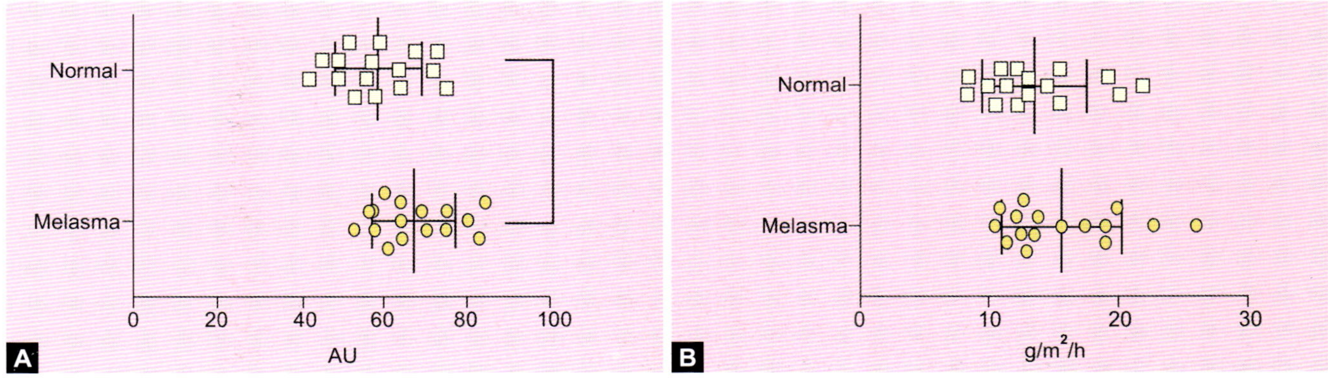

Figs 1A and B: Basal stratum corneum properties. (A) Stratum corneum capacitance was higher in lesional skin than in perilesional normal skin; (B) No significant difference was observed between the TEWL values of these two skin types (p <0.05). (*Source:* Lee DJ et al. Journal of the European Academy of Dermatology and Venereology (JEADV), 2011)

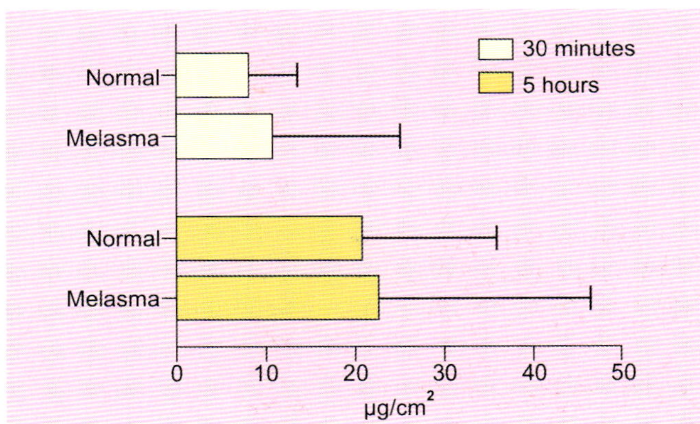

Fig. 2: Difference in amount of sebum. There was no significant difference in sebum amount at both 30 minutes and 5 hours after facial degreasing (*Source:* Lee DJ et al. JEADV, 2011)

BASAL STRATUM CORNEUM PROPERTIES

The SC hydration was significantly increased in lesional skin compared to perilesional normal skin (66.9 ± 9.9 vs 58.4 ± 10.1; p <0.029). However, the basal TEWL showed no significant difference between lesional and perilesional normal skin (15.6 ± 4.6 vs 13.5 ± 4.0, p <0.210) **(Figs 1A and B)**.

SEBUM CONTENT

Sebum amount measurement showed no significant difference between lesional skin and perilesional normal skin at 30 minutes after facial washing (μg/cm², 7.9 ± 5.8 vs 10.6 ± 14.5, p = 0.897). After 5 hours for acclimatization, the amount of sebum and the sebum excretion rate during 5 hours showed no significant difference (μg/cm², 5 hours after degreasing: 20.5±15.4 vs 22.4±24.1, p=0.752) **(Fig. 2)**.

SEBUM CONTENT THICKNESS AND EXPRESSION OF PPAR-α AND ALOX15B

Because lipid metabolism related genes, such as *PPARA* and *ALOX15B*, were found to be down-regulated in melasma, we examined their protein levels. There was no significant difference in immunoreactivity of PPAR-α and ALOX15B between lesional and perilesional normal skin. However, we found that the SC thickness was reduced in the lesional skin of melasma in comparison with perilesional normal skin (μm, 10.4 ± 2.9 vs 14.5 ± 5.5, p = 0.052) **(Figs 3A and B)**.

DISCUSSION

The present study demonstrated that melasma skin showed a normal hydration state and sebaceous gland activity. However, the SC integrity and barrier function were impaired in the lesional skin of melasma. The SC thickness was reduced in lesional skin and it positively correlated with the barrier recovery rate. The melanin index negatively correlated with barrier recovery rate **(Figs 4A and B)**.

The mechanisms underlying abnormal barrier function in melasma are unclear, but there are possible explanations. Recently, it was found the lipid metabolism-associated genes, such as peroxisome proliferators-activated receptor alpha (PPARA), arachidonate 15-lipoxygenase, and type B (ALOX15B), were down-regulated in the lesional skin of melasma. It is well known that the lipids of SC play an important role in maintaining cutaneous barrier homeostasis. PPAR-α is an important regulator of lipid catabolism, mediating fatty acid oxidation, fatty acid uptake, and lipoprotein assembly and transport. Therefore, down-regulated lipid metabolism-associated genes may be a causal

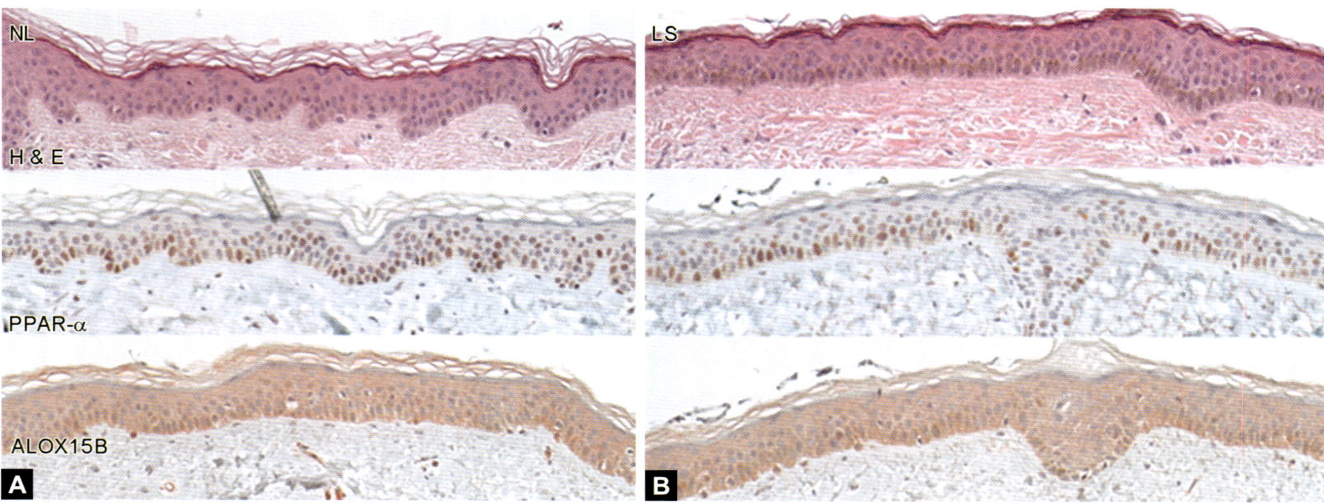

Figs 3A and B: Thickness of stratum corneum in melasma. (A) Stratum corneum thickness was lower in melasma-involved skin compared to perilesional normal skin; (B) There was no significant difference of PPAR-α and ALOX15B expression between lesional and perilesional normal skin (NL: perilesional; LS: melasma involved skin; original magnification X 200). (*Source:* Lee DJ et al. JEADV, 2011)

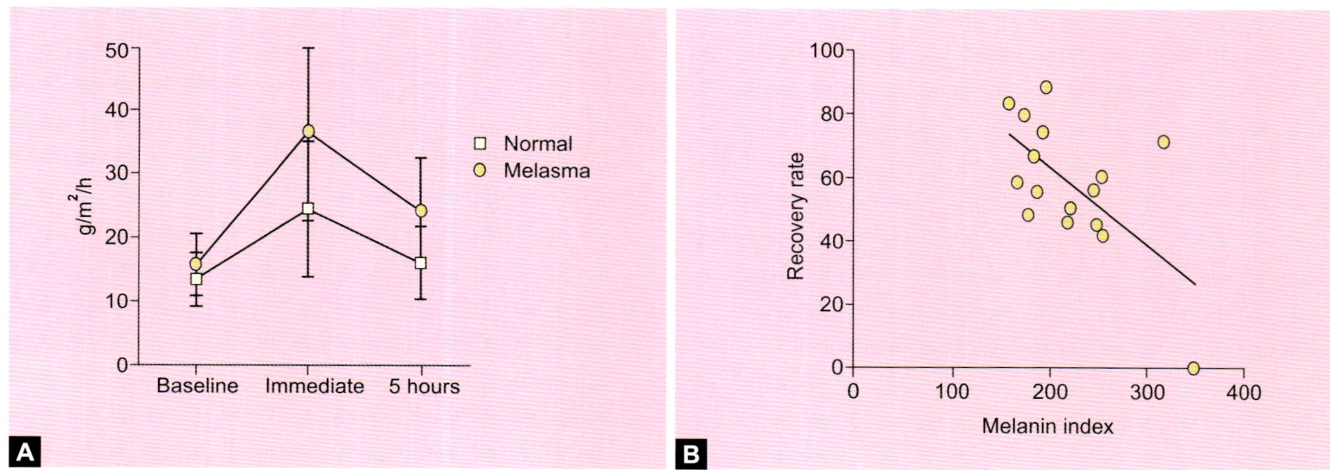

Figs 4A and B: Barrier recovery rate. (A) Immediately after tape-stripping 5 times, the rate of TEWL in melasma-involded skin was significantly higher in comparison to perilesional normal skin. In addition, 5 hours after the tape-stripping, the barrier recovery rate was significantly delayed in melasma-involved skin in comparison to perilesional normal skin ($p < 0.05$); (B) There was negative correlation between the melanin index and barrier recovery rate. (*Source:* Lee DJ et al. JEADV, 2011)

factor of the impairment of epidermal barrier function in melasma, although we could not confirm the down-regulation of these proteins by immunohistochemical staining. The reduced SC thickness may play another role of impairment barrier in lesional skin. We found that SC thickness positively correlated with barrier recovery rate. SC thickness is correlated linearly to the 1/TEWL value. Furthermore, it has been reported that SC thickness is significantly correlated with the objective score of atopic dermatitis. Also, in acute eczematous atopic skin which disrupted barrier function, SC thickness is significantly decreased compared to non-lesional and control healthy skin. That means that SC thickness may influence the epidermal barrier homeostasis. Taken together, it is speculated that reduced SC thickness and down-regulation of lipid metabolism-related genes in melasma influence the impairment barrier function in melasma.

Chronic UV exposure influences cutaneous fatty acid metabolism and barrier function. Also, chronic UV irradiation reduces the epidermal free fatty and triglyceride synthesis that has an important role in epidermal barrier homeostasis. In addition, UVB exposure is detrimental to the epidermal permeability barrier in a dose-dependent and time-dependent manner. In photoaged skin, barrier recovery is significantly delayed. Therefore, an altered barrier function in melasma might be a result of the chronic UV exposure and accompanying epidermal hyperpigmentation. Interestingly, we found a negative correlation between melanin index and barrier recovery rate. It means that patients with severe melasma may be having poor SC function.

Very recently, it has been suggested that barrier function is influenced by pigmentation in the SC. Skin type IV-V subjects have more acidic SC due to more melanosomes than pale-skinned subjects, and these acidic conditions were attributed to enhanced SC integrity and accelerated barrier recovery in darker skins.

This study also demonstrated a significant increase of both the melanin and erythema index in melasma-involved skin. Also, a positive correlation appeared between the melanin index and the erythema index.

In conclusion, in the present study we have demonstrated that the epidermal permeability barrier recovery is delayed, and SC integrity is decreased in melasma-involved skin compared to perilesional normal skin. These results suggested that improving SC function should be considered in treating melasma.

REFERENCE

1. Lee DJ, Lee J, Ha J, et al. Defective barrier function in melasma skin. J Eur Acad Dermatol Venereol. 2012;26: 1533-7.

38

Defective Importance of Pendulous Melanocytes in Melasma

Jean-Paul Ortonne

Key Features

- Melasma is associated with vacuolar degeneration of the basal cells and focal degeneration of the basement region.
- Pendulous cells which are seen in melasma are melanocytes protruding into the dermis.
- Fractional laser may aggravate melasma due to disruption of basement membrane resulting in migration and hyperactivation of melanocytes.
- Treatment of melasma should not damage the basement membrane zone.

DOES ALTERED BASEMENT MEMBRANE OF MELASMA LESIONS AFFECTS TREATMENT OUTCOME IN THE SKIN?

Sanchez et al. reported the presence of vacuolar degeneration of the basal cells and focal vacuolar degeneration of the basement region with melasma.[1] With electron microscopy, they observed melanocytes in the basal layer of the lesional epidermis, which frequently protrude into the dermis and suggested an increased activity of them.

Fontana-Masson stain showed that epidermal basal cells protruded into the dermis of melasma lesions (66%). These cells could be melanocytes because with immunohistochemistry we observed basal epidermal cell (c-kit positive) protruded into the dermis **(Fig. 1)**. The protrusion of basal cells was reported previously in two women with melasma. In this report, they found that epidermal melanocytes protruded into the dermis using an immunohistochemical marker to melanocyte, melanonoma antigen specific Mab NK1-beteb (Monosan, Uden, Netherlands). Regarding these protrusions of melanocytes, it had been reported that they are hyperactive melanocytes. Once in the dermis, the melanocytes could be "active" and allow the persistence of melasma lesions **(Figs 2 and 3)**.[2]

Therefore, other factors like hormones, progesterone and estrogen, and their receptors in epidermis and dermis could contribute as trigger or a persistent stimulus to hyperpigmentation. Unexpectedly, with periodic acid-Schiff (PAS) stain, we found damage on the basal membrane in 95.8% of melasma lesions versus 58.3% of perilesional skin, and with antibody to collagen type IV, we observed damage in 83% of melasma lesions versus 66% of perilesional skin; this damage was observed as total absence of BM and absence of disruption along the BM.[2] Because we only use one type of collagen, it is possible that either another type of collagen like type VII or laminins were affected. This damage could facilitate the fall of melanin and the migration of active melanocytes

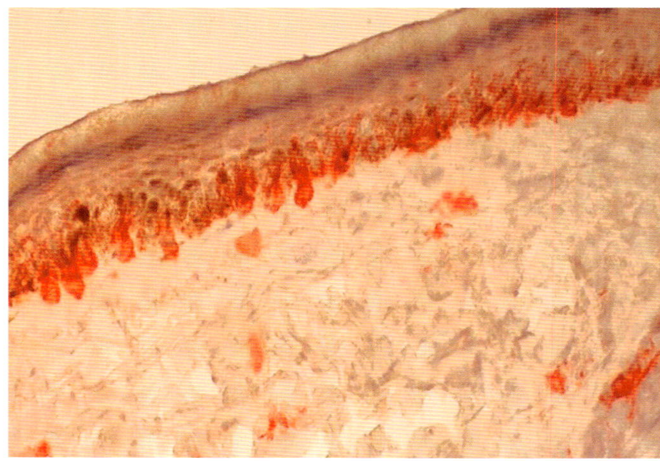

Fig. 1: Pendulous melanocytes: Basal positive c-kit cells protrude into the dermis. (*Source:* Reference number 2)

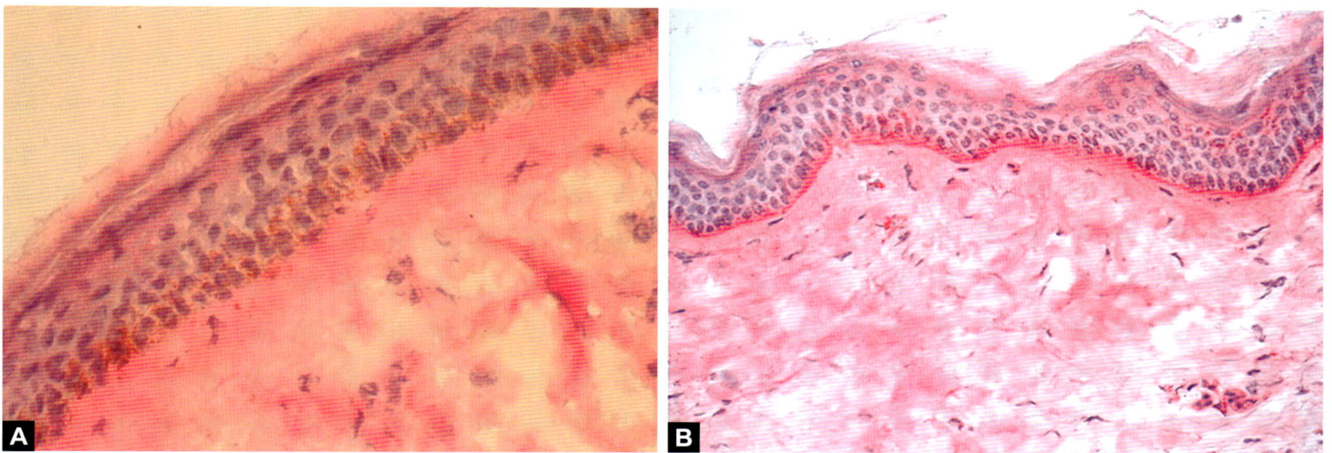

Figs 2A and B: Evidence of damage in the basal membrane: (A) PAS stain section showing absence of basal membrane in melasma skin; (B) Integrity of the basal membrane in perilesional skin of the same patient. (*Source:* Reference number 2)

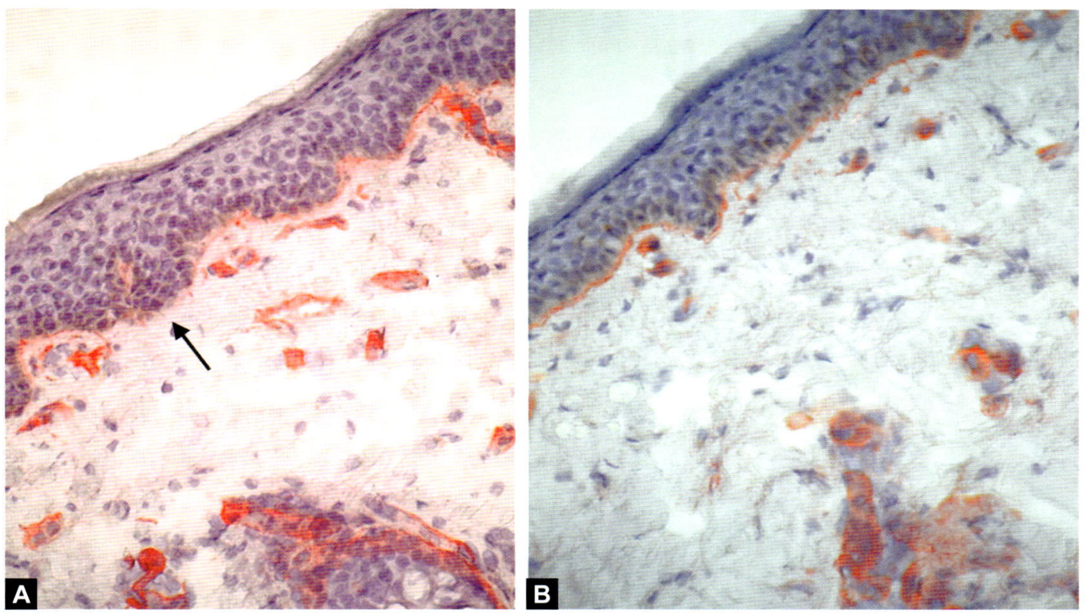

Figs 3A and B: Evidence of damage in the basal membrane: (A) Immunohistochemistry with antibody to collagen IV showing disruption of basal membrane (arrow) in melasma skin; (B) Integrity of the basal membrane in perilesional skin of the same patient. (*Source:* Reference number 2)

into the dermis leading to the constant hyperpigmentation in melasma. The damage of BM could be produced through an increase in the activity of matrix metalloproteinases (MMPs) like MMP-2 and MMP-9, causing the degradation of type IV collagen and type VII collagen in the skin during chronic ultraviolet (UV) exposure in a microenvironment of cutaneous photoaging **(Figs 4A and B)**.

Does Altered Basement of Melasma Lesion Affects Treatment in Asian Skin?

JR Choi thought that the possibility of migrating melanocytes with disrupted basement membrane is associated with an aggravation of melasma after a fractional laser which is sometimes encountered in the melasma patients of Asian skin.[3]

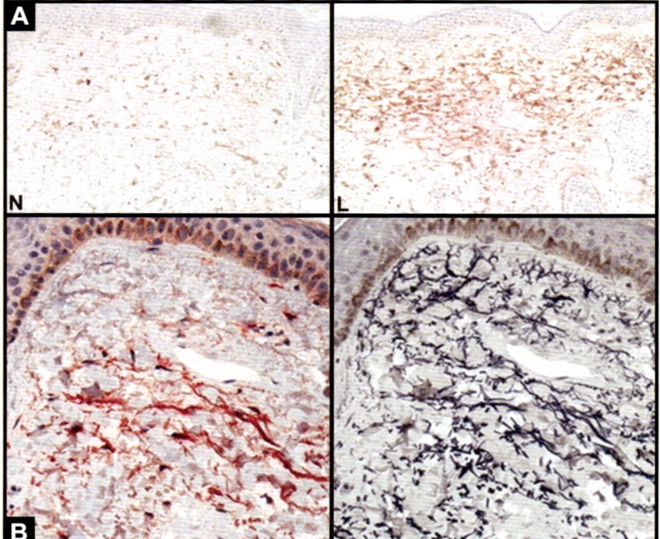

Figs 4A and B: Pendulous melanocytes. A characteristic feature of melasma and how it may occur. (A) Matrix metalloproteinase (MMP-2) expression was significantly increased in lesional skin (L) compared with perilesional normal skin (N); (B) Lesional skin MMP2 expression was colocalized with elastotic material (left: MMP immunostaining; right: Verhoeff-Van Gieson stain). (*Source:* Reference number 4. Available from *http://onlinelibrary.wiley.com/doi/10.1111/j.1365-2133.2011.10648.x/full#f2* [Accessed October, 2013])

Recently, it has been found that the extracellular domain of syundecan-2 (SDC-2) as cell surface receptor was associated with soluble and/or unsoluble factors in the extracellular matrix. Some of them previously demonstrated that SDC-2 was associated with melanin synthesis and migration of melanocytes. SDC-2 was not expressed in normal basement membrane. The authors observed the expression of SDC-2 in the lesional melasma of two Korean women before and after the fractional laser.

In patient one, who showed clinical improvement, Fontana-Masson staining of lesional melasma showed decrease of melanosomes while SDC-2 was decreased along the BM area. In Fontana-Masson-stained melasma sections, the amount of melanin was significantly increased in all epidermal layers, and free melanin and dermal melanophages were seen in lesional skin before the treatment. In patient two, who showed clinical aggravation of melasma lesion, Fontana-Masson staining of lesional melasma showed increase of melanosomes while SDC-2 was increased along the BM area. Moreover, in lesional skin, we detected a protrusion of pigmented cells into the dermis. In two paired nonlesional skin samples, no evidence of damage was shown in BM.

Taken together, it seems that a laser, which can make further BM damage, may make melanocytes hyperactive and migratory. The abnormality of the BM could be produced through an increase in the activity of MMPs, causing the degradation of type IV collagen and type VII collagen or replacement by abnormal deposition of extracellular matrix such as SDC-2. Therefore, gentle treatment not to affect BM, is mandatory to get satisfactory and safe outcome in the treatment of melasma.

PENDULOUS MELANOCYTES: A CHARACTERISTIC FEATURE OF MELASMA AND HOW IT OCCURRED

Melasma, a commonly acquired hyperpigmentary disorder of the face, is characterized by epidermal hyperpigmentation. The melanocytes within the lesional skin are larger, intensely NK1/beteb immunostained cells with prominent dendrites than melanocytes in the unaffected skin, suggesting that melanocytes are active in melasma **(Figs 5A and B)**. Some melanocytes have shown the feature of protruding into the dermis, so-called pendulous cells.[4] *In vivo* reflectance confocal microscopy examination showed that 6 out of 25 patients had activated dendritic melanocytes in the melasma lesional skin, corresponding to pendulous melanocytes seen in histology. The feature has also been described not only in melasma, but also in other hyperpigmentary disorders such as café-au-lait spots and senile lentigo and in the intense UV-A irradiated skin even in normal black skin. These findings suggested that pendulous melanocytes seem to occur in epidermal hypermelanosis related to hyperactivity of the melanocytes **(Figs 6A to D)**.

The present study showed that pendulous melanocytes seem to be a characteristic feature of melasma; the exact mechanism of pendulous change of the melanocytes in melasma is unclear. However, our results suggested that loosening of basement membrane by increased MMP-2 expression may facilitate the pendulous changes of the melanocytes. The expression of E-cadherin or $\alpha 6$ integrin showed little difference, suggesting cellular adherence does not influence the pendulous change.

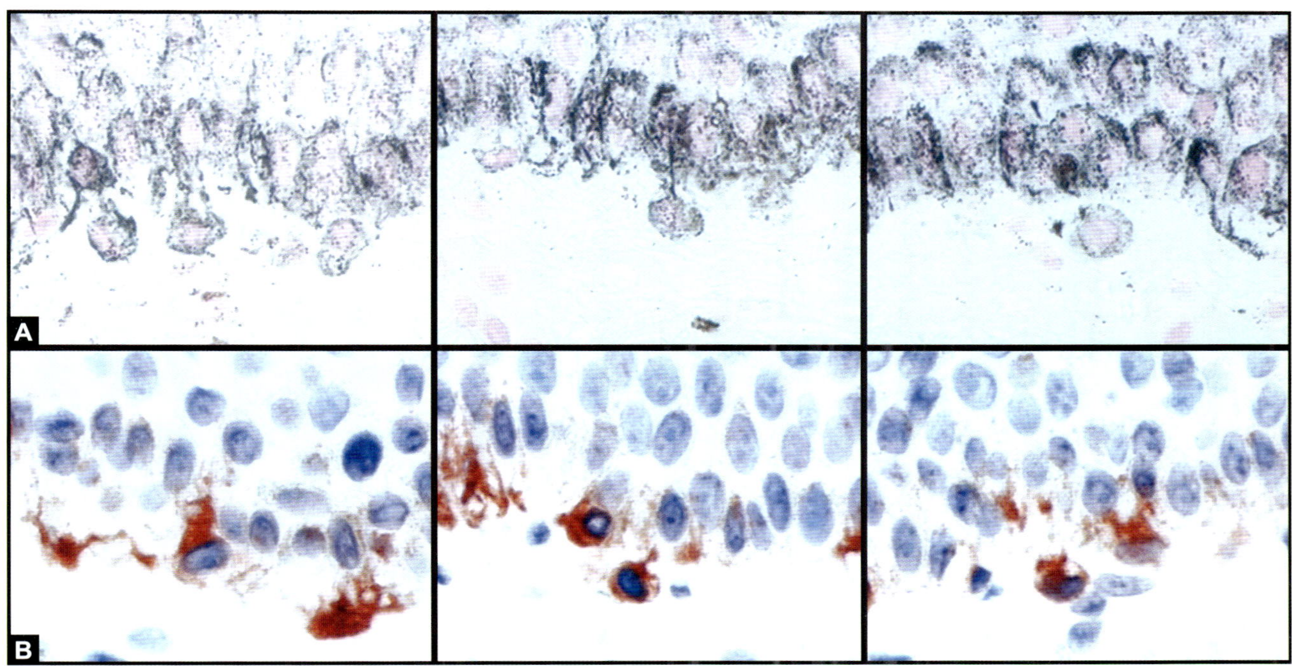

Figs 5A and B: Pendulous melanocytes. (A and B) Pendulous positive for Fontana-Masson staining (these cells were positive by NKI/beteb immunostaining): (*Source:* Reference number 4. Available from *http://onlinelibrary.wiley.com/doi/10.1111/j.1365-2133.2011.10648.x/full#f2.* [Accessed October, 2013].)

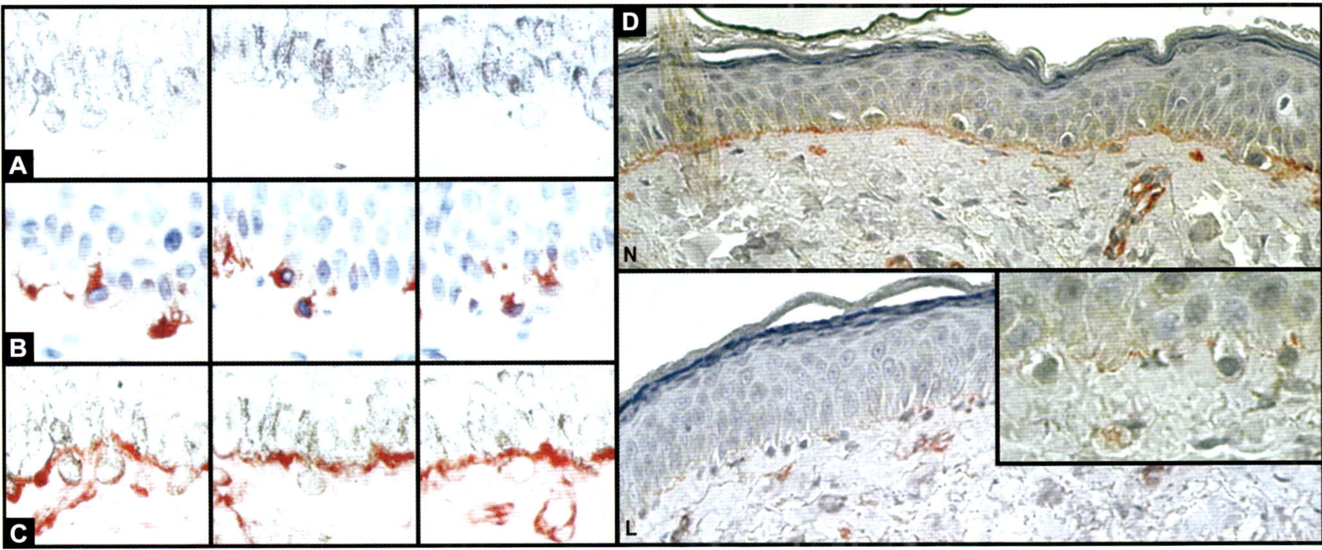

Figs 6A to D: (A) Characteristic feature of melasma and how it occurred; (B) Pendulous melanocytes are surrounded by weakly stained type IV collagen; (C) Overall type IV collagen expression was significantly reduced in the lesional skin; (D) Conclusion: Loosening of basement membrane by increased MMP2 expression in melasma (N, normal skin; L, lesional skin). (*Source:* Lee LJ, et al. Br J Dermatol. 2011)

Increased MMP-2 expression would be a causal factor of the loosening basement membrane. Interestingly, recent transcriptomics study of melasma showed that MMP-2 mRNA levels were significantly upregulated in melasma. MMPs derived by UV-B irradiation were considered to be contributing in the destruction of basement membrane structure *in vivo*. It was also suggested that MMPs overexpression may be associated with the elastotic material in the sun-damaged skin. Melasma skin has shown features of solar damaged skin such as the increased solar elastosis and vasculature. In the present study, we showed that MMP-2 immunoreactivity was clearly colocalized with elastotic materials. Therefore, it is speculated that chronic sun exposure may increase MMP-2 expression, which loose basement membrane in melasma. These would be responsible for the pendulous change of melanocytes in melasma.

Considering high-dose UV-A irradiation could induce a shift of melanocytes from the epidermis into the dermis, it may be possible that the pendulous cells may easily drop into the dermis or become destroyed by trauma including laser treatment. The destructed melanocytes would leave heavy pigmentation in the dermis resulting postinflammatory hyperpigmentation or hypopigmentation after treatment. Therefore, it would be needed to consider this distinguishing histological feature in treatment.

REFERENCES

1. Sanchez NP, Pathak MA, Syozo S, et al. Melasma: a clinical light microscopic ultrastructural and immunofluorescence study. J Am Acad Dermatol. 1981;4(6):698-710.
2. Torres-Alvarez B, Mesa-Garza IG, Castanedo-Cazaves JP, et al. Histochemical and immunohistochemical study in melasma: evidence of damage in the basal membrane. Am J Dermatopathol. 2011;33(3):291-5.
3. Choi JR, Won CM, Oh ES, et al. Does altered basement membrane of melasma lesion affect treatment outcome in Asia skin? Am J Dermatopathol. 2013;35(1):137-8.
4. Lee DJ, Park KC, Ortonne JP, et al. Pendulous melanocytes: a characteristic feature of melasma and how it occurred. Br J Dermatol. 2012;166(3):684-6.

39

Classification and Clinical Features of Melasma

Kiran Godse, Shweta Agarwal

Key Features

- It is found more commonly in women probably due to association with hormonal changes.
- Characterized by presence of brown macules symmetrically distributed on both sides, usually on the face.
- Racial prevalence: seen more in Hispanics, Asians and Africans.
- Recurrences are common.

INTRODUCTION

Melasma ("melas" in Greek means black) is a common hyperpigmentary disorder characterized by the appearance of light to dark brown or brown-gray macules with irregular borders appearing symmetrically primarily on the face. When seen during pregnancy, it is also called chloasma (derived from the Greek word "chloazein" which means to be green) or the mask of pregnancy.

CLINICAL FEATURES

The areas of hypermelanosis are centrofacial, malar and mandibular. Additional sites of involvement are extensor forearms, mid-upper chest[1] and neck.[2] Hana Bak et al. found that the lesions of melasma occur symmetrically in the distribution related to the trigeminal nerve. They performed biopsies on lesional and non-lesional skin which showed markedly greater expression of nerve growth factor receptor (NGFR) and neuropeptidase (NEP) than non-lesional skin. Hence, it was suggested that these neuroactive molecules may play an important role in regulation of melanogenesis.[3] The lesions may appear first or are accentuated following excessive sunlight exposure or during pregnancy. In fair skinned patients, the pigmentation may reduce or resolve completely after parturition, whereas, it may persist in women with darker skin (Fitzpatrick skin types III–V). It rarely appears before puberty. Up to 70% pregnant women and 10% men are affected with it.[4-6] Melasma is a common condition in Latino men and is associated with a poor quality of life (QoL) in some affected individuals.[7] It has an adverse impact on the health related quality of life (HRQoL), i.e. social life, emotional well-being, physical health and money matters in Hispanic woman.[8] It has been reported that African-Americans are more likely to have a positive history of melasma.[9] It is more common in Hispanics and Asians.[2] The causative and exacerbating factors are exposure to sunlight, pregnancy, genetic factors,[9] oral contraceptive pills, estrogen replacement therapy, ovarian or thyroid dysfunction, ovarian tumors, cosmetics, nutritional, phototoxic and photoallergic medications, anti-epileptics like phenytoin, infections like of chikungunya fever.[10,11] The main causative factors among the male patients appeared to be sun-exposure and family history with hormones not playing a major role.[6,12] In a case-control study done by Adalatkhah Hassan et al., 120 female melasma patients and 120 control patients were enrolled after matching for age. The study showed that existence of freckles, lentigines and more than three melanocytic nevi were positively related to developing melasma. The chance of melasma increased up to 23 times for patients having more than three melanocytic nevi. Campbell de morgan angiomas were seen among 26 patients (21.8%) in case group compared to 6 patients (5%) in control group.[13]

CLASSIFICATION

The classification of melasma can be done on the basis of:

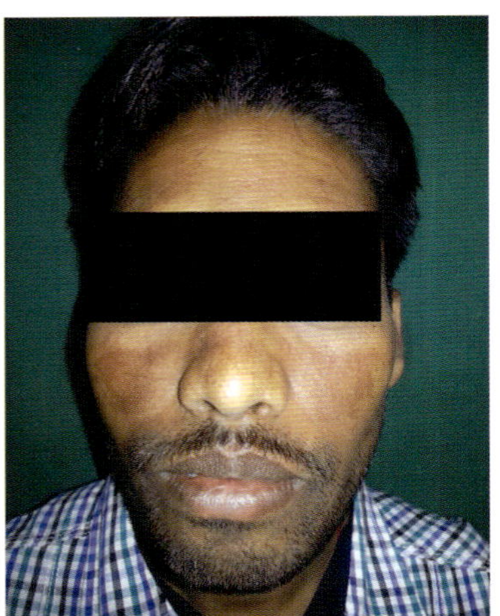

Fig. 1: Malar pattern in males

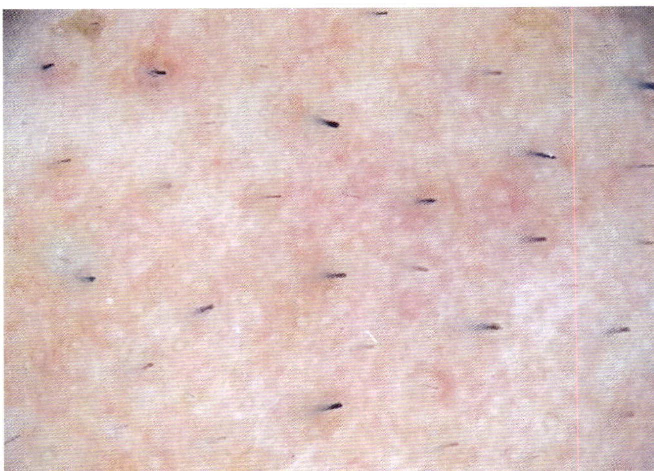

Fig. 2: Dermatoscopic picture showing diffuse reticular pigmentation and follicular sparring characteristic of melasma

Distribution of Lesions

- *Centrofacial (63%):* It is the most common presentation. The lesions are seen on the lateral forehead, cheeks, nose, upper lip (sparing the philtrum) and chin.
- *Malar (21%):* Cheeks and nose
- *Mandibular (16%):* Mandibular ramus
- In women, the centrofacial pattern is more common[12,14-16] and in men, the malar pattern is more common **(Fig. 1)**.[16-18]

Lateral cheek pattern, reddened or inflamed forms of melasma (also called erythrosis pigmentosa faciei), Poikiloderma of Civatte (reddened, photoaging changes seen on the sides of the neck, mostly affecting patients older than 50 years), brachial type of melasma affecting shoulders and upper arms (also called acquired brachial cutaneous dyschromatosis) are other distributions mentioned by Vazquez M et al.[6]

Based on Wood's Lamp Examination

- Epidermal
- Dermal-lesions may be seen as slightly bluish due to Tyndall effect
- Mixed
- Indeterminate
  - The indeterminate type is seen in very dark patients.

Histopathology[14,15]

- Epidermal
- Dermal
- Mixed

Course

Depending on the natural history of the lesions, melasma may also be classified into:

- *Transient type:* It disappears within a year of withdrawal of hormonal stimulus.
- *Persistent type:* It persists for more than a year after withdrawal of hormonal stimulus and is maintained by ultraviolet radiation (UVR) and other factors.[19]

In theory, lesions due to increased epidermal melanin are accentuated and those due to increased dermal melanin are not accentuated in Wood's lamp examination. But, this does not correlate with the histological findings. Therefore, the use of Wood's lamp for distinguishing epidermal from dermal pigmentation is questionable. Reflectance confocal microscopy (RCM) *in vivo* was used to determine the depth of melanin and co-related with the histopathological findings by Liu H et al. and based on those findings, the lesions were classified into epidermal and mixed.[20]

Dermoscopy of melasma shows diffuse reticular pigmentation, follicular sparing, sparing of acrosyringium, uniform globules or blotches of pigmentation as compared to ochronosis which shows no follicular sparing, brown amorphous areas, multiple arciform structures, thick globular structures over melasma patch **(Fig. 2)**.[21]

CONCLUSION

Melasma is a common cosmetic problem among females since it mainly affects the face and thereby causing considerable physical and psychological distress.

It is easy to diagnose clinically but must also be classified on the basis of the distribution (centrofacial, malar and mandibular or extrafacial) and depth of pigment (epidermal, dermal and mixed). The depth can be evaluated clinically by Wood's lamp and also histopathologically.

Dermatoscopy is a newer non-invasive tool which can be used to differentiate melasma from other conditions.

REFERENCES

1. Pandya AG, Guevara IL. Disorders of hyperpigmentation. Dermatol Clin. 2000;18:91-8.
2. Newcomer VD, Linderberg MC, Sternberg TH. A melanosis of the face (cholasma) Arch. Dermatol. 1961;83:284-99.
3. Bak H, Lee HJ, Chang SE, et al. Increased Expression of Nerve Growth Factor Receptor and Neural Endopeptidase in the Lesional Skin of Melasma. Dermatologic Surgery. 2009;35:1244-50.
4. Dominguez AR, Balkrishnan R, Ellzey AR, et al. Melasma in Latin patients: Cross-cultural adaptation and validation of quality of life questionnaire in Spanish language. J Am Acad Dermatol. 2006;55:59-66.
5. Moin A, Jabery Z, Fallah N. Prevalence and awareness of melasma during pregnancy. Int J Dermatol. 2006;45:285-8.
6. Vazquez M, Maldonado H, Benmaman C, et al. Melasma in men: A clinical and histologic study. Int J Dermatol. 1988;27:25-7.
7. Pichardo R, Vallejos Q, Feldman SR, et al. The prevalence of melasma and its association with quality of life in adult male Latino migrant workers. Int J Dermatol. 2009;48:22-6.
8. Pawaskar Manjiri D, Parikh Parth, Markowski Tania, et al. Melasma and its impact on health-related quality of life in Hispanic women. J Dermatol Treat. 2007;18:15-9.
9. Ortonne JP, Arellno I, Berneburg M, et al. A global survey of the role of ultraviolet radiation and hormonal influences in the development of melasma. J Eur Acad Dermatol Venerol. 2009;23:1254-62.
10. Kandhari R, Khunger N, Singh A. Flagellate pigmentation and exacerbation of melasma following chikungunya fever: A less frequently reported finding. Indian J Dermatol Venereol Leprol. 2012;78:774.
11. Inamadar AC, Palit A, Sampagavi VV, et al. Cutaneous manifestations of chikungunya fever: Observations made during a recent outbreak in south India. Int J Dermatol. 2008;47:154-9.
12. Sarkar R, Puri P, Jain RK, et al. Melasma in men: a clinical, aetiological and histological study. J Eur Acad Dermatol Venereol. 2010;24:768-72.
13. Adalatkhah Hassan, Sadeghi-bazargani Homayoun, Aminisani Nayereh. Melasma and its association with different types of nevi in women: A case-control study. BMC Dermatology. 2008;8:1-5.
14. Sanchez NP, Pathak MA, Sato S. Melasma: a clinical, light microscopic, ultrastructural and immunofluorescence study. J Am Acad Dermatol. 1981;4:698-710.
15. Kang WH, Yoon KH, Lee ES, et al. Melasma: histopathological characteristics in 56 Korean patients. Br J Dermatol. 2002;146:228-37.
16. Sarkar R, Jain RK, Puri P. Melasma in Indian males. Dermatol Surg. 2003;29:204.
17. Vazquez M, Maldonado H, Benmaman C, et al. Melasma in men. A clinical and histologic study. Int J Dermatol. 198;27:25-7.
18. Khanna N, Rasool S. Facial melanoses: Indian perspective. Indian J Dermatol Venereol Leprol. 2011;77:552-64.
19. Ardigo M, Cameli N, Berardesca E, et al. Characterization and evaluation of pigment distribution and response to therapy in melasma using *in vivo* reflectance confocal microscopy: a preliminary study. J Eur Acad Dermatol Venereol. 2010;24:1296-303.
20. Liu H, Lin Y, Nie X, et al. Histological classification of melasma with reflectance confocal microscopy: a pilot study in Chinese patients. Skin Res Technol. 2011;17:398-403.
21. Uday SK. Dermoscopy and Trichoscopy in Diseases of the Brown Skin: Atlas and Short Text, 1st edn. Jaypee Brothers Medical Publishers; 2013.

40

Medical Management of Melasma

Rashmi Sarkar, Shivani Bansal

Key Features

- Melasma is an acquired hypermelanosis of sun-exposed skin which presents as symmetric, light to dark brown colored macules.
- Different therapeutic modalities, especially the gold standard hydroquinone have been used in the treatment of melasma.
- First-line therapy for melasma should consist of effective topical therapies; mainly fixed triple combinations.
- Multiple novel topical agents are being investigated for their potential as hypopigmenting agents with unique mode of action.

INTRODUCTION

Melasma is derived from the Greek word, "melas" meaning black. It is an acquired hypermelanosis of sun-exposed skin which presents as symmetric, light to dark brown colored macules having irregular, serrated and geographic borders. Although melasma may affect any race, it is the most common pigmentary disorder among Asians. It is more common in women, especially in their reproductive years, but about 10% cases occur in men. In an Indian study by Sarkar et al. 20.5% patients of melasma were men and it showed no difference clinically and histopathologically as compared to melasma in females.[1]

The pathophysiology of melasma is multifactorial. Before starting therapy, various factors like hormonal, ovarian or thyroid dysfunction, history of any medications or cosmetics should be ruled out. By causing cosmetic disfigurement of the face, melasma is frequently associated with significant emotional and psychological stress. Different therapeutic modalities, especially the gold standard hydroquinone have been used in the treatment of melasma. However, treatment continues to be a challenge as the pathogenesis is not yet clear and there is paucity of trials. The existing modalities which are used are topical depigmenting agents, used alone, or in combinations and peeling agents like glycolic acid (GA), trichloroacetic acid, salicylic acid and lactic acid. Physical agents like lasers and dermabrasion have also been tried with limited success.[2] Photoprotective measures like the avoidance of direct sun-exposure and the regular use of a broad-spectrum sunscreen are always advised, although clinical studies on their role are lacking.

First-line therapy for melasma should consist of effective topical therapies **(Table 1)**; mainly fixed triple combinations.[2] Topical agents are much more effective in the epidermal type of melasma.[3] Treatment with these agents must be continued for several months before significant clinical benefits become

Table 1: Topical therapies for melasma

Mechanism of action	*Compound*
Tyrosinase inhibition	Hydroquinone, kojic acid, azelaic acid, and arbutin
Reduces the transfer of melanosomes from melanocytes to keratinocytes	Niacinamide
Facilitates rapid pigment loss through induction of desquamation	Retinoids and glycolic acid
Destruction of melanocytes	Azelaic acid
Antioxidants	Kojic acid, ascorbic acid, zinc, and pycnogenol
Decrease of alpha-melanocyte-stimulating hormone, which stimulates melanin synthesis	Tranexamic acid

noticeable. These may consist of phenolic and non-phenolic compounds.

HYDROQUINONE

Hydroquinone (HQ) is a hydroxyphenolic compound and is most commonly used for treatment of melasma. It inhibits the conversion of dihydroxyphenylalanine (DOPA) to melanin by inhibition of the enzyme, tyrosinase. Other proposed mechanisms are the inhibition of DNA and RNA synthesis, degradation of melanosomes and destruction of melanocytes.[4] It is used as monotherapy in concentrations of 2–5%, though 4% is the preferred one especially in the Indian set-up. In a double-blind placebo-controlled trial involving 48 patients with melasma on the face, HQ 4% or placebo was applied twice daily for 12 weeks. Results indicated total improvement of melasma in 38% of patients treated with HQ as well as partial improvement as well as no treatment failures in 57% of patients. In contrast, in the placebo group, 8% of patients had total improvement, 58% had partial improvement, but 17% were classified as treatment failures.[5]

Hydroquinone can be combined with tretinoin and steroid as triple combination therapy or can also be used in conjunction with chemical peels. HQ is also used in combination with GA and kojic acid (KA) for added benefits but in a split-faced prospective trial in 21 Hispanic women with bilateral epidermal and mixed melasma lasting 8 weeks study found that combination of 4% HQ and GA improved melasma which was not significant.[6] A recent study in 15 Latin American women incorporated hyaluronic acid with HQ and GA as a novel cream preparation and found it well tolerated and with a significant decrease in melasma area and severity index (MASI) scores of 64% at the end of study in the treatment of melasma.[7]

Adverse reactions of HQ are related to its dose and the duration of treatment. Irritation is the most common complication; other adverse effects include erythema, stinging, colloid milium, irritant and allergic contact dermatitis, nail discoloration, transient hypochromia, and paradoxical postinflammatory hypermelanosis. Prolonged use of HQ can result in blue-black pigmentation of treated areas known as ochronosis. There was a proposed ban on HQ in 2006 due to concerns of ochronosis and carcinogenicity, but subsequently it was observed that the evidence of carcinogenicity due to topical application in human beings was not substantial.

Under no circumstances should monobenzylether, or any other ethers of HQ, be used to treat melasma as they can lead to a permanent loss of melanocytes with the development of a disfiguring confetti-like leukoderma.

RETINOIDS

Retinoids, such as tretinoin, is thought to have an inhibitory effect on tyrosinase by inhibiting the enzyme's transcription, as well as on dopachrome conversion factor, with a resulting interruption of melanin synthesis and also reduces hyperpigmentation through the induction of desquamation.[8] Compared with phenolic compounds like HQ, it typically takes at least 24 weeks with retinoid to see clinical improvement. Retinoic acid concentrations ranging from 0.05% to 0.1% have been used. They can be used as monotherapy or in combination with HQ as penetration enhancers.

Topical retinoic acid monotherapy resulted good therapeutic response in clinical trials but better results are seen in combination with other agents like HQ and corticosteroids.[9] Associated side effects are erythema and peeling in the area of application; postinflammatory hyperpigmentation has also been reported.[8]

TOPICAL STEROIDS

Steroids act by decreasing the irritative effects of the hypopigmenting agents, as well as inhibiting melanin synthesis by decreasing cellular metabolism.

Potent or superpotent steroids, when used alone for a period of 8 weeks only, have been associated with good therapeutic responses, but monotherapy is not recommended due to their frequent untoward effects.[10] But these are usually not used alone in practice. Various combinations with HQ and retinoic acid have given good cosmetic results in clinical trials.[11] Adverse effects of topical steroids include irritation, rosacea-like dermatosis, atrophy, telangiectasia, and hypertrichosis.

TRIPLE COMBINATION THERAPY

The preferred topical application is in the form of triple combination (TC) where HQ is used along with a topical steroid and a retinoid. The addition of tretinoin eliminates pigment and increases keratinocyte proliferation by preventing the oxidation of HQ and improving epidermal penetration. Further, adding topical corticosteroids reduces the irritative effects of hypopigmenting agents, and inhibits melanin synthesis by decreasing cellular metabolism. This combination, HQ 5%, tretinoin 0.1%, and dexamethasone 0.1%, was first introduced in 1975 and termed the Kligman formula (KF) after its inventor. It has been the most extensively used combination therapy for melasma worldwide in various different combinations and modifications.[12]

Taylor SC et al. compared the efficacy and safety of a hydrophilic cream formulation containing tretinoin 0.05%, hydroquinone 4.0%, and fluocinolone acetonide 0.01% (RA+HQ+FA) with the dual-combination agents tretinoin plus hydroquinone (RA+HQ), tretinoin plus fluocinolone acetonide (RA+FA), and hydroquinone plus fluocinolone acetonide (HQ+FA) in a multicenter, randomized, investigator-blind study in 641 adult patients of moderate to severe melasma in Fitzpatrick skin types I–IV.[13] It was found that significantly more of the patients treated with RA+HQ+FA

(26.1%) experienced complete clearing compared with the other treatment groups (4.6%) at the end of week 8 (P <.0001) and also 75% reduction pigmentation was observed in more than 70% of patients treated with RA+HQ+FA compared with 30% in patients treated with the dual-combination agents.

Amongst the medical therapies analyzed by a recent Cochrane review, TC creams have been found to be the best topical therapy.[14] In a recent multicenter trial by Chan et al. 260 South East Asian patients were randomized to TC (FA 0.01%, HQ 4%, tretinoin 0.05%) cream or 4% HQ cream for 8 weeks. Significantly more participants in the TC group (87/125) compared to the 4% HQ group (57/129) achieved a score of 0 (clear) or 1 (minor hyperpigmentation).[15] A similar study on 120 patients demonstrated significantly lower melasma severity scores in the triple therapy groups than in the HQ group.[16]

Triple combination cream exhibits a safe profile with low potential for adverse events. In a long-term, multicenter and open-label, study in 173 patients of once-daily application of TC therapy (FA 0.01%, HQ 4%, tretinoin 0.05%), no cases of skin atrophy or skin thinning were seen after 6–12 months of treatment (one or two course). Only 6 cases showed telangiectasia, most of which had improved by the end of the study. Most adverse effects were expected: application-site reactions that were mild and transient in nature and did not require remedial therapy.[11] In an another study of same TC for 24 weeks in 62 patients with moderate to severe melasma, the atrophogenic potential of TC cream was evaluated through serial histopathological examination of skin biopsies. No statistically significant histopathologic signs of atrophy of the epidermis or dermis were noted at any time point throughout the study.[17] To maintain safety profile, TC creams can be used continuously for 12 weeks then can be maintained twice per week for another 12 weeks if no relapse occurs.[18]

Triple combination creams can be combined with chemical peels or used as priming agents before chemical peels. Forty Indian patients with Fitzpatrick skin types III-IV with moderate to severe melasma were randomized to treatment with the modified KF (hydrocortisone 1%, HQ 2%, tretinoin 0.05%) daily plus 6 serial GA 30–40% (chemical peel) treatments at 3-week intervals or to modified KF alone.[19] A significant decrease in the MASI score at 21 weeks compared with baseline was observed in both groups. But the group receiving GA showed a trend toward more rapid and greater improvements than the other group.

OTHER RETINOIDS

Various other retinoids like adapalene, tazarotene and topical isotretinoin have also been used. Adapalene, a naphthoic acid derivative with retinoid activity, was found to be equally efficacious as 0.05% tretinoin cream in a randomized split face trial in Indian patients but with significantly less side effects than tretinoin.[20] In another randomized study in 30 Thai patients, topical isotretinoin combined with sunscreen versus vehicle plus sunscreen showed no significant difference in clinical effects till 40 weeks.[21]

KOJIC ACID

Kojic acid (KA) 2% is produced by the fungus, *Aspergillus oryzae*. It also inhibits tyrosinase and is also a potent antioxidant. KA may be effective if a patient has difficulty in tolerating other first-line therapies. It is used at concentrations ranging from 1% to 4%. It has been found equivalent to other therapies but it may cause more irritation.

In a split-face design in 39 patients with melasma, GA 5% combined with either 4% HQ or 4% KA daily for 3 months has been compared. Both combinations proved equally effective with a reduction of pigmentation in 52% of the patients although complete clearing was not noted in any patient.[22] In one double-blind study, KA 2% combined with HQ 2% was shown to be superior to GA 10% and HQ 2%.[23] It may cause contact dermatitis and erythema.

AZELAIC ACID

Azelaic acid, a C9 dicarboxylic acid, is a weak competitive inhibitor of tyrosinase and may also have both cytotoxic and antiproliferative effects on melanocytes.[24] Topical azelaic acid has selective effects on abnormal melanocytes with no depigmentation effect on normally pigmented skin. It can also be used for postinflammatory hyperpigmentation in acne. It is available as a cream at a concentration of 15–20%. It can be used alone or with steroid as a sequential therapy but under strict supervision [25] or with tretinoin.[26]

In a double-blind randomized study, 20% azelaic acid was found to be equivalent to 4% HQ in the treatment of melasma, without the latter's undesirable side-effects.[27] Another controlled study has found azelaic acid to be superior to 2% HQ.[28] Adverse effects are mild, include pruritus, mild erythema, scaling, and burning. It is a good alternative in those patients who cannot tolerate HQ, according to the author's personal experience.

GLYCOLIC ACID

Glycolic acid 5–10% is an alpha-hydroxy acid and has been studied in combination with other agents. It decreases pigment by many mechanisms including thinning the stratum corneum, enhancing epidermolysis, dispersing melanin in the basal layer of the epidermis, and increasing collagen synthesis in the dermis.[29]

In a randomized controlled trial, 10% GA plus 4% HQ in a cream containing vitamins C and E and sunscreen was compared with a cream containing sunscreen alone in group of Hispanic patients. Results indicated a significant decrease (75%) in the degree of pigmentation using the study cream compared with sunscreen alone (13%); (P\0001). Irritation was a common side effect which resolved with the temporary cessation of application and application of moisturizers.[23]

ARBUTIN

Arbutin, the *beta*-D-glucopyranoside derivative of HQ, is a naturally occurring plant product. The glycosidic bond is hydrolyzed *in vivo* leading to the controlled release of HQ but its action is dose-dependent and less toxic than HQ. Arbutin acts by the inhibition of tyrosinase, thereby decreasing melanin formation. *Deoxyarbutin* is a recently developed derivative of arbutin which has been produced by removing the hydroxyl groups from the molecule. This produces reversible skin-lightening by direct inhibition of tyrosinase.[30] Although good controlled clinical trials are lacking, initial experimental studies have demonstrated that it could be a safe and effective treatment for hypermelanotic disorders.[31]

OTHER AGENTS

Ascorbic Acid

It affects melanogenesis by reducing dopaquinone to DOPA, by antiradical and antioxidant properties. Ascorbic acid, however, is highly unstable in aqueous solution and stable esters like magnesium ascorbyl-2-phosphate (MAP) have been synthesized. Ascorbic acid could be used alone or in combination therapy. In a double-blind clinical trial of 16 patients of melasma, 4% HQ showed a better response than 5% ascorbic acid but almost no side effects of latter.[32] A formulation containing 25% L-ascorbic acid and chemical penetration enhancer was also found to be efficacious and stable in melasma patients.[33]

Zinc

It is another oral antioxidant, anti-inflammatory agent, which has peeling and exfoliating properties. In an open clinical trial, 28 patients of melasma applied 10% zinc sulfate ($ZnSO_4$) solution twice daily for 8 weeks and were followed for MASI scoring every 2 weeks till 3 months after stopping the treatment. There was 49.78% improvement in the mean MASI scores ($P < 0.005$), which was maintained in most of the patients at even 3 months follow-up visit. Few patients noted mild burning sensation.[34] Thus, zinc might serve as a new, effective, safe, non-costly formulation for melasma with long-lasting effects.

Tranexamic Acid

It is a lysine analog, plasmin inhibitor and hence decreases alpha-melanocyte-stimulating hormone, which stimulates melanin synthesis. In an open study by Lee et al. on 100 Korean women with melasma, tranexamic acid (TA) given intradermally (4 mg/mL) weekly for 12 weeks caused significant decrease in MASI score (P value < 0.05), and 76.5% subjects reported lightening of melasma with minimal side effects.[35] TA can be applied as cream preparation also. But in a recent double blind, randomized, split face trial in 23 patients, 5% TA cream applied daily did not show any significant results as compared to vehicle after 12 weeks study period.[36]

Oral Agents

Pycnogenol

It is a plant extract obtained from the bark of the French maritime pine (*Pinus pinaster*). Procyanidins constitute 65% and 75% of pycnogenol, which has antioxidant and anti-inflammatory properties. In addition, it recycles vitamin C, regenerates vitamin E and also protects against ultraviolet (UV) radiation.

A clinical study on efficacy of pycnogenol with 75 mg daily oral intake (25 mg 3 times a day) for a total of 30 days in 30 melasma patients showed a decrease in pigmentary intensity ($P < 0.001$) and melasma area index ($P < 0.001$) in 80% of the patients. No side effect was noted, and blood and urinary parameters were within normal range before and after study. Moreover, several other associated symptoms such as fatigue, constipation, pains in the body and anxiety also improved.[37]

Proanthocyanidin

In a randomized, double bind, placebo-controlled trial, in 60 Phillipino females with bilateral epidermal melasma, a combination of oral proanthocyanidin plus vitamin A, C, and E taken twice daily for 8 weeks were compared with placebo intake by mexametric and MASI score analysis. There was significant reduction in MASI scores ($P = 0.001$) and pigmentation by mexametry ($P < 0.0001$) in malar regions. The combination was also found to be safe.[38]

Tranexamic Acid

Tranexamic acid (TA) tablets were prescribed at a dosage of 250 mg twice daily for 6 months in 74 Chinese patients. Around 48 patients had good to excellent response after treatment and poor response in only 3 patients. Side effects of TA such as gastrointestinal discomfort (5.4%) and hypomenorrhea (8.1%) were observed, but no severe complications were found. Thus oral TA is an effective and safe therapy for the treatment of melasma.[39]

Other New and Experimental Agents

Multiple novel topical agents are being investigated for their potential as hypopigmenting agents with unique mode of action.[40] But, further trials are required to study their efficacy and safety before they can be further recommended.

Aloesin

It is derived from aloe vera. Currently, it is used in several over-the-counter cosmeceutical preparations. It competitively inhibits hydroxylation of tyrosinase to DOPA and oxidation of DOPA to dopachrome. Although human studies are lacking but in a recent study it has been found to suppress pigmentation by 34%.[41]

Flavonoids

Flavonoids are naturally occurring benzopyrene derivatives which can be classified into flavones, flavonols, isoflavones, flavanones and anthocyanidins. They have well-known anti-inflammatory, antioxidant, antiviral, and anticarcinogenic properties.[42] They have the advantage of formulation into nanocapsules so that they are protected until they reach an active site of melanin synthesis where they exert a powerful reducing action, have antiradical activity, and act as a substrate competitor for the tyrosinases.

Mequinol (4-Hydroxyanisole)

It is a derivative of HQ, which is a more effective competitor of tyrosinase and has lesser side effects. It is currently marketed in the USA at a concentration of 2% in combination with 0.01% tretinoin as a penetration enhancer. In a pilot, small case series of five men with melasma by Keeling et al., the topical solution of 2% mequinol and 0.01% tretinoin was applied twice daily for 12 weeks and patients followed for 16 weeks. Four out of five patients achieved complete clearance at 12 weeks, and one patient showed moderate improvement, and the results were maintained at follow-up 4 weeks after discontinuation of drug.[43]

Alpha-Lipoic Acid

Due to its both fat and water-solubility properties, it can act both in lipid cell membrane and aqueous compartment of melanocytes. Thus it may act as a novel skin lightening agent for melasma, provided human trials are undertaken.

Niacinamide (Nicotinamide)

This biologically active amide form of niacin (vitamin B_3); can reduce pigmentation by reversibly preventing the transfer of melanosomes from melanocytes to the keratinocytes. It has no effect on tyrosinase activity.[44]

Rucinol

It is a phenolic derivative, which inhibits both tyrosinase and tyrosinase related protein. In a prospective double-blind randomized vehicle-controlled split-face comparative trial in 32 female patients with melasma, rucinol serum 0.3% showed statistically significant effect as compared to vehicle-treated site.[45]

Green Tea

Green tea extracts has anti-inflammatory properties and modulate melanin production in dose-dependent manner. It has been found to down regulate microphthalmia-associated transcription factor (MITF) and tyrosinase production in one *in vitro* study.[46] However, the studies of its effects in human beings are limited because of stability and penetration issues.

Hydroxycoumarins

The hydroxycoumarins are novel antioxidants, which have alpha tocopherol like structure. They act by inhibiting tyrosinase in cultured human melanocytes and cell homogenates, and also have scavenging and quenching activities.[47]

Liquorice Derivatives

Liquorice is the root of the perennial herb *Glycyrrhiza glabra*. Glabridin is an oil-soluble derivative of liquorice extract. Although human studies are lacking, Glabridin has been shown to have tyrosinase inhibitory as well as anti-inflammatory properties in experimental studies.[48]

N-acetyl-4-S-cysteaminylphenol

N-acetyl-4-S-cysteaminylphenol (NCAP) is a phenolic agent which inhibits the tyrosinase activity. It is more stable and causes less irritation than HQ. Clinical changes were evident after 2–4 weeks of daily application. In a study of 12 patients with melasma with 4% NCAP, 66% of patients showed marked improvement and 8% showed a complete resolution of melasma lesions.[49]

Soy

It is a plant derivative found in tofu products as well as in soybeans and soy milk. Soy trypsin inhibitor (STI) and Bowman-Birk inhibitor (BBI) are its active ingredients which have antioxidant properties, and also inhibit melanosome transfer to keratinocytes. It has been shown to improve mottled pigmentation in 12 weeks.[50] Although not used in melasma, it could be a promising agent.

Other agents which can also inhibit melanin pigmentation are ellagic acid, gentisic acid, silymarin, naturally derived botanical extracts, dioic acid, octadecenedioic acid, linoleic acid and cinnamic acid. However, treatment of melasma still remains largely unsatisfactory.

CONCLUSION

Management of melasma is challenging and requires long-term treatment with topical agents. The results are often unsatisfactory. The existing and most tried topical therapy is hydroquinone and the triple combination with tretinoin and corticosteroids, which is considered the gold standard for melasma. Many new agents that inhibit melanogenesis have been developed. But, further trials are required to study their efficacy and safety before they can be further recommended.

REFERENCES

1. Sarkar R, Puri P, Jain RK, et al. Melasma in men: a clinical, etiological and histological study. J Eur Acad Dermatol Venereol. 2010;24(7):768-72.
2. Rendon M, Berneburg M, Arellano I, et al. Treatment of melasma. J Am Acad Dermatol. 2006;54(5 Suppl 2):S272-81.
3. Prignano F, Ortonne JP, Buggiani G, et al. Therapeutical approaches in melasma. Dermatol Clin. 2007;25(3):337-42.
4. Jimbow K, Obata H, Pathak MA, et al. Mechanism of depigmentation by hydroquinone. J Invest Dermatol. 1974; 62(4):436-49.
5. Ennes SBP, Paschoalick RC, Mota De Avelar Alchorne M. A double-blind, comparative, placebo-controlled study of the efficacy and tolerability of 4% hydroquinone as a depigmenting agent in melasma. J Dermatolog Treat. 2000; 11:173-9.
6. Hurley ME, Guevara IL, Gonzales RM, et al. Efficacy of glycolic acid peels in the treatment of melasma. Arch Dermatol. 2002;138(12):1578-82.
7. Guevara IL, Werlinger KD, Pandya AG. Tolerability and efficacy of a novel formulation in the treatment of melasma. J Drugs Dermatol. 2010;9(3):215-8.
8. Romero C, Aberdam E, Larnier C, et al. Retinoic acid as modulator of UVB-induced melanocyte differentiation: Involvement of the melanogenic enzymes expression. J Cell Sci. 1994;107(pt 4):1095-103.
9. Griffiths CE, Finkel LJ, Ditre CM, et al. Topical tretinoin (retinoid acid) improves melasma: a vehicle-controlled, clinical trial. Br J Dermatol. 1993;129(4):415-21.
10. Kanwar AJ, Dhar S, Kaur S. Treatment of melasma with potent topical corticosteroids. Dermatology. 1994;188(2):170.
11. Torok HM, Jones T, Rich P, et al. Hydroquinone 4%, tretinoin 0.05%, fluocinolone acetonide 0.01%: a safe and efficacious 12-month treatment for melasma. Cutis. 2005;75(1):57-62.
12. Kligman AM, Willis I. A new formula for depigmenting human skin. Arch Dermatol. 1975;111(1):40-8.
13. Taylor SC, Torok H, Jones T, et al. Efficacy and safety of a new triple-combination agent for the treatment of facial melasma. Cutis. 2003;72(1):67-72.
14. Rajaratnam R, Halpern J, Salim A, et al. Interventions for melasma. Cochrane Database Syst Rev. 2010;(7):CD003583.
15. Chan R, Park KC, Lee MH, et al. A randomized controlled trial of the efficacy and safety of a fixed triple combination (fluocinolone acetonide 0.01%, hydroquinone 4%, tretinoin 0.05%) compared with hydroquinone 4% cream in Asian patients with moderate to severe melasma. Bri J Dermatol. 2008;159(3):697-703.
16. Ferreira Cestari T, Hassun K, Sittart A, et al. A comparison of triple combination cream and hydroquinone 4% cream for the treatment of moderate to severe facial melasma. J Cosmet Dermatol. 2007;6(1):36-9.
17. Bhawan J, Grimes P, Pandya AG, et al. A histological examination for skin atrophy after 6 months of treatment with fluocinolone acetonide 0.01%, hydroquinone 4%, and tretinoin 0.05% cream. Am J Dermatopathol. 2009;31(8):794-8.
18. Grimes PE, Bhawan J, Guevara IL, et al. Continuous therapy followed by a maintenance therapy regimen with a triple combination cream for melasma. J Am Acad Dermatol. 2010;62(6):962-7.
19. Sarkar R, Kaur C, Bhalla M, et al. The combination of glycolic acid peels with a topical regimen in the treatment of melasma in dark-skinned patients: a comparative study. Dermatol Surg. 2002;28(9):828-32.
20. Dogra S, Kanwar AJ, Parsad D. Adapalene in the treatment of melasma: a preliminary report. J Dermatol. 2002;29(8): 539-40.
21. Leenutaphong V, Nettakul A, Rattanasuwon P. Topical isotretinoin for melasma in Thai patients: a vehicle controlled clinical trial. J Med Assoc Thai. 1999;82(9):868-75.
22. Guevara IL, Pandya AG. Safety and efficacy of 4% hydroquinone combined with 10% glycolic acid, antioxidants, and sunscreen in the treatment of melasma. Int J Dermatol. 2003;42(12):966-72.
23. Garcia A, Fulton JE Jr. The combination of glycolic acid and hydroquinone or kojic acid for the treatment of melasma and related conditions. Dermatol Surg. 1996;22(5):443-7.
24. Fitton A, Goa KL. Azelaic acid. A review of its pharmacological properties and therapeutic efficacy in acne and hyperpigmentary skin disorders. Drugs. 1991;41(5):780-98.
25. Sarkar R, Bhalla M, Kanwar AJ. A comparative study of 20% azelaic acid cream monotherapy versus a sequential therapy in the treatment of melasma in dark-skinned patients. Dermatology. 2002;205(3):249-54.
26. Zaumseil RP, Graupe K. Topical azelaic acid in the treatment of melasma: pharmacological and clinical considerations. In: Melasma—New Approaches to Therapy. London: Martin-Dunitz; 1995. pp. 19-41.
27. Baliña LM, Graupe K. The treatment of melasma 20% azelaic acid versus 4% hydroquinone cream. Int J Dermatol. 1991;30(12):893-5.
28. Verallo-Rowell VM, Verallo V, Graupe K, et al. Double blind comparison of azelaic acid and hydroquinone in the treatment of melasma. Acta Derm Venereol. 1989;143:58-61.
29. Usuki A, Ohashi A, Sato H, et al. The inhibitory effect of glycolic acid and lactic acid on melanin synthesis in melanoma cells. Exp Dermatol. 2003;12(Suppl 2):43-50.
30. Chawla S, deLong MA, Visscher MO, et al. Mechanism of tyrosinase inhibition by deoxyArbutin and its second-generation derivatives. Br J Dermatol. 2008;159(6):1267-74.
31. Boissy RE, Visscher M, DeLong MA. DeoxyArbutin: a novel reversible tyrosinase inhibitor with effective *in vivo* skin lightening potency. Exp Dermatol. 2005;14(8):601-8.
32. Espinal-Perez LE, Moncada B, Castanedo-Cazares JP. A double-blind randomized trial of 5% ascorbic acid vs 4%

hydroquinone in melasma. Int J Dermatol. 2004;43(8): 604-7.
33. Hwang SW, Oh DJ, Lee D, et al. Clinical efficacy of 25% L-ascorbic acid (C'ensil) in the treatment of melasma. J Cutan Med Surg. 2009;13(2):74-81.
34. Sharquie KE, Al-Mashhadani SA, Salman HA. Topical 10% zinc sulfate solution for treatment of melasma. Dermatol Surg. 2008;34(10):1346-9.
35. Lee JH, Park JG, Lim SH, et al. Localized intradermal microinjection of tranexemic acid for treatment of melasma in Asian patients: a preliminary clinical report. Dermatol Surg. 2006;32(5):626-31.
36. Kanechorn Na Ayuthaya P, Niumphradit N, Manosroi A, et al. Topical 5% tranexamic acid for the treatment of melasma in Asians: a double-blind randomized controlled clinical trial. J Cosmet Laser Ther. 2012;14(3):150-4.
37. Ni Z, Mu Y, Gulati O. Treatment of melasma with pycnogenol. Phytother Res. 2002;16(6):567-71.
38. Handog EB, Galang DA, de Leon Godinez MA, et al. A randomized, double-blind, placebo-controlled trial of oral procyanidin with vitamins A, C, E for melasma among Filipino women. Int J Dermatol. 2009;48(8):896-901.
39. Wu S, Shi H, Wu H, et al. Treatment of melasma with oral administration of tranexamic acid. Aesthetic Plast Surg. 2012;36(4):964-70.
40. Sarkar R, Chugh S, Garg VK. Newer and upcoming therapies for melasma. Indian J Dermatol Venereol Leprol. 2012;78(4):417-28.
41. Choi S, Lee SK, Kim JE, et al. Aloesin inhibits hyperpigmentation induced by UV radiation. Clin Exp Dermatol. 2002;27(6):513-5.
42. Bandyopadhyay D. Topical treatment of melasma. Indian J Dermatol. 2009;54(4):303-9.
43. Keeling J, Cardona L, Benitez A, et al. Mequinol 2%/tretinoin 0.01% topical solution for the treatment of melasma in men: a case series and review of the literature. Cutis. 2008;81(2):179-83.
44. Greatens A, Hakozaki T, Koshoffer A, et al. Effective inhibition of melanosome transfer to keratinocytes by lectins and niacinamide is reversible. Exp Dermatol. 2005;14(7):498-508.
45. Khemis A, Kaiafa A, Queille-Roussel C, et al. Evaluation of efficacy and safety of rucinol in patients with melasma: a randomized controlled trial. Br J Dermatol. 2007;156(5):997-1004.
46. Kim DS, Park SH, Kwon SB, et al. Epigallocatechin-3-gallate and hinokitiol reduce melanin synthesis via decreased MITF Production. Arch Pharm Res. 2004;27(3):334-9.
47. Yamamura T, Onishi J, Nishiyama T. Antimelanogenic activity of hydrocoumarins in cultured normal human melanocytes by stimulating intracellular glutathione synthesis. Arch Dermatol Res. 2002;294(8):349-54.
48. Yokota T, Nishio H, Kubota Y, et al. The inhibitory effect of glabridin from licorice extracts on melanogenesis and inflammation. Pigment Cell Res. 1998;11(6):355-61.
49. Jimbow K. N-acetyl-4-S-cysteaminylphenol as a new type of depigmenting agent for the melanoderma of patients with melasma. Arch Dermatol. 1991;127(10):1528-34.
50. Wallo W, Nebus J, Leyden JJ. Efficacy of soy moisturizer in photoaging: a double blind vehicle controlled 12-week study. J Drugs Dermatol. 2007;6(9):917-22.

41

Photoprotection for Melasma

Narendra Gokhale

Key Features

- Ultraviolet and visible light can induce melanin formation.
- The regular use of broadspectrum sunscreen is effective in preventing melasma.
- Broadspectrum sunscreens enhance the efficacy of other topical therapies.
- Use protective clothing in addition to sunscreens.

INTRODUCTION

The sun is a gigantic powerhouse emitting high level of energy that reaches out into the solar system. The earth receives a fair share of this energy in the form of electromagnetic radiation. The sunlight reaching the earth's surface has many beneficial effects as mentioned in **Box 1**.

Box 1

Beneficial effects of sunlight

- Vision
- Photosynthesis
- Vitamin D synthesis
- Killing of germs
- Mood elevator

However, this radiation also has deleterious effects on the skin like causing and aggravating inflammatory reactions, malignancies and hyperpigmentary disorders.[1]

ELECTROMAGNETIC RADIATION

The energy from the sun reaches us as electromagnetic waves. It is a wide spectrum varying from X-rays at one end to infrared at other end as shown in **Table 1**. We are primarily concerned with the wavelength between 200 nm and 1200 nm, which includes ultraviolet (UV), visible and infrared. Ultraviolet is divided into UVA, UVB and UVC. UVA is further subdivided into UVA1 and UVA2.

The UV radiation (UVR) reaching the Earth's surface is only 5% of the terrestrial radiation as most of it is absorbed by the ozone layer in the atmosphere. At any given time and meteorological condition, UVA is at least 17 times UVB, i.e. 90–95% of UVR is UVA. The factors that affect the amount and type of UVR are summarized in **Table 2**.[2,3]

Table 1: Spectrum of electromagnetic radiation

Wavelength	200–290	290–320	320–340	340–400	400–700	>700
Name	UVC	UVB	UVA2	UVA1	Visible	Infrared

Table 2: Factors affecting type and amount of ultraviolet radiation

S. No.	*Factor*	*Effect*
1.	Solar zenith angle—an angle between an imaginary perpendicular line and a line from its base to the sun	Shorter UVB rays are maximum at noon and least at dawn and dusk
2.	Ozone layer	Filters UVC completely, but a concern where it is getting damaged
3.	Pollution	Dust over cities filters UV radiation
4.	Cloud cover	Filters UVB and infrared but not UVA
5.	Altitude	More UV at higher altitudes
6.	Reflecting surfaces	Snow, water and sand reflect UV light

Effects of Ultraviolet Radiation on the Skin

The UV light on reaching the skin is reflected, absorbed and passed through. It is absorbed primarily by the melanin pigment and has numerous effects on the epidermal keratinocytes and melanocytes. It produces effects on the dermal components including collagen, elastin and the immune system of the skin.[3,4] Different effects are produced by different wavelengths as outlined in **Table 3**.

Some of the effects are produced in a short span of time while others take place slowly as shown in **Table 4**.

Pigmentation Following Ultraviolet Exposure

Pigment production occurs in skin following both UVA and UVB exposure. UVA induces three types of pigmentation.[4] Immediate pigment darkening develops rapidly in minutes and it also fades rapidly. The second type persistent pigment darkening (PPD) occurs due to oxidation of melanin. It may persist for many weeks depending on UVA dose and skin type. The third type, delayed pigmentation, which is a long lasting (several months) tan, starts some days after UV exposure. It is due to increased melanin synthesis in response to intense UVA exposure or repeated suberythemal doses.[4]

Ultraviolet B-induced tanning is a delayed pigmentation due to melanin synthesis. This usually follows burn and usually disappears with epidermal turnover after 1 month. The melanin so produced provides a uniform tan as a protection against future burns. In dark-skinned individuals, UVA has greater pigmenting effects than UVB. In Asian skin, an irregular pigmentation can occur following sun exposure as in melasma. In fact, pigmentary changes are one of the principal signs of photoaging in Asian skin.[4,5]

Table 3: Effect of different ultraviolet wavelengths on skin

Type	*UVB*	*UVA*
Effect	Absorbed by deoxyribonucleic acid (DNA) and proteins	Not absorbed by DNA
	Direct damage	Penetrates deeper
	Sunburn	Aging
	Cancer	Tanning
		Immunosuppression
		Photocarcinogenesis
		Exogenous photodermatitis
		Idiopathic photodermatoses

Table 4: Time-dependent effects of ultraviolet radiation on skin

Immediate	Delayed
Sunburn-UVB	Tanning-UVA + UVB
Tanning-UVA	Aging-UVA
Vitamin D synthesis	Malignancy UVB
Thickening	Immunological changes

PHOTOPROTECTION

Any measure which is aimed at preventing the sunlight from reaching the skin helps in minimizing the deleterious effects of sunlight. It includes general measures including lifestyle changes, use of sunscreens, use of protective clothing and glass.[3]

General Measures

The patient should be counseled about general measures as outlined in **Box 2**. They should be advised to avoid sunlight as much as possible. As melasma is aggravated by exposure to all the wavelengths including UVB, UVA and visible, any time of the day has enough sunlight, not necessarily hot afternoon hours, when only UVB and heat are more. Wearing of broad-brimmed hats, other head gears and scarves should be encouraged as, if properly worn they provide better photo protection than the best sunscreens. Patients should be asked to keep to the shade of buildings and trees when sun avoidance is not possible. The patients should also be asked to avoid applying cosmetics containing perfumes, which are potent photo sensitizers, to any part of the body.

Box 2

General measures of sun protection

- Avoid sun throughout the day
- Wear broad hats, scarves, ***dupattas*** whenever going out
- Keep to the shade when outside
- Avoid scented cosmetics and wet wipes

SUNSCREENS

Sunscreens are over the counter drugs which are applied with the intention to prevent sunlight from reaching the skin.[2,3,6,7] They may reflect, or scatter the UV light like inorganic ones or like organic filters they may absorb the UVR and emit back a longer wavelength.[4,7,8] Words like sunblock are not acceptable and should be avoided.[2]

The sunscreen because of reflection, scattering or absorbing the UVR reduces the amount of UVR reaching the skin and the effects produced by it. Hence, it prevents DNA damage, decreases melanin production and also decreases the damage to collagen and elastic fibers.[9,10]

Table 5: Criteria for an ideal sunscreen
• Broad spectrum (covers UVB + UVA II + UVA I)
• Photostable
• Good substantivity
• Cosmetically acceptable
• Water resistant
• Nonsensitizing
• Fragrance free
• Cost effective

The Ideal Sunscreen

The ideal sunscreen which satisfies all the criteria outlined in **Table 5** remains elusive.[8]

Classification of Ingredients

Sunscreens are divided into organic and inorganic depending on their mechanism of action. The terms physical and chemical are no longer used. There are three commonly used nomenclatures for sunscreen agents in the world. These are International Nomenclature Cosmetic Ingredient (INCI) name, US adopted name (USAN) and trade name.[11]

The inorganic sunscreens act by reflecting and scattering UVR. The organic ones act by absorbing UVR and release lower energy by emitting out a longer wavelength which is not harmful.

Inorganic sunscreens: The list of inorganic sunscreens is outlined in **Box 3**.

Box 3

Inorganic sunscreens

- Zinc oxide
- Titanium oxide
- Magnesium oxide
- Iron oxide
- Red veterinary petrolatum

Inorganic sunscreens reflect or scatter UV rays. They are excellent sunscreens for heavy exposures as well as melasma as they act on UV, visible as well as the infrared spectrums and are opaque so provide a good camouflage effect. They have the added advantage of not causing contact sensitivity.

But these products are messy to apply, are comedogenic and there are concerns regarding free radical production, especially titanium dioxide. To add to it, when applied on the skin they look white, because of diffuse scattering of visible light.[4] To address these issues, they are now being formulated in micronized forms which are coated with dimethicone or silica. Nano-sized titanium dioxide shows synergistic effect with organic filters. But micronized titanium dioxide shifts its protection spectrum to UVB.[11] They may be absorbed into the blood when applied in large quantities over large surface areas.

Among the commonly used ones, zinc oxide has greater protection in UVA1 spectrum, while titanium dioxide has more protection in UVB and UVA2. Titanium dioxide is more white and photoactive so more likely to produce free radicals.

Organic sunscreens: These are aromatic compounds with a carboxyl group, that absorb UV light of a specific wavelength, depending on their chemical structure, and then emit a longer wavelength of lesser energy, usually in the form of insensible heat.[3,7,8,10] The molecular structure responsible for absorbing UV energy is called a chromophore.

A chromophore consists of electrons engaged into multiple bond sequences between atoms, generally conjugated double bonds. On absorbing the energy of a photon, the electron is shifted to a higher energy orbit in the molecule. The filter that was in a low energy state transforms to a higher energy state (excited). From the excited state, the filter molecule can simply deactivate and resume its ground state while releasing the absorbed energy as unnoticeable heat. If it structurally degrades because of the high energy state then it is labeled as photo unstable.[10]

Organic filters are rarely used alone, but usually in combination with inorganic as they may not provide satisfactory UVA1 protection. These are generally odorless and colorless. There is a risk of contact dermatitis, specially benzophenones and older ones like para-aminobenzoic acid (PABA). They may be photo unstable like avobenzones and cinnamates and hence are combined with octocrylene and tinosorb S to stabilize them. They are absorbed systemically.

Some of the ingredients may show synergistic effect, viz. terephthalylidene dicamphor sulfonic acid (TDSA) and drometrizole trisiloxane (DTS) and TDSA and bis-ethylhexyloxyphenol methoxyphenyl triazine (BEMT).[10]

A list of organic filters is provided in **Tables 6 and 7**.

Table 6: Organic UVB filters[2]

USAN name	*INCI name*	*Peak absorption wavelength*
Aminobenzoates		
PABA	PABA	283
Padimate O	Ethyl dimethyl PABA	311
Cinnamates		
Octinoxate	Ethylhexyl methoxycinnamate	311
Cinoxate	Cinoxate	289
Salicylates'		
Octisalate	Ethylhexyl salicylate	307
Homosalate	Homosalate	306
Trolamine salicylate	Time and extend application salicylate	260, 355
Benzophenones		
Others		
Octocrlene	Octocrylene	303
Ensulizole	Phenylbenzimidazole sulfonic acid	310
Mexoryl XL	DTS	303, 344

Abbreviations: PABA, para-aminobenzoic acid; DTS, drometrizole trisiloxane

Table 7: Organic UVA filters[2,7]

Class	Name	Peak absorption wavelength
Benzophenones		
Oxybenzone	Benzophenone 3	288, 325
Sulisobenzone	Benzophenone 4	366
Dioxybenzone	Benzophenone 8	352
Tinosorb M	MBBT	305, 306
Tinosorb S	BEMT	310, 343
Other		
Methylanthranilate	Meradimate	355
Avobenzone/Parsol 1789	BMDM	360
Mexoryl SX	TDSA	345
Mexoryl XL	DTS	303, 344
Uvinul A+	DHHB	354
Neo-Heliopan AP	DPDT	335

Abbreviations: TDSA, terephthalylidene dicamphor sulfonic acid; DTS, drometrizole trisiloxane; DHHB, diethylamino hydroxybenzoyl hexyl benzoate; DPDT, disodium phenyl dibenzimidazole tetrasulfonate; BEMT, bis-ethylhexyloxyphenol methoxyphenyl triazine; MBBT, methylene bis-benzotriazolyl tetramethylbutylphenol; BMDM, butylmethoxy dibenzoyl methane.
To summarize the filters with good UVA1 protection are zinc oxide, sulisobenzone, tinosorb M, avobenzone, mexoryl SX, mexoryl XL, uvinul A+ and Neo-Heliopan AP.

Sunscreen Protection Criteria

There is much confusion and ignorance about judging the efficacy of sunscreens. It stems from the fact that even dermatologists are not aware about the protection spectra of different ingredients and the hype created in the media and by pharmaceutical companies about sun protection factor (SPF) adds to the confusion. The criteria outlined in **Box 4** are generally used.

Box 4

Criteria for evaluation of sunscreen protection

- SPF
- PA Factor Japanese standard
- Australian/New Zealand standard
- European union rating
- Boots star rating
- Critical wavelength

Abbreviations: SPF, sun protection factor; PA, protection grade of UVA.

Sun Protection Factor

It is the most widely used term in relation to sunscreens. Originally, an acronym for SPF, the FDA has expanded the term to sunburn protection factor. It tells us about how much longer the skin covered with sunscreen takes to burn as compared to unprotected skin. It is defined as the ratio of the least amount of ultraviolet energy (UVB) required to produce minimal erythema dose (MED) on sunscreen-protected skin to the amount of energy required to produce the same erythema on unprotected skin. For the skin to be labeled protected, 2 mg/cm^2 layer of sunscreen has to be applied.[2-4,6-8] A sunscreen with an SPF of 15 blocks 93% of UVB radiation, while one with an SPF of 30 blocks about 97% of UVB radiation.

What it means for the patient is that it helps him to know how much longer that individual can stay out in the sun with minimal damage to his skin. For example, if a person develops minimal erythema after 30 minutes of unprotected sun exposure and develops a burn on 90 minutes (three times MED) of sun exposure, the same person can stay in the sun for 90 minutes and get just 10% of the MED, if he applies a SPF 30 sunscreen. If the same person applies a SPF 15 sunscreen, he shall be exposed to 20% MED on 90 minutes of sun exposure. With chronic exposure, the damage caused by UVR is halved by a sunscreen having a SPF 30 as compared to a sunscreen of SPF 15. So although the percentage energy absorption increases by just 4% on doubling the SPF from 15 to 30, the cumulative sun damage is reduced by half.[2]

Since burn and erythema are primarily caused by UVB, SPF is a measure of UVB protection and does not provide information regarding UVA protection, which is mainly responsible for pigment production, photoallergic dermatitis and aging **(Table 8)**.[3,4,7,8,10]

Products having SPF greater than 50 can only write SPF 50+ on the packaging and are not allowed to mention the exact SPF.[7]

PA Rating

This method was developed by the Japanese Cosmetic Industry Association.[12] It studies the PPD, i.e. the persistent pigment darkening caused by UVA radiation. It is the ratio of the UVA dose required to produce PPD after 2–24 hours of exposure on protected skin, to the UVA dose required to produce the same effect on unprotected skin. The ratio thus arrived is graded into categories as outlined in **Table 9**. It essentially measures the ability to prevent tanning, hence is more useful index for the darker skin types and the one which is useful when selecting a sunscreen for a patient with melasma. Since PPD response requires more than 10 J/cm^2 doses which is roughly equivalent to 40 minutes of mid-day

Table 8: Grading system for sun protection factor[6]	
Grade	*SPF*
Low	2–15
Medium	15–30
High	30–50
Highest	> 50

Table 9: PA rating according to degree of persistent pigment darkening ratio	
PA	*SPF*
+	2–4
++	4–8
+++	> 8

summer sunlight, it also tests the photo stability of the sunscreen.[7,9,10]

Australia/New Zealand Standard

This is an *in vitro* method where ultraviolet light of wavelength 320 to 360 nm is passed through a layer of the sunscreen and the amount transmitted through the layer is measured on the other side. An 8 um layer of the product should not transmit more than 10% of the radiation, and a 20 um layer should not transmit more than 1% of the radiation.[2]

European Standard

In 2006 the minimum requirements of UVA protection were approved in Europe.[13] The UVAPF should be at least one-third of the SPF of the product, which translates to a SPF/UVAPF ratio less than or equal to three. This criterion has also been recently adopted by Australia and the Mercosur countries (*viz*. Argentina, Brazil, Paraguay and Uruguay).

Ultraviolet A radiation at 15 J/cm^2, which is reached in about 45 minutes of sun exposure, is able to induce PPD. This PPD is induced very easily on dark skin types (III, IV, V). Since most Indians have Fitzpatrick skin phototypes IV to V, the criteria of a SPF/UVAPF ratio of less than 3 for a sunscreen should be made applicable to India too. Also worth remembering is the fact that UVA damage can occur after acute or repeated UVA exposure below 15 J/cm^2.[4]

In fact few studies have reported the reduction in pigmentation due to the use of a sunscreen having an SPF/UVAPF value of less than three.[4]

Boots Star Rating

This is an *in vitro* method where the ratio of UVA to UVB absorbance before and after irradiation is calculated as shown in **Table 10**. It is also a measure of UVA protection.[8]

Table 10: Boots star rating[8]		
Ratio of UVA:UVB absorbance		
Before	*After*	*Boots star rating*
< 0.6	< 0.56	None
> 0.6	> 57	***
> 0.8	> 76	****
> 0.9	> 86	*****

Substantivity

The substantivity of a sunscreen refers to its ability to retain its effectiveness under the stress of exercise, sweating and swimming.[3,8] The older terminology of water proof is no longer to be used. **Box 5** lists the terms commonly used.

Box 5

Terms referring to substantivity

- Water resistant
- Very water resistant
- Sweat resistant

Water resistant: A sunscreen is labeled water resistant if it is able to retain its efficiency after two sequential immersions in water of 20 minutes each.

Very water resistant: A sunscreen is labeled water resistant if it is able to retain its efficacy after four sequential immersions in water of 20 minutes each.

A water resistant sunscreen is also sweat resistant.

Application of Sunscreens

The sunscreens need to be applied liberally to form a thick layer to be effective. Since they do not stay long enough, they need to be reapplied repeatedly.

The ideal amount to be applied is 2 mg/cm^2.[3,8,14] So an average adult with 1.73 m^2 surface area requires 35 mL in one application! This can be achieved by the "teaspoon rule" shown in **Table 11**.

Ideally the sunscreen needs to be reapplied 2 hourly, which is practically not possible for most of the patients.

Since most patients apply less than the desired quantity and less frequently, the recent trend is to prescribe sunscreens

Table 11: Teaspoon rule[14]	
3 mL or just more than half teaspoon	Each arm face and neck
5 mL or just more than one teaspoon	Each leg chest back

with higher protection, i.e. SPF 50+ and PA+++ to partially compensate for the lacuna.

Selecting the Right Sunscreen for a Patient with Melasma

The patient of melasma requires a broad-spectrum sunscreen which covers UVA, UVB as well as the visible spectrum.[15] Inorganic sunscreens are the preferred ones as they provide protection from the entire spectrum and provide a camouflage effect also, especially the ones containing ferric oxide. Since inorganic alone in high concentrations are not cosmetically acceptable, a blend of inorganic and organic are the best. Those patients who would like a less visible sunscreen, should be prescribed only organic sunscreens.

The sunscreen needs to be applied liberally as explained above and repeatedly throughout the day. It needs to be emphasized to the patient that even when they stay indoors they should continue to use the sunscreen as the indirect sunlight can also aggravate melasma.

A note should also be made of the coexistent conditions like acne and the general hydration of the skin of the patient, their occupation, their needs and expectations from the product prescribed. Gel-based products and sprays are better for oily and acne prone skin and people involved in heavy physical labor and those who sweat a lot, like sportspersons. Water in oil emulsion will be a good option during harsh winters and for the aging skin.

Lakhdar et al.[16] reported the use of a broad-spectrum sunscreen with a SPF of 50+ and UVA protection factor of 28 to prevent the development of melasma in pregnant women. In this study, 200 Moroccan women less than 3 months pregnant were asked to apply this sunscreen 2 hourly irrespective of the sun exposure. Melasma occurred in only 2.7% of these women, while the prevalence of melasma in the same population is 53%. In this study 8 of the 12 patients with pre-existing melasma also improved.

In another study the difference in efficacy between hydroquinone containing agent in combination with a vehicle versus the same cream in combination with a broad protection sunscreen was compared. In those patients who used sunscreen 96.2% showed improvement while in the other group 80.7% showed improvement.[17]

Sadly, there are no randomized controlled trials proving the efficacy of sunscreens in melasma. But the authors strongly believe that they should be prescribed to all patients of melasma because of the overwhelming evidence of their efficacy in preventing and reducing melanin production.

PROTECTIVE CLOTHING

Since the best of sunscreens do not provide 100% protection from UV rays and do not last long enough, patients of melasma should be encouraged to wear protective clothing like broad hats and scarves to increase the protection level specially when going out in the sun.

The efficacy of fabrics to protect from sunlight is expressed as UPF or ultraviolet protection factor. It is the ratio of average effective UV irradiance transmitted without fabric to the average effective UV irradiance transmitted through fabric. The UPF value calculated therefore indicates how much longer a person can stay in the sun when fabric covers the skin to produce the same degree of erythema than if he had not worn the fabric.[18,19] The fabric is then classified as good or very good for UV protection as shown in **Table 12**.

Different types of fibers provide varying levels of UV protection as shown in **Table 13**.

Many factors influence the protection provided by clothes. The factors that affect the UV protection of fibers are outlined in **Table 14**. Generally a fiber with a tighter weave will allow less UV light to pass through it. Washing causes the material to shrink reducing the distance between fibers, thus enhancing the protection. But a wet cloth is less protective because of the water causing separation of the fibers and also because the water reduces the scattering of light.[2] A fabric that is stretchable allows more sunlight to go through. Colored

Table 12: Levels of protection according to ultraviolet protection factor

UPF	*Level*
15–24	Good protection
40–50	Very good protection

Table 13: Ultraviolet protection of different fibers[18,19]

Best absorbers	Polyester
Moderate absorbers	Wool, silk, nylon
Poor absorbers	Cotton

Table 14: Factors affecting ultraviolet protection of fibers[2]

Factor	*Effect*
Layers	More the number of layers, better the protection
Style of garment	
Weave	Tighter the weave, more the protection
Washing	Increases
Hydration	Decreases
Stretchable	Less protection
Bleaching agents	Increase protection
Color	Increases protection
Distance from skin	More the better

clothes absorb some sunlight increasing the protection, but also heat up in the process. The further a cloth is from the skin, the greater is the UV protection. So loose fitting clothes offer higher protection than clothes clinging to the patient's skin.

CONCLUSION

Photoprotection forms the cornerstone of any therapeutic regimen for melasma and increases the effectiveness of other therapeutic modalities. It helps in preventing the synthesis of new melanin by melanocytes and helps in improving the overall texture and feel of the skin. Dermatologists should be aware of the various options available and choose a product wisely.

REFERENCES

1. Matts PJ. Solar ultraviolet radiation: Definitions and terminology. Dermatol Clin. 2006;24(1):1-8.
2. Lim HW. Photoprotection and sun-protective agents. In: Wolff K, Goldsmith LA, Katz SI, Gilchrest BA, Paller AS, Leffell DJ (Eds). Fitzpatrick's dermatology in general medicine. 7th edn. New York: McGraw-Hill; 2008. pp. 2137-41.
3. Rai R, Srinivas CR. Photoprotection. Indian J Dermatol Venereol Leprol. 2007;73(2):73-9.
4. Moyal D. Need for a well-balanced sunscreen to protect human skin from both Ultraviolet A and Ultraviolet B damage. Indian J Dermatol Venereol Leprol. 2012;78(Suppl 1): 24-30.
5. Rai VM, Shenoi SD, Balachandran C, et al. Minimal erythema response (MED) to solar simulated irradiation in normal Indian skin. Indian J Dermatol Venereol Leprol. 2004;70(5):277-9.
6. Levy SB. Sunscreens. In: Wolverton SE (Ed). Comprehensive dermatologic drug therapy. 2nd edn. Philadelphia: Saunders; 2007. pp. 703-18.
7. Moyal D, Galdi A, Oresajo C. Sunscreens. In: Zoe Diana Draelos (Ed). Cosmetic Dermatology Products and Procedures. Wiley-Blackwell; 2010. pp. 144-9.
8. Kaimal S, Abraham A. Sunscreens. Indian J Dermatol Venereol Leprol. 2011;77(2):238-43.
9. Moyal D. Prevention of ultraviolet-induced skin pigmentation. Photodermatol Photoimmunol Photomed. 2004;20(5): 243-7.
10. Moyal D. The development of efficient sunscreens. Indian J Dermatol Venereol Leprol. 2012;78(Suppl 1):31-4
11. Hexsel CL, Bangert SD, Hebert AA, et al. Current sunscreen issues: 2007 Food and Drug Administration sunscreen labelling recommendations and combination sunscreen/insect repellent products. J Am Acad Dermatol. 2008;59(2):316-23.
12. Japan Cosmetic Industry Association (JCIA). Measurements standard for UVA protection efficacy. Tokyo, Japan: JCIA; 1996.
13. European Commission recommendation. On the efficacy of sunscreen products and the claims made relating thereto. Official J Eur Union. 2006;265;39-43.
14. Schneider J. The teaspoon rule of applying sunscreen. Arch Dermatol. 2002;138(6):838-9.
15. Sheth VM, Pandya AG. Melasma: a comprehensive update: part II. J Am Acad Dermatol. 2011;65(4):699-714.
16. Lakhdar H, Zouhair K, Khadir K, et al. Evaluation of the effectiveness of a broad-spectrum sunscreen in the prevention of chloasma in pregnant women. J Eur Acad Dermatol Venereol. 2007;21(7):738-42.
17. Vazquez M, Sanchez JL. The efficacy of broad-spectrum sunscreen in the treatment of melasma. Cutis. 1983;32(1): 92,95-6
18. American Society for Testing and Materials (ASTM International). Standard D 6603-00, Standard guide for labeling of UV-protective textiles. In: Bailey SJ, Baldwin NC, McElrone EK, et al (Eds). ASTM Standard; 2004. pp. 1187-91.
19. Crews PC, Kachman S, Beyer AG. Influence on UVR transmission of undyed woven fabrics. Textile Chem Colorist. 1993;31:17-26.

42

Chemical Peeling for Melasma

Annyce Treherne, Valerie D Callender

Key Features

- A promising and successful second-line modality or adjunctive treatment for melasma is chemical peeling
- Superficial peels are the most commonly used peels to treat melasma
- The safest and most effective chemical peeling agent for melasma is glycolic acid
- Proper peeling technique and caution must be used to minimize the incidence or risk of dyspigmentation, especially in darker skin patients.

INTRODUCTION

Melasma is an acquired disorder of hypermelanosis that is symmetrically distributed mainly on the face, but can rarely occur on other areas of the body such as the neck and upper extremities.[1] It occurs mainly in women with darker skin types (Fitzpatrick IV–VI) and is associated with several risk factors, which include ultraviolet radiation exposure, hormonal influences, genetics, thyroid disease, anti-seizure and phototoxic medications.[1] In addition, quality of life studies have shown a negative impact and psychological distress in individuals affected by melasma, and therefore treatment is imperative.[2,3]

Currently, there is no definitive modality of treatment available for melasma, especially given the refractory and recurrent nature of the condition and because of this, management can be very frustrating for the both the patient, as well as the treating physician. A promising and successful second-line modality or adjunctive treatment for melasma is chemical peeling. Chemical peeling is an effective method of removing excess pigment in the epidermis, which works well for both epidermal and mixed type melasma. In addition, efficacy can be increased by combining chemical peeling with topical skin lightening agents and sun protective measures.

CHEMICAL PEELS

Chemical peeling is a skin resurfacing procedure in which a chemical agent is applied to the skin to cause a controlled destruction of a portion or the entire epidermis, with or without the dermis.[4] This controlled destruction leads to exfoliation, which improves the skin surface appearance, texture and stimulates new skin growth. Chemical peeling works in the treatment of melasma by the removal of unwanted melanin.[5]

Chemical peels may be divided by depth of injury into superficial, medium-depth and deep peels.[6] Superficial peels are the most commonly used peel to treat melasma. Medium-depth peels are rarely used because of the risk of dyschromias. While deep peels should be avoided in melasma patients because of the risk of postinflammatory dyschromias, keloid formation, and scarring.[7] Superficial peels penetrate the stratum corneum to the papillary dermis. Following a superficial peel epidermal regeneration with desquamation can be expected within 3–5 days.[8] Superficial peels include glycolic acid (GA), salicylic acid (SA), lactic acid (LA), tretinoin, Jessner's solution and trichloroacetic acid (TCA) in low concentrations between 10% and 20%.

Glycolic Acid Peel

Glycolic acid is a food derived alpha hydroxy acid. GA improves the skin surface by weakening the intercellular cohesion of the stratum corneum causing thinning of the stratum corneum and desquamation.[9] It is considered a superficial peeling agent that varies in strength from 20% to 70% and pH between 1 and 3. The efficacy of the peel depends on the strength, pH and application time.

Glycolic acid peels are the most commonly used peel for the treatment of melasma. The mechanism of action of GA to treat melasma is believed to be by inhibiting tyrosinase activity in a pH-independent manner.[5] Multiple studies have shown GA to be effective in the treatment of melasma.[10-13]

Lim and Tham[10] performed a small-scale study with ten Asian women with melasma and fine wrinkles treated with 2% hydroquinone and 10% GA applied to both sides of the face. One side of the face had a series of GA peels from 20% to 70% applied every 3 weeks for 26 weeks. At the end of the study the melasma treated with GA improved to a greater degree.

Javaheri et al.[11] also assessed the safety and efficacy of a series of GA peels in 25 Indian women with melasma. Patients were treated with 50% GA cream peels once per month for three consecutive months. The improvement of pigmentation was measured by the melasma area and severity index (MASI) at regular intervals, and at the end of the 3-month follow-up period. Reduction in the MASI score was observed in 91% of the patients and epidermal-type of melasma showed a better response when compared to the mixed type.

Glycolic acid peels have also been studied in combination with topical regimens. A study of 40 Indian patients assessed the efficacy of a series of GA peels used in combination with a topical bleaching formula versus topical bleaching formula alone in the treatment of melasma.[14] Both groups applied a modified Kligman's formula (hydroquinone 5%, tretinoin 0.05% and hydrocortisone acetate 1% in a cream base) daily. In addition to the modified Kligman's formula one group also received six serial GA peels every 3 weeks. The first three peels were with 30% GA and the last three peels used 40% GA. Both groups demonstrated a statistically significant improvement of the MASI score. However, the group receiving the GA peels showed a faster and greater degree of improvement. Other studies have also shown a significant improvement by adding GA peels to topical bleaching combinations.[15,16]

Rendon et al.[16] studied the addition of GA to the only US Food and Drug Administration approved triple combination (TC) cream containing fluocinolone acetonide 0.01%, hydroquinone 4% and tretinoin 0.05%. The participants were pretreated with TC for 2 weeks then received five serial GA peels every 2 weeks. By week 12, significant improvement of pigmentation was achieved. Suggesting the use of TC cream in sequence with GA peels may enhance their effect leading to better results than using either agent alone.

Glycolic acid peels alone and in conjunction with TC creams have proven to be beneficial in the treatment of melasma with minimal side effects. Adverse effects of GA shown in studies have included erythema, hyperpigmentation, hypopigmentation, and at higher concentrations burns and scarring have occurred. Side effects associated with GA peels are usually mild and may be minimized by slowly increasing the GA from lower concentrations of 20–35% up to higher concentrations of 70%.

Lactic Acid Peel

Lactic acid is also an alpha hydroxy acid and has a similar mechanism of action to GA. LA similar to glycolic causes thinning of the stratum corneum by reducing corneocyte adhesion.[17] LA is rarely used in the treatment of melasma despite the fact that it is inexpensive and readily available. Sharquie et al[18] performed a study with 20 patients to evaluate the efficacy and safety of LA for the treatment of melasma. Serial LA peels using pure LA (92%; pH 3.5) were performed every 3 weeks until the desired response was achieved or six sessions were performed. All 12 patients who completed the treatment showed a statistically significant decrease in the MASI score by 56% and no relapse was appreciated at the 6 month follow-up.

A later study compared LA peels for melasma to Jessner's solution.[19] A split face design was employed with the application of Jessner's solution to one side and LA to the other side. The results of the study revealed LA and Jessner's solution were equally effective in the treatment of melasma. Both studies by Sharquie et al. failed to demonstrate adverse effects associated with LA peels.

Salicylic Acid Peel

Salicylic acid, a beta hydroxy acid, is a hydroxyl derivative of benzoic acid and represents a carboxylic acid attached to an aromatic alcohol, phenol. SA is a lipophilic agent, which produces desquamation of the upper lipophilic layers of the stratum corneum.[20] SA also exhibits anti-inflammatory capabilities secondary to its effects on the arachidonic cascade.[21] Common indications for SA peels include acne vulgaris, photoaging, postinflammatory hyperpigmentation and melasma. SA is available in concentrations from 20% to 30% in a hydroethanolic solution for peeling.

Grimes[20] performed a pilot study to assess the safety and efficacy of SA peels in skin types V and VI. The study included 25 patients, 6 of whom had melasma. The patients were pre-treated with hydroquinone 4% for 2 weeks prior to undergoing a series of five SA peels. Two 20% and then three 30% peels were performed at 2-week intervals. Moderate to significant improvement occurred in 66% of the patients with melasma. Sixteen percent of the patients experienced mild side effects, which included temporary crusting, hypopigmentation, transient dryness, and hyperpigmentation which all resolved within 7–14 days. Residual hypopigmentation or hyperpigmentation did not occur.

A prospective randomized split face trial of SA peels for the treatment of melasma in Latin American women was performed to determine the efficacy of SA peels when added to hydroquinone.[22] Twenty Latin American women with moderate to severe bilateral melasma were treated with 4% hydroquinone to both sides of the face twice daily. One half of the face was also treated with two 20% then two 30% SA peels performed at 2-week intervals. Both sides showed significant improvement in pigment intensity; however, there was no difference in the amount of improvement between the peeled side and unpeeled side. Mild adverse events occurred in 20% of the patients, which included erythema, burning, and peeling. SA appears to be safe in the treatment of melasma but efficacy varies by study. At this time larger studies and comparison trials are necessary to determine the efficacy of SA peels in the treatment of melasma.

Jessner's Peel

Jessner's solution is a superficial peeling agent containing resorcinol 14 g, SA 14 g, 85% LA 14 g, and 95% ethanol to a sufficient quantity up to 100 mL. Jessner's solution is an intense keratolytic agent, which causes the loss of corneocyte cohesion within the stratum corneum. This loss of corneocyte cohesion leads to an intercellular and intracellular edema within the upper layer of the dermis.[23] Jessner's is used in the treatment of melasma, postinflammatory hyperpigmentation, acne, photo damage and lentigines.

A study of 16 women with melasma by Lawrence et al.[24] evaluated the clinical efficacy of Jessner's peel versus GA peel in the treatment of melasma. The patients were first treated with tretinoin 0.05% cream for 1–2 weeks prior to the initiation of the chemical peels. After the initial treatment of tretinoin cream, 3 peels were performed at 1-month intervals. During the peel treatments, 70% GA was applied to the right side of the face and Jessner's solution was applied to the left side. At the end of the trial a statistically significant decrease of the MASI score by 63% was achieved. There was no statistically significant difference in the two sides of the face. No adverse reactions were appreciated with Jessner's solution. While 1 patient treated with GA developed extensive epidermolysis with postinflammatory hyperpigmentation. Two additional patients treated with GA developed crusting and erythema; and an additional 4 patients developed persistent erythema. At 6 months follow-up only the patients who continued their topical regimen partially maintained improvement while the patients who did not relapsed.

As previously discussed Jessner's peels have also been compared to LA peels revealing that the Jessner's peel had equal efficacy to LA peel for the treatment of melasma.[19] These patients also maintained their improvement at long-term follow-up.

Jessner's solution appears as safe and effective for the treatment of melasma as GA and LA. However, long-term follow-up of the studies involving Jessner's solution differ in its ability to maintain improvement.

Trichloroacetic Acid Peel

Trichloroacetic acid may be used as a superficial, medium-depth, or deep peel. Superficial peeling may be achieved with concentrations of 10–25%. Increasing concentrations (>35%) of TCA increases the risk for scarring and post-inflammatory dyschromias. The mechanism of action of TCA is by epidermal protein precipitation causing necrosis.[23,25] In the treatment of melasma TCA may be used in low concentrations alone or in combination with other agents, most commonly Jessner's solution.

TCA (10–20%) peels have been tested against GA (20–35%) peels in a comparative study of 40 patients with melasma.[26] The study concluded that both TCA and GA significantly reduced MASI scores and with no statistically significant difference in them. In this study more adverse effects were associated with TCA as compared to GA. Both peels showed adverse effects including erythema and burning. The burning was more pronounced with TCA and post-peel cracking was also observed. A similar comparison study by Puri[27] of 15% TCA peel versus 35% GA peel for treatment of melasma yielded similar results. In addition another comparative study TCA versus GA revealed a quicker and better response in chronic pigmentation with TCA.[28]

TCA may also be used in combination with Jessner's solution. Jessner's solution is applied prior to the TCA to act as a pretreatment keratolytic, which alters the epidermal barrier allowing for even and controlled penetration of the TCA.[29] In a study of 20 female patients with melasma by Safoury et al.[30] a combination of modified Jessner's solution with 15% TCA was compared to 15% TCA alone. The study concluded that Jessner's improved the efficacy of TCA while minimizing the postinflammatory hyperpigmentation associated with TCA.

In summary, from available data, TCA appears to be as efficacious in treating melasma as GA. However, TCA also has an increased risk of adverse effects as compared to GA and caution should be taken especially in skin types IV–VI because of the increased risk of dyschromias.

Tretinoin Peel

Topical tretinoin is commonly used alone or in conjunction with Kligman's formula for the treatment of melasma. However, this does not seem to be true for tretinoin peels. Tretinoin peels are a superficial peeling agent. It is believed that the mechanism of action for tretinoin peels is similar to that of tretinoin cream, which modifies the epidermis and causes dispersion of melanin.[31,32] A study of 10 Indian patients with melasma by Khunger et al.[13] evaluated the efficacy and safety of tretinoin peels versus GA peels. This was a split-face comparison study in which weekly applications of 1% tretinoin peel and 70% GA peel for a total of 12 weeks. At the end of the study period a statistically significant decrease in the MASI score was noted for both sides of the face. There was also no statistically significant difference between the two sides of the face indicating 1% tretinoin peels are as efficacious as 70% GA peels. Tretinoin peels were also well tolerated and the side effects were minimal with only 2 patients experiencing erythema and superficial desquamation.

TECHNIQUE

Chemical peels are performed as an in-office procedure, and the frequency of application varies, occurring every 2–4 weeks for multiple treatment sessions.[33] The concentration of the peeling agent should begin low and titrated up based upon the response to the treatment. Topical preparations, such as hydroquinone, retinoids, and cosmeceuticals are commonly used prior to the procedure, so a careful and detailed history must be obtained prior to the peel application. Topical retinoids and other exfoliating agents should be discontinued 3–7 days prior to the peel. Prophylactic anti-viral therapy is necessary in patients with a history of herpes simplex. A test spot is recommended in all patients to determine tolerance and minimize the risk of adverse events, particularly in patients with darker skin types.

The treatment area should be properly cleansed with a gentle cleanser and all makeup removed. Acetone or alcohol is used to degrease the skin which will enhance the penetration of the peeling agent.

The eyes should be protected and covered with moisten gauze, disposable adhesive pads or eye shields. Petrolatum should be applied to sensitive skin areas including the lateral canthal creases, perinasal area, oral commissures and lips. The peeling agent is evenly applied with a sponge or cotton tip applicator and left on for several minutes. The application time varies and is based on the type and concentration of the peel used. A handheld fan may be used to minimize any discomfort. Frosting of the skin is seen with TCA which denotes the end point which is in contrast to the white precipitation or crystallization seen with SA peels. Neutralization of the peeling agent is necessary for AHA and TCA peels. However, the chemical peel procedure should be immediately terminated (neutralized) if intense erythema, blistering, vesiculation or excessive patient discomfort occurs, regardless of the peel used.

POST-PEEL INSTRUCTIONS

Emollients and sunscreen protection should be applied immediately after the procedure and continued during the exfoliation period for 1–2 weeks. If intense erythema is evident, then an application of a moderate-high potency topical corticosteroid should be applied to the affected area to minimize the risk of postinflammatory hyperpigmentation or hypopigmentation.[33] Gentle cleansing and moisturizing agents should be used daily to promote healing.

Home maintenance products, including skin lightening agents and sunscreen, can be initiated in 2–3 days post-procedure.

CONCLUSION

Chemical peels are proving to be a promising treatment for melasma. They should certainly be considered as either a second line treatment or adjunct to topical bleaching agents. It is important to choose an appropriate peeling agent and concentration to achieve optimum results. The safest and most effective chemical peel for melasma to date is GA. LA and tretinoin peels have also shown good results with minimal side effects; however, more studies are warranted to recommend their use. TCA peels at concentrations between 10% and 20% have been efficacious in studies but should be used with caution in skin types IV–VI because of the risk of postinflammatory hyperpigmentation and hypopigmentation. Proper peeling technique and post-peel care counseling to include photoprotection is also important to achieve optimum results.

REFERENCES

1. Ball Arefiev KL, Hantash BM. Advances in the treatment of melasma: a review of the recent literature. Dermatol Surg. 2012;38:971-84.
2. Balkrishnan R, McMichael AJ, Camacho FT, et al. Development and validation of a health-related quality of life instrument for women with melasma. Br J Dermatol. 2003;149(3):572-7.
3. Pawaskar AR, Parikh P, Markowski T, et al. Melasma and its impact on health-related quality of life in Hispanic women. J Dermatol Treat. 2007;18:5-9.
4. Khunger N. Standard guidelines of care for chemical peels. Indian J Dermatol Venereol Leprol. 2008;74(Suppl):S5-12.
5. Sheth VM, Pandya AG. Melasma: a comprehensive update: part II. J Am Acad Dermatol. 2011;65:699-714.
6. Coleman WP, Brody HJ. Advances in chemical peeling. Dermatol Clin. 1997;15:19-26.
7. Pandya AG, Guerva IL. Disorders of hyperpigmentation. Dermatol Clin. 2000;18;91-8.
8. Rendon MI, Berson DS, Cohen JL, et al. Evidence and considerations in the application of chemical peels in skin disorders and aesthetic resurfacing. J Clin Aesthet Dermatol. 2010;3:32-43.
9. Song JY, Kang HA, Kim MY, et al. Damage and recovery of skin barrier function after glycolic acid chemical peeling and crystal microdermabrasion. Dermatol Surg. 2004;30:390-4.
10. Lim JT, Tham SN. Glycolic acid peels in the treatment of melasma among Asian women. Dermatol Surg. 1997;23:177-9.
11. Javaheri SM, Handa S, Kaur I, et al. Safety and efficacy of glycolic acid facial peel in Indian women with melasma. Int J Dermatol. 2001;40:354-7.
12. Grover C, Reddu BS. The therapeutic value of glycolic acid peels in dermatology. Indian J Dermatol Venereol Leprol. 2003;69:148-50.
13. Khunger N, Sarkar R, Jain RK. Tretinoin peels versus glycolic acid peels in the treatment of melasma in dark skinned patients. Dermatol Surg. 2004;30:756-60.
14. Sarkar R, Kaur C, Bhalla M, et al. The combination of glycolic acid peels with a topical regimen in the treatment of melasma in dark-skinned patients: a comparative study. Dermatol Surg. 2002;28:828-32.
15. Godse KV, Sakhia J. Triple combination and glycolic acid peels in melasma in Indian patients. J Cosmet Dermatol. 2011;10:68-9.

16. Rendon M, Cardona LM, Bussear EW, et al. Successful treatment of moderate to severe melasma with triple combination cream and glycolic acid peels: a pilot study. Cutis. 2008;82(5):372-8.
17. Van Scott EJ, Yu RJ. Hyperkeratinazation, corneocyte cohesion and alpha-hydroxy acid. J Am Acad Dermatol. 1984;11(5 Pt 1):867-79.
18. Sharquie KE, Al-Tikreety MM, Al-Mashhadani SA. Lactic acid as a new therapeutic peeling agent in melasma. Dermatol Surg. 2005;31:149-54.
19. Sharquie KE, Al-Tikreety MM, Al-Mashhadani SA. Lactic acid chemical peels as a new therapeutic modality in melasma in comparison to Jessner's solution chemical peels. Dermatol Surg. 2006;32:1429-36.
20. Grimes PE. The safety and efficacy of salicylic acid chemical peels in darker-racial ethinic groups. Dermatol Surg. 1999;25;18-22.
21. Lee HS, Kim IH. Salicyclic acid peels for the treatment of acne vulgaris in Asian patients. Dermatol Surg. 2003;29:1196-9.
22. Kodali S, Guevara IL, Carrigan CR, et al. A prospective, randomized, split face, controlled trial of salicylic acid peels in the treatment of melasma in Latin American women. J Am Acad Dermatol. 2010;63(6):1030-5.
23. Bolognia JL, Jorizzo JL, Schaffer JV, et al. Dermatology, 3rd edn. Philadelphia: Elsevier Saunders; 2012.
24. Lawrence N, Cox SE, Brody HJ. Treatment of melasma with Jessner's solution versus glycolic acid: a comparison of clinical efficacy and evaluation of the predictive ability of Wood's light examination. J Am Acad Dermatol. 1997;36: 589-93.
25. Roegnigk RK, Brodland DG. A primer of facial chemical peel. Dermatol Clin 1993:11:349-59.
26. Kumari R, Thappa DM. Comparative study of trichloroacetic acid versus glycolic acid chemical peels in the treatment of melasma. Indian J Dermatol Venereol Leprol. 2010;76: 447.
27. Puri N. Comparative study of 15% TCA peel versus 35% glycolic acid peel for the treatment of melasma. Indian Dermatol Online J. 2012;3(2):109-13.
28. Kalla G, Garg A, Kachhawa D. Chemical peeling-glycolic acid versus trichloroacetic acid in melasma. Indian J Dermatol Venereol Leprol. 2001;67:82-4.
29. Monheit GD. The Jessner's-trichloroacetic acid peels: an enhanced medium depth peel. Dermatol Clin. 1995;13:277-83.
30. Safoury OS, Zaki NM, El Nabarawy EA, et al. A study comparing chemical peeling using modified Jessner's solution and 15% trichloroacetic acid versus 15% trichloroacetic acid in the treatment of melasma. Indian J Dermatol. 2009;54:41-5.
31. Grimes PE. Melasma: etiologic and therapeutic considerations. Arch Dermatol. 1995;131:1453-7.
32. Bulengo-Ransby SM, Griffiths CE, Kimbrough-Green CK, et al. Topical tretinoin (retinoic acid) therapy for hyperpigmented lesions caused by inflammation of the skin in black patients. N Eng J Med. 1993;328(20):1438-43.
33. Callender VD, Narurkar VA, Davis EC. Cosmetic treatments. In: Taylor SC, Badreshia-Bansal S, Callender VD, et al. (Eds). Treatments for Skin of Color. Elsevier Sanders; 2011. pp. 309-47.

43

Cosmetics, Cosmeceuticals and Camouflage for the Treatment of Melasma

Vic A Narurkar

Key Features

- Monotherapy has a limited role in management of melasma.
- Combination therapy with cosmeceuticals and chemical peels works well in treating melasma.
- Cosmetic camouflage can significantly improve the quality of life of the patients.

INTRODUCTION

The treatment of melasma is challenging as it is a fluid condition whose exact pathogenesis is still uncertain, with exaggeration of the condition with UV light, and correlation of the condition to hormonal treatments, photosensitizing agents, autoimmune thyroid disorders and environmental factors. The condition typically affects women, usually during pregnancy or with the use of oral contraceptives, and shows a higher predilection in skin of color. The majority of melasma is centrofacial, with variations of malar and mandibular types, as well as extra facial involvement. First line therapy has generally been limited to the use of topical hydroquinones, alone or in combination with prescription topical retinoids and topical corticosteroids. Over the last few years, advancements in non-hydroquinone agents, chemical peeling and energy based devices have been made. This chapter reviews such advancements, as patients are continually seeking alteranative treatments to topical hydroquinone therapy for melasma.

NON-HYDROQUINONE PRESCRIPTION AGENTS

Table 1 summarizes the classes of various non-hydroquinone formulations which have been reported to be successful in the treatment of melasma. Topical azelaic acid has been reported to be a successful agent, and studies have compared the efficacy of 20% topical azelaic acid with 4% hydroquinone with comparable results.[1,2] Darker skin can be treated safely with this product without concerns of excessive irritation leading to postinflammatory hyperpigmentation. Topical retinoic acid of prescription strength as monotherapy is also an excellent non-hydroquinone option for the treatment of melasma and has been studied in skin of color. Most studies are limited to comparison with vehicle alone and show excellent clearance of melasma.[3,4] One study reported the successful use of adapalene for the treatment of melasma, with higher clearance in patients on adapalene compared to topical tretinoin.[5]

Table 1: Prescription agents for the treatment of melasma
• Hydroquinone (4%)
• Azelaic acid (20%)
• Adapalene
• Tretinoin

COSMECEUTICAL AGENTS

Table 2 summarizes the various cosmeceutical agents which have been reported to be successful in the treatment of melasma. Typical second line treatments for melasma include azelaic acid and kojic acid as monotherapy. Double blind studies of 20% azelaic acid to 4% hydroquinone have shown comparable results in darker skinned patients.[6,7] There are little or no controlled clinical trials in the use of kojic acid, and most reports are anecdotal. Third line therapies for melasma with cosmeceuticals include topical vitamin C, glycolic acid, topical resorcinol and retinoic acid combinations and

Table 2: Non-hydroquinone non-prescription agents useful in the treatment of melasma
• Arbutin
• Ellagic acid
• Kojic acid
• Licorice extract
• Ascorbic acid
• Niacinamide
• Melanozyme
• Soy proteins
• Retinoids
• Resorcinol

melanozyme containing products.[8-10] Most studies are limited to small sample size and therefore should be interpreted with caution.

ENERGY BASED DEVICES

Table 3 summarizes the various energy based devices which have been reported to be successful in the treatment of melasma. Initial reports of intense pulsed light and traditional laser resurfacing[11,12] as options for treatment of melasma later proved to be unsuccessful, with high rates of recurrence and possible exacerbation in darker skin types. Low fluence and low treatment density non-ablative fractional lasers[13,14] are now generally considered the treatment of choice for refractory melasma which has not responded to traditional treatments **(Figs 1A and B)**. Low fluence Q switched 1064 nm laser treatments have also been reported as a safer alternative in darker skin.[15] As a general rule, the majority of studies show that lasers may exacerbate the condition and extra caution should be taken in treatment of darker skin types, with significantly lower energy and treatment density settings **(Figs 2A and D)**.

Table 3: Energy based devices useful in the treatment of melasma
• Intense pulsed light/broadband light sources
• Non-ablative 1,440 nm fractional laser
• Non-ablative 1,540 nm fractional laser
• Non-ablative 1,550 nm fractional laser
• Non-ablative 1,927 nm fractional laser
• Ablative 2,940 nm laser
• Q switched 755 nm laser
• Q switched 1,064 nm laser

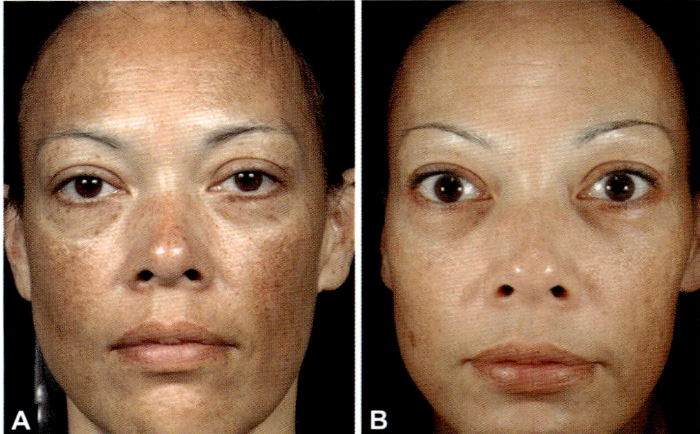

Figs 1A and B: Treatment of melasma with low wattage non-ablative 1,927 nm fractional laser

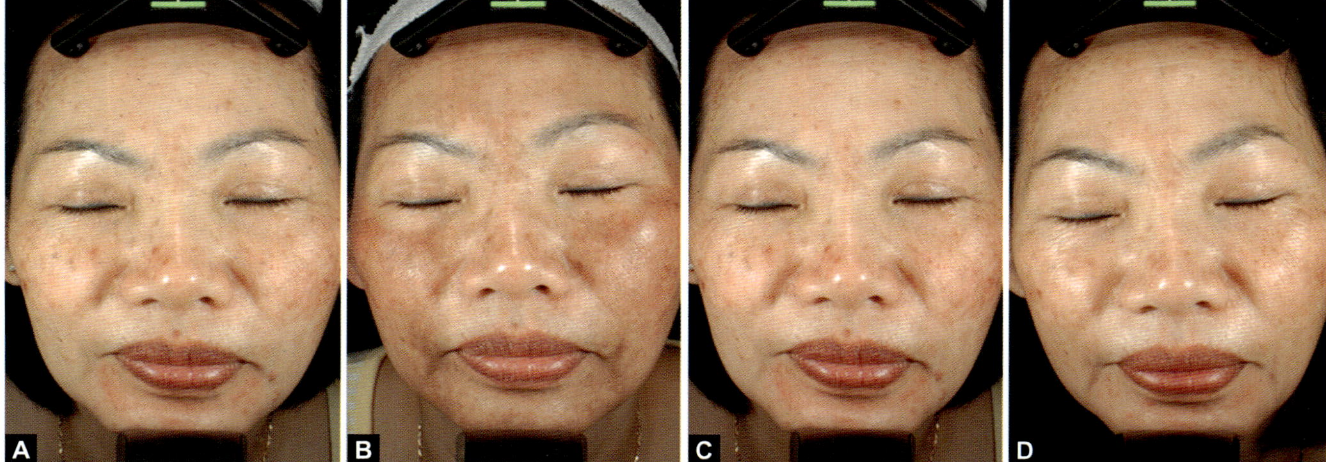

Figs 2A to D: Exacerbation of melasma in skin type V with non-ablative fractional laser and correction with 4% hydroquinone and tretinoin

Table 4: Chemical peels useful in the treatment of melasma
• Glycolic acid peels
• Tretinoin peels
• Jessner's solution
• Trichloroacetic acid peels

CHEMICAL PEELING

Table 4 summarizes the various types of peeling agents which can be used for the treatment of melasma. As with lasers and light sources, extra caution should be utilized when using chemical peeling for melasma, especially in skin of color, as exacerbation and recurrence is quite common. The safest peeling agents are low strength glycolic acid peels of 20%, which can be titrated to higher concentrations based on tissue response. Several studies show the efficacy of these peels in darker skinned individuals.[14,16] Tretinoin peels, alone or in combination with low strength resorcinol are also a safe option for melasma treatment in darker skin. Trichloroacetic acid peels of low concentration may be an option, but extra caution should be used when considering higher concentrations, as there is both a risk of hypopigmentation and hyperpigmentation.

COMBINATION TREATMENTS

While the literature does not have randomized controlled clinical trials on the combination treatment of melasma, most practitioners perform this on a daily basis. The rationale for combination therapies is based on the fact that melasma is a fluid condition and shows a high rate of recurrence. Monotherapies for melasma generally treat melasma in a finite time space. The strategy of combination therapies for melasma involves the use of topical agents to prime the skin prior to any energy based device treatments or chemical peeling as well as treat melasma with topical therapy. Energy based devices and chemical peeling are performed several weeks after starting topical treatments. Thereafter, topical treatments are continued to prevent recurrence. There are several studies that support the use of combination therapies. Comparative evaluation of topical treatments with 2% hydroquinone and 0.025% retinoic acid in combination with glycolic peels achieved the best results than topical treatment or peels alone in Indian patients skin types IV to VI.[15] In one study of skin type III patients, combination treatments with topical ascorbic acid and trichloroacetic acid peel produced better results than either regimen alone.[17] With energy based devices, most of the evidence is anecdotal. Most physicians prime the skin with topical hydroquinone, retinoic acid and cosmeceutical agents prior to non-ablative fractional laser resurfacing for melasma and continue this regimen after treatment. More clinical trials are necessary to prove these results.

CAMOUFLAGE TREATMENTS

Cosmetic camouflage is an effective way to disguise hyperpigmentation resulting from melasma and can also alleviate patient anxiety and distress over the condition. It can also be used during the recovery aspects of treatments of melasma which may lead to temporary hyperpigmentation. Studies have shown that camouflage can improve quality of life for a variety of skin conditions where medical and surgical treatment is challenging. Ideal cosmetic camouflage approaches for melasma necessitate the use of waterproof, non-translucent and long lasting agents, with appropriate color blending and color corrections.

CONCLUSION

Melasma is a very challenging condition that shows a high rate of recurrence. It is particularly challenging in darker skin types, as many modalities of treatment have the potential of exacerbation of the underlying condition. Monotherapy is rarely successful in the treatment of melasma, and most physicians advocate the use of combination therapies. Topical treatments in combination with chemical peeling and energy based devices offer the most effective treatment for melasma. More large scale and double blinded clinical trials of combination therapy of melasma are necessary in the future.

REFERENCES

1. Verallo-Rowell VM, Verallo V, Graupe K, et al. Double blind comparison of azelaic acid and hydroquinone in the treatment of melasma. Acta Derm Venereol Suppl (Stockh). 1989;143:58-61.
2. Balina LM, Graupe K. The treatment of melasma. 20% azelaic acid versus 4% hydroquinone cream. Int J Dermatol. 1991;30(12):893-5.
3. Kimbrough-Green CK, Griffiths CE, Finkel LJ, et al. Topical retinoic acid (tretinoin) for melasma in black patients. A verhicle controlled clinical trial. Arch Dermatol. 1994;130(6):727-33.
4. Griffiths CE, Finkel LJ, Ditre CM, et al. Topical retinoin (retinoic acid) improves melasma. A vehicle controlled, clinical trial. Br J Dermatol. 1993;129(4):415-21.
5. Dogra S, Kanwar AJ, Prasad D. Adapalene in the treatment of melasma: a preliminary report. J Dermatol. 2002;29(8):539-40.
6. Huh C, Seo K, Park J, et al. A randomized, double blind placebo controlled trial of vitamin C iontophoresis in melasma. Dermatology. 2003;206(4):316-20.
7. Negishi K, Kushikata N, Takeuchi K, et al. Photorejuvenation by intense pulsed light with objective measurement of skin color in Japanese patients. Dermatol Surg. 2006;32(11):1380-7.
8. Naito SK. Fractional photothermolysis treatment for resistant melasma in Chinese females. J Cosmet Laser Ther. 2007;9(3):161-3.

9. Rokhsar CK, Fitzpatrick RE. The treatment of melasma with fractional photothermolysis: a pilot study. Dermatol Surg. 2005;31(12):1645-50.
10. Lee HS, Won CH, Lee DH, et al. Treatment of melasma in Asian skin using a fractional 1550 nm laser: an open clinical study. Dermatol Surg. 2009;35(10):1499-504.
11. Kim HS. A split-face comparison of low fluence Q-switched Nd:YAG laser plus 1550 nm fractional laser vs Q switched Nd:YAG monotherapy for facial melasma in Asian skin. J Cosmet Lase Ther. 2013;15(3):143-9.
12. Javaheri SM, Handa S, Kaur I, et al. Safety and efficacy of glycolic acid facial peel in Indian women with melasma. Int J Dermatol. 2001;40(5):354-7.
13. Lim JT, Tham SN. Glycolic acid peels in the treatment of melasma among Asian women. Dermatol Surg. 1997;23(3):177-9.
14. Khunger N, Sarkar R, Jain RK. Tretinoin peels versus glycolic acid peels in the treatment of melasma in dark skinned patients. Dermatol Surg. 2004;30(5):756-60.
15. Garg VK, Sarkar R, Agarwal R. Comparative evaluation of beneficiary effects of priming agents (2% hydroquinone and 0.25% retinoic acid) in the treatment of melasma with glycolic acid peels. Dermatol Surg. 2008;34(8):1032-9.
16. Sarkar R, Kaur C, Bhalla M, et al. The combination of glycolic acid peels with a topical regimen in the treatment of melasma in dark skinned patients: a comparative study. Dermatol Surg. 2002;28(9):828-32.
17. Soliman MM, Ramadan SA, Bassiouny DA, et al. Combined tricholoroacetic acid peel and topical ascorbic acid versus tricholoroacetic acid alone in the treatment of melasma: a comparative study. J Cosmetic Dermatol. 2007;6(2): 89-94.

44

Recent Trends and Future Treatment Paradigms of Melasma Based on Current Understanding of Pathophysiology

Saumya Panda

Key Features

- It is time to move forward from the erstwhile linear, structured, static conception of pathophysiology of melasma to a more fluid and dynamic model that acknowledges the interaction of epidermal keratinocytes and melanocytes with dermal vasculature and fibroblasts.
- A novel management perspective that addresses this conceptual sea change and moves beyond melanocytes as the only therapeutic target is the need of the hour.
- Independent clinical trials of these newer agents with a long follow-up period must take place if melasma patients have to have flare-free lives beyond the triple combination.

INTRODUCTION

Our understanding of the pathophysiology of melasma has undergone a sea change in the past decade. The classic model of the disease was outlined in a landmark paper by Sanchez et al.[1] in 1981. With the aid of Wood's lamp and light microscopy, melasma was classified into three types, based on the location and extent of the abnormal deposits of pigment:

1. Epidermal
2. Dermal
3. Mixed.

With the employment of newer investigative techniques, such as *in vivo* reflectance confocal microscopy (RCM), immunohistochemistry and electron microscopy, the static, linear model of melasma has given way to a conceptual revolution, where melasma is not just about the deposition of melanin and the disposition of melanocytes, but the result of dynamic interaction of melanocytes with diverse cellular elements, viz. keratinocytes, dermal fibroblasts and vascular endothelium. The rigid structural dichotomy of epidermal and dermal melasma is also passe, with current evidence strongly favoring the hypothesis that melasma is the result of complex epidermal-dermal interactions.

The concepts about the traditionally known major etiologic agents, namely sun exposure, female sex hormones, and genetic influences, have also been fine tuned in recent years, making available to us significant new knowledge that should be of major relevance to the management of this condition.

The treatment of melasma remains challenging. The triple combination formula consisting of hydroquinone, tretinoin and topical steroid, devised by Kligman and Willis in 1975[2] remains the gold-standard of melasma therapy despite concern being raised about the safety of this combination in long-term usage. Light-based therapies and numerous cosmeceuticals, mainly botanicals and phytochemicals, have been claimed to improve melasma, but either these promises have been ill-founded, or these treatments have been found to have inherent risk, such as postinflammatory hyperpigmentation, particularly in darker-skinned individuals.

In this chapter, we shall summarize those aspects of our newer understanding of the pathophysiology of melasma that could significant impact upon management of this condition. We shall also delineate developing treatment options as also the changing role of established therapies in the light of these novel advances in basic research. The idea is to provide an understanding of the unfolding changes in the management of melasma in the light of the conceptual evolution.

THE OLD CLASSIFICATION SCHEME IS NOT VALID

The classic classification schema proposed by Sanchez et al.[1] took into account the depth of melanin pigment deposition in melasma. They utilized Wood's lamp for the purpose of depth distinction. However, they themselves acknowledged the limitation of this method in patients of dark complexion, in whom the lesions are frequently not discernible. This was hypothesized to be due to an increased number of melanosomes in the normal skin of these individuals. Wood's lamp actually utilizes the physical phenomenon of Tyndall effect (differential scattering) and thus requires a background of relatively low ambient pigmentation so that the contrast between an area of melanotic pigmentation, like that in melasma, and normally pigmented skin, may be perceived as an intensification of pigmentation.[3] An Indian study borne out this fact when as many as 69.24% (36/52) of the patients had to be classified as indeterminate on Wood's lamp examination, which simply means that no type according the depth could be reliably established in a significant proportion of cases.[4] However, long back it had been established that regardless of skin type, Wood's lamp examination did not help predict treatment outcome, as it did not correlate well enough with histologic types.[5]

The classical classification scheme had assumed great prognostic significance due to the fact that hydroquinone, the gold standard among topical bleaching agents, is a tyrosinase inhibitor that targets melanocytes, and not melanophages. Thus melasma with deeper melanin deposition within dermal melanophages, namely dermal and mixed melasma, became synonymous with bad prognosis.

A recent study has suggested that even histologic classification using single skin biopsy is nonrepresentative.[6] When complete melasma lesions were examined using *in vivo* RCM, it was seen that the topographic distribution of melanophages was highly heterogeneous among and within the different regions. This finding suggested that a reliable classification scheme should be based on the ratio of total epidermal to dermal melanin involving the whole lesional skin, as represented by the melanin index. However, even now therapeutic outcome studies are being reported stratifying the subjects according to the conventional classification scheme.[7]

A Caveat

Much of our novel understanding of the pathophysiology of melasma hinges upon various studies carried out by RCM. Before we attempt to integrate the RCM findings into emerging management models, we should be aware of its main technical limitation, that is narrow thickness of the field of imaging.[8] This inherent technical liability might have biased some of the RCM studies toward stressing melasma more as an epidermal disease than a dermal one. The awareness of this basic technical shortcoming would enable us to take a balanced view of the recent RCM findings vis-à-vis established histopathologic facts about melasma.

IS THERE A TRUE DERMAL MELASMA?

A departure from the conventional histopathologic model of melasma was announced in a 2002 study by Kang et al.[9] They found that dermal melanophages were present in both lesional and perilesional normal-appearing skin in 36% of patients in their series. They also found that there was no statistically significant difference in dermal free melanin in lesional compared to perilesional normal skin. They also found more severe solar elastosis, a greater number of epidermal melanocytes, and significantly increased melanin in all layers of the epidermis. These findings first hinted that there might not be clear cut differentiating features between epidermal and dermal melasma.

Grimes et al.[10] corroborated some of these findings in their study on patients with Fitzpatrick's phototypes IV to VI having epidermal and mixed melasma on Wood's lamp examination. They found that all lesional biopsy specimens had increased melanin in epidermis and dermis, including in those patients having epidermal melasma as per Wood's lamp examination. On Mel-5 staining, there was no increase in the number of melanocytes, but the melanocytes were larger with more prominent dendritic processes. These findings suggested that the patients having epidermal melasma on Wood's lamp examination might have a significant amount of dermal melanin too.

These results suggest that true dermal melasma is probably nonexistent. All melasma are, in essence, mixed. These findings put a serious question mark upon the erstwhile conventional wisdom of attaching prognostic significance to the putative depth of the individual melasma cases, as there is now overwhelming evidence that the conventional notions of alluding depth to the cases of melasma are not valid any more.

ROLE OF EPIDERMAL MELANIN IN MELASMA

Histological studies of melasma over the past decade have consistently shown that the lesional skin demonstrates increased melanin deposition in all layers of the epidermis. The detected increase has varied from 35% in 26 patients of skin types II to V in one study,[6] and 61% in 11 patients of skin types IV to VI in another,[10] to as much as 83% in 56 patients in a Korean study.[9] Furthermore, an interesting paper has shown that a significant number of melasma patients (11/30) display degraded molecules of melanin in the stratum corneum of lesional skin.[11] This finding has been hypothesized to explain the variable success rate of hydroquinone which might not be effective at all against these modified melanin molecules. A recent transcriptomic study in 12 Korean melasma patients has suggested that higher amounts of epidermal melanin are due to activation of melanogenesis in epidermal melanocytes.[12]

These new findings seem to suggest that the true primary histologic target in melasma is the epidermal melanin in the lesional skin. These findings also provide a clue to the lack of efficacy of the long wavelength lasers that primarily target dermal melanin. The crux of the paradox of using lasers in melasma lies in the twin facts of longer wavelengths penetrating deeper to ostensibly target dermal melanin on one hand, and on the other melanin absorption being better with shorter wavelengths.[13] Simply put, most of the light gets absorbed by the increased epidermal melanin in the lesional skin, rendering this technology relatively ineffective. Laser therapy in melasma becomes yet more challenging a proposition considering the discovery of modified melanin molecules in the epidermis, raising the question whether we have the lasers effective against the modified melanin with quite different Raman spectra.

HYPERACTIVE MELANOCYTES

There is upregulation of many genes related with melanin synthesis and melanocyte markers [tyrosinase, *tyrosinase-related protein* (TRP)-1, TRP-2, *microphthalmia-associated transcription factor (*MITF)] in lesional skin of melasma patients.[13] It is still unclear whether there is an increase in the number of melanocytes in melasma. NKI/beteb immunostaining showed an increase in the number of melanocytes in the lesional skin, while Mel-5 and MITF staining did not.[9,10,12] Furthermore, melanocytes in lesional skin were more dendritic, contained more mitochondria, Golgi bodies, and rough endoplasmic reticulum, suggesting that they were more biologically active than their counterparts in normal skin.[9]

Taken together, these findings suggest that heightened biological activity of melanocytes rather than an absolute increase in their number is responsible for hyperpigmentation in melasma. The implication is that agents inhibiting activity of melanocytes rather than only the production of melanin would be effective, at least in a subset of melasma patients, probably those who are resistant to therapy. Thus, agents on the horizon, like 2,5-dimethyl-4-hydroxy-3(2H)-furanone (DMHF), that can inhibit production of MITF and reduce the production of TRP-1, besides inhibiting production of tyrosinase, seem promising in this regard.[14]

However, it is difficult to assess the real promise of these agents for which no published clinical trials are available, in the light of our previous experiences regarding such molecules. A couple of examples will suffice. Tretinoin inhibits TRP-1 and TRP-2, and decreases post-transcriptional levels of tyrosinase and TRP-1 after ultraviolet (UV) B exposure,[15] besides inhibiting tyrosinase transcription.[16] But such *in vitro* evidence of acting upon hyperactive melanocytes does not get translated in clinical trials, where tretinoin requires months to show improvement in monotherapy, irrespective of the skin phototypes of the patients.[17,18] Azelaic acid is another example. Among its many pharmacodynamic properties, azelaic acid appears to have selective effects on hyperactive and abnormal melanocytes.[19] The cytotoxic and antiproliferative effects may be mediated via inhibition of mitochondrial oxidoreductase activity and DNA synthesis in the melanocyte.[20] As a result, cellular mitochondrial respiration and anaerobic glycolysis are inhibited.[21] Azelaic acid may exhibit some inhibitory effect on tyrosinase activity but this action does not appear to be primary by any means.[22] Yet there are clinical trials that maintain that azelaic acid is not better than hydroquinone as a hypopigmenting agent in melasma.[23]

PENDULOUS MELANOCYTES AND SPECTRUM OF RADIATION RESPONSIBLE IN MELASMA

Some melanocytes in melasma show the feature of protrusion from the basement membrane into the upper dermis, and are thus named pendulous melanocytes. These cells are positive on NKI/beteb immunostaining, confirming that these are melanocytes.[6] *In vivo* RCM evaluation showed that 6/25 patients in a series had prominent dendritic melanocytes in the lesional skin, corresponding to pendulous melanocytes seen in histology. The findings suggested that pendulous melanocytes occur in epidermal hypermelanosis displaying hyperactivity of melanocytes.[24]

Matrix metalloproteinase (MMP)-2, but not MMP-9, was significantly upregulated in the lesional skin demonstrating pendulous melanocytes. The MMP-2 overactivity also colocalized with elastotic degeneration. It has been hypothesized that loosening of basement membrane by MMP-2 overexpression may cause the pendulous nature of the melanocytes. A transcriptomic study showed that MMP-2 messenger ribonucleic acid (mRNA) levels were significantly elevated in melasma.[25] The study also showed that α-6 integrin, through which melanocytes bind to basement membrane, or E-cadherin, through which the former bind to keratinocytes, were not overexpressed, suggesting that cellular adhesion, or the lack of it, does not influence the pendulous nature of the melanocytes.

Matrix metalloproteinases induced by UVB irradiation has been suggested to contribute to the destruction of basement membrane *in vivo*.[26] Thus, it has been speculated that chronic sun exposure may increase MMP-2 expression, which loosens the basement membrane in melasma.

High-dose UVA irradiation is also known to induce a shift of melanocytes from the epidermis into the dermis.[27] Thus, it may be hypothesized that the pendulous cells easily drop down on to the dermis or become destroyed by phototrauma, including that caused by lasers. This phenomenon would then be responsible for intense pigmentation in the dermis, resulting in postinflammatory dyschromia.

Recently, it has been shown that although both long wavelength UVA (UVA1) and visible light can induce pigmentation in skin types IV to VI, pigmentation induced by the latter is darker and more sustained. No such pigmentation is observed in skin type II.[28] This gives a clue why treating melasma in darker skin poses a formidable challenge, and also underscores the need for development of filters that protect against visible light. Such ultra-spectral filters (encompassing UVA1, 340–400 nm and visible light, 400–700 nm) are currently not available.

Organic sunscreens usually offer no protection against visible light. Inorganic filters, such as iron oxide, titanium oxide and zinc oxide can offer some visible light protection, and are to an extent useful in treating melasma in darker-skinned individuals. However, the spectral protection of these agents varies according to their particle size, larger particles of titanium dioxide and zinc oxide offering some protection in the visible range.[29] The difference in visible light protection afforded by high sun protection factor (SPF) sunscreens with inorganic agents was illustrated in a recent study that compared two inorganic sunscreens containing titanium dioxide, zinc oxide and iron oxide for their ability to protect against blue light sensitivity induced by aminolevulinic acid application. The sunscreen containing 3.2% iron oxide afforded a protection factor of 22:1 (i.e. the ratio of the lower blue light fluence that induced erythema on sunscreen protected skin to the lower blue light fluence that induced erythema on skin that was unprotected), whereas the sunscreen with a lower concentration of 0.3% iron oxide afforded only a protection factor of 2:1.[30] Studies like this could be our guide to decide which sunscreen to opt for in our melasma patients, as the most recent overarching systemic review on melasma informs us that there is yet to be a single trial of any sunscreen versus placebo in melasma, although in most trials the use of a sunscreen is recommended.[31]

Another interesting recent finding in this regard is that the temperature of human skin can increase to more than 40°C in direct sunlight, following the conversion of absorbed infrared (IR) rays into heat.[32] It has also been demonstrated that heat shock induced the expression of MMP-1 and MMP-3, but not MMP-2 at the mRNA and protein levels in a dose-dependent manner, in cultured normal human skin fibroblasts through activation of extracellular signal-related kinase and c-Jun N-terminal kinase and an autocrine *interleukin*-6 loop.[33] This increased expression of MMPs by heat leads to degradation of extracellular matrix proteins such as collagen (viz. type I procollagen) and elastic fibers (viz. tropoelastin, fibrillin-1). Heat also induces MMP-12, which is capable of destroying the pre-existing elastic fiber network, thereby contributing to the accumulation of elastotic material.[34] Therefore, heat, like UV, is a major environmental stimulus that probably plays an important role in the development of solar elastosis that is one of the major histopathological characteristics of melasma.[9] It has been known since long that chronic IR exposure can cause pronounced elastosis in mouse skin, mimicking the damage caused by UV.[35] Like UV, heat shock generates both H_2O_2 and O_2^-.[36] Heat shock induced O_2^- is responsible for MMP-9 expression, whereas H_2O_2 is involved in the induction of both MMP-1 and -9.[37] In addition to UV radiation, IR plus visible light and the heat energy generated by natural sunlight exposure induce MMP-1 expression after exposing human skin.[38] IR plus visible light also increase MMP-9 expression and decrease type I procollagen synthesis after exposure to natural sunlight.[39]

Thus, not only UV irradiation, but also visible light and heat in the form of IR, are responsible for the molecular and ultrastructural changes brought about by sun exposure in melasma. The effect of heat delivered through the visible part of the spectrum is particularly interesting, because that would render even the ultra-spectral sunscreens including filter for the complete visible spectrum (something that is not available at present, anyway) only partially useful in the treatment and prevention of melasma. The findings also corroborate the importance of habits and activities, like smoking[40] and cooking in the etiology of melasma, which were hitherto always suspected yet did not have a clear explanation.

Furthermore, these findings underscore the need for the development of molecules that go beyond mere tyrosinase inhibition, and are able to reduce and suppress harmful effects of solar radiation (UV, visible light and IR), such as generation of reactive oxygen species, immune responses and induction of apoptosis. Silymarin, derived from milk thistle (*Silybum marianum*), which is a natural polyphenolic flavonoid, and its main constituent silybin (silibinin), demonstrate these properties.[41] In a combined human and animal study, silymarin showed tremendous improvement of melasma in a dose-dependent manner.[42] Similarly, it has been demonstrated that topical application of genistein or N-acetylcysteine can interrupt the UV-signaling cascade.[43]

DEFECTIVE BARRIER FUNCTION IN MELASMA SKIN

In another interesting development, melasma lesional skin was demonstrated to have impaired stratum corneum integrity and delayed barrier recovery rate.[44] Lipid metabolism was identified in this study as one of the most affected biological processes in melasma, and microarray analysis found most of the lipid metabolism-associated genes, such as peroxisome proliferator-activated receptor alpha (PPARA), arachidonate 15-lipoxygenase type B, diacylglycerol O-acyltransferase 2-like 3 and PPAR-gamma coactivator 1-alpha, to be down regulated.

This study puts in perspective earlier clinical findings, viz. statistically significant association of melasma with adult atopics (74/196) and significantly higher MASI score among the latter compared to nonatopics.[45] These findings should also necessitate sufficient caution in incorporating potent topical corticosteroids like mometasone in the triple combination creams,[46] which by virtue of enhanced penetrability in melasma skin compared to normal skin, can readily produce unacceptable side-effects like "topical steroid-dependent face".[47] A tapering regimen of the triple combination cream[48] is justified not only on account of the "relapsing" nature of melasma, but also to counteract the serious issue of topical steroid dependence or addiction,[49] that is more relevant to melasma skin because of the impaired barrier function.

DERMAL-EPIDERMAL INTERACTION AND PARACRINE REGULATION

The relationship between melanocytes and keratinocytes, and the relationship of the latter with melanin biosynthesis, has been known since long, from the time that the epidermal melanin unit was first described in the early 1960s.[50] In the past few years, however, the paracrine linkages among keratinocytes, fibroblasts and melanocytes have been highlighted in the context of UV radiation. In response to UV radiation, human keratinocytes secrete one of the melanogenic cytokines, namely the stem cell factor (SCF).[51] Dermal fibroblasts also secrete SCF; this suggests the possibility that overexpression of these cytokines by the fibroblasts may activate melanocytes in the overlying epidermis.[52] SCF expression in the lesional skin of melasma was demonstrated to be significantly increased around dermal fibroblasts compared to the non-lesional skin.[53] Melasma skin also showed a greater expression of c-kit, the receptor for SCF, in the basal layer of the epidermis.[54] Grichnik et al.[55] revealed some time back that the SCF/c-kit pathway can increase melanocyte number, size, and dendricity when injected into human skin explants. The fibroblast-derived cytokines stimulate the proliferation and melanogenesis of melanocytes in culture.[56] Therefore, there is a possibility that the dermal inflammation induced by accumulation of UV radiation may be associated with activation of fibroblasts, which may result in upregulation of SCF in the dermis of melasma patients leading to increased melanogenesis.[12] CD117 (c-kit) the receptor for SCF, is a receptor tyrosine kinase[57] that is located mainly in the basal layer of the epidermis, associated with keratinocytes, mast cells and melanocytes. The relationship between c-kit and pendulous melanocytes was established when the protrusion of c-kit-positive basal cells into the dermis was evident in 70% of lesional melasma versus that in 29% of perilesional skin.[58] The damage to the basement membrane is mediated through MMPs (MMP-2 and -9) causing the degradation of collagen types IV and VII, besides producing pigmentation.[26] Other than visible light and UV radiation, heat plays its part in MMP-1 expression in keratinocytes through transient receptor potential vanilloid, part of a large family of nonselective cation channels present in keratinocytes.[59]

Classically, increased epidermal melanin in melasma has been reported in the basal/suprabasal cells as pigmentary caps,[1] but later on the increased melanization was noted in all layers of the epidermis,[9] that is in keeping with the recent findings mentioned above. This current outlook is reinforced by recent elucidation of melanosome processing, where pigment globules containing multiple melanosomes were found to be released from various areas of the dendrites of normal melanocytes that were then captured by the microvilli of normal keratinocytes, which incorporated than in a protease-activated receptor-2 (PAR-2)-dependent manner. The melanocytes and keratinocytes demonstrating this efficient transfer mechanism were both obtained from darkly pigmented skin, thus rendering this finding all the more relevant to our clinical perspective.[60]

The identification of c-kit in the melanization process gave rise to attempts to therapeutically target tyrosine kinase, a large subclass of protein kinase that includes tyrosinase and TRP-1. Such attempts gained ground after imatinib mesylate, an ABL protein-tyrosine kinase inhibitor, that inhibits signal transduction mediated by c-kit and platelet-derived growth factor (PDGF) receptors,[61] was found to cause hypopigmentation in the skin.[62] It was postulated that this was due to SCF ligand-binding of tyrosine kinase receptor (KIT) and downstream activation of mitogen-activated protein (MAP) kinase (Erk-2). Microphthalmia (Mi), a basic helix-loop-helix leucine zipper transcription factor, is phosphorylated by MAP kinase at a serine residue (S73). Once phosphorylated, Mi transactivates the tyrosine pigmentation gene promoter and affects pigment production.[63] The enthusiasm was dampened when it was found that tyrosine kinase inhibition with imatinib also results in persistent cutaneous hyperpigmentation.[64] The clinical paradox of imatinib causing both hypo- and hyperpigmentation appears to relate to the simultaneous inhibition of c-kit and PDGF receptors.[65]

Another important development is the finding that soybean trypsin inhibitor (STI), derived from genistein, reversibly inhibits the PAR-2 pathway,[66] recently described as being necessary for melanosome transfer and phagocytosis by keratinocytes in the darker-skinned individuals.[60] It has been additionally demonstrated that STI as well as Bowman-Birk inhibitor (BBI), derived from daidzein, can inhibit both baseline and UVB-induced pigmentation *in vitro*,[67] by the same mechanism of inhibition of keratinocyte phagocytosis of melanosomes. However, as of now, no trials of STI/BBI in melasma are there in the literature.

In a crucial discovery on paracrine regulation of melanogenesis, Western blotting revealed that treatment with phorbol 12-myristate-13-acetate and 4-amino-phenylmercuric acetate (APMA) induced the production of a soluble from of KIT, released from the cell surface of cultured human melanocytes, s-kit that in turn abolishes SCF-induced melanogenesis in human melanocytes.[68] Thus, s-kit functions as a decoy receptor to inhibit the signaling of SCF and its receptor, the membrane-bound KIT (m-KIT).[69] The production of s-kit was increased by the addition of tumor necrosis factor-alpha-converting enzyme, APMA and other MMP activators in both the cultured supernatant of human melanocytes *in vitro* and intact epidermis in a dose-dependent manner, and that s-kit production abolished SCF/m-KIT signaling, resulting in complete inhibition of SCF-induced melanogenesis.[68] This has opened potentially a new vista of development of hypopigmenting agents having a novel mechanism and targets.

Niacinamide and lectins are the other groups of agents that have been shown to reduce skin hyperpigmentation by reversibly inhibiting melanosome transfer to keratinocytes.[70] Unfortunately, there is yet to be a placebo-controlled trial that has employed niacinamide alone in melasma.

ROLE OF VASCULAR ENDOTHELIUM

Recent data showed with factor VIII-related antigen staining that melasma lesions have more vascularization compared to the perilesional normal skin.[71] Increased expression of vascular endothelial growth factor (VEGF) in keratinocytes was suggested as the major angiogenic factor for altered vessels in melasma.[72] Exposure of human skin to UVB as well as near-IR induces dermal angiogenesis and alters the balance between epidermal angiogenic factor (i.e. VEGF) and endogenous angiogenic inhibitor (i.e. TSP-2).[73] This is one more explanation why heat along with sun exposure is now considered to be important in the causation of melasma. It is also shown that there is an increase in inducible nitric oxide synthase expression in melasma lesions, providing another perspective to the pathogenesis of increased vasculature in melasma.[74]

At least one novel molecule has been tried in melasma based on its effect on the vascular characteristics of melasma lesions. This is tranexamic acid (TXA). It is a plasmin inhibitor and a lysine analogue. Plasmin converts extracellular matrix-bound VEGF into freely diffusible forms.[75] Thus TXA suppresses angiogenesis, and also inhibits neovascularization induced by basic fibroblast growth factor (FGF).[76] In addition, TXA can decrease the activity of mast cells, as evidenced by the almost complete abolition of mast cell activation after ischemia and reperfusion injury.[77] Mast cells are related to various histological changes associated with melasma. Repetitive UV irradiation increases the number of mast cells and mast cell tryptase. Tryptase degrades type IV collagen.[78] Thus, increased numbers of mast cells and tryptase might be the cause of weak basement membrane zone and pendulous melanocytes in melasma. Mast cells also play an important role in the development of solar elastosis in melasma. Mast cells can also induce vascular proliferation by secreting various angiogenic factors, viz. VEGF, FGF-2, and transforming growth factor-β.[79] Another mechanism of action for TXA has been suggested whereby in keratinocytes it prevents the binding of plasminogen to keratinocytes, leading to less free arachidonic acid and subsequent decreased production of prostaglandins, which in turn leads to a decrease in tyrosinase activity in melanocytes.[80] A histological evaluation in melasma showed that TXA decreased epidermal pigmentation as well as dermal changes, such as vessel number and increase in mast cells.[81] But no long-term follow-up study is available as yet.

In this regard, it is worth speculating upon the probable effect of tyrosine kinase inhibitors that inhibit c-kit as well as VEGF. Sunitinib is one such oral tyrosine kinase inhibitor that acts upon VEGF receptors, PDGF receptor, c-kit and colony stimulating factor-1 receptor.[82] Vatalanib is another oral protein tyrosine kinase inhibitor, which inhibits all known VEGF receptors, as well as PDGF receptor-β and c-kit but most specifically VEGF receptor-2.[83] However, it is too early to predict whether and what kind of effect these agents might have on pigmentation.

The unraveling of the vascular factors in melasma has given a shot in the arm to various laser and light-based therapies that has now got a target in addition to melanin. For example, the quality-switched neodymium-doped yttrium-aluminum garnet (QS-Nd:YAG) laser, that induces sublethal injury to melanosomes at low dose,[84] also causes subcellular damage to the upper dermal vascular plexus that is one of the pathogenetic factors in melasma.[85] The use of pulsed dye laser (PDL) in melasma is purely based on the theory that vascularization plays an important role in its pathogenesis. Melanocytes express VEGF receptors-1 and -2.[86] Thus PDL purportedly decreases melanocyte stimulation by its antiangiogenic mechanism. However, the use of lasers, of whatever variety, is fraught with the challenge of postinflammatory hyperpigmentation that is particularly persistent and resistant in the darker population. Thus, their use in melasma is problematic in our clinical scenario. The use of lasers in melasma in the deeply pigmented population needs be reviewed afresh in the light of a very recent documentation of formation of new melasma lesions following high-fluence, 1064-nm, QS-Nd:YAG laser in an Asian patient[87] that has conventionally been recommended as a laser of choice in individuals with darker skin tones having pigmentary lesions.[88]

ENDOCRINE CORRELATES OF MELASMA

The fact that melasma has some correlation with the sex hormones simply follows from some demographic details: women are much more affected (90%) than men (10%).[89] Also, melasma occurs in 50–75% of pregnant women,[90] and in 10–25% percent of women taking oral contraceptives.[91] Elevated levels of estrogen, progesterone, and melanocyte stimulating hormone (MSH), especially in the third trimester, have been found in association with melasma.[92] Estradiol increases the levels of melanogenic enzymes, particularly TRP-2, in normal human melanocytes.[93] Additional supporting evidences include the demonstration of increased estrogen receptors (ERs) in lesional skin of melasma[94] and also a statistically significant increase in the expression of α-MSH.[95] Two distinct intracellular ERs (ER-α and ER-β) have been identified that belong to the superfamily of nuclear hormone receptors.[96] Among them, ER-β is the predominant ER in melanocytic lesions.[97] Even in male melasma, the expression of ER-β, and progesterone receptor were slightly increased in the lesional skin compared to the nonlesional skin, though the difference was not statistically significant.[53]

Among the newer agents, TXA is known to decrease α-MSH by virtue of its antiplasmin activity.[98] Another promising agent, DMHF, has been shown to decrease α-MSH-induced melanin content and tyrosinase activity without being cytotoxic.[14]

Strong ER-β expression is seen in human epidermis, with cells situated in the stratum basale and stratum spinosum being more immunoreactive than those in the stratum granulosum, while the stratum corneum is devoid of immunoreactivity. In contrast, there is no specific nuclear staining for ER-α. Strong nuclear staining for ER-β is also seen in the papillary dermis and the blood vessels.[99] A novel selective estrogen receptor modulator[100] acting on the ER-β in the epidermis and dermis would definitely be a boon to, at least, a significant subset of female melasma patients.

DEPIGMENTING AGENTS WITH NOVEL MECHANISMS OF ACTION

Hydroquinone, that had for long borne the mantle of being the gold standard among the bleaching agents, happens to have a shortcoming that is quite well-known. That is the marked lack of effect of hydroquinone at dermal-epidermal junction (DEJ) and dermis. Hydroquinone, that reversibly inhibits tyrosinase, and thus, melanin synthesis, can hardly be expected to have any effect on the dermal pigment, as the origin of that pigment is in the DEJ, and following the capture of that pigment by the dermal macrophages, the turnover of elimination is slow and absolutely insensitive to inhibition of synthesis as dermal macrophages do not synthesize melanin.[101] Thus the search for novel depigmenting agents is always on, agents which would purportedly not depend only on tyrosinase inhibition to achieve the diminution of pigmentation. A few of them will be summarized here:

- *Ascorbic acid:* Decreases pigment by interacting with copper at the active site of tyrosinase and by reducing dopaquinone by blocking dihydrochinindol-2-carboxyl acid oxidation.[102] Disadvantages are that the molecule is rapidly oxidized, and highly unstable.
- *Arbutin/deoxyarbutin:* Inhibits tyrosinase and 5,6-dihydroxyindole-2-carboylic acid polymerase and also inhibits melanosome maturation. Disadvantage is that there is no clinical trial in melasma.
- *Glutathione:* Dose-dependently inhibits melanin synthesis and aggregation by inhibiting the binding between tyrosinase and L-DOPA.[103] Only *in vitro* study has been done.
- *Rucinol:* Inhibits tyrosinase and TRP-1.[104]
- *Oligopeptides (e.g. decapeptide-12):* Melanocytotoxic.[105]
- *Coffeeberry extract:* Protects against UVB-induced pyrimidine dimer formation and inflammation.[106] No clinical trial in melasma has been done.
- *Green tea polyphenols:* Chief active ingredient is epigallocatechin-3-gallate.[107] These have anti-inflammatory and antioxidant properties. There is no *in vivo* clinical study.
- *Gentisic acid:* Smaller esters of gentisic acid inhibit melanogenesis without cytotoxicity and mutagenesis.[108]
- *Hydroxycoumarins:* Strongly inhibits tyrosinase, besides having scavenging and quenching activities.[109]
- *Alpha lipoic acid:* Inhibits dopachrome formation.[110] No *in vivo* trial has been done.
- *Linoleic acid:* Accelerates tyrosinase degradation and stratum corneum turnover.
- *Dioic acid:* Acts as agonist of PPAR, which regulates tyrosinase transcription and melanosome transfer.[111]
- *Lincomycin:* Inhibits melanogenesis post-transcriptionally.
- *Magnolignan:* Decreases maturation of tyrosinase and accelerates its degradation.[112]
- *Antisense oligonucleotides:* Modulate the synthesis of key enzymes of melanogenesis, including tyrosinase, TRP-1 and TRP-2.[113] No clinical trial in melasma has been conducted.

As can be seen, a large majority of these agents have not been tested in a clinical trial on melasma patients. Even those that have been put through trials, the latter have been too short to be of significant value to inform our clinical practice. Considering the natural history of the condition, a systematic review has recommended that clinical trials in melasma should have an intervention period of at least 6 months and there should be long-term follow-up for at least 12 months following the intervention to assess the maintenance of response.[31]

CONCLUSION

The pathogenesis of melasma has now taken a much different shape compared to what it was even two decades back **(Fig. 1)**. In tune with the new advances in the delineation of the pathophysiology of the condition, new directions in the management of the condition have become imperative **(Table 1)**.

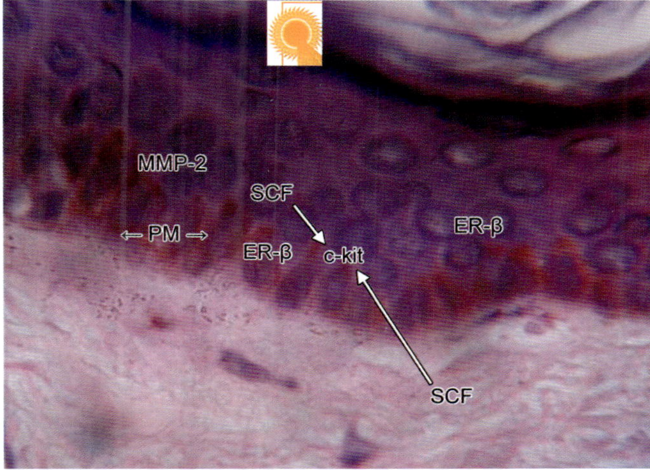

Fig. 1: The current model of pathogenesis of melasma underscoring epidermal-dermal interactions. Note the interaction between stem cell factor (SCF), present mainly in the dermal fibroblasts, but also in smaller amount in the epidermis, with its receptor, c-kit. Upregulation of mediators like matrix metalloproteinase-2 (MMP-2) in response to heat and light leads to formation of pendulous melanocytes (PM), and a series of other cascading effects. The increased presence of estrogen receptor-beta (ER-β) in stratum basale and spinosum also plays its part

Table 1: Newer findings of melasma pathophysiology and concomitant advances in management

Sl. No.	*Current pathophysiologic concept*	*Corresponding management strategy or new molecular development*
1.	The classical classification system of melasma (epidermal/ dermal/mixed) is superseded by novel concept of epidermal dermal interaction	Wood's lamp has no role in classification or prognostication RCM is a valuable tool for assessing melasma lesions
2.	True primary histologic target is epidermal melanin	Current trend of using long-wavelength laser needs be revisited
3.	Stratum corneum contains degraded, modified melanin	Superficial modified melanin with unique Raman spectra is different from ordinary melanin and it is questionable whether pigment lasers can be successfully directed at these chromophores
4.	Hyperactive melanocytes are important in pathogenesis	Agents that inhibit activity of melanocytes rather than the production of melanin would be more useful, e.g. DMHF
5.	Pendulous melanocytes are the source of dermal melanin in melasma	Pendulous cells are destroyed by phototrauma, including that caused by lasers, releasing dermal melanin, and resulting in postinflammatory dyschromia. This is one more reason of not using lasers in melasma
6.	Visible light induces persistent deep hyperpigmentation in skin types IV to VI	Organic sunscreens are not useful in type IV to VI skin. Inorganic filters can offer some visible light protection. No sunscreen at present provides complete visible light protection
7.	Heat (infrared rays) can give rise to molecular changes resulting in melasma	Patients should be advised to quit smoking
8.	Generation of ROS results from ultraviolet signaling cascade	The cascade is inhibited by silymarin, n-acetylcysteine, genistein, etc.
9.	Impaired stratum corneum integrity results in delayed barrier recovery rate in melasma	Triple combination creams should be used as short-term Tapering regimen would be useful Higher concentration of hydroquinone for long period should be avoided too to prevent exogenous ochronosis
10.	Lipid metabolism-associated genes, viz. PPARA, ALOX15B, DGAT2L3 etc. are down regulated	Dioic acid and its congeners are agonists of PPAR
11.	The SCF/c-kit pathway is instrumental for the paracrine linkages among keratinocytes, melanocytes and fibroblasts, mediated by MMPs	C-kit being a receptor tyrosine kinase, inhibitors of tyrosine kinase could be explored for hypopigmenting activity; s-kit, TACE and APMA also abolish SCF/c-kit signaling
12.	PAR-2 dependent melanosome transfer mechanism is relevant in darker skin	Soy protein reversibly inhibits PAR-2
13.	VEGF is responsible for neovascularization in melasma	Tranexamic acid acts in melasma mainly by virtue of its antiangiogenic activity Vascular lasers, like PDL, copper bromide laser, or even QS-Nd:YAG act by virtue of damage to blood vessels
14.	ER-β and α-MSH are increased in lesional skin. Estradiol also increases TRP-2	A novel SERM acting on ER-β in skin could be useful Tranexamic acid and DMHF decrease α-MSH

Abbreviations: RCM, reflectance confocal microscopy; DMHF, 2,5-dimethyl-4-hydroxy-3(2H)-furanone; ROS, reactive oxygen species; PPARA, peroxisome proliferator-activated receptor alpha; ALOX15B, arachidonate 15-lipoxygenase, type B; DGAT2L3, diacylglycerol O-acyltransferase 2-like 3; SCF, stem cell factor; MMP, matrix metalloproteinase; TACE, tumor necrosis factor-alpha-converting enzyme; APMA, 4-aminophenylmercuric acetate; PAR-2, protease-activated receptor-2; VEGF, vascular endothelial growth factor; PDL, pulsed dye laser; QS-Nd:YAG, quality-switched neodymium-doped yttrium-aluminum garnet; ER-β, estrogen receptors beta; α-MSH, alpha melanocyte stimulating hormone; TRP, tyrosinase-related protein; SERM, selective estrogen receptor modulator.

Still, there are quite a few loose ends, missing links and unanswered questions that promise to keep this condition as recidivist as it is now until the time these questions are answered and those loose ends tied up satisfactorily. For example, we are still in the dark why only certain areas of face are selectively more involved than others. What is the exact link between the hormonal receptors and UV-induced cytokines? How far significant, in reality, is the role of the melanophages? How to situate the pendulous melanocytes accurately in the current model of pathophysiology? Is the dermal activity involving fibroblasts and blood vessels a primary event or an epiphenomenon? How far necessary is it to target blood vessels along with melanin and melanocytes?

Despite these uncertainties, it is clear that we should move forward from the erstwhile static, structured, linear model of pathophysiology of melasma to the more fluid and dynamic model that acknowledges the interaction of epidermal keratinocytes and melanocytes with dermal vasculature and fibroblasts. Newer treatment options that address the conceptual sea change and move beyond only targeting the melanocytes should be looked forward to. At the same time, it must be acknowledged that independent clinical trials with a long follow-up period must take place if the patients of melasma hope to have lives beyond the triple combination.

REFERENCES

1. Sanchez NP, Pathak MA, Sato S, et al. Melasma: a clinical, light microscopic, ultrastructural, and immunofluorescence study. J Am Acad Dermatol. 1981;4(6):698-710.
2. Kligman AM, Willis I. A new formula for depigmenting human skin. Arch Dermatol. 1975;111(1):40-8.
3. Panda S. Melasma study: methodological problems. Indian J Dermatol. 2011;56(6):772-3.
4. Panda S. A comparative study of superficial facial peeling with trichloroacetic acid and glycolic acid in the cases of resistant melasma. Unpublished MD dissertation, Ranchi University, Ranchi; 1999. p. 62.
5. Lawrence N, Cox SE, Brody HJ. Treatment of melasma with Jessner's solution versus glycolic acid: a comparison of clinical efficacy and evaluation of the predictive ability of Wood's light examination. J Am Acad Dermatol. 1997;36(4):589-93.
6. Kang HY, Bahadoran P, Suzuki I, et al. *In vivo* reflectance confocal microscopy detects pigmentary changes in melasma at a cellular level resolution. Exp Dermatol. 2010;19(8):e228-33.
7. Wanitphakdeedecha R, Keoprasom N, Eimpunth S, et al. The efficacy in melasma treatment using a 1410 nm fractional photothermolysis laser. J Eur Acad Dermatol Venereol; 2013.
8. Debarbieux S, Depaepe L, Poulalhon N, et al. Reflectance confocal microscopy characteristics of eight cases of pustular eruptions and histopathological correlations. Skin Res Technol. 2013;19(1):e444-52.
9. Kang WH, Yoon KH, Lee ES, et al. Melasma: histopathological characteristics in 56 Korean patients. Br J Dermatol. 2002;146(2):228-37.
10. Grimes PE, Yamada N, Bhawan J. Light microscopic, immunohistochemical, and ultrastructural alterations in patients with melasma. Am J Dermatopathol. 2005;27(2):96-101.
11. Moncada B, Sahagún-Sánchez LK, et al. Molecular structure and concentration of melanin in the stratum corneum of patients with melasma. Photodermatol Photoimmunol Photomed. 2009;25(3):159-60.
12. Kang HY, Ortonne JP. What should be considered in treatment of melasma. Ann Dermatol. 2010;22(4):373-8.
13. Alster TS, Lupton JR. Laser therapy for cutaneous hyperpigmentation and pigmented lesions. Dermatol Ther. 2001;14:46-54.
14. Lee J, Jung E, Lee J, et al. Mechanisms of melanogenesis inhibition by 2,5-dimethyl-4-hydroxy-3(2H)-furanone. Br J Dermatol. 2007;157(2):242-8.
15. Ortonne JP. Retinoid therapy of pigmented disorders. Dermatol Ther. 2006;19(5):280-8.
16. Roméro C, Aberdam E, Lernier C, et al. Retinoic acid as modulator of UVB-induced melanocyte differentiation. Involvement of the melanogenic enzymes expression. J Cell Sci. 1994;107 (Pt 4):1095-103.
17. Griffiths CE, Finkel LJ, Ditre CM, et al. Topical tretinoin (retinoic acid) improves melasma. A vehicle-controlled, clinical trial. Br J Dermatol. 1993;129(4):415-21.
18. Kimbrough-Green CK, Griffiths CE, Finkel LJ, et al. Topical retinoic acid (tretinoin) for melasma in black patients. A vehicle-controlled clinical trial. Arch Dermatol. 1994;130(6):727-33.
19. Fitton A, Goa KL. Azelaic acid. A review of its pharmacological properties and therapeutic efficacy in acne and hyperpigmentary skin disorders. Drugs. 1991;41(5):780-98.
20. Grimes PE. Melasma. Etiologic and therapeutic considerations. Arch Dermatol. 1995;131(12):1453-7.
21. Nazzaro-Porro M. Azelaic acid. J Am Acad Dermatol. 1987; 17(6):1033-41.
22. Breathnach AS. Melanin hyperpigmentation of skin: melasma, topical treatment with azelaic acid, and other therapies. Cutis. 1996;57(1 Suppl):36-45.
23. Piquero Martín J, Rothe de Arocha J, Beniamini Loker D. [Double-blind clinical study of the treatment of melasma with azelaic acid versus hydroquinone]. Med Cutan Ibero Lat Am. 1988;16(6):511-4.
24. Lee DJ, Park KC, Ortonne JP, et al. Pendulous melanocytes: a characteristic feature of melasma and how it may occur. Br J Dermatol. 2012;166(3):684-6.
25. Kang HY, Suzuki I, Lee DJ, et al. Transcriptional profiling shows altered expression of wnt pathway- and lipid metabolism-related genes as well as melanogenesis-related genes in melasma. J Invest Dermatol. 2011;131(8): 1692-700.

26. Inomata S, Matsunaga Y, Amano S, et al. Possible involvement of gelatinases in basement membrane damage and wrinkle formation in chronically ultraviolet B-exposed hairless mouse. J Invest Dermatol. 2003;120(1):128-34.
27. Bacharach-Buhles M, Lubowietzki M, Altmeyer P. Dose-dependent shift of apoptotic and unaltered melanocytes into the dermis after irradiation with UVA 1. Dermatology. 1999;198(1):5-10.
28. Mahmoud BH, Ruvolo E, Hexsel CL, et. al. Impact of long-wavelength UVA and visible light on melanocompetent skin. J Invest Dermatol. 2010;130(8):2092-7.
29. Bissonnette R. Update on sunscreens. Skin Therapy Lett. 2008;13(6):5-7.
30. Bissonnette R, Nigen S, Bolduc C, et al. Protection afforded by sunscreens containing inorganic sunscreening agents against blue light sensitivity induced by aminolevulinic acid. Dermatol Surg. 2008;34(11):1469-76.
31. Rajaratnam R, Halpern J, Salim A, et al. Interventions for melasma. Cochrane Database Syst Rev. 2010;7:CD003583.
32. Lee HS, Lee DH, Cho S, et al. Minimal heating dose: a novel biological unit to measure infrared irradiation. Photodermatol Photoimmunol Photomed. 2006;22(3): 148-52.
33. Park CH, Lee MJ, Ahn J, et al. Heat shock-induced matrix metalloproteinase (MMP)-1 and MMP-3 are mediated through ERK and JNK activation and via an autocrine interleukin-6 loop. J Invest Dermatol. 2004;123(6):1012-9.
34. Chen Z, Seo JY, Kim YK, et al. Heat modulation of tropoelastin, fibrillin-1, and matrix metalloproteinase-12 in human skin *in vivo*. J Invest Dermatol. 2005;124(1):70-8.
35. Kligman LH. Intensification of ultraviolet-induced dermal damage by infrared radiation. Arch Dermatol Res. 1982;272(3-4):229-38.
36. Zhang HJ, Xu L, Drake VJ, et al. Heat-induced liver injury in old rats is associated with exaggerated oxidative stress and altered transcription factor activation. FASEB J. 2003;17(15):2293-5.
37. Shin MH, Moon YJ, Seo JE, et al. Reactive oxygen species produced by NADPH oxidase, xanthine oxidase, and mitochondrial electron transport system mediate heat shock-induced MMP-1 and MMP-9 expression. Free Radic Biol Med. 2008;44(4):635-45.
38. Cho S, Lee MJ, Kim MS, et al. Infrared plus visible light and heat from natural sunlight participate in the expression of MMPs and type I procollagen as well as infiltration of inflammatory cell in human skin *in vivo*. J Dermatol Sci. 2008;50(2):123-33.
39. Cho S, Shin MH, Kim YK, et al. Effects of infrared radiation and heat on human skin aging *in vivo*. J Investig Dermatol Symp Proc. 2009;14(1):15-9.
40. Ertam I, Mutlu B, Unal I, et al. Efficiency of ellagic acid and arbutin in melasma: a randomized, prospective, open-label study. J Dermatol. 2008;35(9):570-4.
41. Kren V, Walterová D. Silybin and silymarin—new effects and applications. Biomed Pap Med Fac Univ Palacky Olomouc Czech Repub. 2005;149(1):29-41.
42. Altaei T. The treatment of melasma by silymarin cream. BMC Dermatol. 2012;12:18.
43. Kang S, Chung JH, Lee JH, et al. Topical N-acetyl cysteine and genistein prevent ultraviolet-light-induced signaling that leads to photoaging in human skin *in vivo*. J Invest Dermatol. 2003;120(5):835-41.
44. Lee DJ, Lee J, Ha J, et al. Defective barrier function in melasma skin. J Eur Acad Dermatol Venereol. 2012;26(12):1533-7.
45. Singh AK, Panda S. Melasma and atopic dermatitis—a significant association? Abstract Book, First South Asian Regional Conference of Dermatology, Kathmandu; 1999.
46. Godse KV, Zawar V. Mometasone menace in melasma. Indian J Dermatol. 2012;57:324-6.
47. Saraswat A, Lahiri K, Chatterjee M, et al. Topical corticosteroid abuse on the face: a prospective, multicenter study of dermatology outpatients. Indian J Dermatol Venereol Leprol. 2011;77(2):160-6.
48. Arellano I, Cestari T, Ocampo-Candiani J, et al. Preventing melasma recurrence: prescribing a maintenance regimen with an effective triple combination cream based on long-standing clinical severity. J Eur Acad Dermatol Venereol. 2012;26(5):611-8.
49. Kligman AM, Frosch PJ. Steroid addiction. Int J Dermatol. 1979;18(1):23-31.
50. Fitzpatrick TB, Breathnach AS. The epidermal melanin unit system. Dermatol Wochenschr. 1963;147:481-9.
51. Hachiya A, Kobayashi A, Ohuchi A, et al. The paracrine role of stem cell factor/c-kit signaling in the activation of human melanocytes in ultraviolet-B-induced pigmentation. J Invest Dermatol. 2001;116(4):578-86.
52. Imokawa G, Yada Y, Morisaki N, et al. Biological characterization of human fibroblast-derived mitogenic factors for human melanocytes. Biochem J. 1998;330(Pt 3): 1235-9.
53. Jang YH, Sim JH, Kang HY, et al. The histopathological characteristics of male melasma: comparison with female melasma and lentigo. J Am Acad Dermatol. 2012;66(4): 642-9.
54. Kang HY, Hwang JS, Lee JY, et al. The dermal stem cell factor and c-kit are overexpressed in melasma. Br J Dermatol. 2006;154(6):1094-9.
55. Grichnik JM, Burch JA, Burchette J, et al. The SCF/KIT pathway plays a critical role in the control of normal human melanocyte homeostasis. J Invest Dermatol. 1998;111(2):233-8.
56. Imokawa G. Autocrine and paracrine regulation of melanocytes in human skin and in pigmentary disorders. Pigment Cell Res. 2004;17(2):96-110.
57. Rönnstrand L. Signal transduction via the stem cell factor receptor /c-kit. Cell Mol Life Sci. 2004;61(19-20):2535-48.

58. Torres-Álvarez B, Mesa-Garza IG, Castanedo-Cázares JP, et al. Histochemical and immunohistochemical study in melasma: evidence of damage in the basal membrane. Am J Dermatopathol. 2011;33(3):291-5.
59. Lee YM, Li WH, Kim YK, et al. Heat-induced MMP-1 expression is mediated by TRPV1 through PKCalpha signaling in HaCaT cells. Exp Dermatol. 2008;17(10):864-70.
60. Ando H, Niki Y, Ito M, et al. Melanosomes are transferred from melanocytes to keratinocytes through the processes of packaging, release, uptake, and dispersion. J Invest Dermatol. 2012;132(4):1222-9.
61. Buchdunger E, Cioffi CL, Law N, et al. Abl protein-tyrosine kinase inhibitor STI571 inhibits *in vitro* signal transduction mediated by c-kit and platelet-derived growth factor receptors. J Pharmacol Exp Ther. 2000;295(1):139-45.
62. Tsao AS, Kantarjian H, Cortes J, et al. Imatinib mesylate causes hypopigmentation in the skin. Cancer. 2003;98(11):2483-7.
63. Hemesath TJ, Price ER, Takemoto C, et al. MAP kinase links the transcription factor Microphthalmia to c-Kit signalling in melanocytes. Nature. 1998;391(6664):298-301.
64. Alexandrescu DT, Dasanu CA, Farzanmehr H, et al. Persistent cutaneous hyperpigmentation after tyrosine kinase inhibition with imatinib for GIST. Dermatol Online J. 2008;14(7):7.
65. Valeyrie L, Bastuji-Garin S, Revuz J, et al. Adverse cutaneous reactions to imatinib (STI571) in Philadelphia chromosome-positive leukemias: a prospective study of 54 patients. J Am Acad Dermatol. 2003;48(2):201-6.
66. Rendon M, Berneburg M, Arellano I, et al. Treatment of melasma. J Am Acad Dermatol. 2006;54:S272-81.
67. Prime C, Sharlow E, Liebel F, et al. An alternative approach to depigmentation by soybean extracts via inhibition of the PAR-2 pathway. J Invest Dermatol. 2001;116:587-95.
68. Kasamatsu S, Hachiya A, Higuchi K, et al. Production of the soluble form of KIT, s-KIT, abolishes stem cell factor-induced melanogenesis in human melanocytes. J Invest Dermatol. 2008;128(7):1763-72.
69. Dahlen DD, Lin NL, Liu YC, et al. Soluble kit receptor blocks stem cell factor bioactivity *in vitro*. Leuk Res. 2001;25(5):413-21.
70. Greatens A, Hakozaki T, Koshoffer A, et al. Effective inhibition of melanosome transfer to keratinocytes by lectins and niacinamide is reversible. Exp Dermatol. 2005;14(7):498-508.
71. Kim Eh, Kim YC, Lee ES, et al. The vascular characteristics of melasma. J Dermatol Sci. 2007;46(2):111-6.
72. Kim EJ, Park HY, Yaar M, et al. Modulation of vascular endothelial growth factor receptors in melanocytes. Exp Dermatol. 2005;14(8):625-33.
73. Kim MS, Kim YK, Cho KH, et al. Infrared exposure induces an angiogenic switch in human skin that is partially mediated by heat. Br J Dermatol. 2006;155(6):1131-8.
74. Jo Hy, Kim CK, Suh IB, et al. Co-localization of inducible nitric oxide synthase and phosphorylated Akt in the lesional skins of patients with melasma. J Dermatol. 2009;36(1):10-6.
75. Ferrara N. Binding to the extracellular matrix and proteolytic processing: two key mechanisms regulating vascular endothelial growth factor action. Mol Biol Cell. 2010;21(5):687-90.
76. Bastaki M, Nelli EE, Dell'Era P, et al. Basic fibroblast growth factor induced angiogenic phenotype in mouse endothelium. A study of aortic and microvascular endothelial cell lines. Arterioscler Thromb Vasc Biol. 1997;17(3):454-64.
77. Reichel CA, Lerchenberger M, Uhl B, et al. Plasmin inhibitors prevent leukocyte accumulation and remodeling events in the postischemic microvasculature. PLoS One. 2011;6(2):e17229.
78. Iddamalgoda A, Le QT, Ito K, et al. Mast cell tryptase and photoaging: possible involvement in the degradation of extra cellular matrix and basement membrane proteins. Arch Dermatol Res. 2008;300(Suppl 1):S69-76.
79. Crivellato E, Nico B, Ribatti D. Mast cells and tumour angiogenesis: new insight from experimental carcinogenesis. Cancer Lett. 2008;269(1):1-6.
80. Sheth VM, Pandya AG. Melasma: a comprehensive update. Part II. J Am Acad Dermatol. 2011;65:699-714.
81. Na JI, Choi SY, Yang SH, et al. Effect of tranexamic acid on melasma: a clinical trial with histological evaluation. J Eur Acad Dermatol Venereol. 2013;27(8):1035-9.
82. Burstein HJ, Elias AD, Rugo HS, et al. Phase II study of sunitinib malate, an oral multitargeted tyrosine kinase inhibitor, in patients with metastatic breast cancer previously treated with an anthracycline and a taxane. J Clin Oncol. 2008;26:1810-6.
83. Wood JM, Bold G, Buchdunger E, et al. PTK787/ZK 222584, a novel and potent inhibitor of vascular endothelial growth factor receptor tyrosine kinases, impairs vascular endothelial growth factor-induced responses and tumor growth after oral administration. Cancer Res. 2000;60(8):2178-89.
84. Lee MW. Combination 532-nm and 1064-nm lasers for noninvasive skin rejuvenation and toning. Arch Dermatol. 2003;139(10):1265-76.
85. Arora P, Sarkar R, Garg VK, et al. Lasers for treatment of melasma and post-inflammatory hyperpigmentation. J Cut Aesthet Surg. 2012;5(2):93-103.
86. Plonka PM, Passeron T, Brenner M, et al. What are melanocytes really doing all day long......? Exp Dermatol. 2009;18(9):799-819.
87. Lee WJ, Kim YJ, Noh TK, et al. Formation of new melasma lesions in the periorbital area following high fluence, 1064-nm, Q-switched Nd/YAG laser. J Cosmet Laser Ther. 2013;15(3):163-5.
88. Goldberg DJ. Laser treatment of pigmented lesions. Dermatol Clin. 1997;15(3):397-407.

89. Guevara IL, Pandya AG. Safety and efficacy of 4% hydroquinone combined with 10% glycolic acid, antioxidants, and sunscreen in the treatment of melasma. Int J Dermatol. 2003;42(12):966-72.
90. Wong RC, Ellis CN. Physiologic skin changes in pregnancy. J Am Acad Dermatol. 1984;10(6):929-40.
91. Moin A, Jabery Z, Fallah N. Prevalence and awareness of melasma during pregnancy. Int J Dermatol. 2006;45(3):285-8.
92. Pérez M, Sánchez JL, Aguiló F. Endocrinologic profile of patients with idiopathic melasma. J Invest Dermatol. 1983;81(6):543-5.
93. Kippenberger S, Loitsch S, Solano F, et al. Quantification of tyrosinase, TRP-1, and Trp-2 transcripts in human melanocytes by reverse transcriptase-competitive multiplex PCR—regulation by steroid hormones. J Invest Dermatol. 1998;110(4):364-7.
94. Lieberman R, Moy L. Estrogen receptor expression in melasma: results from facial skin of affected patients. J Drugs Dermatol. 2008;7(5):463-5.
95. Im S, Kim J, On WY, et al. Increased expression of alpha-melanocyte-stimulating hormone in the lesional skin of melasma. Br J Dermatol. 2002;146(1):165-7.
96. Verdier-Sévrain S, Bonté F, Gilchrest B. Biology of estrogens in skin: implications for skin aging. Exp Dermatol. 2006; 15(2):83-94.
97. Schmidt AN, Nanney LB, Boyd AS, et al. Oestrogen receptor-beta expression in melanocytic lesions. Exp Dermatol. 2006;15(12):971-80.
98. Sarkar R, Chugh S, Garg VK. Newer and upcoming therapies for melasma. Indian J Dermatol Venereol Leprol. 2012;78(4):417-28.
99. Thornton MJ. The biological actions of estrogens on skin. Exp Dermatol. 2002;11(6):487-502.
100. Saudagar RB, Dighe NS, Musmade DS, et al. SERMs in treatment of breast cancer. Asian J Pharm Res. 2011;1:81-6.
101. Ardigo M, Cameli N, Berardesca E, et al. Characterization and evaluation of pigment distribution and response to therapy in melasma using *in vivo* reflectance confocal microscopy: a preliminary study. J Eur Acad Dermatol Venereol. 2010;24(11):1296-303.
102. Draelos ZD. Skin lightening preparations and the hydroquinone controversy. Dermatol Ther. 2007;20(5):308-13.
103. Matsuki M, Watanabe T, Ogasawara A, et al. [Inhibitory mechanism of melanin synthesis by glutathione]. Yakugaku Zasshi. 2008;128(8):1203-7.
104. Kim DS, Kim SY, Park SH, et al. Inhibitory effects of 4-n-butylresorcinol on tyrosinase activity and melanin synthesis. Biol Pharm Bull. 2005;28(12):2216-9.
105. Abu Ubeid A, Zhao L, Wang Y, et al. Short-sequence oligopeptides with inhibitory activity against mushroom and human tyrosinase. J Invest Dermatol. 2009;129(9): 2242-9.
106. Leyden JJ, Shergill B, Micali G, et al. Natural options for the management of hyperpigmentation. J Eur Acad Dermatol Venereol. 2011;25(10):1140-5.
107. Katiyar SK, Ahmad N, Mukhtar H. Green tea and skin. Arch Dermatol. 2000;136(8):989-94.
108. Curto EV, Kwong C, Hermersdörfer H, et al. Inhibitors of mammalian melanocyte tyrosinase: *in vitro* comparisons of alkyl esters of gentisic acid with other putative inhibitors. Biochem Pharmacol. 1999;57(6):663-72.
109. Yamamura T, Onishi J, Nishiyama T. Antimelanogenic activity of hydrocoumarins in cultured normal human melanocytes by stimulating intracellular glutathione synthesis. Arch Dermatol Res. 2002;294(8):349-54.
110. Tsuji-Naito K, Hatani K, Okada K. Modulating effects of a novel skin lightening agent, alpha-lipoic acid derivative, on melanin production by the formation of DOPA conjugate products. Bioorg Med Chem. 2007;15(5):1967-75.
111. Wiechers JW, Rawlings AV, Garcia C, et al. A new mechanism of action for skin whitening agents: binding to the peroxisome proliferator-activated receptor. Int J Cosmet Sci. 2005;27(2):123-32.
112. Nakamura K, Yoshida M, Uchiwa H, et al. Down-regulation of melanin synthesis by a biphenyl derivative and its mechanism. Pigment Cell Res. 2003;16(5):494-500.
113. Lazou K, Sadick NS, Kurfurst R, et al. The use of antisense strategy to modulate human melanogenesis. J Drugs Dermatol. 2007;6(6 Suppl):s2-7.

45

Exogenous Ochronosis

Vijay Zawar, SK Tan

Key Features

- Clinicians must be aware of exogenous ochronosis (EO) as it could be missed be easily by those ignorant of this condition.
- Avoid using hydroquinone (HQ) for long time and in concentrations higher than 2%. Sun protection is mandatory.
- Therapeutic success in established cases of EO is not certain. It is, therefore, important to recognize in time to stop further progress.

INTRODUCTION

The Term

Ochre = Old French *ocre,* from Latin *ōchra,* from Greek *ōkhra,* from *ōkhros* pale yellow late 14c. As a color name, "brownish-yellow"

(*Source:* Online Etymology Dictionary, © 2010 Douglas Harper)

Definition

Ochronosis refers to a clinical condition of blue-gray-black shades or their combination of pigmentation, which histologically represents yellow-brown deposits in the dermis.

Ochronosis could be endogenous or exogenous. Endogenous ochronosis also known as alkaptonuria, is the inborn error of metabolism, autosomal recessive, causing cutaneous pigmentation due to deficiency of the enzyme homogentisate 1, 2-dioxygenase. It was first described by Garrod[1] in 1902. It refers to the deposition of polymerized homogentisic acid (HGA; 2, 5-dihydroxyphenylacetic acid) as a grossly blue-black pigment in all collagen-containing structures.[2] Apart from cutaneous pigmentation, it often involves musculoskeletal system, ocular pigmentation, calculi in genitourinary system and cardiac disease.

Exogenous ochronosis is an acquired pigmentary disorder simulating endogenous ochronosis clinically and histologically, albeit without systemic manifestations. It manifests as tissue deposition of microscopic, ochre-colored pigment in the dermis, imparting a blue-black hue to the skin **(Fig. 1)**.[3] It frequently involves face and neck.

The condition has been most commonly reported following the topical application of HQ,[4-6] but can occasionally occur from exposure to various substances such as phenol, trinitrophenol, resorcinol, mercury, picric acid, benzene, and systemic treatment with antimalarials and L-3,4-dihydroxyphenylalanine (L-DOPA).[7-10]

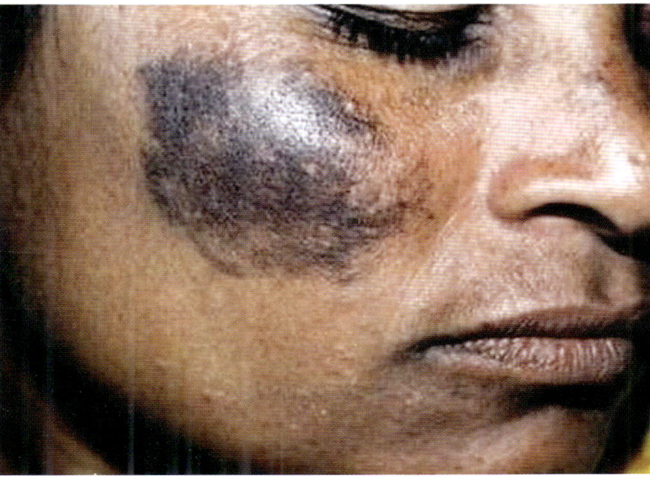

Fig. 1: Prolonged unsupervised hydroquinone application for melasma in a woman without adequate sun protection resulted into progressive blue-black pigmentation

In its early stages, it often mimics melasma hyperchromia, especially in fairer skin-type III and IV patients.[11,12]

HISTORICAL ASPECTS

- *Beddard and Plumtre (1902):* Exogenous ochronosis in a patient that used phenol on a leg ulcer[13]
- *Woolley (1952):* Exogenous ochronosis due to the application of carbolic acid compresses[14]
- *Findlay (1975):* Who several south African patients following HQ application,[15] who developed ochronosis and "colloid mili" gradually after a few years of HQ use
- Subsequent reports were mainly from South Africa and it was thought that this condition was confined to dark-skinned individuals, who used high concentrations of HQ.[16-26]

EPIDEMIOLOGICAL ASPECTS

Several reports of this condition were published in recent times involving patients apart from Africans and Americans of African descent were hailing from Brazil,[25,26] Puerto Rico,[27] Spain,[28] Bulgaria,[28] India,[4] Thailand[29] and Singapore,[6,11,12] indicating that EO may occur across a wide spectrum of skin-types, from type II or III[28] to type V,[4] and is not limited to only to the darker skin-types.

Thus, geographical and ethnic data indicate that EO is not exclusively limited to the darker skin races. Misdiagnosis in early stages or gross under-reporting was likely. Confirmed diagnosis requires skin biopsies and that may have resulted in under-reporting.

PREDISPOSING FACTORS

Hull and Procter[30] reported that, in addition to HQ use, the presence of viable melanocytes and sun-exposure were necessary factors. They reported a case of EO developing in a patient in areas of normal skin but not in adjacent vitiliginous skin where melanocytes were absent.

It was earlier believed that EO developed mainly in patients who had used HQ in high concentrations or in products mixed with other compounds, which enhanced its absorption. Findlay[15] reported that his series of patients used strong HQ-containing creams continuously for several (up to 8) years, and developed the dermatosis gradually over 6 months to 3 years or longer. This view has been also observed by many other authors.[20,21,30-38]

However, other reports state that the condition may develop even with low concentrations of HQ, and even in those who have used the product for relatively short periods. This suggests that our knowledge of the pathogenesis of EO is still incomplete and there could exist different aggravating factors and an individual susceptibility for development of EO too.[31-36]

CLINICAL FEATURES AND STAGING

Dogliotti[40] in 1979, classified EO into three clinical stages:

1. Erythema and mild hyperpigmentation **(Fig. 2)**
2. Hyperpigmentation, pigmented colloid milium (caviar-like lesions) and atrophy **(Fig. 3)**
3. Papulonodular lesions **(Fig. 4)**.

Hardwick et al.[19] graded the condition into five grades, based on the severity of the condition. It should be noted

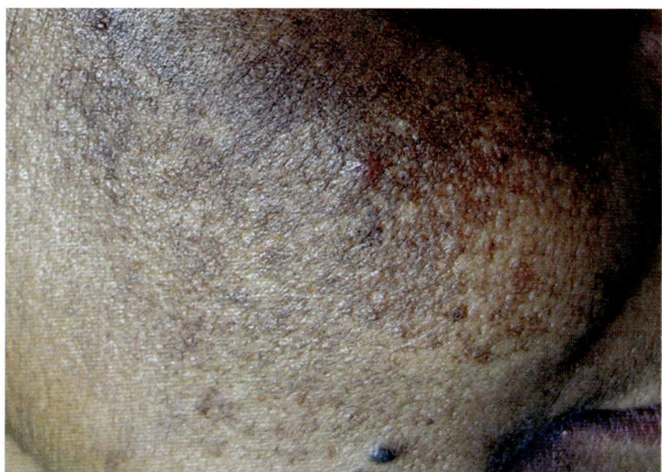

Fig. 2: Melasma with early exogenous ochronosis (Dogliotti's stage I)

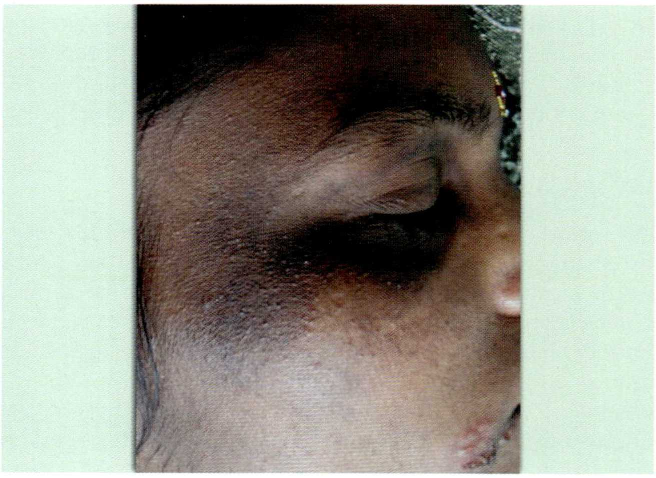

Fig. 3: Colloid milia in a case of advanced exogenous ochronosis (Dogliotti's stage II)

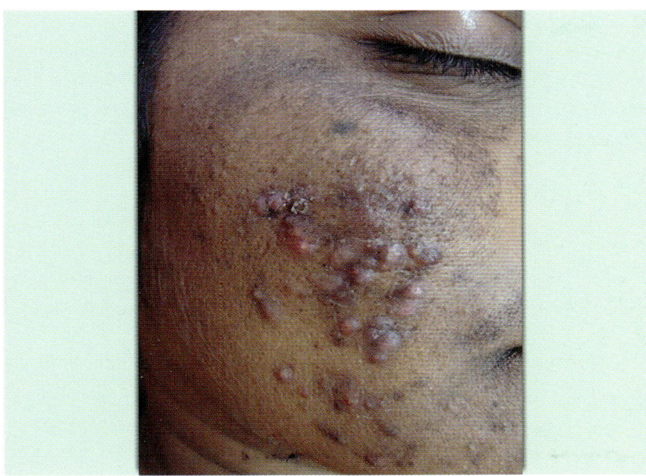

Fig. 4: Papulonodular lesions in a case of advanced exogenous ochronosis (Dogliotti's stage III)

that Hardwick's series was based only on clinical diagnosis whereas Dogliotti had histopathological confirmation from biopsies taken from the patients.

Phillips et al.[31] graded the condition into mild, moderate and severe in a large series of 395 cases.

Several reports and textbooks described the condition under different headings as "blue-black or slate-gray hyperpigmentation", "darkening and coarsening of the skin, followed by a hyperpigmented papular condition", and "mild ochronosis is characterized clinically by coarsening and darkening of the skin; severe ochronosis, by coalescing, caviar-like black papules and atrophy". "Coarsening of skin texture by the appearance of many tiny papules which gradually enlarge to coalescent pitch-black caviar-like excrescences" **(Figs 5A and B)**.[30-38]

Diagnostic doubts arise when EO presents in the early stages—in ethnic Chinese Asians it is easily mistaken for melasma[6,11,12] and often further treated with HQ-containing products, sometimes in increasing concentrations, aggravating the condition.

In differentiating EO from melasma, one of the features we noticed fairly consistently in some patients was "speckling" in EO as opposed to a more diffuse light brown hyperchromia in melasma. This "speckling" probably corresponds to the minute black papules that were just discernible on close inspection described as "mild EO" by Phillips et al.[31]

DIAGNOSIS

An attempt should be made in every suspected case of ochronosis to rule out the intrinsic cause (i.e. alkaptonuria) by a simple urine test, if other sophisticated laboratory support for analysis of homogentisic acid oxidase (HGAO) levels in blood is unavailable.

Current techniques in use include Wood's lamp (ultraviolet) examination and photography, which have not been very reliable[4,6,11,12] in differentiating melasma from EO. Dermatoscopy has shown to be of some value in some studies.[25,39,41]

Histopathological examination of skin biopsy is the gold standard to diagnose EO by virtue of seeing ochre-colored, banana-shaped, cavalier like deposits in the dermis due to degenerated collagen fibers. However, every suspected patient may not be willing to undergo facial skin biopsy. The pathognomonic histological feature appears to be the presence of "ochre-colored and banana-shaped fibers"—this finding is universal in all published reports **(Fig. 6)**.[31-40]

The most recent reports describe reflectance confocal microscopy (RCM)[42] as an important tool in making diagnosis by non-invasive method, which, however, is not available at every physician's office.

Reflectance confocal microscopy features described by Gil et al.[42] included a normal honeycombed epidermal pattern, with typical refractile basal cells corresponding to physiologic hyperpigmentation of the basal layer at the

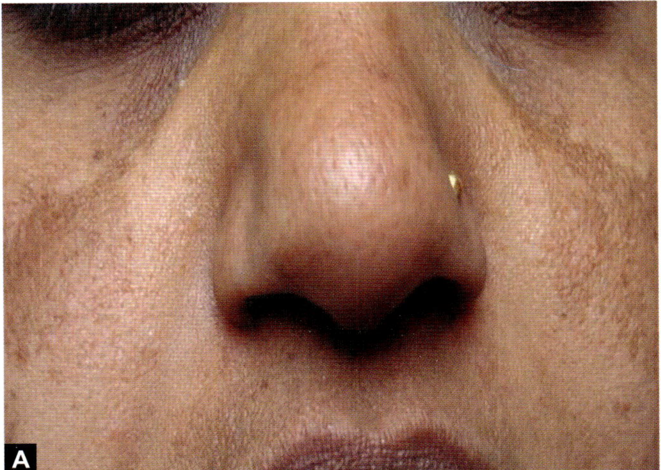

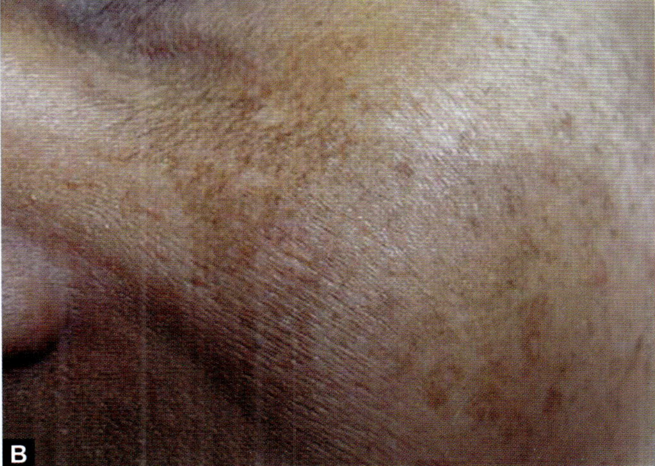

Figs 5A and B: (A) Coarse-speckled pigmentation in a patient with melasma. This should arouse a suspicion of exogenous ochronosis; (B) A close view of the same patient. Caviar-like pigmented papules are also seen

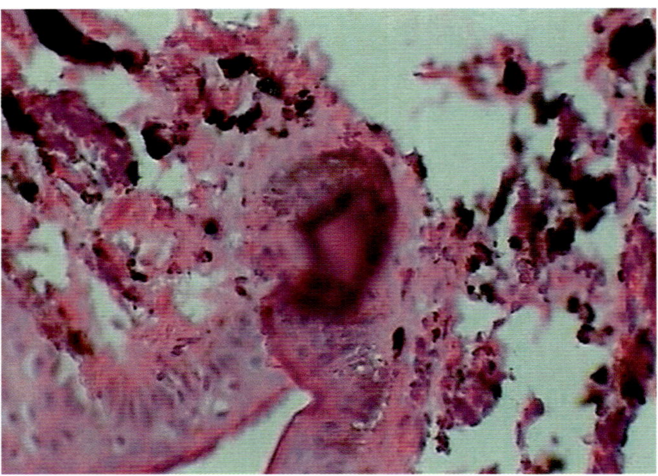

Fig. 6: Histological study revealed in the same patient the classical ochre-colored banana-shaped bodies in dermis. This was possibly the first confirmed case in India and was published in J Cosmet Dermatol in 2004

dermoepidermal level. At the dermal level, there were widespread hyporefractile oval to banana-shaped spaces that corresponded to the banana-shaped bodies observed on histologic sections. Although these features were from a single patient in the study and unconfirmed by other studies, it is a foundation on which other future studies may be based. An interesting association of sarcoidosis has been described in background of EO.[43]

TREATMENT OF EXOGENOUS OCHRONOSIS

Treatment of EO is challenging and often disappointing. The most important initial step is immediate cessation of HQ use upon confirming the diagnosis. Early EO, mimicking mild melasma, may not be a major cosmetic problem and is best left alone after stopping HQ therapy. Further treatment of the existing melasma, if required, would require non-HQ based skin-lighteners. Moderate-to-severe cases of EO are cosmetically disfiguring and patients often request treatment. Various modalities of treatment have been described, including chemical peels, dermabrasion and CO_2 laser resurfacing,[43,44] although the results have not been very consistent and encouraging. Q-switched neodymium-doped yttrium aluminum garnet laser utilizing a collimated handpiece with large spot sizes and low fluence may show promising results.[12] This may also treat underlying melasma.[45-48] However, more work needs to be carried out to confirm the efficacy of such treatments.

The United States Food and Drug Administration (US FDA) now proposes that skin bleaching drug products should not be available OTC. FDA also suspected carcinogenic potential of HQ being used in various skin bleaching products for long-term. Therefore, it recommends sell of HQ restricted to prescription of registered medical practitioners only and also recommends close medical supervision in patients receiving HQ.[49-51]

REFERENCES

1. Garrod AE. The incidence of alkaptonuria: a study in chemical individuality. 1902 [classical article]. Yale J Biol Med. 2002;75(4):221-31.
2. O'Brien WM. Biochemical, pathologic and clinical aspects of alkaptonuria, ochronosis and ochronotic arthropathy. Am J Med. 1963;34:813-9.
3. Dubin DB, Barba AR, Sober AJ. Drug-induced or-related pigmentation-Ochronosis. In: Nordlund JJ, Boissy RE, Hearing VJ, King RA, Ortonne JP (Eds). The Pigmentary System. Physiology and Pathophysiology, 1st edn. Oxford: Oxford University Press; 1998. pp. 924-5.
4. Zawar V, Mhaskar ST. Exogenous ochronosis following hydroquinone for melasma. J Cosmet Dermatol. 2004;3(4):234-6.
5. Westerhof W, Kooyers TJ. Hydroquinone and its analogues in dermatology: a potential health risk. J Cosmet Dermatol. 2005;4(2):55-9.
6. Tan SK, Sim CS, Goh CL. Hydroquinone-induced exogenous ochronosis in Chinese—two case reports and a review. Int J Dermatol. 2008;47(6):639-40.
7. Rausing A, Rosen U. Black cartilage after therapy with levodopa and methyldopa. Arch Pathol Lab Med. 1994; 118(5):531-5.
8. Kaufmann B, Wegmann W. Exogenous ochronosis after L-dopa treatment. Pathologe. 1992;13(3):164-6.
9. Bruce S, Tschen JA, Chow D. Exogenous ochronosis resulting from quinine injections. J Am Acad Dermatol. 1986;15(2 Pt 2):357-61.
10. Thomas AE, Gisburn MA. Exogenous ochronosis and myxoedema from resorcinol. Br J Dermatol. 1961;73:378-81.
11. Tan SK. Exogenous Ochronosis—a Diagnostic Challenge. J Cosmet Dermatol. 2010;9(4):313-7.
12. Tan SK. Exogenous ochronosis in ethnic Chinese Asians: a clinicopathological study, diagnosis and treatment. J Eur Acad Dermatol Venereol. 2011;25(7):842-50.
13. Beddard AP, Plumtre CM. A further note on ochronosis associated with carboluria. Q S Med 1912;5:505-7.
14. Woolley PB. Exogenous ochronosis. Br Med J. 1952;2(4787): 760-1.
15. Findlay GH, Morrison JG, Simson IW. Exogenous ochronosis and pigmented colloid milium from hydroquinone bleaching creams. Br J Dermatol. 1975;93(6):613-22.
16. Findlay GH, De Beer HA. Chronic hydroquinone poisoning of the skin from skin-lightening cosmetics. A South African epidemics of ochronosis of the face in dark-skinned individuals. S Afr Med J. 1980;57(6):187-90.

17. Tidman MJ, Horton JJ, MacDonald DM. Hydroquinone-induced ochronosis—light and electron microscopic features. Clin Exp Dermatol. 1986;11(3):224-8.
18. Connor T, Braunstein B. Hyperpigmentation following the use of bleaching creams. Localized exogenous ochronosis. Arch Dermatol. 1987;123(1):105-6,108.
19. Hardwick N, Van Gelder LW, Van der Merwe CA, et al. Exogenous ochronosis: an epidemiological study. Br J Dermatol. 1989;120(2):229-38.
20. Burke PA, Maibach H. Exogenous ochronosis: an overview. J Dermatol Treatment. 1997;8:21-6.
21. Levin CY, Maibach H. Exogenous ochronosis. An update on clinical features, causative agents and treatment options. Am J Clin Dermatol. 2001;2(4):213-7.
22. Mahé A, Ly F, Aymard G, et al. Skin diseases associated with the cosmetic use of bleaching products in women from Dakar, Senegal. Br J Dermatol. 2003;148(3):493-500.
23. Olumide YM, Akinkugbe AO, Altraide D, et al. Complications of chronic use of skin-lightening cosmetics. Int J Dermatol. 2008;47(4):344-53.
24. Petit A, Cohen-Ludman C, Clevenbergh P, et al. Skin lightening and its complications among African people living in Paris. J Am Acad Dermatol. 2006;55(5):873-8.
25. Charlín R, Barcaui CB, Kac BK, et al. Hydroquinone-induced exogenous ochronosis: a report of four cases and usefulness of dermascopy. Int J Dermatol. 2008;47(1):19-23.
26. Ribas J, Scettini AP, Cavalcante Mde S. Exogenous ochronosis hydroquinone induced: a report of four cases. An Bras Dermatol. 2010;85(5):699-703.
27. Martín RF, Sánchez JL, González A, et al. Exogenous ochronosis. P R Health Sci J. 1992;11(1):23-6.
28. Kadurina M, Dimitrov B, Tonev S. Hydroquinone-induced exogenous ochronosis. Journal of Plastic Dermatology. 2009;5(2):197-201.
29. Kullavanijaya P, Ophaswongse S, Silprachawong S. Exogenous ochronosis and pigmented colloid milium induced by bleaching skin cream. Environ Dermatol. 1998;5(1):20-5.
30. Hull PR, Procter PR. The melanocyte: an essential link in hydroquinone-induced ochronosis. J Am Acad Dematol. 1990;22(3):529-31.
31. Phillips JI, Isaacson C, Carman H. Ochronosis in black South Africans who used skin lighteners. Am J Dermatopathol. 1986;8(1):14-21.
32. Howard I. Maibach. Pigmentary disorders from exogenous causes. In: Levine N (Ed). Pigmentation and Pigmentary Disorders, 1st edn. Boca Raton: CRC Press;1993. pp. 417-38.
33. Jordaan HF, Van Niekerk DJ. Transepidermal elimination in exogenous ochronosis. A report of two cases. Am J Dermatopathol. 1991;13(4):418-24.
34. Hoshaw RA, Zimmerman KG, Menter A. Ochronosislike pigmentation from hydroquinone bleaching creams in American blacks. Arch Dermatol. 1985;121(1):105-8.
35. Penneys NS. Ochronosis like Pigmentation from hydroquinone bleaching creams. Arch Dermatol. 1985;121(10): 1239-40.
36. Lawrence N, Bligard CA, Reed R, et al. Exogenous ochronosis in the United States. J Am Acad Dermatol. 1988;18(5 Pt 2):1207-11.
37. Weiss RM, del Fabbro E, Kolisang P. Cosmetic ochronosis caused by bleaching creams containing 2% hydroquinone. S Afr Med J. 1990;77(7):373.
38. Kramer KE, Lopez A, Stefanato CM, et al. Exogenous Ochronosis. J Am Acad Dermatol. 2000;42(5 pt 2):869-71.
39. Zawar V, Tan SK. Exogenous Ochronosis-a review for clinicians. Expert Rev. Dermatol. 2012;7(2):171-80.
40. Dogliotti M, Leibowitz M. Granulomatous ochronosis-cosmetic induced skin disorder in blacks. S Afr Med J. 1979;56(19):757-60.
41. Berman B, Ricotti C, Viera M, Amini S. Differentiation of exogenous ochronosis from melasma by dermascopy. Poster Abstracts—American Academy of Dermatology 67th Annual Meeting, March 6-10, 2009, San Francisco, California
42. Gil I, Segura S, Martinez-Escala E, et al. Dermascopic and reflectance confocal microscopic features of exogenous ochronosis. Arch Dermatol. 2010;146(9);1021-5.
43. Moche MJ, Glassman SJ, Modi D, et al. Cutaneous annular sarcoidosis developing on a background of exogenous ochronosis: a report of two cases and review of the literature. Clinical and Experimental Dermatology. 2010;35(4): 399-402.
44. Diven DG, Smith EB, Pupo RA, et al. Hydroquinone-induced localized exogenous ochronosis treated with dermabrasion and CO_2 laser. J Dermatol Surg Oncol. 1990;16(11): 1018-22.
45. Bellew SG, Alster TS. Treatment of exogenous ochronosis with a Q-switched alexandrite (755 nm) laser. Dermatol Surg. 2004;30(4 pt 1):555-8.
46. Polnikorn N. Treatment of refractory dermal melasma with the MedLite C6 Q-switched Nd:YAG laser: two case reports. J Cosmet Laser Ther 2008;10(3):167-73.
47. Wattanakrai P, Mornchan R, Eimpunth S. Low-fluence Q-switched neodymium-doped yttrium aluminum garnet (1,064 nm) laser for the treatment of facial melasma in Asians. Dermatol. Surg. 2010;36(1):76-87.
48. Brown AS, Hussain M, Goldberg DJ. Treatment of melasma with low fluence, large spot size, 1064-nm Q-switched neodymium-doped yttrium aluminum garnet (Nd:YAG) laser for the treatment of melasma in Fitzpatrick skin Types II-IV. J. Cosmet Laser Ther. 2011;13(6):280-2.
49. Levitt J. The safety of hydroquinone: a dermatologist's response to the 2006 Federal Register. J Am Acad Dematol. 2007;57(5):854-72.
50. DeCaprio AP. The toxicology of hydroquinone—relevance to occupational and environmental exposure. Crit Rev Toxicol. 1999;29(3):283-330.
51. USFDA (1998). Comments RPT 4 and RPT 5.[online]. Available from: http://www.fda.gov/ohrms/dockets/dockets/78n0065/78n-0065-let0016-vol4.pdf [Accessed, october, 2013].

46

Periocular Pigmentation

Manas Chatterjee

Key Features

- Periocular darkening is a condition with multifactorial etiology.
- It is more common in Indians.
- Though multiple etiologies may be responsible for this condition, there are basically five pathophysiologic mechanisms: melanin or other sources of pigment, thin skin with visible veins (the latter could occur with venous congestion as well), cutaneous laxity, prominent tear trough and periorbital edema.
- The stretch test is able to distinguish whether the condition is due to pigment (no change on stretching the lower eyelid skin downward at the level of the cheek), laxity (improvement) and vascular (worsening).
- In addition to aging and altered subcutaneous fat distribution, sun exposure is a common aggravating factor.
- Treatment depends on the cause and consists of bleaching agents, chemical peels, light sourced devices such as pigment lasers, intense pulsed light (IPL) and fractional photothermolysis for pigment-induced darkening; vascular lasers, vitamin K included topical agents and IPL in addition to fillers for vascular etiology and blepharoplasty, ablative lasers and volumetric filling for cutaneous laxity and other structural defects.

INTRODUCTION

Periocular pigmentation has been known by various names such as periorbital melanosis, dark circles, infraorbital pigmentation, idiopathic cutaneous hyperchromia of the orbital region. It is defined as bilateral, round, homogeneous pigment macules on the infraorbital regions. It is worsened by generalized fatigue, especially lack of sleep, in which case, it is associated with puffy eyes/eye bags **(Fig. 1)**. It is associated with fluctuation of intensity, which is regarded as physiologic by some. As a matter of fact, this condition is considered a phenomenon within the limit of physiology.

Certain ethnic groups such as mixed races and those with Jewish inheritance are more severely affected. Multiple members of family may be affected, related to anatomic considerations. By definition, it does not include conditions which also cause facial pigmentation.

Patients, especially women, are really concerned about it, relating dark circles with impairment in their quality of life. It interferes with facial appearance, giving a tired, sad, or hangover look.

EPIDEMIOLOGY

There is no available data on prevalence of this condition due to it being transitory, with lack of etiological explanations and

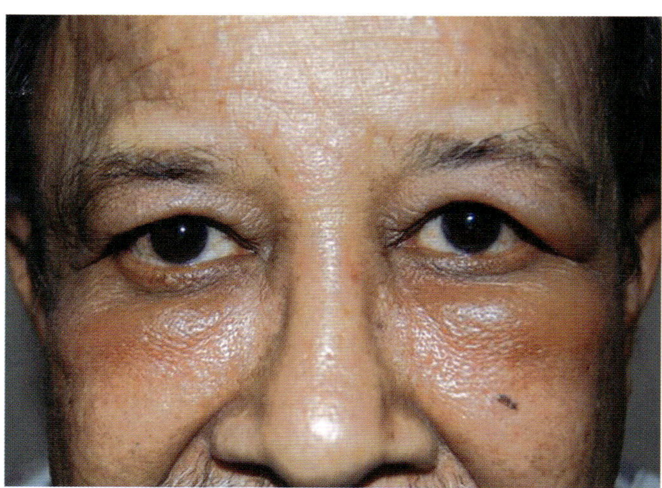

Fig. 1: Puffy eyes leading to periocular darkening

is considered a cosmetic nuisance. About 9% of American women below 30 years of age are concerned about this condition.[1]

HISTORY

There has been little investigation as to the cause of this common disorder. It is stated to occur from a variety of reasons.

One of the first references to this condition was by Touraine in 1937, wherein it was said to be due to prominence of vessels due to loss of subcutaneous fat and muscle tonus in the region. The probable earliest publication dealing exclusively with this condition was by Adlercreutz[2] where he referred to it as being caused by biliary and genitourinary tract diseases. Winkelmann in 1965 attributed this condition to dehydration due to severe systemic disorders. Mark in 1966 associated it to allergic rhinitis.

ETIOLOGY AND DIAGNOSTIC CONSIDERATIONS

Causative factors[3] that are known to play a role in the occurrence of periocular pigmentation are as under:

- Genetic trait
- Sun exposure
- Dermal melanin deposition
- Melanocyte stimulating hormone-induced melanosis
- Post-traumatic
- Post-inflammatory [eczemas: atopic dermatitis **(Fig. 2)**/ allergic contact dermatitis/airborne contact dermatitis **(Fig. 3)**]
- Cosmetics containing phototoxic agents **(Fig. 4)**, usually psoralens, etc.
- Acanthosis nigricans **(Fig. 5)**
- Seborrheic melanosis **(Fig. 6)**
- Bilateral nevus of Ota[4]
- Fixed drug eruptions[5]
- Macular and systemic amyloidosis[6]
- *Lead of Kohl pencils*:[7] Originally antimony trisulfide—the ore stibnite called "ethmid"; scarce and expensive and replaced by galena (lead sulfide) with same gray-black color and shiny appearance;[8] Abnormal pigmentation of eyelid and lacrimal sac seen in patients with eyeliners of lead due to deposition of metal particles in dermis and increased epidermal melanin production; lead may also be tattooed; lead hue with pallor and lividity seen; high blood (twice) and conjunctival (six times) lead levels seen in quoted study; D-penicillamine effective by chelating lead at low dose of 750 mg per day.
- Application of travoprost[9,10] bimatoprost,[11,12] the latter available as 0.3% solution; the prescribing information for bimatoprost includes warnings related to skin changes such as possible lid pigmentation of the periorbital tissue; the most common adverse events caused by Latisse® use are described as eye pruritus, conjunctival hyperemia, skin hyperpigmentation, ocular irritation, dry eye symptoms and erythema of the eyelid; these have been described in less than 4% of patients:
- Free radical/oxidant damage
- Fatigue
- Periorbital edema, subcutaneous fat herniation, gravitational
- Superficial location of vasculature
- Shadowing due to skin laxity.

Systemic factors that play a role in the etiology of this condition are as under:

- Prolonged use of mercurial or silver preparation **(Table 1)**
- Parenteral gold therapy

Table 1: Specific colors of some causes of periocular pigmentation (Adapted from: Feletti F, Vincenzi C, Pazzaglia M, Tosti A. Periocular pigmentation associated with use of travoprost for the treatment of alopecia areata of the eyelashes. JEADV 2007; 21: 423)

Cause	*Color*	*Associated features*
Mercurial or silver preparation	Blue gray	Pigmentation of nasolabial and neck folds
Chrysiasis	Mauve	Slate-blue discoloration of sun-exposed skin
Eczema	Brown	Typical eczema changes
Familial	Brown	—
Hormone induced	Brown	Facial hyperpigmentation
Hypohidrotic ectodermal dysplasia	Dark brown	Frontal bossing, saddle nose, prominent supraorbital ridge, hypohidrosis, dental changes
Lichen planus	Violaceous, sometimes brown	Typical lichen planus changes
Minocycline	Gray	Blue-gray pigmentation within areas of inflammation or scarring, legs, forearms
Nevus of Ota	Blue-gray	Involvement of ocular structures, nasopharynx, auricular mucosa, tympanic membrane, dura mater
Post-inflammatory	Brown	—
Post-traumatic	Brown	—
Psoralens	Brown	Sunburn, nausea and vomiting, itching

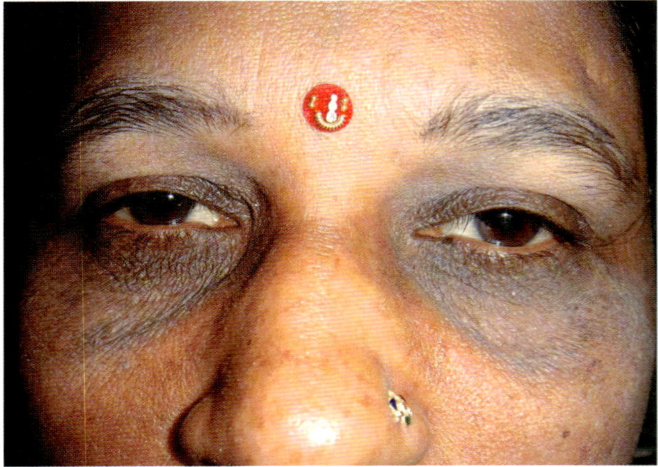

Fig. 2: Post-inflammatory periocular pigmentation following atopic dermatitis

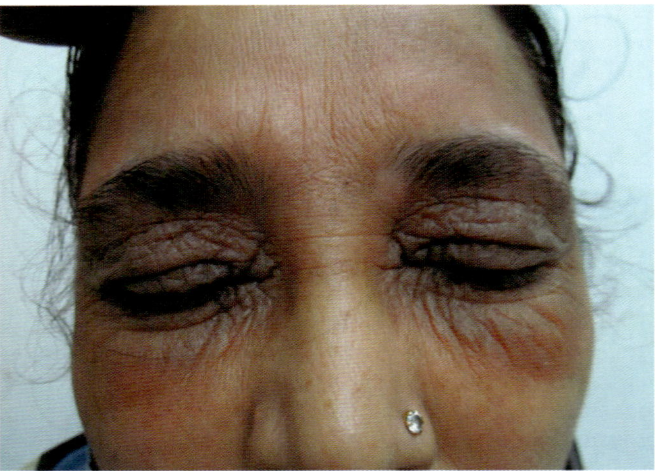

Fig. 3: Inflammatory pigmentation in airborne contact dermatitis

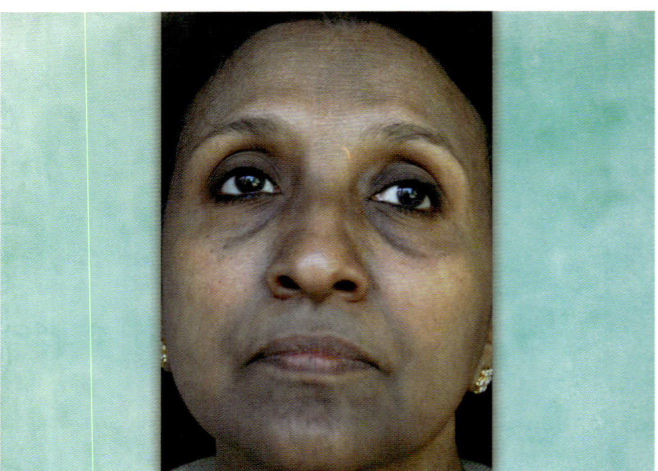

Fig. 4: Pigmented cosmetic contact dermatitis

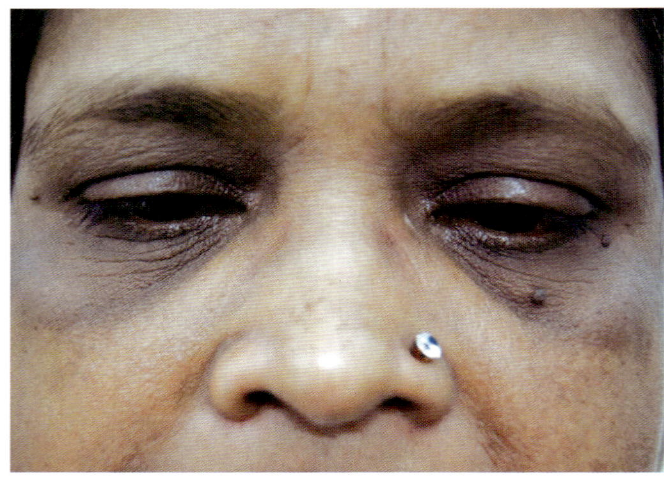

Fig. 5: Periocular acanthosis nigricans with acrochordons

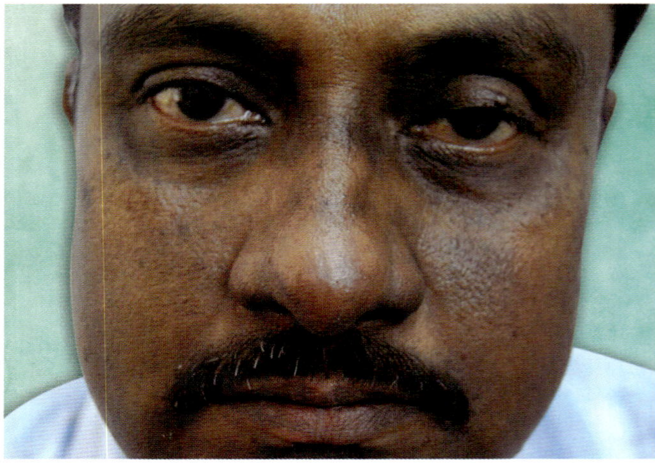

Fig. 6: Periocular and facial seborrheic melanosis

- Long-term minocycline
- Biliary disease, endocrine disturbances (thyroid and menstrual disturbance/hormonal)
- Pregnancy, breastfeeding
- Lichen planus, especially lichen planus pigmentosus
- Peutz-Jeghers syndrome[13]
- Erythema dyschromicum perstans[14]
- Iron deficiency anemia
- Gastrointestinal diseases
- Renal diseases
- Suprarenal disorders
- Vascular disorder associations[15]

Aggravating factors in periocular pigmentation:

- Sun exposure
- Aging process of skin sagging
- Altered subcutaneous fat distribution

Pathomechanisms of Periocular Pigmentation[16]

- *Post-inflammatory*: It is caused by rubbing or scratching of the skin around the eye or by accumulation of fluid due to facial allergy. It presents with irregular patches of brownish or gray pigmentation on the skin on the upper, lower, or both eyelids with features of lichenification, accentuation of skin creases, and eczematous papules or patches in the surrounding areas.
- *Periorbital edema*: Worsens in the morning or after a salty meal. It leads to a purplish color and follows the undefined contours of the underlying fat compartments.
- *Increased melanin deposition*: Caused mainly by dermal melanocytosis and hemosiderin synthesis.
- *Increased visibility of blood vessels*: Caused by visible prominence of subcutaneous vascular plexus or vasculature contained within the orbicularis muscle. This is caused by thin lower eyelid skin overlying the orbicularis oculi muscle. It is associated with erythema, predominantly involving the inner aspect of the lower eyelids, with prominent capillaries or telangiectasia in addition to veins (bluish color).
- *Aging with increased skin laxity (dermatochalasis)*: Caused by combination of dryness of skin, rhytides causing shadowing with overlying pseudoherniation of infraorbital fat. Patients have a dark shadow under an overhanging tarsal muscle, with eye bags.
- *Prominent tear trough*: This is an inherited deformity causing hollowness of the area immediately above the inferior orbital rim. It disappears on direct lighting.

We shall now elucidate some of these pathomechanisms as under:

Pigmentation

Pigmentation is mostly caused by dermal melanocytosis. It is dark brown to blue-gray in color. The most common causes are excessive sun exposure, post-inflammatory due to rubbing, drug ingestion, erythema dyschromicum perstans, fixed drug eruption, familial and nevus of Ota. It sometimes presents as a slightly curved band of brownish skin approximating shape of underlying inferior orbital rim **(Fig. 7)**. It looks darker when present below the bulging lower eyelids induced by pseudoherniation of orbital fat, leading to shadowing. *Stretching of the lower eyelid does not significantly lighten this pigment. This is called the "Stretch test" for periocular pigmentation.*

Genetic (familial or constitutional) factors play an important role in pigmentation. It is associated with a curved band of brownish to black pigmentation on the skin of the lower eyelids with velvety or coarse texture pigment with frequent involvement of the upper eyelids. This form of pigment is most common among Indians. Peters reported a kindred of 20 individuals in five generations and first speculated that this might be an autosomal dominant disorder.[17] Additional large pedigrees have confirmed the heritable nature of this condition. A report in 1969 confirmed that the condition *progressed with age*.[18] This study stated that it usually starts in the lower eyelid and progresses to around the eye **(Fig. 8)**. Fatigue, worry, anxiety, illness worsens this condition and good health and rest tends to improve it. Genetic factors affect the sexes equally. There is wide variation in its ultimate extent and intensity and this condition is seen *more frequently in individuals with dark complexions*.[19] In most of the persons it remains unnoticed from childhood, only to be revealed after any triggering factor(s) such as sun exposure, puberty, pregnancy, use of oral contraceptives, some acute illnesses such as viral hepatitis, typhoid and chickenpox, stress, eye strain, cachexia, etc.[20] In its exaggerated state, it gives the eyes the impression of "raccoon eyes" **(Fig. 9)**.

It is considered that some of these cases may be extensions of *pigmentary demarcation line-F* (PDL-F) of the face **(Fig. 10)**. In 92 (92%) patients out of 100 in a study, periorbital melanosis was found to be an extension of PDL-F.[21]

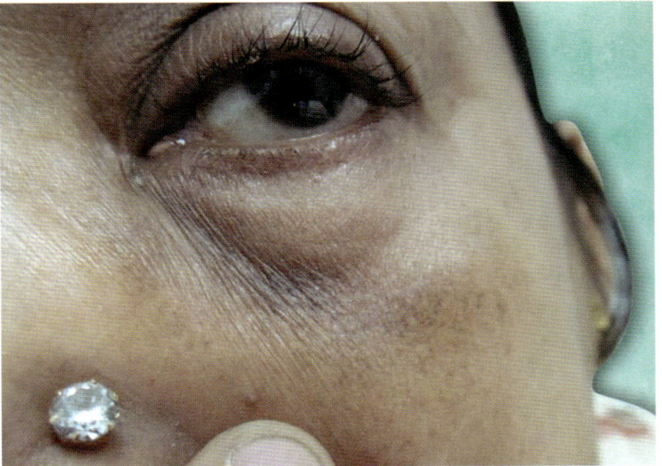

Fig. 7: A curved band of brownish skin approximating shape of underlying inferior orbital rim in periocular pigmentation

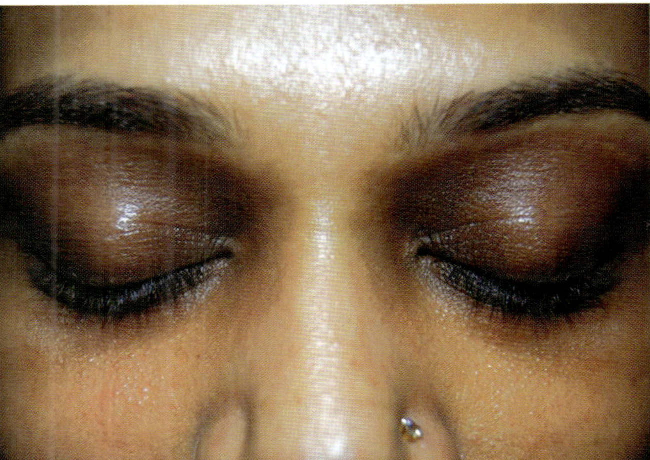

Fig. 8: Autosomal dominant circumocular pigmentation

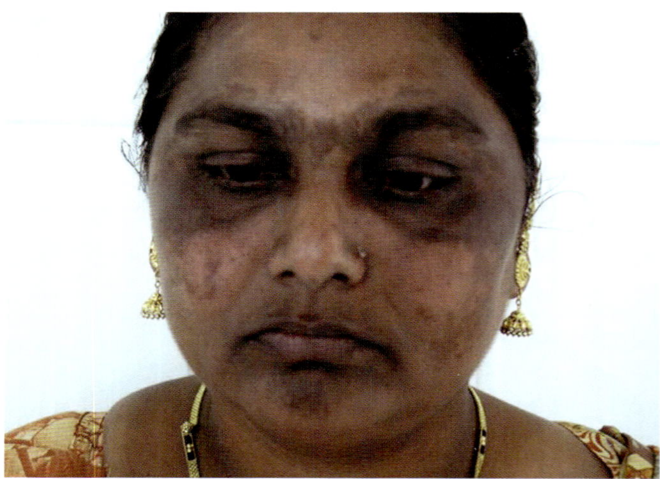

Fig. 9: The raccoon eyes in advanced autosomal dominant periocular pigmentation

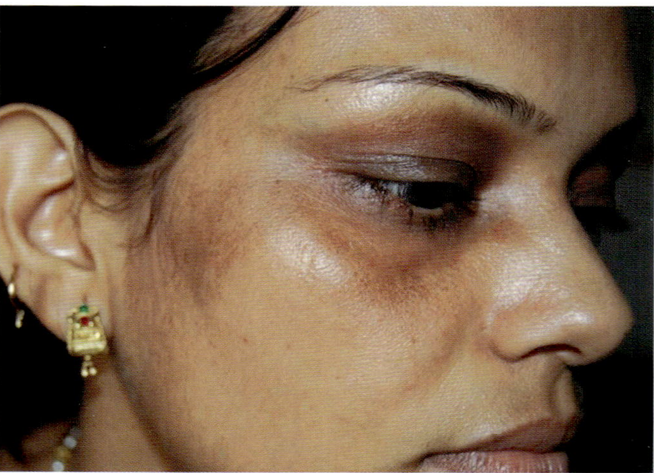

Fig. 10: Periocular pigmentation with pigmentary demarcation line-F (PDL-F)

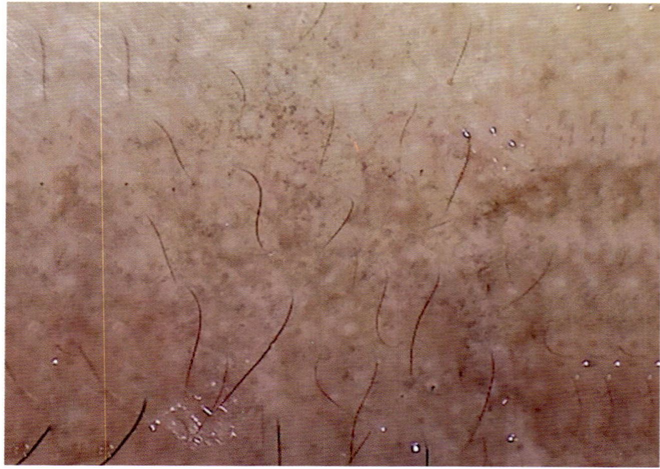

Fig. 11: Dermal granular pigment on dermatoscopy 50X non-polarized

Dermatoscopically, pigment may be perifollicular, reticuloglobular similar to melasma (epidermal and dermal), reticulated or even speckled with dermal granular appearance **(Fig. 11)**. Some cases show blunted reticular appearance similar to erythema dyschromicum perstans (author's observation).

The pigment may be scored as under:

- Light brown
- Dark brown
- Brown-black

If melanocytosis is a fixed finding, what explains the daily fluctuation seen and complained of by patients? Dermal edema leads to Tyndall effect as the eyelid region has a "sponge" property that helps accumulation of fluid in systemic or local edema situations. The evidence for this is the worsening in the morning or after salty meal.[22]

A natural corollary is the differentiation of fat and fluid (edema) over the periocular skin. Compared with normal orbital fat, *edema is still present in downgaze* **(Fig. 12)** *and does not change much in upgaze, whereas fat disappears in downgaze and appears in upgaze* **(Fig. 13)**. This is due to undefined contours of regional fat complements on the face. CO_2 laser causes tightening of dermal tissues and improvement of the skin surface texture in both conditions.

Translucent Skin

This condition is due to thin, translucent lower eyelid skin overlying the orbicularis oculi muscle, with little or no subcutaneous fat. This leads to a visible prominence of the subcutaneous vascular plexus or vasculature contained within the muscle. There is a violaceous appearance of this color, which is more in the inner aspect **(Fig. 14)**. There is *accentuation during menstruation in females. The stretch test deepens the violaceous color* **(Figs 15A and B)**. Improvement with subcutaneous injection of filler/fat indicates that fat is in musculature and not subcutaneous.

Associated venous engorgement accentuates this discoloration. Congestion of nasal and paranasal cavities is a common cause of engorgement of these veins. Venous drainage of this area is by branches of sphenopalatine veins passing backward to the pterygoid plexus **(Fig. 16)**. *Allergic edema of mucous membrane causes pressure effect on veins, interfering with drainage.* This engorgement of lower venous marginal arcades and palpebral veins which drain via angular and inferior ophthalmic vein to same sphenopalatine vein and pterygoid plexus causes the effect of eyelid discoloration. This has been studied and an increased amount of hemoglobin and decreased hemoglobin oxygen saturation has been seen with blood flow rate which was found to be slow at dark eye circles (DEC) in comparison with the cheek. *Blood flow stagnation*

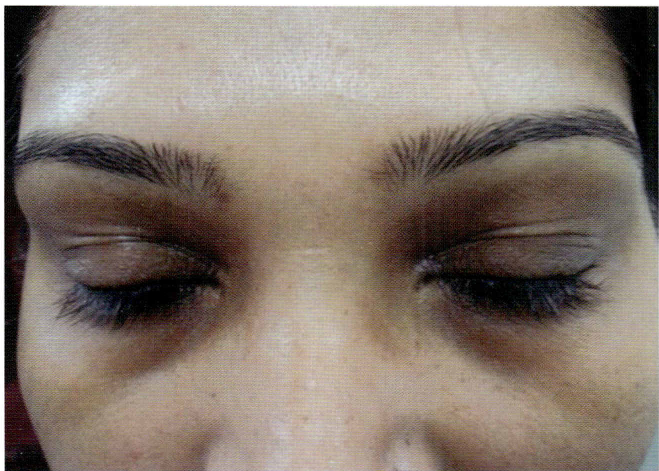

Fig. 12: Periocular edema in a young girl

seems to be one of the factors that could induce DECs.[23] There are other studies that link periorbital hyperchromia (dark circles) to postinflammatory hemodynamic congestion producing a typical bruising aspect on the lower eyelids.[24]

Differentiation between vascular and pigment causes of periorbital pigmentation is also by Wood's lamp and polarized diagnostic light imaging.

Cutaneous Laxity

Collagen and elastin in the thin tissue of the eyelids and periorbital skin undergo *ultraviolet-induced and age-related degeneration*. The damaged epidermis releases collagenases, which further contributes to collagen degeneration. This laxity leads to a shadowing appearance on the lower eyelids which can occur as a *genetic trait* **(Figs 17A and B)**.

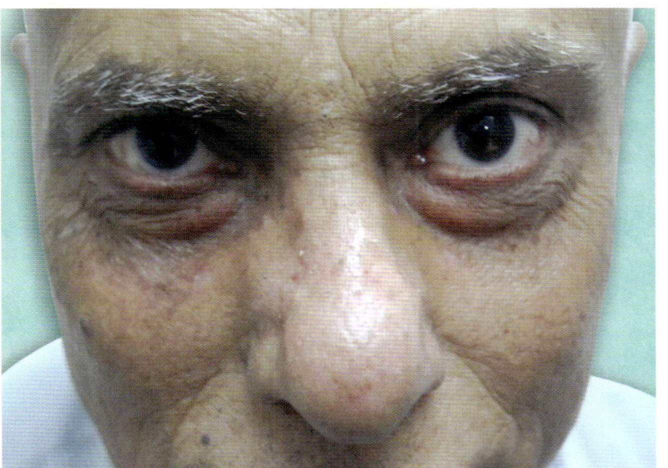

Fig. 13: Periocular fat appears in upgaze

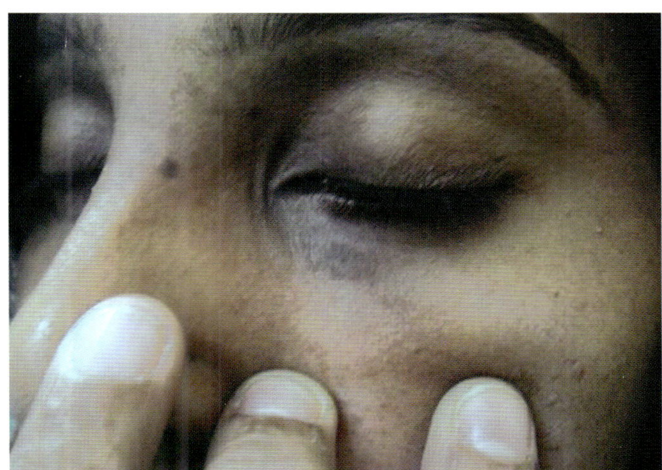

Fig. 14: Violaceous appearance of periocular vasculature, more in the medial aspect

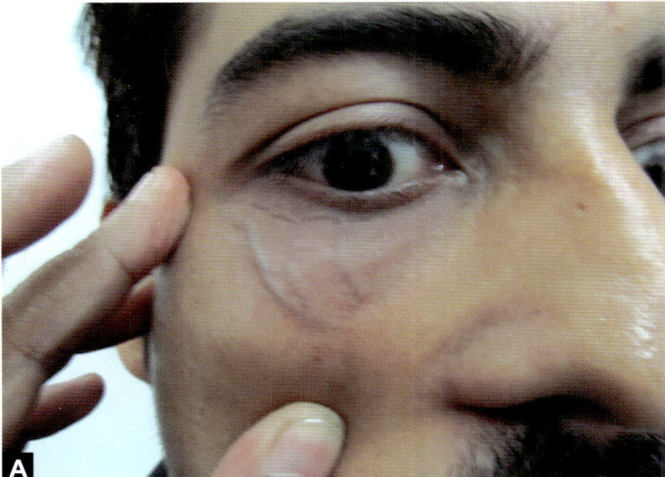

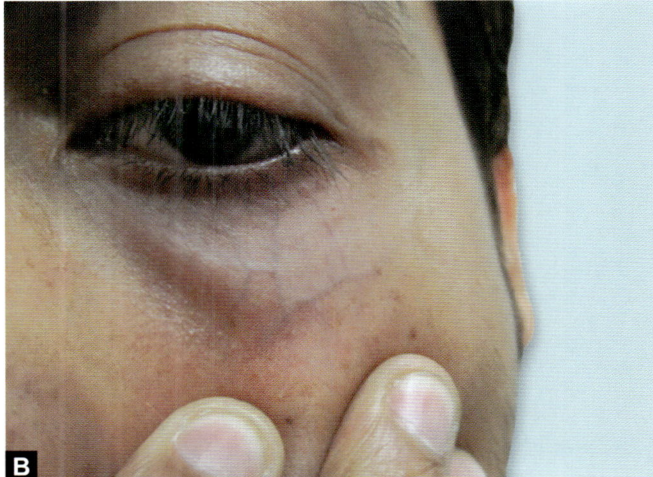

Figs 15A and B: The stretch test in a patient with thin skin and prominent periocular veins

Tear Trough

The tear trough extends from the medial canthus to mid-pupillary line **(Fig. 18)**. It is normally 3 cm or less and continues to the lid-cheek junction (palpebromalar groove). It corresponds to junction of the palpebral and orbital portions of orbicularis oculi muscle. It deepens as patients age because the *infraorbital fat is displaced anteriorly, creating shadowing* below it, depending on lighting conditions, leading to hollowness; also, the orbital bony space increases. The stretch test shows *improvement* of this condition.[25,26]

Tear trough deformity is graded[27] as under:

- *Class I:* Hollowing in medial one-third of orbital rim
- *Class II:* Defect up to midpupillary line
- *Class III:* Full depression extending circumferentially along orbital rim

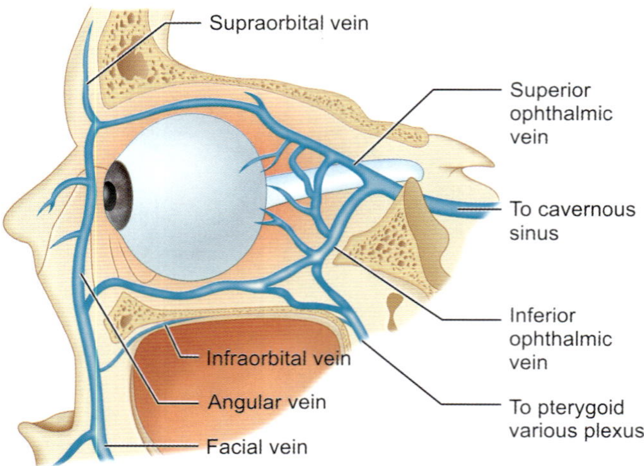

Fig. 16: Venous drainage of the periocular tissues

Multiple etiologies may contribute to dark circles in the same patient.[28] Hyperpigmentation, superficial microvasculature due to engorgement or visibility and slackness of periorbital anatomical structures may all be present in one patient **(Fig. 19)**.

In addition, a number of these patients also have xanthelasma associated with this condition, which the author has found to be more than that in age-matched controls (Unpublished) **(Fig. 20)**.

Studies on Etiological Factors

Several studies have analyzed the proportion of the various etiologies in the genesis of periocular pigmentation. In Asians,[29] in a study of 184 patients, the vascular form of pigmentation was found to be the most common type in 41.8% of patients. The next most common (38.6%) was constitutional, followed by postinflammatory hyperpigmentation (12%). Shadow effects (11.4%) due to an overhanging tarsal muscle, eyebags, or a deep tear trough was fourth. The rest were due to other causes like skin laxity, dry skin, hormonal disturbances, nutritional deficiencies and other chronic illnesses. No significant correlation was found between sleep deprivation or other aggravating factors and periocular hyperpigmentation.

Other studies have been undertaken to establish the cause of periocular pigmentation. Spectrophotometric intracutaneous analysis (SIA) scopy, which is a combination of dermatoscopy, contact remittance spectrophotometry and hyperspectral imaging, enables concentration and distribution of eumelanin, oxyhemoglobin and dermal collagen to be measured *in vivo.*[30] A study to analyze the proportion of hemoglobin and melanin in patients with this condition was conducted with the help of this instrument.[31]

It found no correlation with family history, atopic dermatitis, contact dermatitis, melasma and hormonal

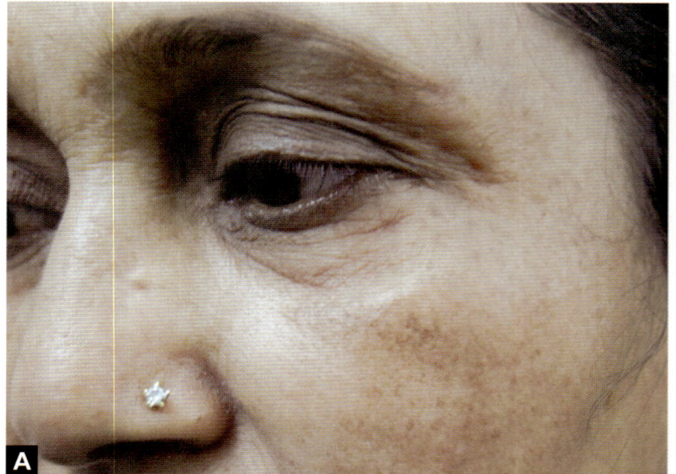

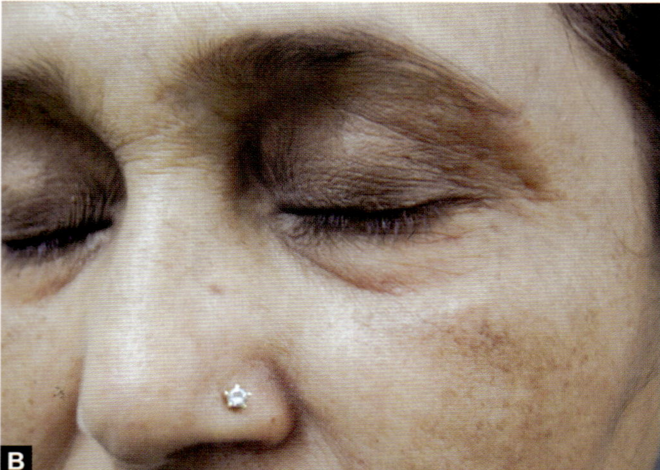

Figs 17A and B: Shadowing due to skin laxity

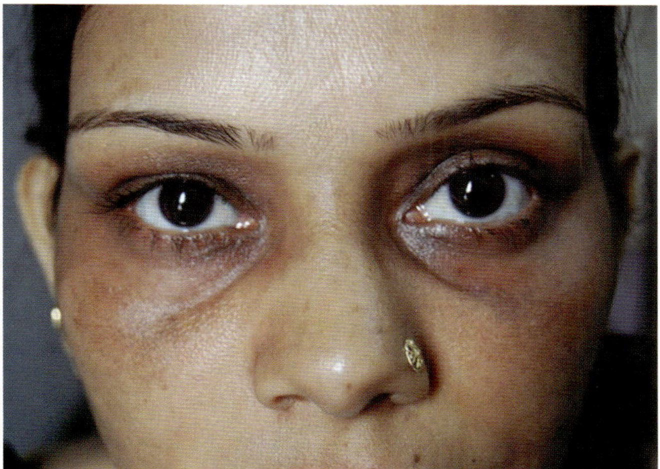

Fig. 18: Class II tear trough

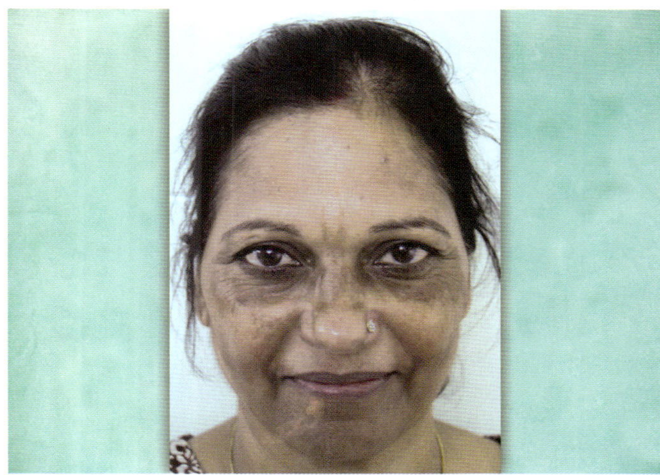

Fig. 19: Hyperpigmentation, cutaneous laxity and vascular etiologies of periocular darkening in the same patient

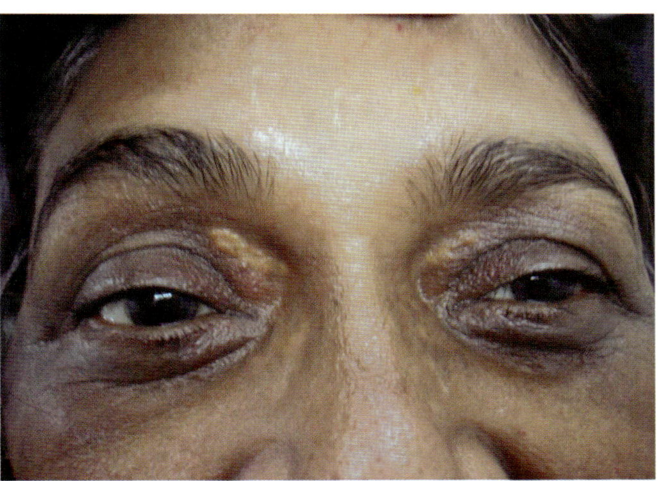

Fig. 20: Periocular pigmentation with associated xanthelasma

factors in periocular pigmentation. It found that the quantity index of total melanin, dermal melanin and hemoglobin to be more in dark circles as compared to normal skin.

The only histopathological[32] study other than the one conducted by the authors [which also included immunohistochemistry **(Figs 21A to C)**, under publication] studied 28 patients with biopsies from the medial lower eyelid with retroauricular skin as control and found that hemosiderin was absent, with increased melanin in papillary dermis correlating with severity of lesions. There was dilatation of blood vessels.

Another clinical analysis[33] reiterated that Wood's lamp can enhance epidermal pigmentation, and established that ultrasonogram can show real-time anatomical structures of eyelids. By ultrasound, the vascular type with periorbital puffiness was found to have increased preseptal thickness of the soft tissue, and infraorbital palpebral bags of the structural type were found to have protruded retroseptal fat pads. It classified DEC into pigmented (brown color), vascular (blue/pink/purple color), structural (skin color), and mixed type pigmented-vascular (PV subtype), pigmented-structural (PS subtype), vascular-structural (VS subtype), and the combined three. Structural included infraorbital palpebral bags, infraorbital grooves, blepharoptosis, and loss of fat or soft tissue volume with bony prominence. It scored DEC by means of Wood's lamp and ultrasound. It revealed that pigmented, vascular, structural, and mixed type of DEC accounted for 5%, 14%, 3% and 78%, respectively. The mixed type, PV (37%), and three-combined type (26%) were most common. The overall mean DEC score was 6.4, while the different types had scores of 4.3, 4.1, 5.0, and 7.0, respectively for pigmented, vascular, structural and mixed forms showing that mixed form was the most common. Though this was, in essence what had already been described, this study formalized the essentially different causes of this entity and that treatment would have to be based on the etiology rather than a "one-size-fits-all" kind of therapy.

TREATMENT

A search of amazon.com revealed 302 products for "dark circles". There are 120,000 videos on youtube dedicated to this entity. Disguising the lesions is almost mandatory for individuals who depend on a well-cared and positive appearance for work or social activities. As individual anatomical basis for dark circles is not clearly defined, treatments may render suboptimal results. Treatment is based on the cause and there is no evidence-based data on use of various medications for periocular pigmentation.

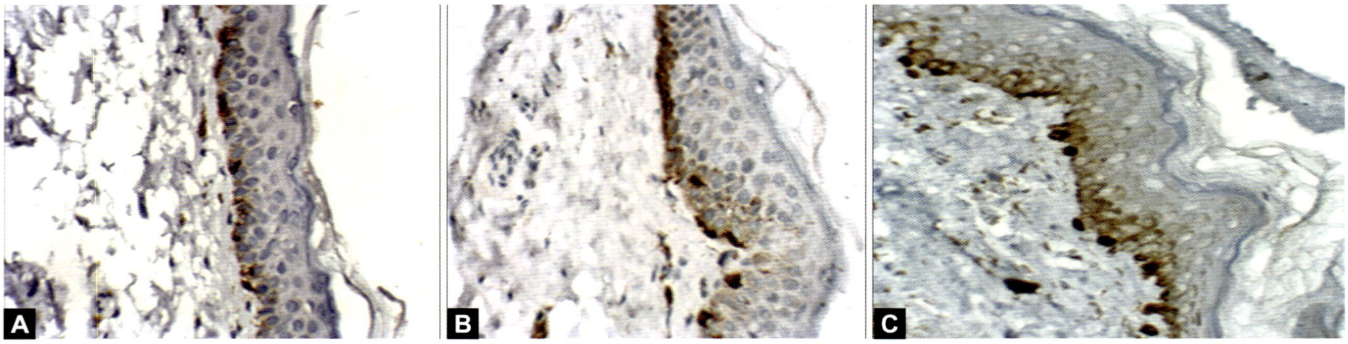

Figs 21A to C: Immunohistochemistry (Melan A) of mild, moderate and severe grades of periocular pigmentation (light brown, dark brown and brown-black respectively

Pigment

If the cause assessed is pigment by stretch testing and other newer investigations described above, treatment needs to be continued for several months. Mechanisms of depigmenting agents include inhibition of tyrosinase activity, inhibition of DNA synthesis in hyperactive melanocytes, reduction of epidermal content of melanin and thickening of epidermis (granular layer). Details of these agents are available in relevant chapters of this text.

Hydroquinone shows effect in 5–7 weeks. Effect is preceded by erythema and scaling. Treatment is continued for 3 months to 1 year. Kligman formula and its modifications are used. Tretinoin leads to thickening of granular layer and among other things, causes melanocyte damage. It shows effect in 24 weeks. Other agents include azelaic acid, steroids, kojic acid, and pidobenzone. There is increasing collagen with vitamin C which may conceal dark discoloration due to congested blood.[34] Some other compounds have been specifically studied for dark circles. These include *Pfaffia paniculata*/*Ptychopetalum olacoides* B/*Lilium candidum* L-associated compound (PPLAC) which is applied as 5% twice a day applied for 28 days. In a study, 90% patients showed improvement on colorimetric testing.[24] Some other products such as a gel containing phytonadione, retinol, vitamin C, vitamin E has been found to be fairly or moderately effective.[35]

Chemical peeling can be used as less or more intense regimen. Trichloroacetic acid, other alpha-hydroxy acids stimulate formation of glycosaminoglycans as an additional mechanism of improvement of periocular darkening in addition to causing reduction of pigment *per se*.

Q-switched ruby lasers have been found to be effective in studies.[3,36] Up to 88.9% of patients have been shown to be improved with two sittings. Reduced dermal melanin post treatment has been demonstrated histologically. Q-switched Nd:YAG laser 1,064 nm reduces deep pigment and vascular component of pigment. West and Alster showed no difference between Q-switched alexandrite (755 nm) and Nd:YAG (1,064 nm) lasers in the therapy of periocular pigmentation. Lasers require metal eye shielding over anterior eye for safe treatment.[37] Q-switched ruby laser with bleaching treatment with tretinoin and hydroquinone has been used in Asians. Initial medical treatment was used to reduce epidermal pigment followed by laser for dermal pigment. Excellent to good response was seen in 15 of 19 patients. Post-inflammatory pigmentation was seen in two patients and reduced dermal pigment in three patients.[28]

Carboxytherapy has also been anecdotally used. Subcutaneous injections of CO_2 were administered once a week for 7 weeks. It led to reduction of facial fine lines and wrinkles as well as a decrease in periorbital hyperpigmentation. Side effects were only transient.[38]

Skin Laxity

Medical therapy has been tried. Human growth factors and cytokines cream, with caffeine, bisabolol and glycyrrhetinic acid and sodium hyaluronate have been used. Wrinkles, lower eyelid bags and sagging, dark circles, skin texture have improved by 14–28% in 6 weeks.[39]

However, the main therapy for these etiologies of periocular darkening is procedural. The basis of these is reversal of age-related changes. They are best treated with ablative and nonablative lasers and surgical methods to improve laxity. Dermatochalasis and periorbital rhytides are significantly improved. However, prolonged dyschromia, scarring, infection are possible sequelae.[40]

CO_2 laser leads to 50% improvement; however, melanin readings post-treatment is not much different compared to pretreatment. This is explained by tightening of dermal tissues and improvement of the skin surface texture.[37] A multistage treatment of two types of lasers has been described. Shadowing occurs secondary to the bulging contour of the lower eyelid. Bluish color occurs secondary to the visible dermal capillary network, and brown color is caused by dermal melanin. Treatment was undertaken by CO_2 laser followed by Q-switched Alexandrite 755 nm. Results were seen in 6–8 weeks.[41] Other lasers that have been used include fractional lasers, pulsed dye laser, diode laser, 1,320 nm Nd: YAG laser, 1,540 nm erbium: glass laser and intense pulse light. Fractional 1,550 nm erbium-doped fiber laser has been used. It is a single case report of four sessions monthly. It is postulated to eliminate melanin pigment from the epidermis and dermis through "melanin shuttle," which exudes the pigment from the skin through microthermal zones. It causes less post-inflammatory hyperpigmentation and removes dermal melanin as well. It also improves laxity of skin.[42]

Tear-trough Depression

Procedures for tear trough deformity include invasive surgical procedures to elevate the soft tissues from the underlying maxilla, fat repositioning or fat extrusion and septal reset.[43] Surgery include transconjunctival blepharoplasty and deep-depth phenol chemical peel simultaneously (for skin laxity/ tear trough and pigment).[44]

Translucent Eyelids and Visible Veins

The principles of therapy are enunciated in the fact that the periocular area contains subcutaneous vascular plexus which are vasculature contained within muscle (orbicularis oculi). The idea is to restore the volume underneath the eyelid.

Autologous fat transplantation or soft tissue fillers are the lines of therapy to create volume between the thin skin and the veins in the musculature. Fat is readily available, safe, noncarcinogenic, easily acquired and autologous. In a study of autologous fat, patients showed an average of 78% improvement.[16] Other studies have also concluded that autologous fat transplantation is an effective method for the treatment of infraorbital dark circles due to thin and translucent lower eyelid skin over the orbicularis oculi muscle.[45] In addition, hyaluronic acid fillers have been used.[26] Non crosslinked hyaluronic acid with glycerol has also been used. Three monthly superficial injections using micropuncture technique led to improvement of between 25% and 50% in skin brightness, texture and turgor. Papules were present after each application, and hematoma was the longest lasting adverse effect.[46]

Issues with the use of injectable fillers in the periorbital tissues include some patients with dark circles noticing dark pigmentation after hyaluronic acid gel filling, palpable nodules with fillers and swelling, bruising, asymmetry, cellulitis, migraine. It is best to use fillers with cannulae rather than needles and deposit the filler just above the periosteum. This would ensure less activity of tissue hyaluronidase leading to increased duration of effect of the filler.[47]

CONCLUSION

It is important to realize that periocular darkening has multiple pathogenetic mechanisms, of which, pigment, vascular, laxity and a prominent tear trough are the broad groups in which they can be divided. Diagnostic modalities include the stretch test, supported by Wood's lamp and ultrasound in addition to more sophisticated methods such as SIA scopy. Treatment depends on the etiology, with pigment managed by pigment reducing agents, laxity managed with lasers, vascular causes managed with fillers and surgery being used in the latter two situations, if less invasive means fail.

REFERENCES

1. Gupta MA, Gupta AK. Dissatisfaction with skin appearance among patients with eating disorders and non-clinical controls. Br J Dermatol. 2001; 145(1):110-3.
2. Aldercreutz E. Periocular hyperpigmentation (Masque Biliaire) and its relation to biliary and genitourinary tract diseases. Acta Medics Scandinavica. 1949;135(1):63-7.
3. Lowe NJ, Wieder JM, Shorr NS, et al. Infraorbital pigmented skin. Dermatol Surg. 1995;21(9):767-70.
4. Kolde G, Schmollack KP, Sterry W. Periorbital hyperpigmentation. Bilateral nevus of Ota. Hautarzt. 2001;52(5):460-3.
5. Tognetti L, Rubegni P, Flori ML, et al. Ocular involvement in generalized fixed drug eruption from nimesulide. Clin Experiment Ophthalmol. 2013. doi: 10.1111/ceo.12103. [Epub ahead of print]
6. Barbhuiya JN, Guha PK, Dutta BN. Primary systemic amyloidosis, presenting as periorbital pigmentation. Ind J Dermatol Venereol Leprol. 1994;60:34-6.
7. El Safoury OS, El Fatah DS, Ibrahim M. Treatment of periocular hyperpigmentation due to lead of kohl (surma) by penicillamine: a single group non-randomized clinical trial. Indian J Dermatol. 2009;54(4):361-3.
8. Omar SS, Inas FG, Laila R, et al. Periorbital pigmentation by lead in kohl. J Egyptian Woman's Dermatol Society. 2006;3:4-18.
9. Schmutz JL, Barbaud A, Tréchot P. [Periocular hyperpigmentation following travoprost application]. Ann Dermatol Venereol. 2008;135(6-7):537.
10. Feletti F, Vincenzi C, Pazzaglia M, et al. Periocular pigmentation associated with use of travoprost for the treatment of alopecia areata of the eyelashes. JEADV. 2007; 21(3):321-3.
11. Kapur R, Osmanovic S, Toyran S, et al. Bimatoprost-induced periocular skin hyperpigmentation. Arch Ophthalmol. 2005;123(11):1541-6.
12. Lee DW. Clinical course of bimatoprost-induced periocular skin hyperpigmentation after stopping bimatoprost treatment. J Kor Ophthalmol Soc. 2007;48:1082-7.
13. Traboulsi EI, Maumenee IH. Periocular pigmentation in the Peutz-Jeghers syndrome. Am J Ophthalmol. 1986;102(1): 126-7.
14. Sardana K, Rajpal M, Garg V, et al. Periorbital hyperpigmentation mimicking fixed drug eruption: a rare presentation of erythema dyschromicum perstans in a paediatric patient. JEADV. 2006; 20(10):1381-2.
15. Sorhage B. Increased pigmentation of the sclera and periorbital region associated with increased cutaneous vascularization of the left arm. J Dtsch Dermatol Ges. 2005;3(4):301-3.
16. Roh MR, Chung KY. Infraorbital dark circles: definition, causes, and treatment options. Dermatol Surg.

2009;35(8):1163-71.
17. Peters R. Auffallende dunkelfarbung der unteren lider als erbliche anomalie. Zbl Prakt Augenheilk. 1918;42:8-11.
18. Goodman RM, Belcher RW. Periorbital hyperpigmentation. Arch Dermatol. 1969;100(2):169-74.
19. Anstey AV. Disorders of skin colour. In: Burns T, Breathnach S, Cox N, Griffiths C (Eds). Rook's Textbook of Dermatology, 8th edn. UK: Wiley-Blackwell; 2010. p. 58.19.
20. Somani VK, Razvi F, Sita VNVL. Pigmentary demarcation lines over the face. Indian J Dermatol Venereol Leprol. 2004;70(6):336-41.
21. Malakar S, Lahiri K, Banarjee U, et al. Periorbital melanosis is an extension of pigmentary demarcation line-F on face. Indian J Dermatol Venereol Leprol. 2007;73(5):323-5.
22. Freitag FM, Cestari TF. What causes dark circles under the eyes? Journal of Cosmetic Dermatology. 2007;6(3):211-5.
23. Masuda Y, Takahashi M, Satou A, et al. Dermatological study on dark eye circles and their improvement with newly developed cosmetics. International Journal of Cosmetic Science. 2004;26:315-6.
24. Eberlin S, Del Carmen Velazquez Pereda M, de Campos Dieamant G, et al. Effects of a Brazilian herbal compound as a cosmetic eye care for periorbital hyperchromia ("dark circles"). J Cosmet Dermatology. 2009;8(2):127-35.
25. Goldberg RA, McCann JD, Fiaschetti D, et al. What causes eyelid bags? Analysis of 144 consecutive patients. Plast Reconstr Surg. 2005;115(5):1395-402.
26. Kane MA. Treatment of tear trough deformity and lower lid bowing with injectable hyaluronic acid. Aesthetic Plast Surg. 2005;29(5):363-7.
27. Hirmand H. Anatomy and nonsurgical correction of tear trough deformity. Plast Reconstr Surg. 2010;125(2):699-708.
28. Momosawa A, Kurita M, Ozaki M, et al. Combined therapy using Q-switched ruby laser and bleaching treatment with tretinoin and hydroquinone for periorbital skin hyperpigmentation in Asians. Plast Reconstr Surg. 2008; 121(1):282-8.
29. Ranu H, Thng S, Goh BK, et al. Periorbital hyperpigmentation in Asians: an epidemiologic study and proposed classification. Dermatol Surg. 2011;37(9):1297-303.
30. Moncrieff M, Cotton SD, Claridge E, et al. Spectrophotometric intracutaneous analysis—a new technique for imaging pigmented skin lesions. Br J Dermatol. 2002;146(3): 448-57.
31. Verschoore M, Gupta S, Sharma VK, et al. Determination of melanin and haemoglobin in the skin of idiopathic cutaneous hyperchromia of the orbital region (ICHOR): A study of Indian patients. J Cutan Aesthet Surg. 2012;5(3):176-82.
32. Graziosi AC, Quaresma MR, Michalany NS, et al. Cutaneous idiopathic hyperchromia of the orbital region (CIHOR): a histopathological study. Aesthetic Plast Surg. 2013;37(2):434-8.
33. Huang YL, Chang SL, Ma L, et al. Clinical analysis and classification of dark eye circle. International Journal of Dermatology. 2013;doi:10.1111/j.1365-4632.2012.05701.x
34. Ohshima H, Mizukoshi K, Oyobikawa M, et al. Effects of vitamin C on dark circles of the lower eyelids: quantitative evaluation using image analysis and echogram. Skin Res Technol. 2009;15(2):214-7.
35. Mitsuishi T, Shimoda T, Mitsui Y, et al. The effects of topical application of phytonadione, retinol and vitamins C and E on infraorbital dark circles and wrinkles of the lower eyelids. J Cosmet Dermatol. 2004;3(2):73-5.
36. Watanabe S, Nakai K, Ohnishi T. Condition known as "dark rings under the eyes" in the Japanese population is a kind of dermal melanocytosis which can be successfully treated by Q-switched ruby laser. Dermatol Surg. 2006;32(6):785-9.
37. West TB, Alster TS. Improvement of infraorbital hyperpigmentation following carbon dioxide laser resurfacing. Dermatol Surg. 1998;24(6):615-6.
38. Paolo F, Nefer F, Paola P, et al. Periorbital area rejuvenation using carbon dioxide therapy. J Cosmet Dermatol. 2012;11(3):223-8.
39. Lupo ML, Cohen JL, Rendon MI. Novel eye cream containing a mixture of human growth factors and cytokines for periorbital skin rejuvenation. J Drugs Dermatol. 2007; 6(7):725-9.
40. Alster TS, Bellew SG. Improvement of dermatochalasis and periorbital rhytides with a high-energy pulsed CO_2 laser: a retrospective study. Dermatol Surg. 2004;30(4 Pt 1):483-7; discussion 87.
41. Manuskiatti W, Fitzpatrick RE, Goldman MP. Treatment of facial skin using combinations of CO_2, Q-switched alexandrite, flashlamp-pumped pulsed dye, and Er:YAG lasers in the same treatment session. Dermatol Surg. 2000; 26(2):114-20.
42. Moody MN, Landau JM, Goldberg LH, et al. Fractionated 1550-nm erbium-doped fiber laser for the treatment of periorbital hyperpigmentation. Dermatologic Surgery. 2012;38(1):139-42.
43. Barton FE, Ha R, Awada M. Fat extrusion and septal reset in patients with the tear trough triad: a critical appraisal. Plast Reconstr Surg. 2004;113(7):2115-21.
44. Epstein JS. Management of infraorbital dark circles. A significant cosmetic concern. Arch Facial Plast Surg. 1999;1(4):303-7.
45. Roh MR, Kim TK, Chung KY. Treatment of infraorbital dark circles by autologous fat transplantation: a pilot study. British Journal of Dermatology. 2009;160(5):1022-5.
46. Succi IB, da Silva RT, Orofino-Costa R. Rejuvenation of periorbital area: treatment with an injectable nonanimal non-crosslinked glycerol added hyaluronic acid preparation. Dermatol Surg. 2012;38:192-8.
47. Goldberg RA, Fiaschetti D. Filling the periorbital hollows with hyaluronic acid gel: initial experience with 244 injections. Ophthal Plast Reconstr Surg. 2006;22(5):335-41; discussion 41-3.

47

Physical Therapies for Periorbital Hyperpigmentation, Chemical Peels and Lasers

Bhavesh Shantilal Devani

Key Features

- Periorbital hyperpigmentation is a very common cosmetological condition that requires multimodal approach to treat which includes peels, laser, topical bleaching agents and lifestyle modification.
- Chemical peeling gives some satisfactory results. Commonly used peels are lactic acid (LA), arginine and low concentration glycolic acid.
- Laser treatment in periorbital hyperpigmentation has been studied and tried very less, even though Q switched Nd:YAG and fractional CO_2 laser (low fluence) gives good results in few patients.

INTRODUCTION

Periorbital hyperpigmentation, also referred to as periorbital melanosis (POM), dark circles or infraorbital pigmentation, is more frequently observed in dark skinned patients, especially Asians. Dark circle is not a formal medical term, but both patients and dermatologists use it to indicate periorbital hyperchromic macules and patches. It is not a medical concern but it can be a cosmetic concern for a large number of individuals, especially for females. It is the second most common dermatological complaint and most common non-hormonal skin problem.

PREVALENCE

This condition affects individuals across a wide range of age, both sexes and all races.

CAUSES OF PERIORBITAL MELANOSIS[1,2]

- Genetic
- Vascular
- Extension of pigmentary demarcation line (PDL-F)[3]
  - Thin and lax skin
  - Pronounced tear trough
  - Postinflammatory hyperpigmentation due to continuous rubbing of eyes in allergic conjunctivitis and because of atopic dermatitis or allergic contact dermatitis
  - Lack of adequate sleep, stress, etc.

Three different conditions contributing to this discoloration:[4]

1. *Shadows:* The shadowing is secondary to the bulging contour of the lower lid (nasojugal groove).
2. *Vessels:* Bluish color secondary to the venous network subcutaneously and/or reddish color secondary to the visible dermal capillary network.
3. *Pigment:* Brown color secondary to superficial melanin or brown/blue secondary to dermal melanin.

These three factors are not always present and any one of them can prevail. Various studies carried have found that histologically, hyperpigmentation is of dermal origin.

CLINICAL PICTURE OF PERIORBITAL MELANOSIS

Dark circles interfere with the facial appearance, giving the patient a tired, sad, or hangover look, which often impact quality of life (**Fig. 1**).

There are various types of treatment modalities available. From the clinical point of view, treatments can be divided into

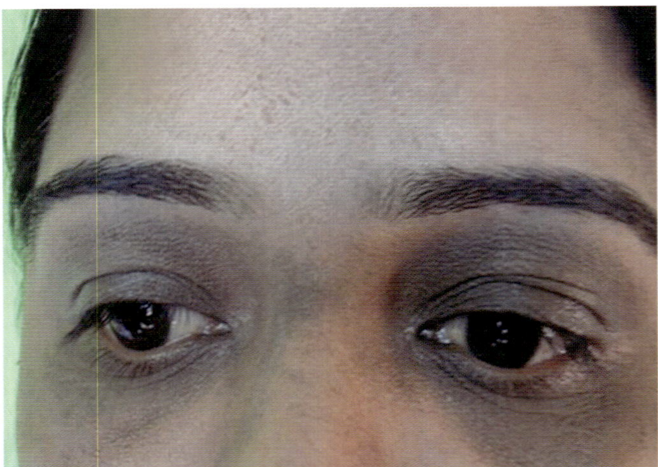

Fig. 1: Periorbital melanosis in Asian skin

five categories: (1) dietary supplement, (2) topical therapy, (3) peeling, (4) lasers and (5) fillers. They can be used either alone or in combination. As per the condition of patient, we have to choose the correct line of treatment.

WHAT IS OUR AIM?

Medications to:

- Decrease leakage and strengthen the capillaries **(Figs 2A and B)**
  - Increase the blood flow to help clearing of oxidized Hb
  - Hydrate the skin in order to decrease the wrinkling
  - Anti-inflammatory agent to decrease the puffiness of the eyes.
  - Increase thickness of skin, increase collagen and elastin to reduce wrinkling around the eyes.

CHEMICAL PEELING FOR PERIORBITAL HYPERPIGMENTATION

It is an application of chemical agent of defined strength to the skin that causes destruction at required depth, followed by remodeling without scarring. It is perhaps the most commonly performed cosmetological office procedure. It is used as adjuvant treatment in POM.

Although there is little support in the literature,[5,6] chemical peeling can be used for the treatment of dark circles. They act through exfoliation, abrasion and shedding of the superficial skin cells. In POM chemical peels reduce pigmentation of the skin significantly, improving some cases of dark circles. Superficial peels used for the treatment of POM are low concentration glycolic acid, salicylic acid, LA, arginine, kojic acid, citric acid and low concentration TCA.[7] The choice of the agent, concentration, number of applications, etc. will depend on each patient's needs. The most frequently used peels for dark circles are arginine and LA peel.

Arginine Peel

Arginine is an amino acid derived from brown sugar. It helps in healing and has a calming action with moisturizing effects. Arginine is the immediate precursor of nitric oxide (NO), urea and ornithine. As a precursor of NO, arginine may have a role in the treatment of conditions where vasodilatation is required. After peel there is dilatation of small arterioles. Vasodilatation in turn increases blood flow that helps in reducing POM. Arginine improves nitrogen balance and has an anti-inflammatory action on macrophages by regulating

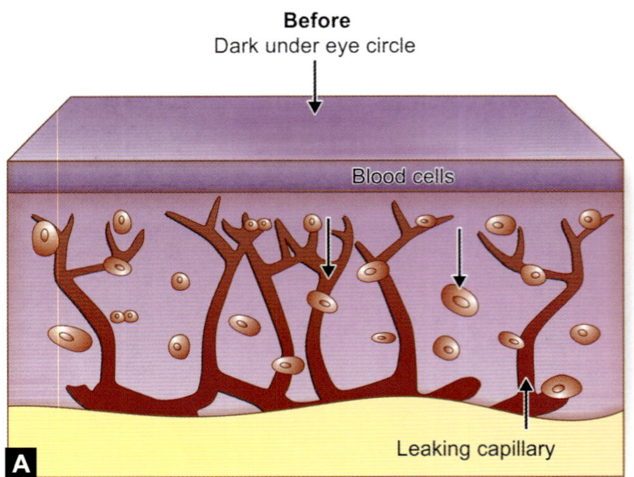

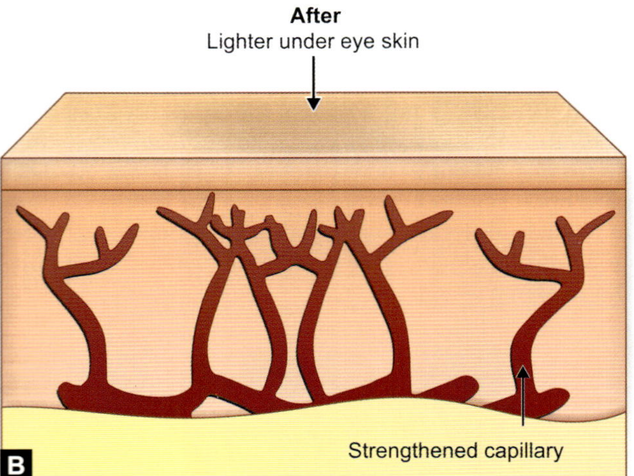

Figs 2A and B: Schematic representation of capillaries before and after chemical peel

NO production, probably through arginase-1 expression. Arginine increases skin hydration and enhances the moisturizing effect of peel. Blood flow resistance is decreased after topical application of arginine. The urea deficit in the stratum corneum in atopic dermatitis and elderly skin is corrected not by applying the moisturizer urea itself but instead by using arginine—its precursor in the Krebs-Henseleit urea cycle. This topical treatment also improves the clinical symptoms of dry skin.

Lactic Acid (LA) Peel [8,9]

Lactic acid (2-hydroxypropanoic acid, α-hydroxypropionic acid) is the next shortest AHA after glycolic acid.[6] A methyl group (CH_3) replaces the terminal hydrogen atom on the alpha carbon.

- Mild AHA
- Derived from sour milk, yogurt, blue berries and tomato juice
- Larger molecule size
- Lactic acid has antimicrobial and anti-inflammatory properties.

Mechanism of Action of Lactic Peel

Similar to glycolic acid main action is to facilitate dissociation of the epidermal cells, desquamation of the stratum corneum and to increase regeneration. It is also said that LA increases the hyaluronic acid content in the skin and acts as a part of skin's natural moisturizing factor. Hence, it improves skin texture and smoothens the skin. It also reduces the wrinkles. One advantage of LA is that it is naturally occurring in the skin so allergic reaction is rare with this molecule.

Argipeel: One of the readily available combination peel for POM.[10]

Argipeel:

- Arginine (20%)
- Lactic acid (20%)
- Aloe vera (1%)
- Allantoin (0.5 %)

Other peels:

- Glycolic acid peel in lower concentration, 15–20% also used in POM. The author's experience is that by adding kojic acid enhancer in low concentration, glycolic acid peel gives good results in POM.
- TCA peel used by western countries in POM; however, there are chances of postinflammatory hyperpigmentation and scarring in Indian skin, so it is not widely used in Asian countries having dark skin people.

Procedure of Arginine Peel

- Patient assessment
- Proper counseling
- Proper informed consent
- Photographic record

A general medical and lifestyle history are evaluated. No specific investigation is advised as it is superficial peel.

The patient is asked to wash face, remove the pre-existing make up and lie down with head elevated to 45° with closed eyes. The hair is pulled back and contact lens removed if patient offer history. Inner canthus is protected with Vaseline. Peeling agent is applied with gauze and kept for 1 hour and patient is asked to wash the face after 1 hour. However, the patient should be told to wash off the face if excessive burning sensation occurs. Author has used this peel by keeping for 1 hour and found no irritation to any of patients. Patient is advised to apply hyaluronic acid and kojic acid along with vitamin C regularly at home. Six to eight sittings are done at interval of 2–3 weeks.

Post-Peel Care

A mild moisturizer and sun block are applied.

Discussion

Counseling and post-peel maintenance are very important in treating POM. Unrealistic expectation is relative contraindication to selecting the patient for chemical peeling. Before doing peel find out the cause of POM and treat accordingly. With chemical peel we did not get much satisfactory result as per patient's expectation but combination of treatment modalities and lifestyle modification gives good results. Argipeel is good option because both Arginine and LA are safe and well tolerated in under eye skin **(Figs 3A and B)**.

LASER TREATMENT FOR PERIORBITAL MELANOSIS

The word "laser" is an acronym which stands for Light Amplification by Stimulated Emission of Radiation (LASER), and uses the principle of selective photothermolysis. Laser that targets pigment and vascularity may be used in POM.[11] Lasers that have been used successfully in periorbital hypermelanosis include the Q switched ruby laser[9,12] and an ablative carbon dioxide (CO_2) resurfacing laser.[13] These lasers may carry a risk of postinflammatory hyperpigmentation. It is

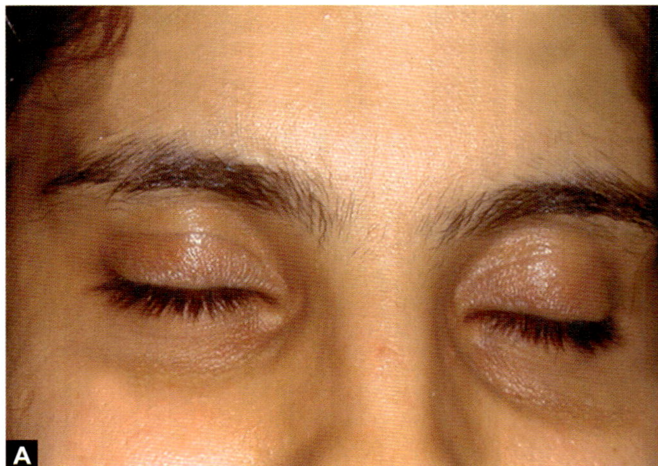
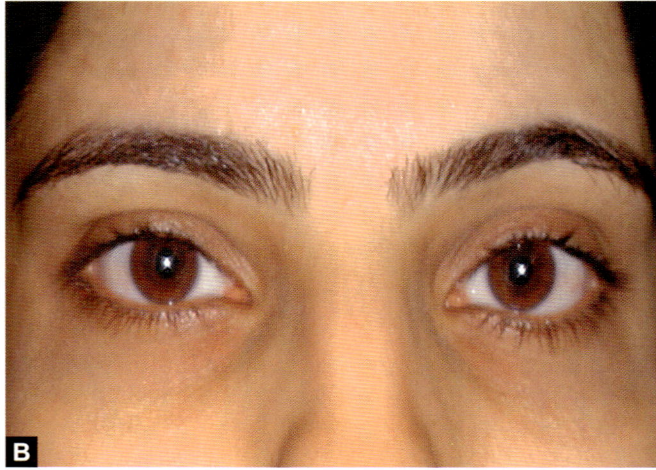

Figs 3A and B: Before and after treatment by Arginine peel (After six sittings). (*Source*: J Sakhiya)

recommended to use appropriate eye protection during laser procedure around eye.[14]

Periorbital melanosis can be treated with 1,550 nm fractionated erbium doped fiber laser.[15,16] Treatment sessions using 1,550 nm fractionated erbium doped fiber laser used 15 mm spot size and four passes with interval of 4–6 weeks. A cooling device should be used during treatment to avoid patient discomfort. After each treatment patient is advised to use at least 30 SPF sunscreens. After four sessions there is significant improvement noted. The non-ablative fractionated 1,550 nm erbium doped fiber laser preserves the stratum corneum while creating microscopic treatment zone (MTZ) of thermal injury in epidermis and dermis.

The laser functions to eliminate melanin pigment from the epidermis through a "melanin shuttle" which excludes the pigment from the skin through the MTZs.[17]

The 1,550 nm fractionated erbium doped fiber laser is safely and effectively used to treat periorbital hyperpigmentation without complication. However, larger studies and ideal parameters are required to treat this common dermatological disease.

Fractional CO_2 laser in very low fluence and in scanner mode helps in reducing wrinkles and pigmentation in periorbital area. Q switched Nd:YAG laser is also proved to be beneficial in POM **(Figs 4A to D)**. During laser the eye should be protected with metal shield.

Woraphong et al. treated eleven patients of periorbital hyperpigmenation with the Q switched alexandrite laser immediately following the use of pulsed CO_2 laser.[18] All patients have distinctively visible brown hyperpigmenation treated with first CO_2 laser followed by QS alexandrite laser. There are three different conditions contributing to periorbital hyperpigmentation:

1. Shadowing secondary to the bulging contour of the lower eyelid.
2. Bluish color secondary to the venous network subcutaneously or red color secondary to the visible dermal capillary network or both.
3. Brown color secondary to melanin superficially or brown/blue secondary to dermal melanin. Only of last group patients where melanin is responsible for hyperpigmentation can be treated with this type of laser. Lesions were treated with 3 mm spot size at the fluence of 8.0 J/cm^2. Pulsed CO_2 laser (ablating laser) was used first because of its efficiency to deliver heat for collagen contraction and then QS Alexandrite laser for better resolving of hyperpigmentation. Epidermal pigment is removed by CO_2 laser and dermal pigment resolved gradually after some time. Melanin is a major skin chromophore of the 755 beam of QS alexandrite laser.[19] The scientific reason for using two lasers in same sitting is that CO_2 laser to ablate the epidermis will eliminate competing epidermal melenocytes and remove epidermis itself, thereby reducing the scattering of beam and physically placing QS alexandrite laser closer to dermal melanin target. In conclusion, the use of multiple lasers in single treatment can be very effective in treating periorbital hyperpigmentation. This combined treatment will not lead to additional adverse sequelae and eliminate the need of multiple sessions which will be beneficial to patients and reduce the number of sitting *per se*.

There is also scientific data suggesting treatment protocol combining Q-switched ruby laser[20] and topical bleaching treatment using retinoic acid and hydroquinone are considered effective for improvement of periorbital hyperpigmentation, with a low incidence of postinflammatory hyperpigmentation.[21]

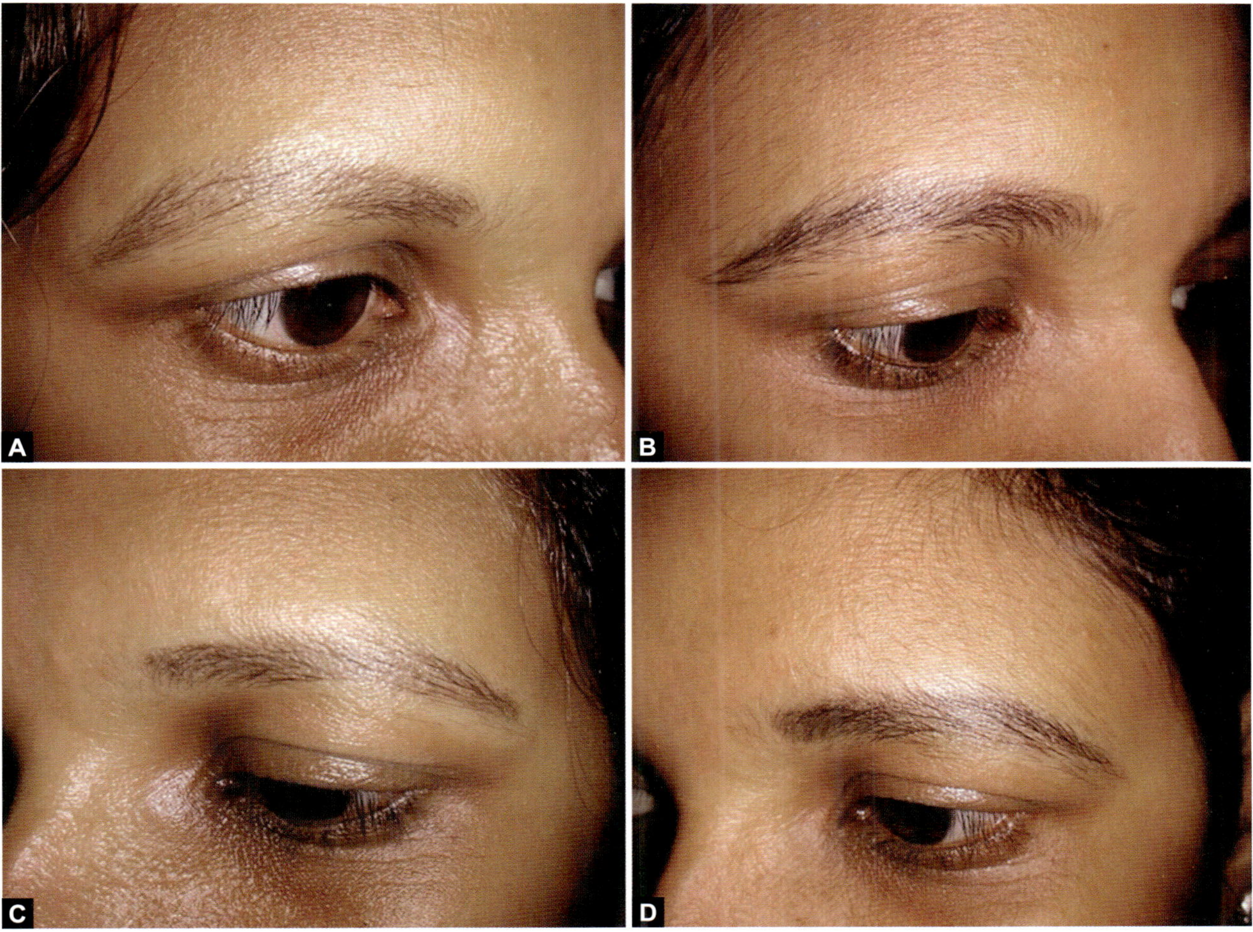

Figs 4A to D: Before and after treatment by low fluence Q-switched Nd:YAG laser. (*Source*: J Sakhiya)

CONCLUSION

Periorbital hyperpigmentation is a complex and challenging dermatological condition for both dermatologist and patients. Management is always a cocktail of treatments. Author found that not all "periorbital hyperpigmentations" are due to melanin pigmentation. Some are vascular and some are postinflammatory and others are due to the anatomical shadowing effects. So it is recommended that different types of periorbital hyperpigmentation should be treated differently. In spite of all treatment, proper counseling is must in each and every patient, and unrealistic patient is a relative contraindication of any procedure or treatment.

ACKNOWLEDGMENTS

Author thanks Dr J Sakhiya for providing photographs for this chapter. The author gratefully acknowledges Dr Manisha Devani, MS (Ophthalmology), for her help in editing this chapter.

REFERENCES

1. Freitag FM, Cestari TF. What causes dark circles under the eyes? J Cosmet Dermatol. 2007;6(3):211-5.
2. Philippe Deprez. Textbook of Chemical Peels:Superficial, Medium and Deep Peels in Cosmetic Practice. Series in Cosmetic and Laser Therapy. CRC Press; 2007 p. 392.
3. Malakar S, Lahiri K, Banerjee U, et al. Periorbital melanosis is an extension of pigmentary demarcation line-F on face. Indian J Dermatol Venereol Leprol. 2007;73(5):323-5.
4. Ranu H, Thng S, Goh BK, et al. Periorbital hyperpigmentation in Asians: an epidemiologic study and a proposed classification. Dermatol Surg. 2011;37(9):1297-303.
5. Gendler EC. Treatment of periorbital hyperpigmenation. Aesthet Surg J. 2005;25(6):618-24.
6. Morrow DM. Chemical peeling of eyelids and periorbital area. J Dermatol Surg Oncol. 1992;18(2):102-10.
7. Brody HJ. Chemical Peeling and Resurfacing, 2nd edition. St. Louis: Mosby; 1997. pp. 137-59.

8. Smith WP. Epidermal and dermal effects of topical lactic acid. J Am Acad Dermatol. 1996;35(3):388-91.
9. Sharquie KE, Al-Tikerrty MM, Al-Mashhadani SA. Lactic acid chemical peels as new therapeutic modality in melasma in comparision to Jessner's solution chemical peel. Dermatol Surg. 2006;32(12):1429-36.
10. Khunger Niti. Combination and sequential peels. Step by Step—Chemical Peels. New Delhi: Jaypee Brothers Medical Publisher; 2009.
11. Shrilatha S Trasi. Periorbital rejuvenation. ACS(I) Textbook on Cutaneous and Aesthetic Surgery. New Delhi: Jaypee Brothers Medical Publishers; 2012. pp. 714-20.
12. West TB, Alsters TS. Improvement of infraorbital hyperpigmentation following carbon dioxide laser resurfacing. Dermatol Surg. 1998;24(6):615-6.
13. Sukal SA, Chapas AM, Bernstein LJ, et al. Eyelid tightening and improved eyelid aperture through nonablative fractional resurfacing. Dermatol Surg. 2008;34(11):1454-8.
14. Lin CC, Tseng PC, Chen CC, et al. Iritis and pupillary distortion after periorbital cosmetic alexandrite laser. Graefes Arch Clin Exp Ophthalmol. 2011;249(5):783-5.
15. Sherling M, Friedman PM, Adrian R, et al. Consensus recommendations on the use of an erbium-doped 1,550-nm fractionated laser and its applications in dermatologic laser surgery. Dermatol Surg. 2010;36(4):461-9.
16. Moody MN, Landau JM, Goldberg LH. Fractionated 1550-nm erbium-doped fiber laser for the treatment of periorbital hyperpigmentation. Dermatol Surg. 2012;38(1): 139-42.
17. Manstein D, Herron GS, Sink RK, et al. Fractional photothermolysis: a new concept for coetaneous remodelling using microscopic patterns of thermal injury. Lasers Surg Med. 2004;34(5):426-38.
18. Manuskiatti W, Fitzpatrick RE, Goldman MP. Treatment of facial skin using combinations of CO_2, Q switched alexandrite, flash lamp-pumped pulsed dye, and Er:YAG laser in the same treatment session. Dermatol Surg. 2000; 26(2):114-20.
19. Anderson RR. Laser tissue interactions. In: Goldman MP, Fitzpatrick RE (Eds). Cutaneous Laser Surgery: The Art and Science of Selective Photothermolysis, 2nd edn. St Louis: Mosby; 1999. pp. 1-18.
20. Watanabe S, Nakai K. Condition known as "dark rings under the eyes" in the Japanese population is a kind of dermal melenocytosis, which can be successfully treated by Q switched ruby laser. Dermatol Surg. 2006;32(6):785-9.
21. Momosawa A, Kurita M, Ozaki M, et al. Combined therapy using Q-switched ruby laser and bleaching treatment with tretinoin and hydroquinone for periorbital skin hyperpigmentation in Asians. Plast Reconstr Surg. 2008;121(1): 282-8.

48

Progressive Macular Hypomelanosis

Prasad Kumarasinghe, Steven Thng

Key Features

- Progressive macular hypomelanosis (PMH) is a common condition among adolescents and young adults.
- It is characterized by asymptomatic hypopigmented ill-defined macules located mostly on the trunk.
- PMH is more often seen in persons with Type II–Type V skin, but it occurs in all ethnic groups.
- According to currently available evidence *Propionibacterium acnes* (*P. acnes*) or a subspecies of *P. acnes* appears to cause PMH.
- Topical benzoyl peroxide and clindamycin with ultraviolet light treatment improves the condition but relapses are common.

INTRODUCTION

Progressive macular hypomelanosis (PMH) is an asymptomatic dermatological condition causing multiple discrete as well as coalescing hypopigmented macules on the skin, predominantly on the posterior trunk and abdomen in young adults. It can cause anxiety and distress in some persons with this condition. The pathogenesis of PMH has been attributed to a subspecies of *Propionibacterium acnes* (*P. acnes*).

Progressive macular hypomelanosis is a common condition in many parts of the world.[1-40] It is often under recognized, misdiagnosed and under-reported. The wording "progressive macular hypomelanosis" is actually a misnomer. While it may progress initially, the progression is not relentless and it tends to improve after many years. This same condition has been described under many different names in the past. The other names used to describe this condition include; cutis trunci variata, progressive macular confluent hypomelanosis, idiopathic macular hypomelanosis of the melanodermic half cast of Guillet-Helenon, Creole dyschromia, nummular and confluent hypomelanosis, idiopathic large macule hypomelanosis and extensive pityriasis alba. We believe that pityriasis alba should be considered a separate entity rather than being confused with PMH.

Currently, there appears to be a consensus for the name "progressive macular hypomelanosis."[3,15,29-31,38,40] Until the etiology and natural history are well established, it is advisable to keep this name rather than change it.

HISTORY

Progressive macular hypomelanosis was first described by Guillet, Gauthier and Helenon as PMH of the trunk (1985) in a publication in French language.[1,3] Borelli (1987) from Venezuela described a similar condition under the name "cutis trunci variata".[2]

Since the 1980s there have been many articles published on this subject.[1-40] Many important papers came from the Netherlands, pioneered by Westerhoff, Menke and Relyveld. Kumarasinghe et al. described PMH for the first time in Asia.[15] In the last 7 years there have been many reports of PMH from other parts of Asia and South America, in people with pigmented skin, as well as in Caucasian populations from many European countries, USA and Australia.[4-14,16-21,24-27,32-37,39,40]

EPIDEMIOLOGY

True prevalence of PMH is unknown. Lesurer et al. (1994) noted 121 PMH cases during systematic screening of 511 patients in Marinique, West Indies.[18] This screening was done to check for leprosy. In an unpublished study carried out at Colombo North Teaching Hospital in Sri Lanka (Kumarasinghe 2000), all patients between 18 and 40 years presenting to the dermatology clinic were screened for PMH irrespective of the presenting complaint, for 8 months. In the cohort screened, up to 10% of the persons were found to have asymptomatic PMH. As such PMH is not uncommon among persons presenting to dermatology clinics for other conditions. Personal observations of the authors at the National Skin Centre in Singapore also suggest a similar picture. Personal observations from Western Australia (PK) suggest a lower prevalence in fair-skinned persons. Many patients with this condition are not very concerned about the patchy pigment variation in this regard. As such many do not see a dermatologist or even a general practitioner. However, some are very distressed and embarrassed about it. Relyveld et al. had identified 48 patients with PMH in one year at The Netherlands Institute for Pigment Disorders, whereas they identified 23 patients with pityriasis versicolor and 17 patients with pityriasis alba during the same period (Relyveld 2007). According to published reports and personal communications, PMH has been reported in the West Indies, the Netherlands, Venezuela, Germany, Spain, Turkey, UK, France, USA, Australia, Sri Lanka, India, Singapore, Malaysia, Ivory Coast, The Philippines, South Korea, Brazil, Senegal and China.[1-40]

Progressive macular hypomelanosis is more commonly detected in Type III, IV, V and VI skin. In fact one author from Senegal mentions that it is a "normal" variation of the skin, which fades away after the fifth decade in life, implying that it is very common in the general population.[19]

Most authors agree that there is a female preponderance. In the Netherlands, it has been reported as 7F:1M among 291 registered PMH patients.[30] However, the degree of female preponderance has been variable in other studies. In the cohort from The Netherlands the mean age was 26.5 years, with an age range between 13 and 45 years. Our cohort from Singapore had a mean age of 25.9 years with an age range between 19 and 45 years.[15] A South Korean study recorded an age range of 14–28 years with a mean of 23.85 years.[12] A Brazilian study[7] recorded mean age of onset of the disease as 20.8 years, in a cohort of 84 patients.

It is almost unbelievable that a common skin disorder such as PMH was not described in the literature before 1985. However, it is unlikely to be a "new" disease. Most likely PMH has existed for many decades or longer but it has not been recognized as a separate condition. However, Relyveld et al. entertain the possibility that it may be due to some mutant strains of *P. acnes* which have evolved over the years.[30,31]

CLINICAL FEATURES

Progressive macular hypomelanosis is characterized by poorly defined nummular hypopigmented macules, localized predominantly on the trunk. Sometimes neck, buttocks and proximal limbs are also affected. Usually the lesions are symmetrically distributed. Posterior trunk is the most commonly affected area, particularly the lower thoracic and lumbar regions. Discrete (e.g. 0.5 cm) and confluent lesions are seen. Sometimes large areas of confluent lesions (e.g. 20 cm) can give rise to a blotchy dyspigmentation. At times it may be difficult to identify the normal areas from hypopigmented areas. This can be resolved by examining the whole body to ascertain the individual patient's normal skin color. Some patients notice non-tanning or minimally tanning pale patches on the trunk after sun exposure (e.g. in summer), as the PMH lesions do not tan as easily as the other areas.

Examination under Wood's Lamp usually enhances the appearance of PMH lesions. This can be particularly useful in light-skinned persons. With a powerful Wood's Lamp, in a totally dark room, red follicular fluorescence can be detected in the hypopigmented areas.[38] In the normally pigmented areas this is not seen. On the contrary, if the room is not darkened sufficiently and the Wood's lamp is weak, one may not see the fluorescent dots. However, we as well as other authors have seen the cases of PMH where the red follicular fluorescence cannot be demonstrated on the hypopigmented macules. One possibility is that such lesions are older lesions, where hypopigmentation remains for many months or years even after the *Propionibacteria* have disappeared or greatly diminished in the area.

Interestingly, acne is not an association with this condition, although acne is etiologically related to infection of the follicles by *P. acnes*.[15,30,38]

The natural history of PMH appears to be occurrence in adolescence or in young adult life, slow progression over many years and a natural decline slowly. One author (PK) has seen some cases of slow resolution over many years. This is further supported by the fact that the mean age of PMH is around 26 years, and PMH is never seen in persons over 50 years.

Figures 1 to 4 show typical appearances of PMH.

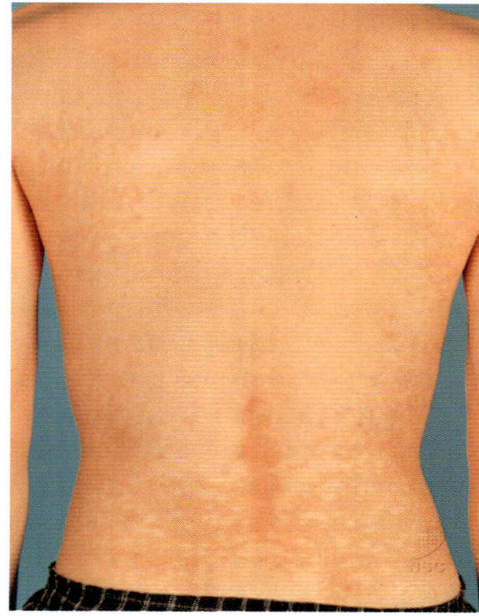

Fig. 1: A Singaporean patient with characteristic hypopigmented ill-defined confluent and discrete macules on the posterior trunk. (*Source:* National Skin Centre, Singapore)

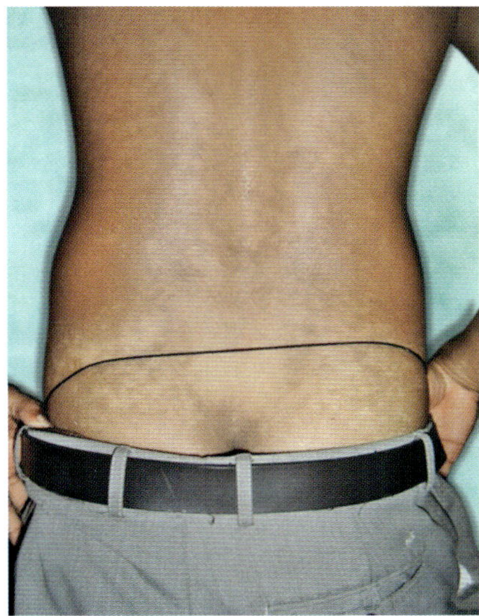

Fig. 2: A Sri Lankan patient with progressive macular hypomelanosis extending to the buttocks. (*Source:* Dr Sathyareka Sivapragasam, Sri Lanka)

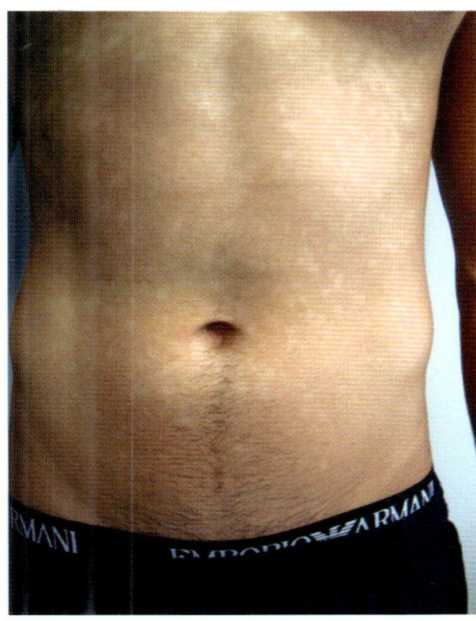

Fig. 3: An Australian patient of Chinese descent with typical hypopigmented macules of PMH on the abdomen and lower chest

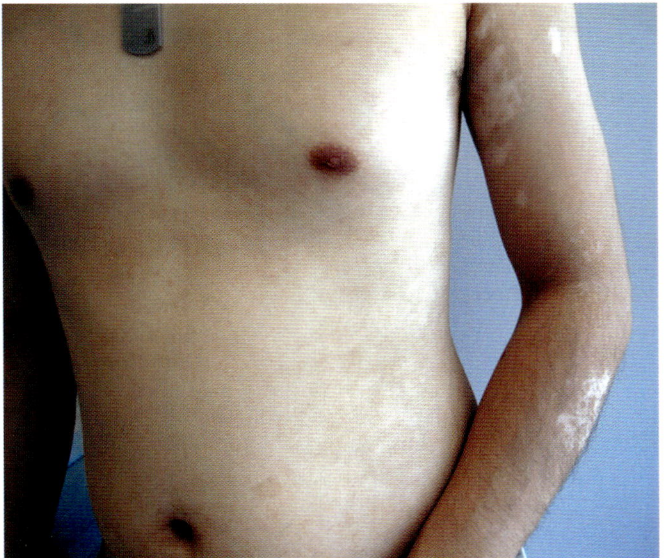

Fig. 4: A patient with co-existing vitiligo of the left upper limb and PMH on the trunk showing the contrast of skin color (vitiligo is not a recognized association; most likely a chance occurrence)

DIFFERENTIAL DIAGNOSES AND PITFALLS IN DIAGNOSIS

Several hypopigmented conditions come to the differential diagnosis of PMH. **Table 1** gives the main differential diagnoses.

Progressive macular hypomelanosis is a clinical diagnosis especially for those experienced clinicians who are familiar with this condition. However, when in doubt certain investigations become helpful.

RELEVANT INVESTIGATIONS

In cases of uncertainty of diagnosis, a skin scrapings test to exclude tinea versicolor, Wood's lamp examination, and skin biopsy could be useful. Confocal scanning laser microscopy examination shows less prominent pigment rings around dermal papillae.[40] Skin scrapings tests are negative for fungi or yeasts. Bacterial culture of the fluorescing follicular areas (under Wood's lamp) would reveal *P. acnes* or a subspecies of *P. acnes*. However, this is not necessary for a diagnosis and it is done only in research settings. Multiple skin biopsies are indicated, if hypopigmented mycosis fungoides is suspected.

DIAGNOSIS

Diagnosis of PMH is mostly clinical. Hypopigmented (but not depigmented) ill-defined normosensitive, discrete and confluent macules, without any significant scaliness on the surface, most prominent on the trunk, without any history of previous inflammation, in an adolescent or an adult up to about 40 years, usually suggests a diagnosis of PMH.

MICROSCOPY AND ELECTRON MICROSCOPY

Light microscopic changes of the hypopigmented skin lesions are often subtle in lighter skin types. If it is not compared with a biopsy of the normal skin of the same patient the appearance

Table 1: Important differential diagnoses, and clues to differentiate them	
Progressive macular hypomelanosis	Hypopigmented ill-defined symmetrically distributed macules mostly on the trunk, rarely on neck, buttocks, arms, non-scaly, non-pruritic. Reddish follicular fluorescence in hypopigmented patches on Wood's lamp examination
Pityriasis versicolor (tinea versicolor)	Well demarcated, neck is a common area affected in addition to the trunk, fine scaling visible in active lesions, scrapings positive for ***Malassezia furfur (M. furfur)***
Hypopigmented mycosis fungoides	Textural change of skin; early lesions atrophic, later infiltrated plaque lesions, buttocks and lower limbs often affected, asymmetric distribution
Tuberculoid leprosy	Sensory impairment of the patches, textural change of skin, thickened peripheral nerves
Post-inflammatory hypopigmentation	Previous history of inflammation, limited to those areas, not progressive
Pityriasis alba	Associated with eczema, face commonly affected
Pseudoleukoderma angiospasticum (Bier's spots)	Due to differential cutaneous vascular dilatation/constriction patterns, more visible on arms than trunk. Less commonly seen in darker skin
Evolving vitiligo	Usually patches are depigmented rather than hypopigmented, face, distal limbs, axillae, groins often affected in vitiligo
Post-kala azar dermal leishmaniasis (PKDL)	Endemic area, past history of leishmaniasis, indurated areas of skin

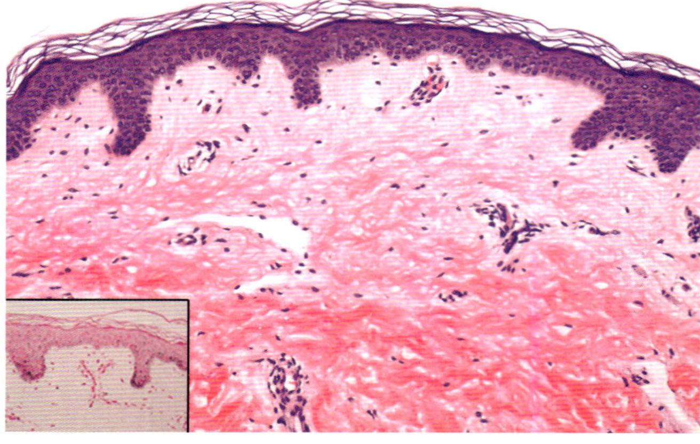

Fig. 5: Hematoxylin and eosin stained sections of a biopsy of a PMH lesion, showing a relatively normal epidermis and dermis on light microscopy. Inset shows slightly reduced melanization on Masson-Fontana stain. (*Source:* National Skin Centre, Singapore)

can be reported as "normal". However, biopsy often rules out or gives clues to other diagnoses in doubtful cases (e.g. leprosy, mycosis fungoides). In many cases, if normal skin of the same person is compared with biopsies from lesional skin a mild reduction of the epidermal melanization can be observed. The dermis does not show any significant changes. **Figure 5** shows microscopic features of hematoxylin and eosin stained sections of lesional skin and normal skin in the same patient.

This histopathological difference in melanization of epidermis is more obvious in darker skinned patients. The number of melanocytes is normal.[15,28,30,38,40] There is no significant inflammatory infiltrate in the dermis. There is no thickening of epidermal keratin layer. There is no spongiosis, fungal hyphae or granulomas. Gram staining of sections of the pilosebaceous units of hypopigmented lesions may show Gram positive material attributed to be bacteria.[30,38]

Electron microscopy of lesional skin shows smaller more immature melanosomes in the melanocytes and the keratinocytes in the epidermis.[3,15,30,38,40] There are melanosome precursors in all stages of development in the lesional melanocytes, but in lesional melanocytes mature melanosomes are distinctly smaller and less melanized than those in lesional skin.[28,30,38] There is a large reduction in the number of Type IV melanosomes in the keratinocytes of PMH lesions, they have smaller Type II–IV melanosomes; they are distributed in clusters in membrane bound groups.[28,40] Wu et al. noted that there was no degradation of melanosomes in the lysosomal compartments.[40] Electron microscopic changes of melanosome size and melanin intensity in the melanosomes are more pronounced in darker skin types, compared to lighter skin types.

Wu et al. reported that melanocytes cultured *in vitro* from the lesional skin showed no obvious differences in morphology, compared to melanocytes cultured from normal skin.[40]

ETIOLOGY

Many theories have been proposed for this dyspigmentation. Borelli considered PMH to be a genodermatosis. He based it on the observation that he noted the disorder among family members.[2]

Guillet et al. thought that PMH occurs only among the mixed races, and postulated that some genes get switched off producing less melanin due to unknown influences.[1,3,11]

Fitzpatrick postulated that it is due to a long-term effect following fungal infection of the skin.[30]

Di Lernia et al. considered the possibility that PMH could be the same condition as extensive pityriasis alba.[41]

However with subsequent worldwide reports it has become clear that PMH occurs in many races, without any ethnic mixing, it does not follow pityriasis versicolor, and it is not the same condition as pityriasis alba.

In 2004, Westerhof et al. reported that many follicles in hypopigmented lesions show red fluorescent dots, corresponding to porphyrins produced by *P. acnes*.[38] His team managed to culture *P. acnes* from the tissue specimens collected from these red fluorescing spots. Subsequently they postulated that PMH is associated with a putative *P. acnes* species.[30,31] In 8 out of 14 patients, they found the species found in the fluorescing dots (on Woods Lamp examination) is slightly different to the *P. acnes* strains found in acne lesions. They used the technique of amplified fragment length polymorphism for genetic mapping. Westerhof et al. proposed that the hypopigmentation in the hypopigmented macules of PMH is due to a pigment lightening factor produced by *P. acnes* or its subspecies. They base their hypotheses on the following facts:[30,38]

- The presence of red follicular fluorescence in the hypopigmented spots and the absence of this phenomenon in the normal skin when viewed under a Wood's light in a dark room.
- Cultivation of *P. acnes* from the follicles in the hypopigmented spots but not from follicles in normal looking skin.
- Improvement of the disorder after elimination of these microorganisms with topical antimicrobial treatment in combination with UVA light.

The same authors reported in 2006 that benzoyl peroxide, clindamycin and UVA improved PMH more than topical fluticazone and UVA.[29]

Several studies from South Korea, Brazil, China and Sri Lanka indicate that treatment with topical Benzoyl peroxide, clindamycin and narrow band UVB therapy also improve PMH.[13,24,33-35,39]

However there are some unanswered questions:

- Why is PMH not common in acne patients?
- Why does PMH not usually occur on the face despite face having the most number of prominent sebaceous glands, and an abundance of *Propionibacteria*?
- Why is it that some patients with PMH do not show any fluorescing follicular dots on Wood's lamp examination?

A few authors (Kuznetsov 2011, Neynaber S et al. 2009) even doubt whether *P. acnes* is the cause of PMH and they think *P. acnes* may be just a "passenger" in the lesions.[16,25]

There may be some age-related hormonal influence on melanogenesis as well, considering that PMH is common in adolescents and young adults. Female preponderance also suggests a hormonal influence.

Overall, we believe that at present there is sufficient evidence to suggest *P. acnes* or its related subspecies are etiologically related to PMH. Even in acne the density of *P. acnes* is not the determining factor of severity of acne, although it is etiologically relevant. Once the inhibitory cellular mechanisms are triggered on in the melanocyte keratinocyte units, they may lead to poor melanization of the epidermis in the downstream effect, due to reduced melanin production by the melanocytes and reduced transfer of melanosomes to the epidermal keratinocytes.

MANAGEMENT

There is no universally accepted method of treatment. Relapses are common. Relyveld et al. recommend once daily 5% benzoyl peroxide and once daily topical clindamycin with UVA irradiation for 20 minutes for 3 times a week.[30] Others have reported success with Lymecycline and topical benzoyl peroxide,[5] oral doxycycline with sun exposure,[27] benzoyl peroxide and narrowband ultraviolet B (NBUVB),[39] NBUVB only,[17] topical benzoyl peroxide and 1% clindamycin without UV treatment,[33] 1% clindamycin, 5% benzoyl peroxide with NBUVB for 3 months[35] and oral isotretinoin.[14]

If it is mild and static we recommend explaining the condition to the patient and simply observing, considering the time and inconvenience of continuing treatment. If the patient is very concerned and wishes to take treatment, our first line is topical 5% benzoyl peroxide and 1% clindamycin lotion topical application and narrowband UVB treatment twice or thrice a week for three months. If a relapse occurs retreatment can be initiated. **Figures 6A and B** show a patient who improved with the above regime of treatment. According

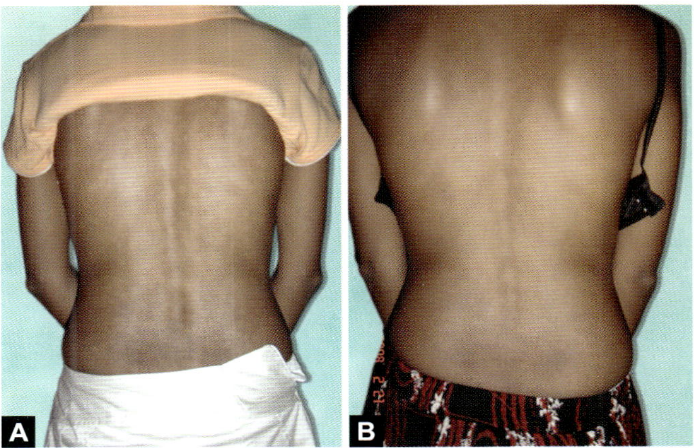

Figs 6A and B: Improvement of PMH lesions after treatment with topical benzoyl peroxide 5%, topical clindamycin 1% and narrowband UVB treatment in a Sri Lankan patient. (*Source:* Dr Sathyareka Sivapragasam, Sri Lanka)

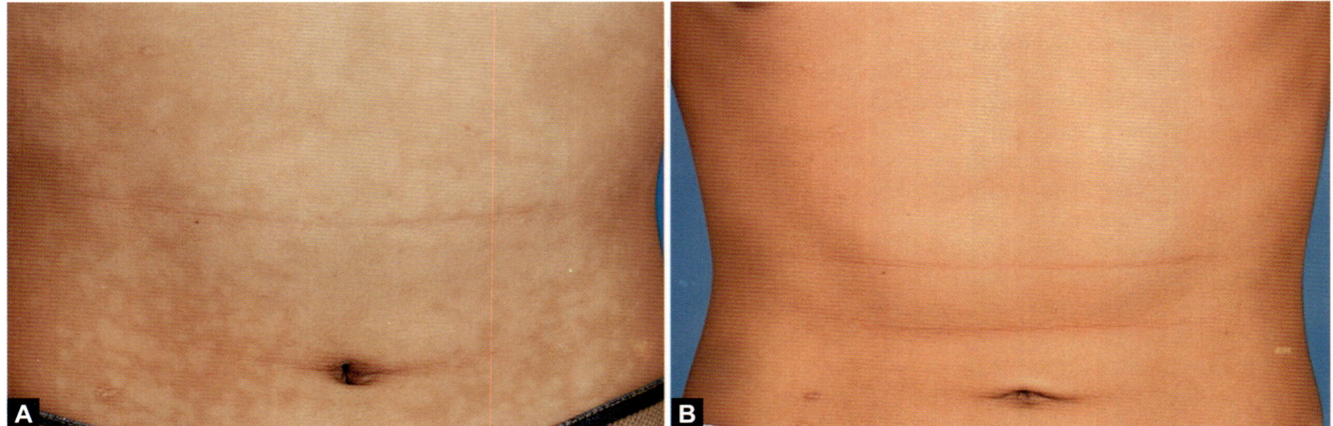

Figs 7A and B: Improvement of PMH lesions in a Singaporean patient after narrowband UVB treatment twice a day for 3 months. (*Source:* National Skin Centre, Singapore)

to the some Singaporean dermatologists (Kwah et al. 2010, ST personal experience) twice a week monotherapy with NBUVB for 3 months also shows very good results.[17] However, relapses are common. **Figures 7A and B** show a patient who improved with narrow band UVB treatment alone.

Kim et al. (2012) reported success with oral isotretinoin in treating PMH.[14] Although oral treatment with isotretinoin will reduce the *Propionibacterium* on the skin by minimizing sebum secretion, it may not be justified considering the significant side effects and the uncertainty about the end point of treatment.

A more effective less cumbersome treatment, with a simpler maintenance regime would be the ideal. But it is yet to come.

FUTURE DIRECTIONS

Further characterization of the subspecies of *P. acnes* that cause PMH, long-term follow-up of PMH to ascertain the natural history of untreated and treated patients, study of hormonal influences on PMH and an easier form of treatment are likely to be the areas where there will be more research in the near future.

CONCLUSION

Progressive macular hypomelanosis is an asymptomatic condition leading to ill-defined hypopigmented symmetrically distributed macules on the trunk. It is more prevalent in young adults. All ethnic groups are affected but it is more apparent in darker skinned races. *Propionebacterium acnes* or a subspecies of *Propionibacterium* appears to be important in the etiology of this condition. It can be treated with topical benzoyl peroxide and clindamycin lotion coupled with ultraviolet light exposure. However relapses are common. It is important to be aware of this condition and make the correct diagnosis.

REFERENCES

1. Guillet G, Gauthier Y, Helenon R. Hypomelanose Maculaire Progressive Du Tronc (Hypopigmentation Primitive Acquise Des Antilles) Paris: Soc Fr Dermatol (Paris) 1985.
2. Borelli D. Cutis 'trunci varieta' a new genetic dermatosis. Med Cutan Ibero Lat Am. 1987;15:317-9.
3. Guillet G, Helenon R, Gauthier Y, et al. Progressive macular hypomelanosis of the trunk: primary acquired hypopigmentation. J Cutan Pathol. 1988;15(5):286-9.
4. Cavalcanti SM, de Franca ER, Lins AK, et al. Investigation of *Propionibacterium acnes* in progressive macular hypomelanosis using real-time PCR and culture. Int J Dermatol. 2011;50(11):1347-52.
5. Cavalcanti SM, Querino MC, Magalhaes V, et al. The use of lymecycline and benzoyl peroxide for the treatment of progressive macular hypomelanosis: a prospective study. Anais brasileiros de dermatologia. 2011;86(4):813-4.
6. Chung YL, Goo B, Chung WS, et al. A case of progressive macular hypomelanosis treated with narrow-band UVB. J Eur Acad Dermatol Venereol. 2007;21(7):1007-9.
7. Duarte I, Nina BI, Gordiano MC, et al. Progressive macular hypomelanosis: an epidemiological study and therapeutic response to phototherapy. Anais brasileiros de dermatologia. 2010;85(5):621-4.
8. Echeverria B, Botella-Estrada R, Escutia B, et al. Progressive macular hypomelanosis successfully treated with topical clindamycin and benzoyl peroxide. Actas dermo-sifiliograficas. 2010;101(6):565-7.
9. Elmariah SB, Kundu RV. Progressive macular hypomelanosis. J Drugs Dermatol. 2011;10(5):502-6.

10. Erpolat S, Gorpelioglu C, Sarifakioglu E. A case of progressive macular hypomelanosis treated with 1% topical clindamycin lotion and narrow-band ultraviolet B. Photodermatol Photoimmunol Photomed. 2010;26(5):277-8.
11. Guillet G, Guillet MH. Creole dyschromia or idiopathic macular hypomelanosis of the melanodermic halfcast of Guillet-Helenon. Bull Soc Pathol Exot. 1997;90(5):333-4.
12. Hwang SW, Hong SK, Kim SH, et al. Progressive macular hypomelanosis in korean patients: a clinicopathologic study. Ann Dermatol. 2009;21(3):261-7.
13. Kim MB, Kim GW, Cho HH, et al. Narrowband UVB treatment of progressive macular hypomelanosis. J Am Acad Dermatol. 2012;66(4):598-605.
14. Kim YJ, Lee DY, Lee JY, et al. Progressive macular hypomelanosis showing excellent response to oral isotretinoin. J Dermatol. 2012;39(11):937-8.
15. Kumarasinghe SP, Tan SH, Thng S, et al. Progressive macular hypomelanosis in Singapore: a clinico-pathological study. Int J Dermatol. 2006;45(6):737-42.
16. Kuznetsov AV, Flaig MJ, Ruzicka T, et al. Progressive macular hypomelanosis Guillet-Helenon: structural and immunohistochemical findings. J Clin Pathol. 2011;64(8):734-6.
17. Kwah YC, Chong WS, Thiam-Seng Theng C, et al. Treatment of progressive macular hypomelanosis with narrow-band ultraviolet B phototherapy. Photodermatol Photoimmunol Photomed. 2010;26(3):153-5.
18. Lesueur A, Garcia-Granel V, Helenon R, et al. Progressive macular confluent hypomelanosis in mixed ethnic melanodermic subjects: an epidemiologic study of 511 patients. Annales de dermatologie et de venereologie. 1994;121(12):880-3.
19. Mahe A. Pigmentary Disorders. In: Tyring SK, Lupi O, Hengge UR (Eds). Tropical Dermatology, 1st edn. Philadelphia: Elsevier; 2006. p. 432.
20. Martinez ML, Azana Defez JM, Lopez Villaescusa MT, et al. Anti-fungal resistant hypopigmented macules in an adolescent. Semergen/Sociedad Espanola de Medicina Rural y Generalista. 2012;38(6):405-7.
21. Martinez-Martinez ML, Azana-Defez JM, Rodriguez-Vazquez M, et al. Progressive macular hypomelanosis. Pediatr Dermatol. 2012;29(4):460-2.
22. Menke HE, Njoo D, Westerhof W. Progressve macular hypomelanosis of the trunk. In: Nordlund JJ (Ed). The Pigmentary Suystem, 1st edn. New York: Oxford University Press; 1988. pp. 686-8.
23. Menke H, Relyveld G, Westerhof W. Comment on the letter by Chung et al. about progressive macular hypomelanosis. J Eur Acad Dermatol Venereol. 2008;22(8):1029-30.
24. Montero LC, Belinchon I, Toledo F, et al. Progressive macular hypomelanosis, excellent response with narrow-band ultraviolet B phototherapy. Photodermatol Photoimmunol Photomed. 2011;27(3):162-3.
25. Neynaber S, Kirschner C, Kamann S, et al. Progressive macular hypomelanosis: a rarely diagnosed hypopigmentation in Caucasians. Dermatol Res Pract. 2009;2009:607682.
26. Pandya AG. Top accessed article: propionibacterium acnes and the pathogenesis of progressive macular hypomelanosis. Arch Dermatol. 2012;148(11):1256.
27. Perman M, Sheth P, Lucky AW. Progressive macular hypomelanosis in a 16-year-old. Pediatr Dermatol. 2008;25(1):63-5.
28. Relyveld GN, Dingemans KP, Menke HE, et al. Ultrastructural findings in progressive macular hypomelanosis indicate decreased melanin production. J Eur Acad Dermatol Venereol. 2008;22(5):568-74.
29. Relyveld GN, Kingswijk MM, Reitsma JB, et al. Benzoyl peroxide/clindamycin/UVA is more effective than fluticasone/UVA in progressive macular hypomelanosis: a randomized study. J Am Acad Dermatol. 2006;55(5):836-43.
30. Relyveld GN, Menke HE, Westerhof W. Progressive macular hypomelanosis: an overview. Am J Clin Dermatol. 2007;8(1):13-9.
31. Relyveld GN, Westerhof W, Woudenberg J, et al. Progressive macular hypomelanosis is associated with a putative Propionibacterium species. J Invest Dermatol. 2010;130(4):1182-4.
32. Rodriguez-Lojo R, Verea MM, Velasco D, et al. Progressive and confluent macular hypomelanosis. Actas dermo-sifiliograficas. 2010;101(3):268-9.
33. Santos JB, Almeida OL, Silva LM, et al. Efficacy of topical combination of benzoyl peroxide 5% and clindamycin 1% for the treatment of progressive macular hypomelanosis: a randomized, doubleblind, placebo-controlled trial. Anais brasileiros de dermatologia. 2011;86(1):50-4.
34. Sim JH, Lee DJ, Lee JS, et al. Comparison of the clinical efficacy of NBUVB and NBUVB with benzoyl peroxide/clindamycin in progressive macular hypomelanosis. J Eur Acad Dermatol Venereol. 2011;25(11):1318-23.
35. Sivapragasam S, Sathgurunathan K. A study of progressive macular hypomelanosis in Sri Lanka. Poster, 68th Annual Conference of American Academy of Dermatology 2010.
36. Tierney EP, Hamzavi I. Progressive macular hypomelanosis arising in a young African American woman in association with pregnancy and a toxic nodular goiter. J Drugs Dermatol. 2010;9(4):393-7.
37. Vermazeren-van Roij JM, Faber WR. A white woman with white skin spots. Nederlands tijdschrift voor geneeskunde. 2011;155(33):A2421.
38. Westerhof W, Relyveld GN, Kingswijk MM, et al. Propionibacterium acnes and the pathogenesis of progressive macular hypomelanosis. Arch Dermatol. 2004;140(2):210-4.
39. Wu XG, Xu AE, Luo XY, et al. A case of progressive macular hypomelanosis successfully treated with benzoyl peroxide plus narrow-band UVB. J Dermatolog Treat. 2010;21(6):367-8.
40. Wu XG, Xu AE, Song XZ, et al. Clinical, pathologic, and ultrastructural studies of progressive macular hypomelanosis. Int J Dermatol. 2010;49(10):1127-32.
41. Di Lernia V, Ricci C. Progressive and extensive hypomelanosis and extensive pityriasis alba:same disease, different names. J Eur Acad Dermatol Venereol. 2005;19(3):370-2.

49

Non-melasma Facial Melanoses

Gautam Kumar Singh

Key Features

- Non-melasma facial melanoses are overlapping, psychologically disturbing and challenging to treat.
- Detailed history, thorough clinical examination, pattern of distribution of pigmentation along with histopathological examination can establish the diagnosis in majority of such cases.
- Avoidance of provoking factors, sun protective measures and additional use of lightening agents may help in management of such dermatoses.

INTRODUCTION

Facial melanoses have always been cosmetically and psychologically disturbing to the patients. Despite of great recent advancement in dermatology as well as cosmetology, treating facial melanoses remains a challenge to the dermatologists, and equally frustrating to the patients. Melasma is the most common facial melanoses which has been studied most comprehenssively in the literature. Hence, most of the treatments of facial melanoses are based upon the response in melasma. This chapter emphasizes upon the other facial melanoses which are sometime challenging to diagnose due to overlapping features and commonly missed in the routine dermatological practices. Although there are numerous causes of facial melanoses which may be either isolated or as component of generalized hypermelanoses or with overlapping features, an attempt is made to give these conditions a classification **(Table 1)**.

Table 1: Proposed classification of facial melanosis

Well-defined facial melanoses:
• Melasma
• Lichen planus pigmentosus (LPP)
• Erythema dyschromicum perstans (EDP)
• Riehl's melanosis (RM)
• Poikiloderma of Civatte (PC)
• Nevus of Ota
• Erythrose peribuccale pigmentaire de BROCQ (EPP)
• Erythromelanosis follicularis of face and neck (EF)
Acquired melanoses which also involve face:
• Friction melanosis
• Tar melanosis
• Berloque dermatitis (BD)
• Idiopathic eruptive macular pigmentation (IEMP)
• Post-chikungunya pigmentation
• Postinflammatory hyperpigmentation (PIH)
• Hyperpigmentation due to drugs and heavy metals
Miscellaneous:
• Periorbital melanosis
• Exogenous ochronosis
• Acanthosis nigricans
• Macular amyloidosis (MA)
• Addisonian pigmentation

WELL-DEFINED FACIAL MELANOSES

Lichen Planus Pigmentosus (LPP)

This entity was first described by Indian authors, Bhutani et al. in Indian population[1] but it has been reported from other racial and ethnic groups such as Latin Americans, Middle Eastern, Japanese and Koreans.[2,3] LPP and erythema dyschromicum perstans (EDP) are now considered distinct entities with different clinical and histopathological features.[4]

It manifests as macular hyperpigmentation mainly involving the face and upper limbs, although it can be more widespread. The lesions initially appear as small, ill-defined oval to round macules, which later become confluent to form large patches of pigmentation **(Fig. 1)**. The disease has chronic course without significant pruritus and without scalp,

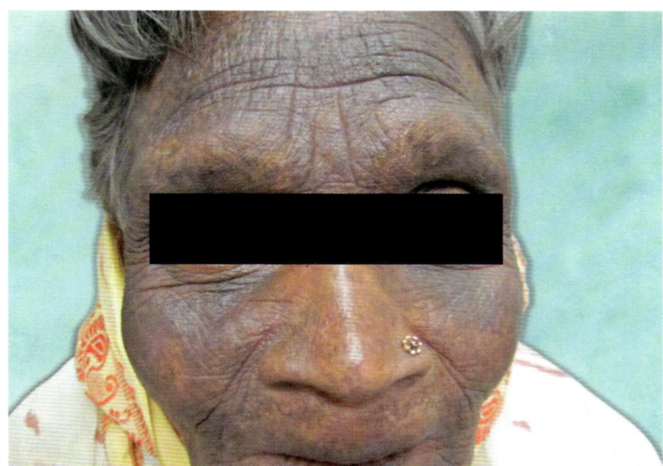

Fig. 1: Diffuse hyperpigmentation of face in lichen planus pigmentosus

nail or mucosal involvement. Lichen planus can be associated features in significant number of LPP.[1,5,6]

It is a condition of unknown etiology. However, mustard oil and amla oil for body massage and/or hair dressing for variable duration have been observed to cause LPP. Mustard oil contains allyl thiocynate, a potential photosensitizer, which could play a role in the pathogenesis of LPP.[7] The association between hepatitis C virus (HCV) infection and lichen planus (LP) has been a subject of controversy. HCV may be one of the factors associated with LPP, in those who have a tendency to develop LPP.[8]

Histopathology of LPP is quite characteristic, having hyperkeratosis, epidermal atrophy, vacuolar degeneration of the basal cell with melanophages, perivascular infiltrate and band-like infiltrate in the upper dermis.[5,8] Topical tacrolimus ointment has been found to be beneficial in the treatment of LPP.[8]

Erythema Dyschromicum Perstans (EDP)

Since the time of first description of this entity by C Oswaldo Ramirez of San Salvador, El Salvador, in 1957, EDP also known as Ashy dermatoses has been a controversial dermatosis.[9] Ramirez called the patients with this eruption Los cenicientos, meaning the ashen ones. The term EDP is credited to Marion B Sulzberger.[10] EDP is most common in Latin America and Asia.

The etiology of EDP is largely unknown. It may be associated with infections, e.g. whipworm, human immunodeficiency virus; the ingestion of toxins, e.g. ammonium nitrate, cobalt, radio contrast media, pesticides, fungicides; medications, e.g. ethambutol, penicillins, benzodiazepines and endocrinopathies like thyroid disease.[11-17] In the majority of patients, an underlying etiology is never detected. In Mexican patients, the presence of the HLA-DR4 allele may be associated with EDP.[15]

Clinically, patients present with oval-to-circular, gray-to-blue-brown macules and patches, which are symmetrically distributed on the trunk, proximal aspects of the extremities, neck and face **(Figs 2A and B)**. In acute phase, may have a thin, erythematous, papular border (piece of string), which is a unique characteristic of EDP. It is usually asymptomatic, but mild pruritus may occur.[16,17]

Zaynoun S et al. do not agree with EDP and Ashy dermatoses as same entity, they have proposed classification to delineate EDP from ashy dermatoses. Ashy dermatosis: patients with idiopathic eruptive hyperpigmented macules, irrespective of the presence or absence of interface dermatitis histologically at the time of examination. EDP: patients with lesions similar to those of ashy dermatosis, but who have or have had lesions with erythematous borders. Simulators: known dermatologic diseases, such as lichen planus (and its variants LPP and actinic lichen planus), postinflammatory hyperpigmentation (PIH), such as pityriasis rosea and erythema multiforme, drug-induced melanodermas, mastocytosis, and others.[18]

Skin biopsy is done to rule out other diagnoses rather than to confirm EDP because of non-specific histologic pattern. Active border may show mild basal cell layer vacuolar degeneration, with a mild perivascular mononuclear cell infiltrate and increased melanophages in upper dermis, adding confusion to the diagnosis of LPP. The immunopathologic study indicates a delayed hypersensitivity reaction. Ultrastructural findings demonstrate immature, small, irregular-shaped melanosomes in melanocytes and peripheral localization of melanosomes in keratinocytes.

There is no consensus guideline for the management of EDP. Spontaneous resolution has been reported in some patients, especially prepubertal children, but many patients with EDP have chronic course.[19] So far, only clofazimine, 100 mg daily for 3 months, has been found most successful.[20,21] The use of dapsone, 100 mg daily for 3 months and oral glucocorticoid therapy also has been suggested anecdotally as beneficial therapies.[22,23] Various other modalities of treatment have been tried with unsatisfactory results which include ultraviolet exposure, antibiotics, antihistamines, griseofulvin, chemical peels, corticosteroids, vitamins, isoniazid, chloroquine and psychotherapy.[18] The use of narrow-band UVB phototherapy has shown success in a few patients.[17] A low-potency topical steroid applied twice a day to the affected areas may be used, with or without a 4% hydroquinone cream for the hyperpigmentation.[22]

Riehl's Melanosis (RM)

It was Riehl, in World War I who first described this entity in people who presented with striking dark-brown to grayish-brown facial pigmentation that was most pronounced on the lateral aspects of the face and neck and primarily

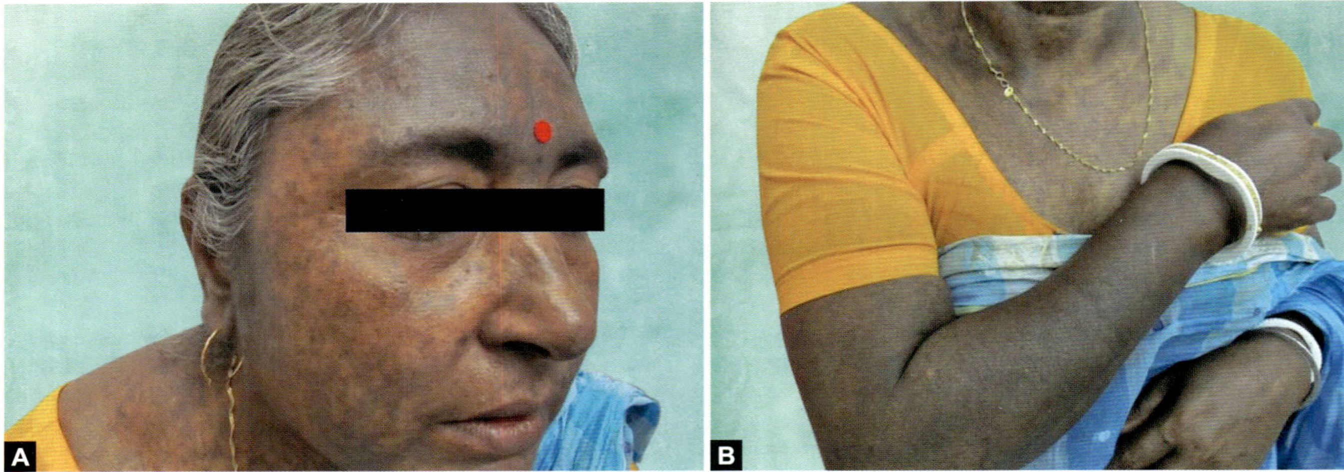

Figs 2A and B: Diffuse hyperpigmentation of face in a lady of erythema dychromium perstans

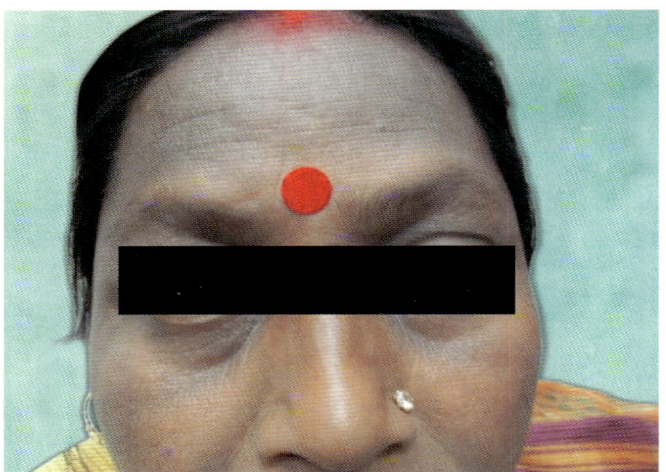

Fig. 3: Slate-gray pigmentation of face, predominantly forehead due to Kumkum application in lady of Riehl's melanosis

concentrated on the forehead, ears, temple and zygomatic regions. Riehl could not explain the cause of this condition with certainty; he attributed it to food substitutes during the time of war.[24] The majority of cases of Riehl melanosis described in the literature differ from the cases of original series of Riehl. Subsequently Osmundsen[25] and Nakayama[26] introduced the term pigmented contact dermatitis (PCD) to describe such melanosis. At present, Riehl's melanosis is considered synonymous with PCD; the common allergen being fragrances and chemicals in cosmetics.[27]

The hyperpigmentation in PCD is postulated to be caused by frequent and repeated contact with small amounts of sensitizing allergens primarily in cosmetic and textile materials. Cosmetic allergens include red and yellow pigments, chromium hydroxide, aniline and azo dyes, bactericidal agents (carbanilides, ricinoleic acid), hair dyes, red kumkum, and fragrances. Textile allergens include optical whiteners, dyes, textile finishes, mercury compounds, formaldehyde and rubber components. Sometimes occupational allergens like coal tar, pitch, asphalt, mineral oil and chromates have been incriminated.[26-36]

Kumkum is the commonest allergen causing RM in India. Commercially available red kumkum contains azo dyes, coal tar dyes, toluidine red, erythrosine, lithal red, calcium salts, fragrances, ground nut oil, tragacanth gum, turmeric powder, paraben and cananga oil.[29,35]

Most biopsy results have shown interface dermatitis with vacuolar basal cells degeneration. The upper dermis often contains a mild-to-moderate lymphohistiocytic infiltrate admixed with melanophages. These findings suggest type IV cytolytic reaction due to repeated exposure of allergens. Findings suggestive of spongiosis are lacking. It is mostly seen in dark complexion people, so pigment-genetic interactions in development of this condition has been postulated.[26-28]

It manifests as varied colored, reticular or diffuse hypermelanosis. There may be preceding erythema, edema and pruritus. The pigmentation can vary from brown, slate-gray, gray-brown, red-brown or blue-brown depending upon incriminating agent **(Fig. 3)**. The site of RM also depends on the allergen responsible for it. Pigmented cosmetic dermatitis due to cosmetics more commonly involves the face, whereas PCD due to textiles more often involves the anterior thighs or the axilla, with sparing of the axillary vault. It is most pronounced in individuals with darker complexions. Pigmentation on sun exposed area is due to photosensitization of allergen by ultraviolet rays.[26-29] Patch test, photopatch test and provocative use test or repeated open application test (ROAT) can be of immense value in finding the allergens.[29]

So far, there is no effective treatment for Riehl's melanosis. Long-term administration of vitamin C, topical application of bleaching agents (e.g. hydroquinone, retinoids and glycolic acid), and sun protection have not achieved satisfactory improvements.[37] Few studies suggest beneficial role of intense pulsed light (IPL).[38,39]

Poikiloderma of Civatte (PC)

"Poikiloderma" is classical triad of linear telangiectasia, mottled hyperpigmentation or depigmentation and superficial atrophy in a reticular pattern.[40] It was first described in 1923 by Civatte.[41] PC is not an uncommon, acquired poikiloderma of the face and neck. It has propensity to involve fair-skinned individuals in their 4–7th decade.[42] It is commonly diagnosed in menopausal females, including iatrogenic menopause.[41-45]

The etiopathogenesis of this condition is still debated. The propensity to involve sun exposed area suggests role of ultraviolet rays. The age and sex distributions of the patients suggest that hormonal factors in combination with the normal aging process may be involved.[43] It has been postulated that PC may be interplay of either photoallergic or phototoxic reaction to the components of perfumes and cosmetics.[43-45] A statistically significant difference of positive patch test reactions to fragrances in PC indicate role of delayed type of hypersensitivity in pathogenesis.[46] Presence of PC in family leads to the speculation that genetic factors may also play a part.[47]

Skin biopsy shows mild to moderate epidermal atrophy, hydropic degeneration of the basal cells and effacement of the rete ridges with band-like inflammatory infiltrate primarily consisting of lymphocytes with few histiocytes in upper dermis along with pigment incontinence. In late stages, a thin flattened epidermis, edema in the upper dermis, and dilated blood vessels are demonstrated. All these features are characteristic but not pathognomatic of PC.[48]

Clinically, it presents as bilaterally symmetrically distributed red to brownish, reticular patches with irregular borders usually involoving V area or sides of neck, the upper chest, and the sides of the face, sparing the anatomically shaded areas. It has a chronic, benign, but irreversible course. Katoulis et al. classified PC into erythematotelangiectatic, pigmented and mixed type depending on the predominating clinical feature.[49] Other causes of poikiloderma, e.g. dermatomyositis, lupus erythematosus, Rothmund-Thomson syndrome, Bloom syndrome, dyskeratosis congenita, etc. should be considered in the differential diagnosis.

The treatment should be targeted to both vascular as well as pigmentary component simultaneously. Various modalities have been tried with varied results. IPL have been found to be effective in the treatment of PC.[50,51] The erythema and telangiectasias respond well to the flashlamp-pumped pulsed-dye laser (585 nm and 595 nm)[52] and to the potassium-titanyl-phosphate laser.[53] Electrosurgery, cryotherapy and argon laser have been unsuccessful. Depigmenting agents can be used as adjuvant in the treatment of the pigmented type of PC. Topical retinoids and chemical peels can improve photoaged skin.[49]

Nevus of Ota

Nevus of Ota (NOO) (nevus fusco-ceruleus ophthalmomaxillaris) is a rare melanocytic hamartoma of the skin along the distribution of the ophthalmic, maxillary and sometimes mandibular branches of trigeminal cranial nerve.[54] It was first described as oculodermal melanosis in 1861 by Hulk[55] followed by Pusey[56] in 1912, as scleral and facial pigmentation. Later, in 1939 a Japanese dermatologist Masao Ota, described bluish-gray irregular hyperpigmentation along the first and second divisions of the trigeminal nerve with frequent mucosal involvement as "Nevus fusco-ceruleus ophthalmomaxillaris".[57] Since then, this melanocytic nevus has been commonly known as NOO.

It usually presents at birth or appears during the first year of life in 50–60% of cases, with a second peak during adolescence. It is more common in Asians and African descent, but very rare in Caucasians. Due to racial differences, genetic factors are thought to be important but familial cases are rare.[54]

Nevus of Ota represents aborted embryonic migration of melanocytes from neural crest to epidermis. Late pubertal onset is explained by pigmentation of the amelanotic nevoid cells present at birth by adolescent spurt of sex hormones.

It manifests clinically with characteristic speckled or mottled coalescing blue-gray pigmentation in the area supplied by ophthalmic and maxillary divisions of trigeminal nerve. It is usually unilateral (90%). It may involve oral mucosa and the eye (conjunctiva, sclera, retrobulbar fat, cornea and retina) in which two levels of pigmentation—brown of conjunctiva and blue of sclera (often not overlapping) are distinct.[58] Based on the extent, Tanino[59] classified NOO into Type I, Type II, Type III and Type IV.

Type IA—mild orbital type: on upper and lower eyelids, periocular and temple region; IB—mild zygomatic type: on the infrapalpebral fold, nasolabial fold and zygomatic region; IC—mild forehead type: on forehead only; ID—on ala nasi only. Type II—on upper and lower eyelids, periocular, zygomatic, cheek and temple regions. Type III—on scalp, forehead, eyebrow and nose. Type IV—bilateral.

Café-au-lait patch, nevus spilus and Hori[60] nevus, or acquired bilateral NOO like macules (ABNOM) are close differential diagnoses. Hori's nevus is probably a distinct variant seen in Koreans and Japanese which has a late onset in adulthood, spares the mucosae, and is clinically characterized by bilaterally symmetrical speckled or confluent brownish-blue or slate-gray pigmentation over the malar regions, temples, root of the nose, ala nasi, the eyelids and forehead.

Hirayama and Suzuki[61] classified NOO according to the distribution of the dermal melanocytes in the dermis as superficial, deep, diffuse, superficial dominant, deep dominant forms. Relevance of such classification is debated as diagnosis of this condition is moreover clinical and skin biopsy is not required to confirm the diagnosis. Histologically, elongated dendritic melanocytes are scattered widely in the papillary to mid reticular dermis. Though NOO persists, it is only rarely complicated by melanoma and is anecdotally associated with ipsilateral glaucoma.[58]

Q-switched (QS) ruby, alexandrite and Nd:YAG lasers have successfully been used in the treatment of NOO. Chan et al.[62] compared the use of QS alexandrite and QS 1064 Nd:YAG lasers, and found that QS alexandrite was better tolerated. However, the QS 1064 Nd:YAG laser was more effective in the lightening of NOO after three or more treatment sessions.[63]

Erythrose Peribuccale Pigmentaire de BROCQ

Erythrose peribuccale pigmentaire de BROCQ (EPP) is a rare facial melanosis, characterized by diffuse brown-red pigmentation distributed symmetrically around the mouth, sparing the vermillion border **(Fig. 4)**. It may involve forehead, temples, and angles of the jaw. The erythema may fluctuate but pigmentation is persistent unless the cause is eliminated when it may fade very gradually. It is commonly seen in middle aged women.[64,65] A similar hyperpigmentation has been reported in patients with subsiding perioral dermatitis due to topical steroids. Exact cause is not known but photodynamic substances in cosmetics are probably responsible.[66]

Erythromelanosis Follicularis of Face and Neck

Erythromelanosis follicularis (EF) is a facial melanosis of unknown origin, characterized by insidious onset, gradually progressive, reddish-brown pigmentation and telangiectasia associated with pale, tiny follicular papules from which vellus hairs are lost. The pigmentation may involve periauricular areas or can extend to the side of neck. It has been mainly reported from Japan. It has been reported to involve mainly young and middle-aged men, but rarely seen in adult females also.[67-69]

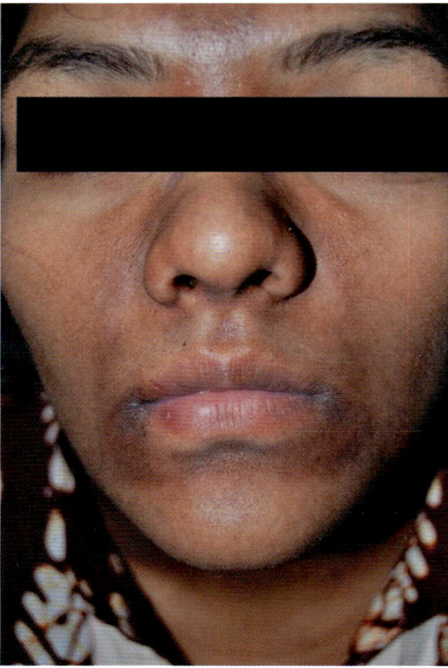

Fig. 4: Diffuse hyperpigmentation around the mouth, with sparing the vermillion border in a lady of Erythrose peribuccale pigmentaire de BROCQ. (*Source*: Col. (Dr) Manas Chatterjee, Senior Advisor and Head, Department of Dermatology, Command Hospital (EC), Kolkata, West Bengal, India)

Histopathological examination has shown enlargement of sebaceous glands and hair follicles with the latter containing lamellar horny masses. The overlying flattened epidermis contains excess melanin and there is an inconspicuous lymphocytic infiltrate around dilated vessels.[68]

ACQUIRED MELANOSES WHICH ALSO INVOLVE FACE

Tar Melanosis

(*Synonyms:* Occupational melanosis; melanodermatitis xerotica or toxic melanodermatitis)

This an occupational dermatosis encountered among workers with tar, coal tar products, mineral oils and other hydrocarbons characterized by the development of asymptomatic small bluish-gray hyperpigmented macules which often coalesce to form large areas involving face trunk and extremities and lesions of the forearm and legs tend to be perifollicular.[70] Substances in coal tar with phototoxic properties are anthracene, benzopyrene, acridine, phenanthrene, pyridine, etc. Initially patients may present with erythema, edema, vesiculation and pruritus of eczema. Gradually they develop hyperpigmentation in a reticulate pattern with variable degree of atrophy, telangiectasia, scaling and follicular keratosis.[71] Histological examination reveals follicular hyperkeratosis, reduced basal cell pigmentation, pigmentary incontinence and perivascular lymphocytic infiltration.[72]

Berloque Dermatitis

(Synonym: Photocontact Dermatitis)

It is a phototoxic reaction to bergapten, or 5-methoxypsoralen, a furocoumarin now known to be the only photoactive component of bergamot oil present in perfume, characterized by deep brown cutaneous pigmentation over the primary sites of application and along the course of its subsequent trickling **(Fig. 5)**.[72] The histopathological findings in berloque dermatitis are identical to other phototoxic reactions, an irritant cutaneous response. The epidermal changes consist of keratinocyte necrosis, intercellular and intracellular edema, and intraepidermal blisters. Changes associated with berloque pigmentation are an increased number and size of melanosomes, with melanocyte hypertrophy.[73]

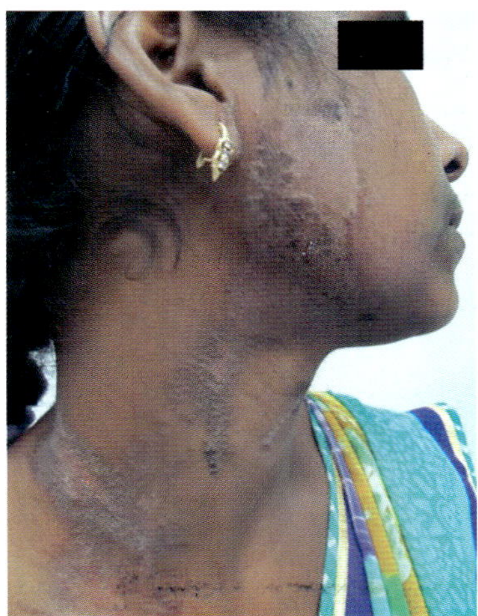

Fig. 5: A case of Barloque dermatitis, a deep dark brown pigmentation seen along the primary sites of application of perfume and along the course of its subsequent trickling

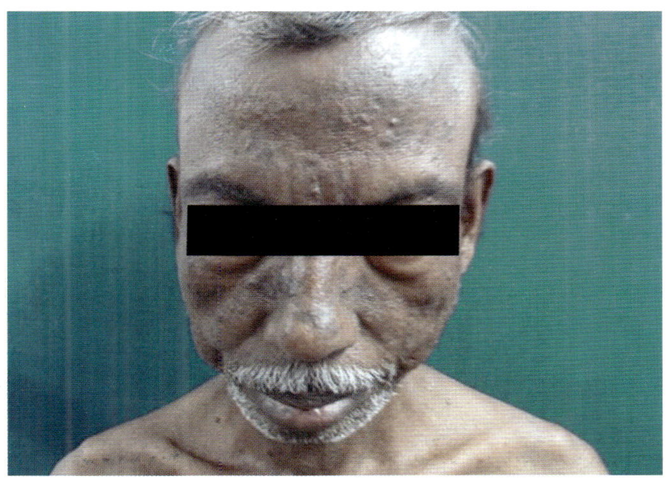

Fig. 6: Postinflammatory hyperpigmentation in a known case of systemic lupus erythematosus

Idiopathic Eruptive Macular Pigmentation

Idiopathic eruptive macular pigmentation (IEMP) is a benign, self-limiting melanosis commonly occurring in children and adolescents. It is characterized by the presence of asymptomatic pigmented macules that involve the face, trunk and proximal extremities.[74] Criteria have been established for diagnosis of IEMP,[75] namely: (a) eruption of brownish, non-confluent, asymptomatic macules involving the trunk, neck and proximal extremities in children and adolescents, (b) absence of preceding inflammatory lesions, (c) no previous drug exposure, (d) basal layer hyperpigmentation of the epidermis and prominent dermal melanophages without visible basal layer damage or lichenoid inflammatory infiltrate and (e) normal mast cell count. In a series of nine cases, an additional histopathological finding of pigmented papillomatosis has been reported.[76] Although histopathological findings are not specific, biopsy is important to exclude the other conditions, which clinically resemble it. The pathogenesis is not known and it is possible that hormonal factors may play a role as the condition is seen in the peripubertal age group.

Postinflammatory Hyperpigmentation

This acquired hyperpigmentation can be attributed to various preceding disease processes that affect the skin such as infections, allergic reactions, mechanical injuries, reactions to medications, phototoxic eruptions, trauma (e.g. burns), and inflammatory diseases, e.g. lichen planus, lupus erythematosus, psoriasis, dermatomyositis, atopic dermatitis, cutaneous T cell lymphoma, etc. It may follow physical procedures like radiofrequency, lasers, light-emitting diodes, and visible light, ultrasound and microdermabrasion.[77,78] Furthermore, lesions of PIH can darken with exposure to UV light. Classically, PIH is most severe in patients whose basal cell layer of the epidermis is disrupted such as lichenoid dermatoses or lupus erythematosus **(Fig. 6)**.

Hyperpigmentation due to Drugs and Heavy Metals

There are many drugs and metals which after ingestion for long time can cause hyperpigmentation. The morphology along with their respective drugs or metals modified from study of KH Mohan[72] is illustrated in **Table 2**.

Post-chikungunya Fever

Chikungunya fever is an acute viral illness caused by an arbovirus of the same name transmitted by the bites of *Aedes* mosquitoes. Clinically dominated by the sudden onset of high fever and the disabling joint symptoms, mucocutaneous manifestations occur in a significant proportion of cases.[79] In a number of patients, hypermelanosis of the skin may develop soon after the rash has resolved. The hyperpigmentation may be of different types including centrofacial and freckle-like, diffuse pigmentation of face **(Fig. 7)**, pinna, and extremities, flagellate pigmentation and pigmentation of existing acne lesions.[79-81]

Table 2: Morphology of drug induced hyperpigmentation, modified from study of KH Mohan[72]

Drugs/metals	*Pattern of pigmentation*
• Amiodarone	Slate-gray to violaceous pigmentation of sun-exposed areas
• Antimalarials	Bluish-black to slate-gray pigmentation on the face, extremities, oral mucosa and nails
• Bleomycin	Flagellate hyperpigmented streaks on the back
• Busulfan, cyclophosphamide, dactinomycin, daunorubicin and 5-fluorouracil	Diffuse hyperpigmentation
• Minocycline	Blue-black to muddy brown pigmentation of face or arms, grayish discoloration of teeth, nails, sclera, oral mucosa
• Chlorpromazine, imipramine	Slate-gray discoloration on photo-exposed area
• Clofazimine	Diffuse brown pigmentation
• Bismuth blue	Gray discoloration of face, neck and hands
• Gold	Blue-gray deposits around eyes
• Mercury	Slate-gray discoloration of skin folds
• Silver	Diffuse slate-gray discoloration of sun-exposed areas
• Arsenic	Diffuse macular bronze pigmentation, most prominent on the trunk, where it may produce the "raindrop" appearance

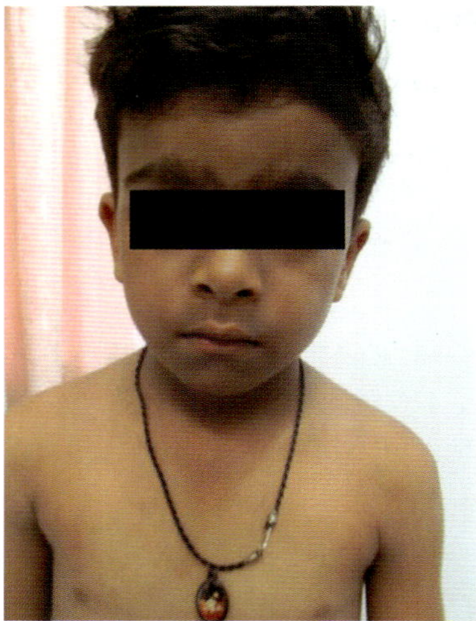

Fig. 7: Post-chikungunya diffuse hyperpigmentation of face in a young boy

MISCELLANEOUS

Periorbital Melanosis (Dark Circle)

As name indicates, it is brown to almost black discoloration around the eyes having great cosmetic concern.[82] Like melasma, it is quite common in middle aged to elderly women. There are not much of studies to know the exact etiology of this condition. However, dermal melanin deposition, PIH (atopic or contact allergic dermatitis), shadowing from lax skin, and infraorbital swelling have been incriminated. It can be familial which is determined by autosomal dominant gene.[83] Study by Malakar S et al. found periorbital pigmentation to be an extension of pigmentary demarcation lines (PDL) over the face also known as (PDL-F).[84] PDL, also known as Futcher's lines or Voigt's lines, are abrupt transition lines from areas of deeper pigmentation to areas with less pigmentation. These are most often observed in darker races and are considered to be normal variants of pigmentation.[65]

Exogenous Ochronosis

Ochronosis is a rare metabolic disease, characterized by speckled and diffuse pigmentation symmetrically distributed over the face, neck and photo-exposed areas **(Fig. 8)**. Exogenous ochronosis is a localized paradoxical hyperpigmentation of the skin due to prolonged use of bleaching agents containing hydroquinone and phenolic compounds.[85,86] This entity was first described by Findlay et al.[87] Topical hydroquinone may inhibit homogentisic acid oxidase in the dermis, with the result of a local accumulation of homogentisic acid that polymerizes to form ochronotic pigment.[88] Histologically, there is a characteristic, yellow-brown banana-shaped fiber in the papillary dermis. Homogenization and swelling of the collagen bundles are noted and a moderate histiocytic infiltrate may be present.[89]

Acanthosis Nigricans

It is characterized by symmetric, hyperpigmented, hyperkeratotic, verrucous plaques that bestow a velvety texture, usually distributed over nape of neck, flexural areas and occasionally mucocutaneous surfaces.[90] It can involve face also. Rapidly progressive and generalized Acanthosis nigricans (AN) should alarm clinician to search for internal malignancies **(Figs 9A and B)**.[91-93] Symptomatic treatments include topical retinoids and keratolytics.[94]

Macular Amyloidosis

It is a second most common form of primary localized cutaneous amyloidosis following lichenoid amyloidosis. It is characterized by macular, grayish-brown, hyperpigmentation predominantly over the interscapular area, buttocks, chest (clavicles, ribs, breast) and shins and forearms.[95] When it is generalized it can involve face and the neck.[96,97] A reticulate or "rippled" pattern of pigmentation is a characteristic diagnostic feature in many cases of macular amyloidosis (MA) **(Figs 10A and B)**. Macules may have mild to moderate pruritus. The condition usually presents in early adult life and persists for many years. Both sexes may be equally affected.

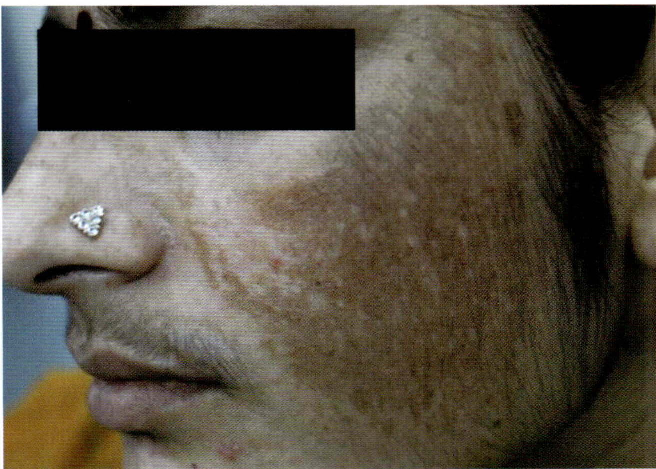

Fig. 8: A paradoxical hyperpigmentation of face in a lady using hydroquinone based cream for long time causing exogenous ochronosis. (*Source*: Col (Dr) Manas Chatterjee, Senior Advisor and HOD, Dermatology, Command Hospital (EC), Kolkata, West Bengal, India)

Histopathology is characteristic which shows amyloid deposition, confined to the papillary dermis. Amyloid exhibit green birefringence with Congo red when viewed under polarizing microscope. Topical dimethyl sulfoxide (DMSO), a chemical solvent, and intralesional or topical steroids are beneficial in the treatment of MA.[72]

Addisonian Pigmentation

It occurs in primary adrenal insufficiency due to autoimmune adrenalitis, tuberculosis or other granulomatous diseases, metastatic malignant disease, sarcoidosis, amyloidosis, and congenital adrenal hypoplasia. Classically, the pigmentation is most pronounced on the light exposed areas, flexures of axillae, plalmar and plantar creases, areas subjected to repeated friction, the normally pigmented sites of nipple, genitalia and mucous membranes. Pigmentation is minimal, if Addison's disease develops rapidly. It is epidermal melanotic hyperpigmentation.[65,98,99]

MANAGEMENT OF NON-MELASMA FACIAL MELANOSIS

Diagnosis

There are many facial melanoses which are clinically distinct, so they are easy to diagnose, e.g. melasma, NOO, Berloque dermatitis, PIH, etc. But many have overlapping features, e.g. LPP, RM, EDP, PC, which pose challenge to diagnosis. Detailed history, thorough clinical examination and skin biopsy will be able to give diagnosis in most of the situations. Addisonian pigmentation may require evaluating adrenal functions. EDP may require HIV test. An approach to diagnose such cases is depicted in **Table 3**.

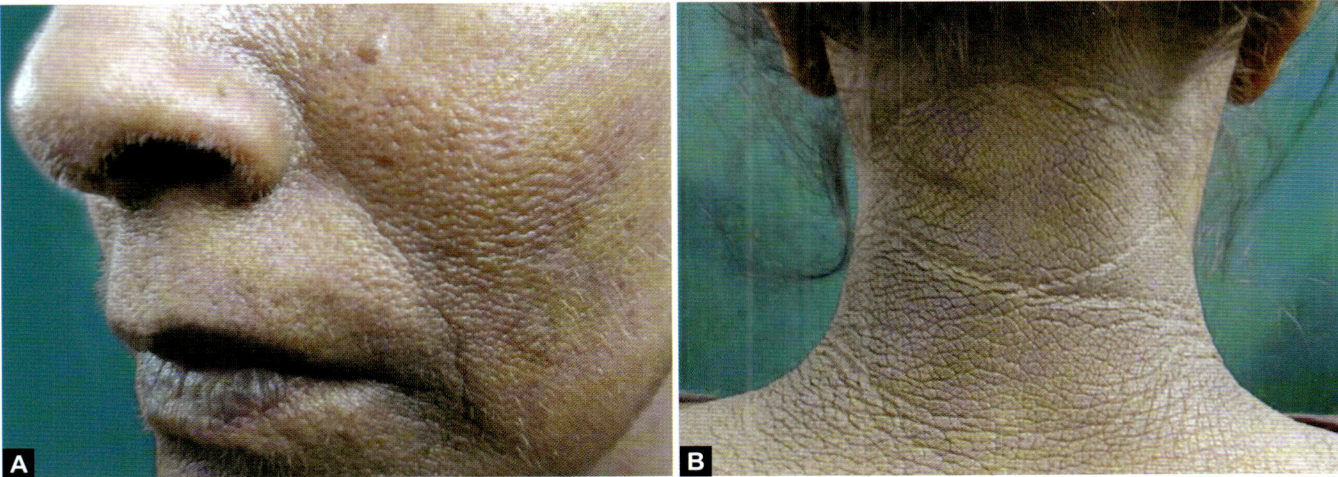

Figs 9A and B: Rapidly progressive extensive acanthosis nigricans in a lady with underlying adenocarcinoma of gallbladder

Table 3: An approach in the management of the facial melanoses

	Clinical picture	*Confirmation if required*	*Treatment*
• Is it clinically very distinct?	Bilaterally symmetrical hyperpigmented macules involving malar areas is typical of melasma	Dermoscopy to type the melasma	Hydroquinone, retinoids, steroids, triple combination, chemical peels, lasers against pigmentation, microdermabrasion
	Speckled or mottled coalescing blue-gray pigmentation in the area supplied by ophthalmic and maxillary divisions of trigeminal nerve is typical of nevus of Ota	Nil	Nd:YAG Laser
	Dark brown, drop like, pendant configuration or place of perfume application with or without preceding erythema	Barloque dermatitis	Remove provoking factor, topical steroid
	Diffuse brown-red pigmentation distributed symmetrically around the mouth, with sparing the vermillion border	Erythrose peribuccale pigmentaire de BROCQ	Withdraw provoking agent
	Reddish-brown pigmentation, telangiectasia associated with follicular papules from which vellus hairs are lost	Erythromelanosis follicularis of face and neck	Photoprotection
• Is it patchy/diffuse hyperpigmentation of face and other body areas?	Previous history of any dermatoses?	Postinflammatory hyperpigmentation	Treat with sunscreen, low potency steroid for short duration or triple combination
	History of intake of any drug or heavy metals?	Hyperpigmentation due to drugs or heavy metals	Discontinue the culprit substances
	History of occupational exposure to tar or tar product; perifollicular pigmentation on exposed area	Tar melanosis	Change the occupation, low potency topical steroid
• Is it confluent hyperpigmentation involving face, trunk and extremities?	If poikiloderma on examination (atrophy, pigmentation and telangiectasia) rule out other poikilodermatous conditions. Menopausal women, pigmentation on sun-exposed area suggest poikiloderma of Civatte	***Characteristic HPE:*** Epidermal atrophy, basal cells degeneration, effacement of the rete ridges, band like inflammatory infiltrate in upper dermis and pigmentary incontinence, confirms poikiloderma of Civatte	Treat pigmentation with IPL/laser while erythema with PDL
	Ash-colored, polycyclic macules with elevated borders (piece of string) suggest EDP	HPE non-specific but mild basal cell degeneration, perivascular inflammatory infiltrate if done from active border	Cap clofazimine for 3 months
	Dark brown patchy pigmentation, history of mustard oil or amla oil application suggest LPP	***Characteristic HPE:*** Atrophic epidermis, vacuolar degeneration of basal cell layer with lichenoid infiltrate of upper dermis, will differentiate from EDP	Tacrolimus ointment
	Pigmentation more on the periphery of face (forehead, temple, mandible) suggests Riehl's melanosis	Interface dermatitis with liquefactive basal cell degeneration, predominant perivascular lymphohistiocytic infiltrate in the upper dermis	Remove offending agents, treat like melasma, IPL can be used
	Rippled pigmentation with pruritus, history of rubbing suggest macular amyloidosis	Amyloid deposition, confined to the papillary dermis which exhibit green birefringence with Congo red when viewed under polarizing microscope	Topical dimethyl sulfoxide (DMSO), intralesional or topical steroids

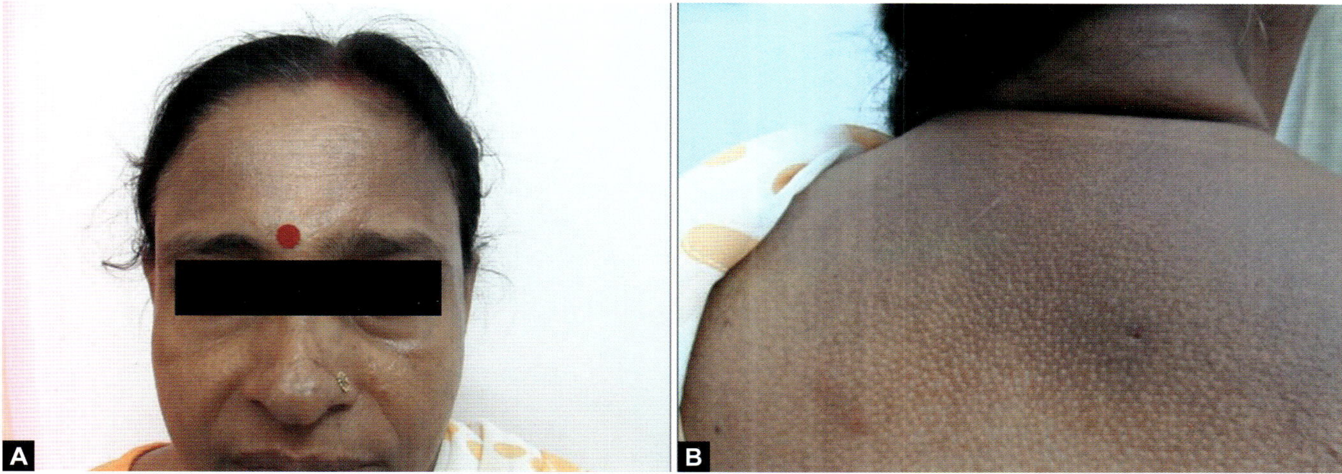

Figs 10A and B: A rippled hyperpigmentation of macular amyloidosis involving back and face

Treatment

There are no universally accepted modalities for most of the facial melanoses. Aim of treatment should include removal of provoking factors by eliciting detailed history, vigorous photoprotection, and some form of active pigment reduction either with topical agents or physical modes of treatment. Photoprotection should include protective covering, reduction of movement in the peak sun hour (10 am to 3 pm) and liberal use of broad spectrum sunscreen in predisposed persons. Avoidance of known provoking factors like causative cosmetic and textile in Riehl's melanosis; perfumes in Berloque dermatitis and mustard oil massage in LPP, etc. are needed.[65]

Lightening agents which have successfully been tried in melasma can be used to treat facial melanoses. These are hydroquinone (2–4%) alone or in combination with retinoid and topical steroids; azelaic acid, kojic acid (1–4%); topically available retinoids, viz. retinoic acid, isotretinoin, adapalene and tazarotene either as monotherapy or combined with HQ, glycolic acid 10%, topical steroids in combination. Physical therapies in the form of different types of chemical peels, lasers against pigmentation and erythema, dermabrasion and microdermabrasion can be utilized depending upon the facial melanoses.[65,72]

REFERENCES

1. Bhutani L, Bedi T, Pandhi R. Lichen planus pigmentosus. Dermatologica. 1974;149:43-50.
2. Kashima A, Tajiri A, Yamashita A, et al. Two Japanese cases of lichen planus pigmentosus-inversus. Int J Dermatol. 2007;46:740-2.
3. Hong S, Shin JH, Kang HY. Two cases of lichen planus pigmentosus presenting with a linear pattern. J Korean Med Sci. 2004;19:152-4.
4. Vega ME, Waxtein L, Arenas R, et al. Ashy dermatosis and lichen planus pigmentosus: a clinicopathologic study of 31 cases. Int J Dermatol. 1992;31:90-4.
5. Kanwar AJ, Dogra S, Handa S, et al. A study of 124 Indian patients with lichen planus pigmentosus. Clin Exp Dermatol. 2003;28:481-5.
6. Namazi MR. Lichen planus pigmentosus presenting as diffuse facial melanosis. J Drugs Dermatol. 2004;3:436-7.
7. Rietschel RL, Fowler JF (Eds). Fisher's Contact Dermatitis, 5th edn. Philadelphia: Lippincott, Williams & Wilkins; 2002. p. 782.
8. Al-Mutairi N, El-Khalawany M. Clinicopathological characteristics of lichen planus pigmentosus and its response to tacrolimus ointment: an open label, non-randomized, prospective study. J Euro Acad of Dermatol and Venereol. 2010; 24:535-40.
9. Ramirez CO. Los cenicientos: problema clinica. Memoria del Primer Congresso Centroamericano de Dermatologica; 1957. pp. 122-30.
10. Convit J, Kerdel-Vegas F. Erythema dyschromicum perstans a hitherto undescribed skin disease. J Invest Dermatol. 1961;36:457-62.
11. Molinero J, Vilata JJ, Nagore E, et al. Ashy dermatosis in an HIV antibody-positive patient. Acta Derm Venereol. 2000;80:78-9.
12. Nelson MR, Lawrence AG, Staughton RC, et al. Erythema dyschromicum perstans in an HIV antibody-positive man. Br J Dermatol. 1992;127:658-9.
13. Penagos H, Jimenez V, Fallas V, et al. Chlorothalonil, a possible cause of erythema dyschromicum perstans (ashy dermatitis). Contact Dermatitis. 1996;35:214-8.

14. Srivastava N, Solanki LS, Chand S, et al. Ashy dermatosis-like pigmentation due to ethambutol. Indian J Dermatol Venereol Leprol. 2008;74;281-2.
15. Correa MC, Memije EV, Vargas-Alarcon G, et al. HLA-DR association with the genetic susceptibility to develop ashy dermatosis in Mexican Mestizo patients. J Am Acad Dermatol. 2007;56:617-20.
16. Chang MW. Disorders of hyperpigmentation. In: Bolognia JL, et al. (Eds). Dermatology, 2nd edn. Mosby, Elsevier Limited; 2008. p. 939.
17. Tlougan BE, Gonzalez ME, Mandal RV, et al. Erythema dyschromicum perstans. Dermatol Online J. 2010;16:17.
18. Zaynoun S, Rubeiz N, Kibbi AG. Ashy dermatoses—a critical review of the literature and a proposed simplified clinical classification. Int J of Dermatol. 2008;47:542-4.
19. Silverberg NB, Herz J, Wagner A, et al. Erythema dyschromicum perstans in prepubertal children. Pediatr Dermatol. 2003;20:398-403.
20. Piquero-Martin J, Pérez-Alfonzo R, Abrusci V, et al. Clinical trial with clofazimine for treating erythema dyschromicum perstans: evaluation of cell-mediated immunity. Int J Dermatol. 1989;28:198-200.
21. Baranda L, Torres-Alvarez B, Cortes-Franco R, et al. Involvement of cell adhesion and activation molecules in the pathogenesis of erythema dyschromicum perstans (ashy dermatitis): the effect of clofazimine therapy. Arch Dermatol. 1997;133:325-9.
22. Kontochristopoulos G, Stavropoulos P, Panteleos D, et al. Erythema dyschromicum perstans: response to dapsone therapy. Int J Dermatol. 1998;37:796-8.
23. Osswald SS, Proffer LH, Sartori CR, et al. Erythema dyschromicum perstans: a case report and review. Cutis. 2001;68:25-8.
24. Riehl G. Uber eine eigenartige melanose. Wien Klin Wochensschr. 1917;30:280-1.
25. Osmundsen PE. Pigmented contact dermatitis. Br J Dermatol. 1970;83(2):296-301.
26. Nakayama H, Harada R, Toda M. Pigmented cosmetic dermatitis. Int J Dermatol. 1976;15(9):673-5.
27. Rorsman H. Riehl's melanosis. Int J Dermatol. 1882;21:75-8.
28. Nakayama H. Pigmented contact dermatitis and chemical depigmentation. In: Rycroft R, Menne T, Frosch P, Lepoittevin J (Eds). Textbook of Contact Dermatitis, 3rd edn. New York: Springer; 2001. pp. 319-33.
29. Shenoi SD, Rao R. Pigmented contact dermatitis. Indian J Dermatol Venereol Leprol. 2007;73:285-7.
30. Serrano G, Pujol C, Cuadra J, et al. Riehl's melanosis: pigmented contact dermatitis caused by fragrances. J Am Acad Dermatol. 1989;21:1057-60.
31. El Sayed F, Manzur F, Bazex J. Pigmented contact dermatitis from cosmetics. Contact Dermatitis. 1995;32:111.
32. Hayakawa R, Matsunaga K, Arima Y. Airborne pigmented contact dermatitis due to musk ambrette in incense. Contact Dermatitis. 1987;16:96-8.
33. Fujimoto K, Hashimoto S, Kozuka T, et al. Occupational pigmented contact dermatitis from azo-dyes. Contact Dermatitis. 1985;12:15-7.
34. Kozuka T, Tashiro M, Sano S, et al. Brilliant Lake Red R as a cause of pigmented contact dermatitis. Contact Dermatitis. 1979;5:297-304.
35. Nath AK, Thappa DM. Kumkum-induced dermatitis: an analysis of 46 cases. Clin Exp Dermatol. 2007;32:385-7.
36. Naganuma M, Hirose S, Nakayama Y, et al. A study of the photo-toxicity of lemon oil. Arch Dermatol Res. 1985;278: 31-6.
37. Pérez-Bernal A, Muñoz-Pérez MA, Camacho F. Management of facial hyperpigmentation. Am J Clin Dermatol. 2000;1: 261-8.
38. Li YH, Liu J, Chen JZ, et al. A pilot study of intense pulsed light in the treatment of Riehl's melanosis. Dermatologic Surgery. 2011;37:119-22.
39. Oiso N, Tsuruta D, Imanishi H, et al. Therapeutic hotline: the effectiveness of intense pulsed light for possible Riehl's melanosis. Dermatologic Therapy. 2010;23:561-63.
40. Grosshans E, Rongioletti F. Diagnostic d'un etat poikilodermique. Pathologica. 1990;82:351-8.
41. Civatte A. Poikilodermie reticuleè pigmentaire du visage et du cou. Ann Dermatol Syph. 1923;6:605-20.
42. Graham R. What is poikiloderma of civatte? Practitioner. 1989;233:1210.
43. Bleehen SS. Disorders of skin colour. In: Champion RH, Burton JL, Burns DA, Breathnach SM (Eds). Rook/Wilkinson/Ebling: Textbook of Dermatology, 6th edn. Oxford: Blackwell Scientific Publications; 1998. pp. 1790-1.
44. Canizares O. Poikiloderma of civatte. Arch Dermatol. 1968;98:429-31.
45. Kang S, Sober AJ. Disturbances in melanin pigmentation. In: Moschella SL, Hurley HJ (Eds). Dermatology, 3rd edn. Philadelphia: WB Saunders Co.; 1992. p. 1458.
46. Katoulis AC, Stavrianeas NG, Katsarou A, et al. Evaluation of the role of contact sensitization and photosensitivity in the pathogenesis of poikiloderma of civatte. Br J Dermatol. 2002;147:493-7.
47. Katoulis AC, Stavrianeas NG, Georgala S, et al. Familial cases of poikiloderma of civatte. Genetic implications in its pathogenesis? Clin Exp Dermatol. 1999;24:385-7.
48. Katoulis AC, Stavrianeas NG, Panayiotides JG, et al. Poikiloderma of civatte: a histopathological and ultrastructural study. Dermatology. 2007;214:177-82.
49. Katoulis A, Stavrianeas N, Georgala S, et al. Poikiloderma of civatte: a clinical and epidemiological study. J Euro Acad of Dermatol and Venereol 2005;19:444-8.
50. Rusciani A, Motta A, Fino P, et al. Treatment of poikiloderma of civatte using intense pulsed light source: 7 years of experience. Dermatol Surg. 2008;34:314-9.
51. Goldman MP, Weiss RA. Treatment of poikiloderma of civatte on the neck with an intense pulsed light source. Plast Reconstr Surg. 2001;107:1376-81.

52. Haywood RM, Monk BE. Treatment of poikiloderma of civatte with the pulsed dye laser: a series of seven cases. J Cutan Laser Ther. 1999;1:45-8.
53. Batta K, Hindson C, Cotterill JA, et al. Treatment of poikiloderma of civatte with the potassium titanyl phosphate (KTP) laser. Br J Dermatol. 1999;140:1191-2.
54. Bhattacharya SK, Girgla HS, Singh G. Naevus of Ota. Int J Dermatol. 1973;12:344-7.
55. Hulke JW. A series of cases of carcinoma of the eyeball. Ophthalmic Hosp Rep. 1861;3:279-86.
56. Pusey WA. Facial pigmented naevus involving the sclera. Ophthal Rec. 1916;25:618-9.
57. Ota M. Fusco-caeruleus ophthalmomaxillaris. Jpn J Dermatol. 1939;46:369-99.
58. Chan H, Kono T. Nevus of ota: clinical aspects and management. SKIN Med: Dermatology for the Clinician. 2003;2:89-98.
59. Tanino H. Uber eine in Japan haufig vorkommende Navusform: "Naevus fusco-caeruleus opthalmo-maxillaris Ota," I: mitteilung: beobachtunguber lokalisation, verfarbung, anordnung and histologische veranderung. Jpn J Dermatol. 1939; 46:435-51.
60. Hori Y, Kawashima M, Oohara K, et al. Acquired, bilateral naevus of Ota-like macules. J Am Acad Dermatol. 1984;10:961-4.
61. Hirayama T, Suzuki T. A new classification of Ota's naevus based on histopathological features. Dermatologica. 1991;183:169-72.
62. Chan HH, King WWK, Chan ESY, et al. *In vivo* trial comparing patients' tolerance of Q-switched Alexandrite (QS Alex) and Q-switched neodymium:yttrium-aluminum-garnet (QS Nd:YAG) lasers in the treatment of nevus of Ota. Lasers Surg Med. 1999;24:24-8.
63. Chan HH, Ying SY, Ho WS, et al. An *in vivo* trial comparing the clinical efficacy and complications of Q-switched 755 nm alexandrite and Q-switched 1064 nm (Nd:YAG) lasers in the treatment of nevus of Ota. Dermatol Surg. 2000;26: 919-22.
64. Belisario JC. Report on a case of erythrose peribuccale de Brocq. Australas J Dermatol. 1954;2:153.
65. Khanna N, Rasool S. Facial melanoses: Indian perspective. Indian J Dermatol Venereol Leprol. 2011;77:552-64.
66. Allen BR, Hunter JA. Abnormal facial pigmentation associated with the prolonged use of topical corticosteroids. Scott Med J. 1975;20:277.
67. Watt TL, Kaiser JS. Erythromelanosis follicularis faciei et colli. A case report. J Am Acad Dermatol. 1981;5:533-4.
68. Anderson BL. Erythromelanosis follicularis faciei et colli. Case reports. Br J Dermatol. 1980;102:323-5.
69. Sardana K, Relhan V, Garg V, et al. An observational analysis of erythromelanosis follicularis faciei et colli. Clin Exp Dermatol. 2008;33:333-6.
70. Mosher DB, Fitzpatrick TB, Ortonne JP et al. Disorders of pigmentation. In: Fitzpatrick TB, Eisen AZ, Wolff K, et al. (Eds). Dermatology in General Medicine, 4th edn. New York: McGraw-Hill; 1993. pp. 903-95.
71. Domínguez-Soto L, Hojyo-Tomoka MT, Memije EV, et al. Pigmentary problems in the tropics. Dermatol Clin. 1994;12:777-84.
72. KH Mohan. Acquired macular hyperpigmentation an overview. Journal of Pakistan Association of Dermatologists. 2011;21:43-54.
73. Elkeeb D, Elkeeb L, Maibach H. Photosensitivity: a current biological overview. Cutan Ocul Toxicol. 2012;31(4):263-72.
74. Grover S, Basu A. Idiopathic eruptive macular pigmentation: report on two cases. Indian J Dermatol. 2010;55:277-8.
75. Sanz de Galdeano C, Léauté-Labrèze C, Bioulac-Sage P, et al. Idiopathic eruptive macular pigmentation: report of five patients. Pediatr Dermatol. 1996;13:274-7.
76. Joshi R. Idiopathic eruptive macular pigmentation with papillomatosis: report of nine cases. Indian J Dermatol Venereol Leprol. 2007;73:402-5.
77. Pandya AG, Guevara IL. Disorders of hyperpigmentation. Dermatol Clin. 2000;18:91-8.
78. Graber EM, Tanzi EL, Alster TS. Side effects and complications of fractional laser photothermolysis: experience with 961 treatments. Dermatol Surg. 2008;34(3):301-5.
79. Bandyopadhyay D, Ghosh SK. Mucocutaneous manifestations of chikungunya fever. Indian J Dermatol. 2010; 55:64-7.
80. Inamadar AC, Palit A, Sampagavi VV, et al. Cutaneous manifestations of chikungunya fever: observations made during a recent outbreak in south India. Int J Dermatol. 2008;47:154-9.
81. Bandyopadhyay D, Ghosh SK. Mucocutaneous features of chikungunya fever: a study from an outbreak in West Bengal, India. Int J Dermatol. 2008;47:1148-52.
82. Lowe NJ, Wieder JM, Shorr N, et al. Infraorbital pigmented skin. Preliminary observations of laser therapy. Dermatol Surg. 1995;21:767-70.
83. Goodman RM, Belcher RW. Periorbital hyperpigmentation. An overlooked genetic disorder of pigmentation. Arch Dermatol. 1969;100:169-74.
84. Malakar S, Lahiri K, Banerjee U, et al. Periorbital melanosis is an extension of pigmentary demarcation line-F on face. Indian J Dermatol Venereol Leprol. 2007;73:323-5.
85. Gandhi V, Verma P, Naik G. Exogenous ochronosis after prolonged use of topical hydroquinone (2%) in a 50-year-old Indian female. Indian J Dermatol. 2012;57:394-5.
86. Zawar VP, Mhaskar ST. Exogenous ochronosis following hydroquinone for melasma. J Cosmet Dermatol. 2004;3: 234-6.
87. Findlay GH, Morrison JGL, Simson IW. Exogenous ochronosis and pigmented colloid milium from hydroquinone bleaching creams. Br J Dermatol. 1975;93:613-22.

88. Levin CY, Maibach H. Exogenous ochronosis: an update on clinical features, causative agents and treatment options. Am J Clin Dermatol. 2001;2:213-7.
89. Engasser PG, Maibach HI. Ochronosis caused by bleaching creams. J Am Acad Dermatol. 1984;10:1072-3.
90. De Witt CA, Buescher LS, Stone SP. Cutaneous manifestations of internal malignant disease: cutaneous para-neoplastic syndromes. In: Wolf K, Lowell A (Eds). Fitzpatric's Dermatology in General Medicine, 7th edn. New York: McGraw Hill publication; 2008. pp. 1493-6.
91. Thiers BH, Sahn RE, Callen JP. Cutaneous manifestations of internal malignancy. CA Cancer J Clin. 2009;59:73-98.
92. Krawczyk M, Mykala-Ciesla J, Kolodziej-Jaskula A. Acanthosis nigricans as a paraneoplastic syndrome. Case reports and review of literature. Pol Arch Med Wewn. 2009;119: 180-3.
93. Singh GK, Sen D, Mulajker DS, et al. Acanthosis nigricans associated with transitional cell carcinoma of the urinary bladder. Indian J Dermatol. 2011;56:722-5.
94. Schwartz RA. Acanthosis nigricans. J Am Acad Dermatol. 1994;31:1-19.
95. Wang WJ. Clinical features of cutaneous amyloidoses. Clin Dermatol. 1990;8:13-9.
96. Brownstein MH, Hashimoto K. Macular amyloidosis. Arch Dermatol. 1972;106:50-7.
97. Wang CK, Lee JYY. Macular amyloidosis with widespread diffuse pigmentation. Britiah fourml of Dermatoiogy. 1996;155:135-8.
98. Braverman IM. Skin signs of systemic disease. Philadelphia: WB Saunders; 1981.
99. Lang PG. Adrenal disroders. In: Callen JP (Ed). Cutaneous Aspects of Internal Disease. London: Year Book Medical Publishers; 1981. pp. 451-62.

50

Pigmentary Abnormalities of Nail

Archana Singal, Namrata Chhabra

Key Features

- A thorough knowledge of the causes of melanonychia and a systematic approach for its evaluation is important as the etiology may vary from benign discoloration due to topical agent to malignant melanoma.
- As the clinical diagnosis of melanonychia is frequently difficult, a biopsy is often necessary, which can be done through punch biopsy, matrix shave biopsy, or lateral longitudinal excision.
- Alteration in the nail unit pigmentation may be a useful marker of the underlying systemic disease.

INTRODUCTION

Pigmentary abnormalities of the nails are a diagnostic challenge for any dermatologist. It may arise from changes in the nail plate, nail bed or nail matrix. Therefore, the differential diagnoses are varied ranging from benign nail plate pigmentation due to a topical agent to a serious pathology such as malignant melanoma arising from the nail matrix.

The normal nail unit **(Fig. 1)**, irrespective of the ethnic background, has a translucent nail plate through which pinkish to reddish nail bed can be seen. Proximally, a crescent-shaped whitish to opaque area of the distal matrix is seen that is referred as lunula. Distally, the nail plate overlies the hyponychium. The surrounding proximal and lateral nail folds should match the adjacent skin color of the patient. Any variation in this morphology, whether it is color, loss of translucency of the nail plate, change in the color of the lunula or nail folds is considered to be a pigment abnormality of the nail unit.

In this chapter, pigmentary abnormalities of the nail unit will be discussed under following headings:

- Melanonychia
- Leukonychia
- Splinter hemorrhages
- Yellow nail
- Greenish-black discoloration of nail
- Abnormalities in color of lunula.

MELANONYCHIA

Melanonychia is a brown or black pigmentation of the nail unit. Melanonychia commonly presents as pigmented band arranged lengthwise along the nail plate, which is known as longitudinal pigment band (LPB)/longitudinal melanonychia (LM) or melanonychia striata **(Fig. 2)**.

Melanonychia most often occurs because of the increased production of melanin by melanocytes present in the nail matrix, usually the distal matrix. A healthy adult has approximately 200 melanocytes per mm^2 in the nail matrix, of which the majority remains dormant. When these melanocytes get activated, melanosomes packed with melanin are transferred to differentiating matrix cells. These then migrate distally to become nail plate onychocytes,[1] resulting in a visible band of pigmentation in the nail plate.

Melanonychia is the clinical sign present in approximately two-thirds of cases of nail apparatus melanoma (NAM). Unfortunately, patients with NAM are often misdiagnosed initially as benign LPB and there is a diagnostic delay of an average of 2 years for NAM, resulting in poor prognosis. Therefore, a thorough knowledge of the causes of melanonychia and a systematic approach for its evaluation is important for an early diagnosis and management.

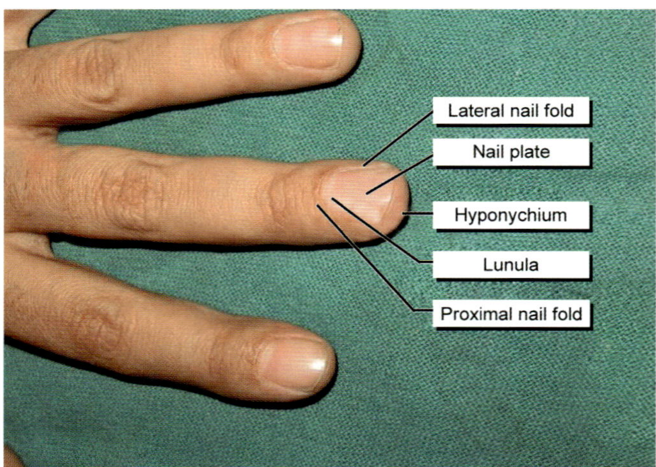

Fig. 1: Gross nail anatomy

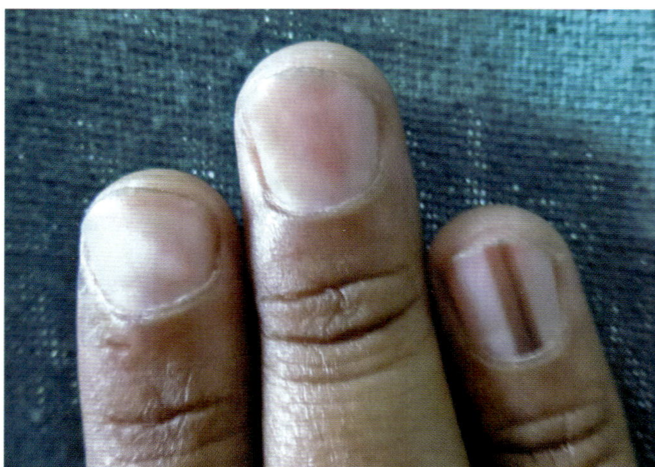

Fig. 2: Longitudinal melanonychia: single band with regular borders

Etiology of Melanonychia

The etiology of melanonychia may be divided into two broad categories:

I. Melanocytic activation
II. Melanocytic hyperplasia

Melanocytic Activation

Melanocytic activation, also termed as melanocytic stimulation or functional melanonychia, describes the process by which melanonychia results from increased melanin pigmentation of the nail matrix epithelium without a concurrent increase in the number of melanocytes.[1] Seventy-three percent of adult cases of single digit LM occur as a result of melanocytic activation.[2] A variety of causes are responsible for melanocytic activation **(Table 1)**.

Table 1: Classification of conditions associated with longitudinal melanonychia

Melanocytic activation	
Physiologic causes	Racial melanonychia Pregnancy
Local and regional causes	• Repeated local trauma from poor footwear or overriding toes • Onychotillomania • Nail biting • Occupational trauma • Carpal tunnel syndrome • Foreign body (subungual) • Radiation therapy • Postinflammatory hyperpigmentation
Dermatologic causes	• Onychomycosis • Chronic paronychia • Psoriasis • Lichen planus • Lichen striatus • Amyloidosis • Chronic radiation dermatitis • Systemic lupus erythematosus • Localized scleroderma • Onychomatricoma • Bowen's disease • Myxoid pseudocyst • Basal cell carcinoma • Subungual fibrous histiocytoma • Periungual verruca • Subungual linear keratosis
Systemic causes	• ***Endocrine:*** Addison's disease, Cushing's syndrome, Nelson's syndrome, hyperthyroidism and acromegaly • Alkaptonuria • Nutritional disorders, Vitamin B_{12} deficiency • Hemosiderosis • Hyperbilirubinemia • Porphyria • Graft versus host disease (lichen planus-type changes accompanied by longitudinal melanonychia) • AIDS
Syndromes	• Laugier-Hunziker syndrome • Peutz-Jeghers syndrome • Touraine syndrome
Melanocytic hyperplasia	
Lentigo	
Nevus	Congenital and acquired
Nail apparatus *in situ* and invasive melanoma	

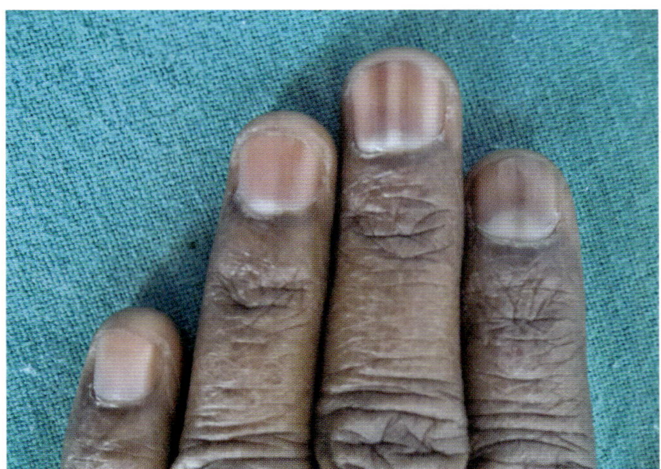

Fig. 3: Racial melanonychia in a man with type V skin type

Table 2: Pigmentary nail abnormalities specific to systemic involvement

Organ system	*Nail changes*
Renal system	Half-and-half nail, Muehrcke's lines, Terry's nail, multiple splinter hemorrhages, Mee's lines
Gastrointestinal system	Terry's nails, Azure lunula, Muehrcke's lines
Cardiovascular system	Splinter hemorrhages, red lunula
Endocrine system	Longitudinal pigment bands, pale blue lunula
Pulmonary system	Yellow nail syndrome, red lunula

Physiologic causes: Physiologic causes of LPB include racial melanonychia and pregnancy. Racial melanonychia is more common in individuals with dark brown skin **(Fig. 3)**, such as African Americans or Hispanics, and affects males and females equally.[3] The number and width of the bands increases with age. Nearly 100% of blacks develop one or more pigmented bands by the age of 50 years.[1] In hands, LPB commonly involves digits used for grasping, such as the thumb, index and middle fingers and in foot, the digits predisposed to trauma such as the great toe.[1]

Systemic causes: Melanonychia due to underlying systemic causes commonly manifests as multiple bands involving both fingernails and toenails. In Addison's disease, nutritional disorders, and AIDS, nail pigmentation is commonly accompanied by cutaneous and mucosal pigmentation.[1] Pigmentary changes of nail can be an important clue to the underlying systemic disease **(Table 2)**.

Iatrogenic causes: Transverse melanonychia, although uncommon, is most commonly reported as a result of iatrogenic causes that include drugs **(Table 3)**, phototherapy,

Table 3: Drugs associated with melanonychia

Chemotherapeutics	*Others*
Bleomycin sulfate	Amodiaquine
Busulfan	Amorolfine, Fluconazole,
Cyclophosphamide	Ketoconazole
Dacarbazine	Arsenic
Daunorubicin hydrochloride	Chloroquine, Mepacrine
Doxorubicin	Clofazimine
Etoposide	Clomipramine
5-Fluorouracil	Diquat
Hydroxyurea	Fluoride
Melphalan hydrochloride	Gold salts, Mercury, Thallium
Methotrexate	Ibuprofen
Nitrogen mustard	Lamivudine, Zidovudine
Nitrosourea	Melanocyte-stimulating hormone
Tegafur	Polychlorinated biphenyl (PCB)
	Phenytoin
	Phenothiazine
	Psoralen
	Roxithromycin, Sulfonamide,
	Tetracycline, Minocycline
	Steroids
	Timolol

X-ray exposure and electron beam therapy.[5] Drug induced melanonychia can result from the involvement of the nail matrix, nail bed, or periungual tissues. Phototoxic, allergic and photo-allergic reactions or simply the metabolism of the drug may result in discolorations, pain, and nail shedding. The pattern of pigmentation and historic time reference of the medication can help determine a cause-effect relationship. The most common drugs causing melanonychia are chemotherapeutic agents **(Fig. 4)** and the pigmentation corresponds to the dosing cycles. Fortunately, drug induced melanonychia undergoes gradual resolution following drug withdrawal.[1]

Local or regional causes: Local causes leading to nail pigmentation include nail cosmetics like nail lacquers, topical medications, fungi, bacteria, neoplasm, occupational and physical agents. Topical agents affect the nail plate most often through adsorption of the substance directly into the nail plate **(Fig. 5)**.

Melanocytic Hyperplasia

Melanocytic hyperplasia, the second broad category of melanonychia, is characterized by an increase in the number of matrix melanocytes and can be either benign or malignant.[1]

Benign melanocytic hyperplasia is subdivided into two categories:

1. Lentigines, when nests of melanocytes are absent
2. Nevi, when at least one melanocytic nest is present

Malignant melanocytic hyperplasia includes both *in situ* and invasive NAM.[1]

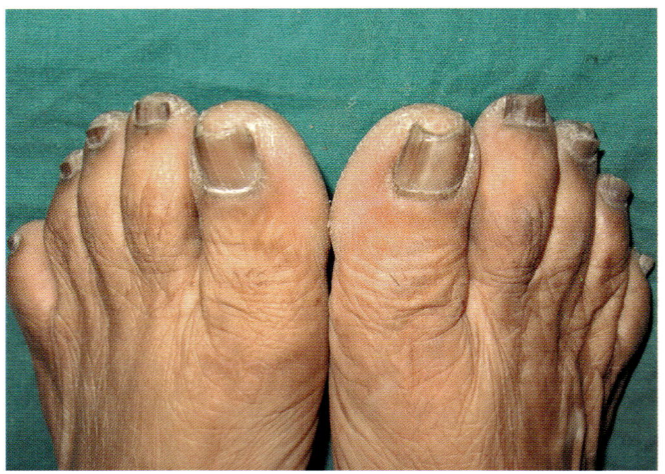

Fig. 4: Diffuse pigmentation involving multiple nails following prolonged cyclophosphamide therapy

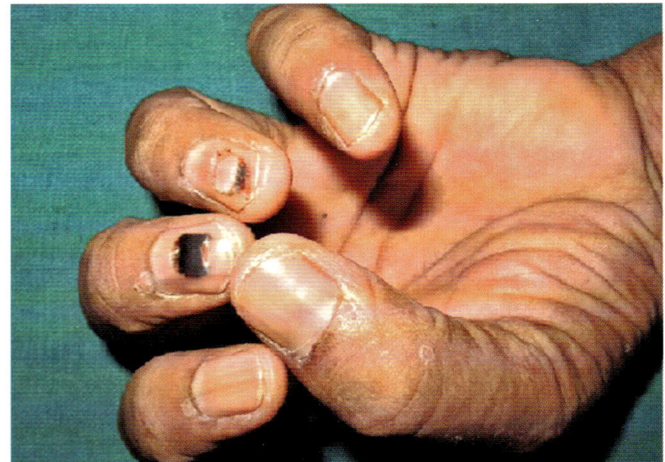

Fig. 5: Melanonychia due to voting ink. Note the pigmentation is moving out with nail growth

Table 4: Modified "ABCDEF" rule for clinical detection of NAM

Age: Peak incidence 5th to 7th decade *Band:* Brown-black band, *Breadth*: > 3 mm *Border*: Irregular/blurred *Change:* Rapid change in growth and/or color or lack of change: Failure of nail dystrophy to improve with treatment *Digit involved:* Thumb > great toe > index finger, single > multiple digits *Dominant*: Hand *Extension:* Extension of pigment to proximal or lateral nail fold *(Hutchinson's sign)* *Family or personal history:* Previous melanoma or dysplastic nevus syndrome
Abbreviation: NAM, nail apparatus melanoma

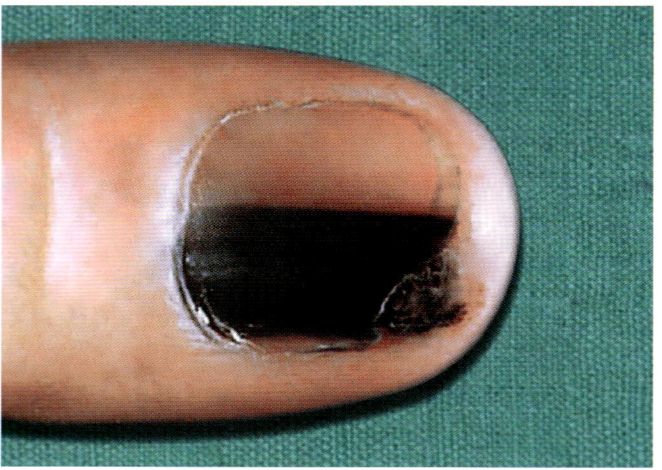

Fig. 6: Malignant melanoma of right thumb with positive Hutchinson's sign

Approach to Evaluation of Melanonychia

History

A thorough history is important if there is no obvious external cause. A careful history should include details of occupational and recreational activities, history of trauma, past illnesses and medications (both systemic and topical), number of nails affected, change in the appearance of the band (or bands) over time, prior history and details of nail clipping or a biopsy sent for histologic examination, results of cultures sent for infectious organisms, racial origin and family history. NAM should be suspected in any patient with unexplained melanonychia with features listed in **Table 4**[6,7] **(Fig. 6)**.

Physical Examination

Following points should be considered while performing examination of melanonychia:

- All 20 nails should be examined
- Nail polish or lacquer should be removed before examination
- Fingernails provide more reliable information than toenails as the clinical signs may get modified in toenails due to trauma of walking and footwear
- Nails should be examined with the digits relaxed and not pressed against any surface[8,9]
- The observer should squeeze the digit tip to see whether the color change is altered substantially. This may help to differentiate discoloration of the nail plate from that caused by a vascular alteration in the underlying nail-bed.
- Examination of the nail plate by looking at it straight on or at cross-section can help identify to some extent if the

pigmentation is originating in the matrix or not. If the pigment is seen on the dorsal side of the nail plate then the pigment is being produced in the proximal matrix; if the pigment is on the ventral surface then its origin is in the distal matrix; if the pigment is in the mid-nail plate then its source is the mid-matrix; if the entire nail plate is involved then it is being produced by the entire matrix.

- As a rule, if nail discoloration follows the shape of the lunula, it is likely to be caused by internal factors because the discoloration is being deposited in the matrix, whereas if it corresponds to the shape of the proximal nail fold, external factors predominate.[10,11]
- Besides examination of nails, careful examination of the oral and genital mucosa may also provide important diagnostic clues to identify etiology of melanonychia especially in syndromes such as Peutz-Jeghers syndrome or Laugier-Hunziker syndrome.[12]

Hutchinson's sign: Extension of pigment from the matrix to the perionychium/proximal nail fold in association with NAM is referred to as Hutchinson's sign **(Fig. 6)**. Though it is helpful in confirming the clinical diagnosis of NAM, it is an inconsistent feature. *Pseudo-Hutchinson's sign* is presence or illusion of pigment in the perionychium, and is associated with both benign and malignant conditions in the absence of melanoma[13] such as:

- Drugs (minocycline)
- AIDS
- Peutz-Jeghers syndrome
- Frictional melanonychia

Dermoscopy: Dermatoscope (dermoscope or epiluminescence microscope) is an important noninvasive tool that can be used to assist the examination of melanonychia. In this procedure, through a drop of oil, the nail unit can be illuminated and seen through a magnifying lens. Dermoscopy may provide clues to decide the need for biopsy.[14] However, dermoscopic findings associated with NAM versus benign melanonychia are not very well defined.

In a study conducted on dermoscopic findings in melanonychia, Ronger et al. reported that NAM was significantly associated with background brown discoloration and presence of irregular longitudinal lines in contrast to benign nevi that showed the presence of regular lines. The study also observed the presence of *micro-Hutchinson's sign* (a Hutchinson's sign that is too small to be seen with the human eye) in cases of melanoma. On the other hand, nail apparatus lentigines, ethnic pigmentation and drug-induced pigmentation were significantly associated with homogeneous longitudinal thin gray lines and gray coloration of the background.[14]

Biopsy of Melanonychia

A variety of biopsy techniques can be used to sample pigmented lesions located within the nail matrix, including punch biopsy, matrix shave biopsy, and lateral longitudinal excision.[15,16] For bands less than 3 mm width, a 3 mm punch biopsy can be used if the origin of the band is located in the distal matrix. The risk of causing a subsequent nail plate dystrophy after the procedure is greater if proximal area of the matrix is sampled. The lateral longitudinal excision is best suited for biopsying suspicious lesions located in the lateral one-third of the nail, as this technique samples all components of the nail unit including the nail matrix, nail bed, nail fold and hyponychium.[6,15] The tangential (shave) biopsy is ideal for sampling an LPB with a lower suspicion of melanoma that is greater than 3 mm in width in the mid-nail plate or of any width originating in the proximal matrix.[6,15,16]

LEUKONYCHIA (WHITE NAIL)

Leukonychia is white discoloration of the nail plate and is divided into three main categories.

1. *True leukonychia*: When pathology originates in the matrix and emerges in the nail plate
2. *Apparent leukonychia:* When pathology is in the nailbed
3. *Pseudoleukonychia:* When pathology is exogenous.

True Leukonychia

True leukonychia occurs when the matrix dyskeratinization, often resulting in parakeratotic foci, imparts a white color to the nail plate. True leukonychia is subdivided as total and partial leukonychia.

Total Leukonychia

Total leukonychia is usually an autosomal dominantly inherited condition but the inheritance may be autosomal recessive in some.[17] In dominantly inherited form, it can be a part of Bart-Pumphrey syndrome in which it is associated with knuckle pads and deafness or Buschkell-Gorlin syndrome in which it is seen in association with sebaceous cysts and renal calculus. Acquired causes of total leukonychia include typhoid fever, leprosy, cirrhosis, nail biting, trichinosis and cytotoxic drugs.

Partial Leukonychia

Partial leukonychia can be punctate, transverse and longitudinal. Punctate leukonychia is common and results from minor nail trauma to the nail in the vicinity of the nail matrix, resulting in nucleated keratinocytes in the nail, which appear as small white areas 1–3 mm in diameter **(Fig. 7)**. An extension of punctate leukonychia is transverse leukonychia, also due to trauma to the matrix, often follows aggressive manicuring **(Fig. 7)**. These narrow white lines runs parallel to the proximal nail fold and grow out with the nail. Another example of transverse leukonychia is *Mee's lines* which are

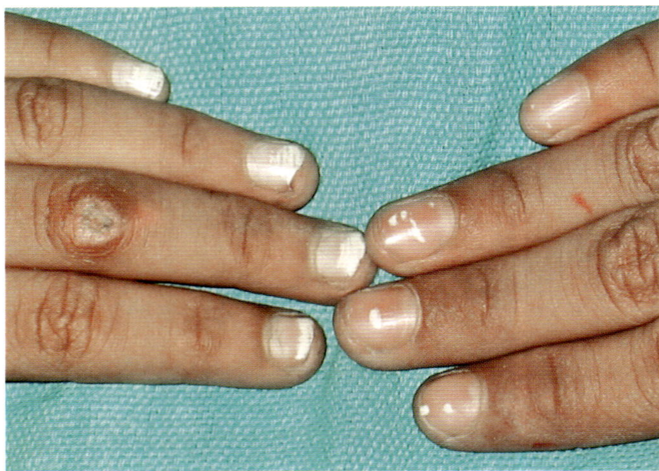

Fig. 7: Trauma induced punctate and transverse leukonychia in two sisters

transverse white bands that frequently affect multiple nails, are characteristically seen in arsenic poisoning, but occur in a number of other conditions **(Table 5)**. Longitudinal leukonychia is 1 mm white longitudinal lines under the nail plate and is associated with Darier's disease.

Apparent Leukonychia

In apparent leukonychia, there is involvement of subungual tissue or subungual hyperkeratosis or pathology of nail bed instead of nail plate.[18] Apparent leukonychia describes a nail that apparently looks white, but is in fact, normal in color. Therefore, when the nail plate is removed in apparent leukonychia, it is of normal color. Onycholysis is an example of apparent leukonychia and the white appearance is due to air beneath the nail.

Three examples of apparent leukonychia seen in association with underlying systemic causes are Terry's nail, Muehrcke's lines and Half-and-half nails **(Table 5)**.

Terry's Nails

Terry's nail appear milky white and opaque from the lunula to the onychodermal band **(Fig. 8)**. Terry's nails are seen in patients with hepatic cirrhosis, chronic congestive heart disease, type 2 diabetes mellitus, and aging. The Terry's nails of congestive heart failure may also be pink, a different presentation from the white nails of liver disease.

Muehrcke's Lines

Muehrcke's lines are paired, white horizontal bands that lie parallel to the lunula and separated by pink bands **(Fig. 9)**. This condition occurs when the serum albumin is low (below 2 g/dL), and disappears when the albumin levels return to normal. Muehrcke's lines occur in patients with renal failure and/or hemodialysis.

Half-and-Half Nail

Half-and-half nail has a proximal, opaque, white portion that obscures the lunula and a distal red/brown color **(Fig. 10)**. It occurs in 9–15% of chronic renal failure patients (Lindsay's nails). They have also been observed in hemodialysis patients, renal transplant recipients and HIV patients.

Table 5: Pigmentary changes of nail other than melanonychia

Color change	*Causes*
Terry's nails	Hepatic failure, cirrhosis, diabetes mellitus, CHF, hyperthyroidism, malnutrition
Yellow nail	Lymphedema, pleural effusion, immunodeficiency, bronchiectasis, sinusitis, rheumatoid arthritis, nephrotic syndrome, thyroiditis, tuberculosis, Raynaud's disease
Half-and-half nails	Specific for renal failure
Muehrcke's lines	Specific for hypoalbuminemia
Mees' lines	Arsenic poisoning, Hodgkin's disease, CHF, leprosy, malaria, chemotherapy, carbon monoxide poisoning
Azure lunula	Hepatolenticular degeneration (Wilson's disease), argyria, bacterial paronychia, quinacrine and zidovudine therapy
Pale-blue lunula	Diabetes mellitus
Red lunula	Cardiovascular disease, COPD, collagen vascular disease, hematologic malignancy
Yellow lunula	Tetracycline therapy
Splinter hemorrhage	Subacute bacterial endocarditis, SLE, rheumatoid arthritis, antiphospholipid syndrome, peptic ulcer disease, malignancies, oral contraceptive use, pregnancy, psoriasis, trauma
Greenish-black nails	Pseudomonas aeruginosa infection

Abbreviations: CHF, congestive heart failure; COPD, chronic obstructive pulmonary disease; SLE, systemic lupus erythematosus

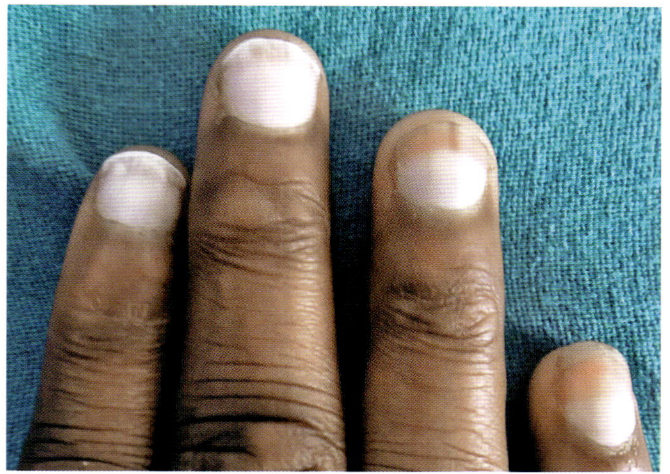

Fig. 8: Terry's nails in a patient with liver cirrhosis

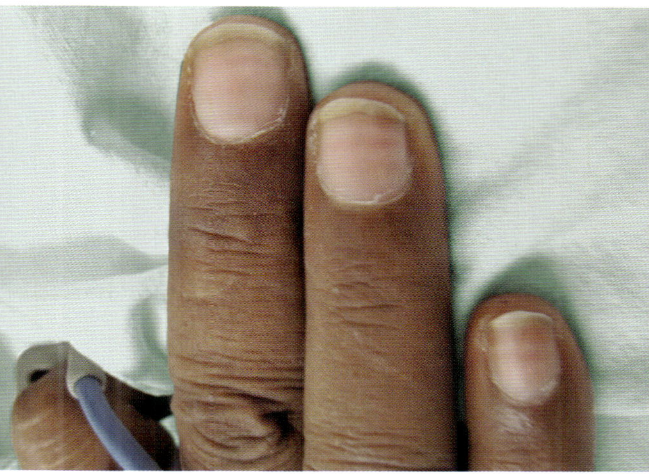

Fig. 9: Muehrcke's lines in a patient of nephritic syndrome with serum albumin of 1.6 gm%

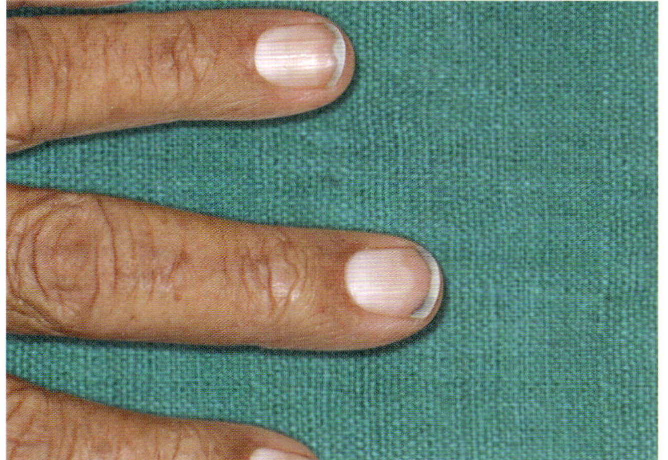

Fig. 10: Half-and-half nail in a patient with renal failure

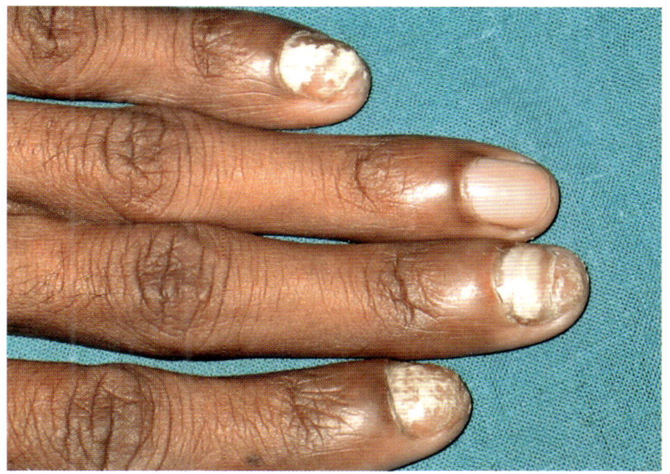

Fig. 11: Superficial white onychomycosis (SWO)

Pseudoleukonychia

Pseudoleukonychia may occur in fungal infection of the nail plate, or when nail varnish produces keratin granulation or may result from trauma. Among fungal infections, superficial white onychomycosis (SWO) cause white nails **(Fig. 11)**. In temperate climates the cause of SWO is usually *Trichophyton mentagrophytes*, but in hot and humid climates, molds, such as *Fusarium species*, may infect the surface of the nail plate. Pseudo leukonychia may also be seen in proximal subungual onychomycosis and endonyx onychomycosis.

Differentiating points between leukonychia associated with systemic disease and secondary to trauma are listed in **Table 6.**

Table 6: Differences between leukonychia associated with systemic disease and secondary to trauma

Leukonychia with systemic disease	*Trauma-induced leukonychia*
Tend to occur on several nails at once	Less frequently involves all nails
Lines are: Homogeneous • Smoother borders • Spread across the entire width of nail plate/bed	Lines are: Irregular • Serrated borders • Does not span across the entire width of the nail plate
Contour parallel to distal lunula	Lines tend to be more linear
History of physical trauma absent	History of physical trauma present

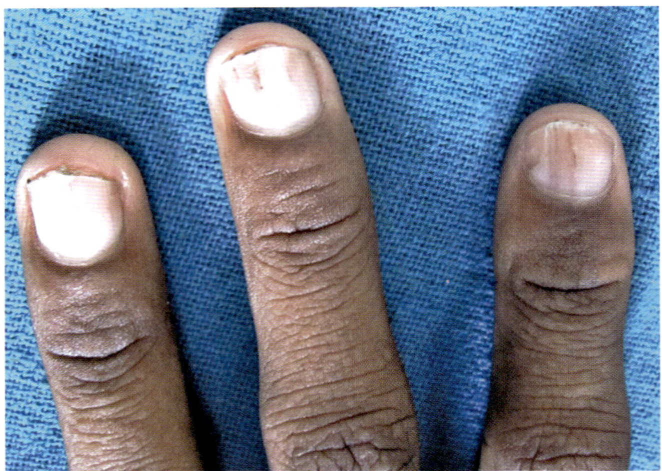

Fig. 12: Splinter hemorrhage in a patient with endocarditis

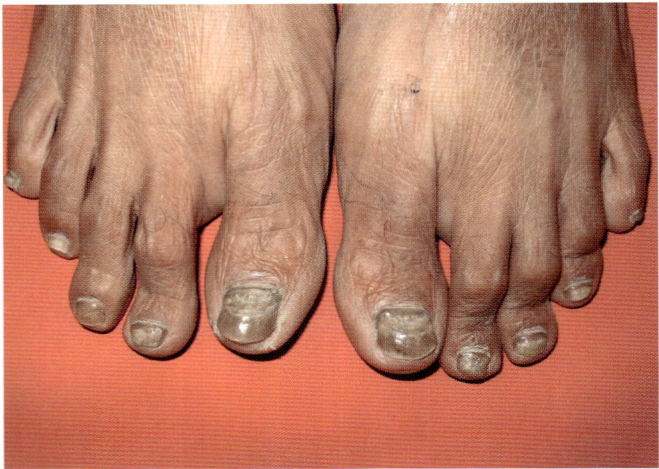

Fig. 13: Yellow toe nails in a patient with bronchiectasis

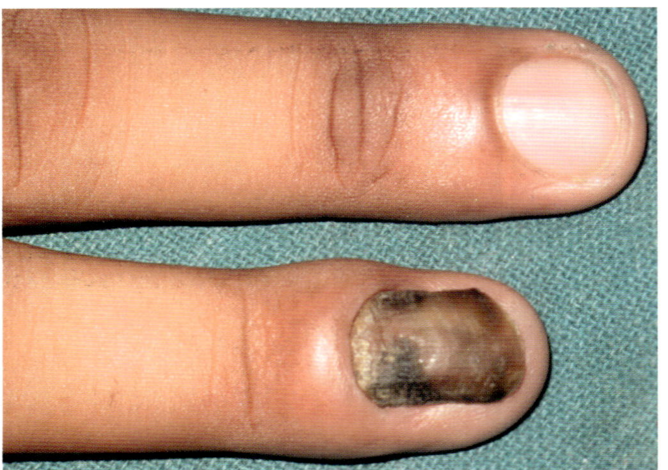

Fig. 14: Greenish-black discoloration due to *Pseudomonas aeruginosa* infection

SPLINTER HEMORRHAGES

Splinter hemorrhages are longitudinal thin lines, red or brown in color beneath the nail plate due to the extravasation of blood from the longitudinally oriented vessels of nailbed **(Fig. 12)**. While the most common cause of splinter hemorrhages is local trauma, they are a classic finding in patients with endocarditis and may be seen in other conditions **(see Table 5)**. Splinter hemorrhages are more specific indicator of endocarditis, if they are present proximally rather than distally on the nail plate and are more common in subacute than acute infection.[19] On the other hand, trauma induced splinter hemorrhages tend to involve few nails, dominant hand and distal end of the nail plate.

YELLOW NAIL

Yellow nail syndrome is a rare syndrome and represents triad of primary lymphedema associated with yellow nails and bronchiectasis. The nails are yellow and slow-growing lunula and cuticle are absent **(Fig. 13)**. Patient may also have associated bronchiectasis or sinusitis, internal malignancies, immunodeficiency syndromes and rheumatoid arthritis **(see Table 5)**.[20] The underlying pathological process is thought to be related to impaired lymphatic drainage. Yellow nails can also be caused by staining of the nail plate by prolonged usage of nail enamel. Drugs like tetracycline can also cause a yellow discoloration of the nail.

GREENISH-BLACK DISCOLORATION

Greenish-black discoloration is typical of *Pseudomonas aeruginosa* infection **(Fig. 14)**. It often starts on one side of a finger nail, growing out from under the proximal nail fold. Treatment is difficult, since part of the infection is hidden and not amenable to topical treatment. Even though the condition is harmless for the patient it may cause life threatening infections in immunocompromised patients.

ABNORMALITY IN COLOR OF LUNULA

Changes in the color of the lunula can be an indication of underlying systemic disorder **(see Table 5)**. In patients with Wilson's disease (hepatolenticular degeneration), the lunula takes on a blue coloration, a phenomenon called azure lunula. Heart failure can turn the lunula red, and tetracycline therapy can turn it yellow. Silver poisoning will turn the nail itself a blue-gray color. Excessive fluoride ingestion can turn nails brown or black.

Thus, alteration in the nail unit pigmentation can provide plethora of information and clue to the underlying systemic disease.

REFERENCES

1. Andre J, Lateur N. Pigmented nail disorders. Dermatol Clin. 2006;24(3):329-39.
2. Tosti A, Baran R, Piraccini BM, et al. Nail matrix nevi: a clinical and histopathologic study of twenty-two patients. J Am Acad Dermatol. 1996;34:765-71.
3. Leung AK, Robson WL, Liu EK, et al. Melanonychia striata in Chinese children and adults. Int J Dermatol. 2007;46(9): 920-2.
4. Cribier B, Mena ML, Rey D, et al. Nail changes in patients infected with human immunodeficiency virus: a prospective controlled study. Arch Dermatol. 1998;134(10): 1216-20.
5. Quinlan KE, Janiga JJ, Baran R, et al. Transverse melanonychia secondary to total skin electron beam therapy: a report of 3 cases. J Am Acad Dermatol. 2005;53:S112-4.
6. Haneke E, Baran R. Longitudinal melanonychia. Dermatol Surg. 2001;27(6):580-4.
7. Rich P. Nail surgery. In: Bolognia JL, Jorizzo JL, Rapini RP (Eds). Dermatology, 2nd edn. New York: Mosby; 2006.
8. Daniel CR, Osment LS. Nail pigmentation abnormalities: Their importance and proper examination. Cutis. 1980; 25(6):595-607.
9. Daniel CR, Osment LS. Nail pigmentation abnormalities: Their importance and proper examination. Cutis. 1982; 30(3):348-60.
10. Zaias N. The Nail in Health and Disease. New York: SP Medical Books: 1980.
11. Zaias N. Disease of the nails. In: Demis J, Dobson RL, Crounse RG (Eds). Clinical Dermatology. New York; Harper & Row: 1974.
12. Braun RP, Baran R, Le Gal FA, et al. Diagnosis and management of nail pigmentations. J Am Acad Dermatol. 2007;56(5):835-47.
13. Baran R, Kechijian P. Hutchinson's sign: a reappraisal. J Am Acad Dermatol. 1996;34(1):87-90.
14. Ronger S, Touzet S, Ligeron C, et al. Dermoscopic examination of nail pigmentation. Arch Dermatol. 2002;138(10): 1327-33.
15. Jellinek N. Nail matrix biopsy of longitudinal melanonychia: diagnostic algorithm including the matrix shave biopsy. J Am Acad Dermatol. 2007;56(5):803-10.
16. Di Chiacchio N, Loureiro WR, Michalany NS, et al. Tangential Biopsy Thickness versus Lesion Depth in Longitudinal Melanonychia: a Pilot Study. Dermatol Res Pract. 2012. p. 353864.
17. Ekmekçi TR, Köşlü A. Lökonişitotalis. Türkderm. 2004;38: 146-7.
18. Bongiorno MR, Aricò M. Idiopathic acquired leukonychia in a 34-year-old patient. Case Rep Med. 2009;2009:495809.
19. Saccente M, Cobbs CG. Clinical approach to infective endocarditis. Cardiol Clin. 1996;14(3):351-62.
20. Scher RK. Acquired immunodeficiency syndrome and yellow nails. J Am Acad Dermatol. 1988;18:758-9.

51

Macular Amyloidosis

Latika Arya

Key Features

- Macular amyloidosis is a chronic, persistent, usually pruritic, pigmentary disorder characterized by rippled pattern of hyperpigmentation usually over scapular area and by presence of amyloid on histology.
- It is one of the protein misfolding disorders. Exact etiopathogenesis of amyloid deposition is not known, but is believed to originate from epidermal keratin. A number of risk factors are associated, among them chronic friction in particular.
- Treatment is challenging and is directed at alleviation of pruritus and removal of amyloid. Recent understandings of the underlying mechanisms of amyloid deposition have provided new concepts for management.

INTRODUCTION

Amyloidosis is a heterogeneous group of diseases characterized by deposition of amyloid—an extracellular proteinaceous substance which has distinctive physical properties and is resistant to proteolytic digestion.[1] It is one of the conformational or protein misfolding diseases, as it is caused by malfunctioning proteins.[2]

Amyloidosis can be systemic, involving several organs and tissues, or localized to a body site.[3,4] Cutaneous amyloidosis is of two types—primary localized cutaneous amyloidosis (PLCA), and secondary cutaneous amyloidosis.[4] PLCA is only localized to the skin without evidence of systemic involvement. It has three clinical variants—the more common macular amyloidosis (MA) and papular or lichen amyloidosis (LA), and the rare nodular amyloidosis[3,4] **(Box 1)**. MA and LA are referred to as "keratinic" amyloidosis, with reference to their origin from epidermal keratin.[5]

Macular amyloidosis was first described by Palitz and Peck in 1952.[6] Its exact etiopathogenesis is still unknown.[4]

Box 1

Classification of amyloidosis

- Systemic
- Cutaneous
  - Primary
    - Macular amyloidosis
    - Lichen amyloidosis
    - Nodular amyloidosis
  - Secondary

Its diagnosis is usually clinical, based on its characteristic rippled pattern of hyperpigmentation, but may frequently require histopathological confirmation.

EPIDEMIOLOGY

Macular amyloidosis is a major cause of skin pigmentation with a higher prevalence in Asia, Middle-East and Central and South America, but rarely reported in Europe and North America.[7-9] PLCA affects the Chinese more frequently, but MA is more common in Indians.[10]

The disease is more prevalent in females as compared to males, as reported in studies from Indonesia, India, Malaysia and South America.[11-14] Most of the cases are sporadic, although 10% cases are reported to be familial.[11] The preponderant age of patients is generally between 40 years and 60 years with age of onset between 30 years and 50 years.[10,11]

PATHOGENESIS

The exact pathogenesis of amyloid deposition in MA is still not clear, although it is believed that it originates from epidermal keratin,[15] and therefore the term "k-amyloid" was proposed.[16] This view is based on ultrastructural findings,[17,18] as well as the fact that amyloid deposits have been shown to contain disulfide bonds that are present in keratin.[19] Also, immunofluorescence studies have shown intense staining of the amyloid for the antikeratin antibody further confirming the keratin origin.[20]

There are different theories explaining the mechanism of amyloid deposition **(Table 1)**. One view is that degenerated keratin peptides of damaged and apoptotic keratinocytes, are transformed into amyloid fibrils by dermal macrophages and fibroblasts. This is known as the fibrillar body theory.[21-24]

Another theory, known as the secretion theory, states that amyloid is produced in the interface of the epidermis and dermis by living basal keratinocytes, which produce the precursor of amyloid because of disturbed keratin metabolism.[25]

Recent research has detected prefibrillar amyloids—small, misfolded intracellular protein oligomers—in the basal cell layer of the epidermis and the surrounding cells in the dermis. These oligomers give rise to large amyloid fibrillar aggregates and have been shown to be the toxic agents in amyloid diseases, by impairing fundamental cellular processes and eventually leading to necrotic cell death.[26,27]

Based on these findings, a mixed theory of amyloid deposition has been proposed.[26] According to this theory, oligomers are formed intracellularly in the basal layer of cells and can either cause immediate cell death or can be released into the dermis and be engulfed by dermal macrophages and fibroblasts, thus transforming into amyloid aggregates. It is proposed that factors, like oxidative stress, low pH, metal ions, or chaperones can cause proteins to develop an abnormal structure and as a result misfold to form amyloid.[28]

It has also been demonstrated that MA has a similar mechanism of amyloidogenesis as other well characterized protein misfolding diseases, like Alzheimer's disease.[29] However, the mechanism of amyloid formation and toxicity is still unknown.

ETIOLOGICAL FACTORS

Macular amyloidosis is believed to be multifactorial in origin. Frictional and environmental epidermal damage, genetic, immunological and other factors are found to be associated in a proportion of patients[30] **(Box 2)**.

Persistent scratching or rubbing is believed to play a major role in its occurrence, as probably the epidermal trauma caused by it results in keratinocyte degradation and formation of amyloid[12] as evident from various case reports of MA associated with the use of nylon brushes and towels. This has been labeled by various names, like friction amyloidosis, towel melanosis and nylon clothes friction dermatitis.[31-35] There is also an association of MA with notalgia paresthetica, further confirming the role of scratching in inducing MA.[36,37]

Various other risk factors may be associated, like race,[3,12] genetic predisposition,[13,38] female gender,[10-13] sun exposure[33,34] and atopy.[39,40]

Genetic factors seem to be involved as evident by its prevalence in Central and South Americans, Middle-East

Box 2

Etiological factors in macular amyloidosis

- Racial—Asia, the Middle-East, Central and Southern America
- Genetic—Most cases sporadic, autosomal dominant in 10%
- Sunlight
- Atopy
- Diabetes mellitus/insulin resistance—oxidative stress, byproduct during formation of advanced glycation end-products
- Chronic friction—nylon brush, bath sponge or towel—epidermal damage (friction amyloidosis)
- Chronic pruritus—In nodular prurigo, Lichen simplex chronicus, notalgia paresthetica
- Associated autoimmune/immune disorders—with extensive involvement
- Epstein-Barr virus

Table 1: Amyloid histogenesis theories

Fibrillary body theory (Hashimoto)[21-24]	*Secretory theory (Yanagihara et al)*[25]	*Mixed theory (Clos AL et al)*[26]
Focal epidermal damage → Apoptosis → filamentous degeneration of keratinocytes (colloid bodies) by dermal fibroblasts and histiocytes, into amyloid depositing in the upper papillary dermis	Amyloid secreted by disrupted basal cells and assembled at the dermoepidermal junction	Oligomers formed intracellularly in the basal layer of cells → • Either cause immediate cell death • Or can be released into the dermis → engulfed by dermal macrophages and fibroblasts → transformed into amyloid aggregates

population and Asians who have dark skin, its familial occurrence in some cases[41] and its association with an autosomal dominant-syndrome[42] (Sipple syndrome or multiple endocrine neoplasia type 2a). Recently, oncostatin M receptor-β mutations along with overexpression of interleukin (IL)-31 receptor have been identified in cases of familial PLCA that results in severe pruritus.[43,44]

Immune mediated factors are thought to play a role in causation of MA, especially in cases with widespread disease.[45] MA has been reported in association with several connective tissue diseases like systemic sclerosis,[46,47] CREST syndrome,[48] rheumatoid arthritis,[49] systemic lupus erythematosus,[49] dermatomyositis,[50] primary biliary cirrhosis,[51] autoimmune cholangitis,[52] sarcoidosis[45] and immunoglobulin (Ig) A nephropathy.[45]

Epstein-Barr virus has been demonstrated in a significant number of cases of PLCA and is postulated to contribute to keratinocyte degeneration.[53]

Patients with PLCA have been reported to have a higher comorbidity of hyperlipidemia and diabetes mellitus. Stress in tissues can be aggravated by diabetes and hyperglycemia that contributes to increased amyloid and oxidative stress-related protein expression and formation of protein deposits as well as producing further oxidative stress.[54]

PATHOLOGY

In MA, no significant changes are seen in the epidermis apart from may be mild thinning or mild hyperkeratosis with acanthosis. Necrotic and apoptotic keratinocytes are sometimes seen in the suprabasal or the basal layers of the epidermis. Focal basal cell layer degeneration with pigment incontinence and melanophages in the papillary dermis may be seen in some cases. Predominant perivascular lymphocytic infiltrate is present.[15,55]

Amyloid deposits are localized to the papillary dermis and not scattered or localized around blood vessels or appendages. They are seen as small amorphous eosinophilic masses on routine hematoxylin and eosin staining **(Figs 1A and B)**, but sometimes can be easily missed without the use of special stains.[4]

The congo-red stain gives an orange-red staining reaction to amyloid, and shows an apple-green birefringence under a polarizing microscope, which is the most confirmatory test **(Fig. 2)**. The staining characteristic is due to the cross-beta-pleated sheet conformation of the polypeptide backbones of the amyloid fibrils.[4,12,55,56] Other special stains for amyloid include the triphenyl methane dyes, methyl and cresyl violet for the demonstration of metachromasia, the periodic acid Schiff's method and fluorescence with thiazole dyes such as thioflavin T.[56]

Direct immunofluorescence usually shows focal IgG, IgM and C3 in the amyloid.[57]

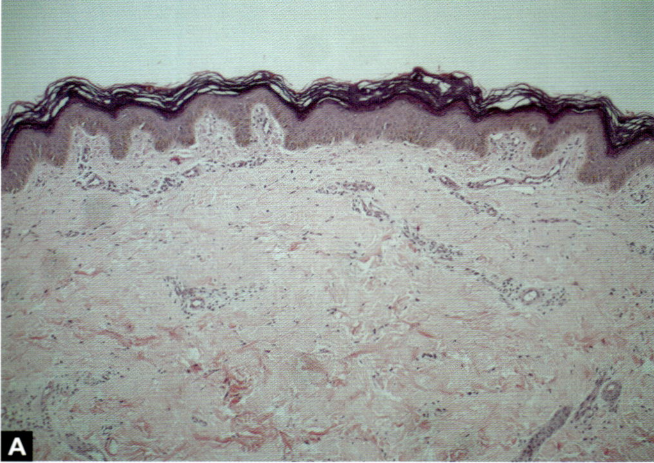

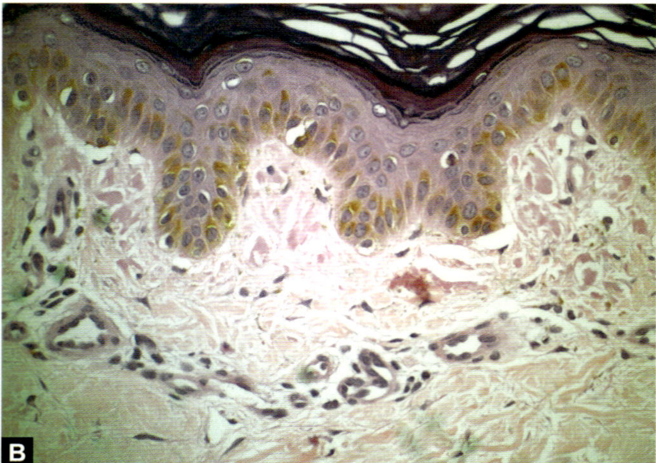

Figs 1A and B: Photomicrograph of macular amyloidosis showing pale pink amorphous amyloid deposits in the papillary dermis. (A) Hematoxylin and eosin (H&E) ×100; (B) H&E ×400. (*Source:* Dr Asha Kubba, Delhi Dermpath Laboratory)

Immunohistochemistry, using antibodies against various cytokeratins, especially CK5, has proved superior to congo-red in the diagnosis of PLCA.[5]

Although electron microscopy is seldom used in the diagnosis of amyloidosis, it can be of value in selected cases, when special stains fail to demonstrate the amyloid deposit or for research purposes.[17] Amyloid deposits are seen as island like aggregations in the dermis and as a network of linear, non-branching, paired, 6–10 nm wide fibrils of indefinite length with hollow cores on profile.[18]

DERMOSCOPY

In addition to history and physical examination, dermoscopy may assist in achieving an accurate diagnosis of PLCA for

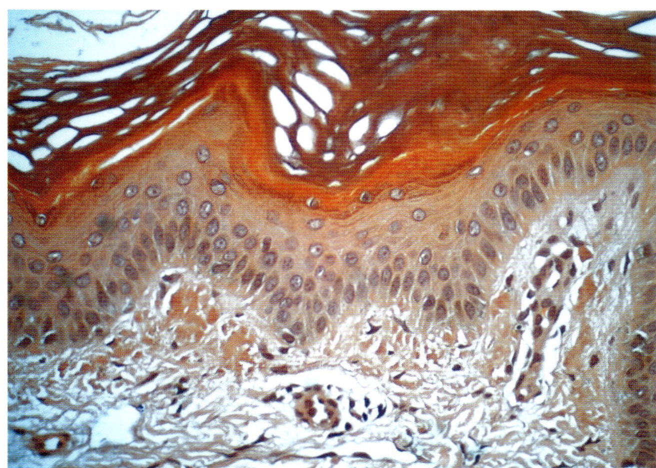

Fig. 2: Photomicrograph of macular amyloidosis showing orange-red deposits of amyloid in papillary dermis. (Congo red ×400). (*Source:* Dr Asha Kubba, Delhi Dermpath Laboratory)

patients with atypical presentations, perhaps avoiding the need for an invasive skin biopsy.

The most common dermoscopic finding of MA is that each "macule" is composed of a central hub surrounded by brownish pigmentation. The color of the central hub can be white or brown, and the configuration of brownish pigmentation around the central hubs can be of three types—fine radiating streaks, leaf-like projections and bulbous projections[58] **(Figs 3B, E and G)**.

The dermoscopic features correlate with the histopathological findings, with the brown pigmentation under dermoscopy being due to basal hyperpigmentation, pigment incontinence and melanin granules within amyloid deposition in the dermal papilla **(Figs 3B and C)**.

Dermoscopy aids in differentiating MA from other disorders such as friction melanosis and lichen simplex chronicus.

CLINICAL FEATURES

Macular amyloidosis **(Figs 3A, D and F)** is a chronic persistent disorder which clinically presents as small (2-4 mm) grayish brownish macules that coalesce to form poorly delineated hyperpigmented patches with a characteristic reticulated or rippled pattern. The patches are distributed asymmetrically over the upper back[12,59] (interscapular areas) **(Fig. 4)**, and extremities (shins and forearms) **(Figs 5 and 6)** predominantly. The buttocks[12,60] clavicles, breast, face, neck, axilla[61] and ribs are less commonly involved.[4,62] Macules may be associated with mild to moderate pruritus, but may be absent in 18% of patients.[50] The disease is progressive in a majority of patients.[12]

Macular and lichen amyloidosis may coexist frequently, which is known as biphasic amyloidosis.[62,63] Unusual variants of MA include diffuse hyperpigmentation,[64] nevoid like hyperpigmentation,[65] a poikilodermatous form,[66] incontinentia pigment like,[67] causing periocular hyperpigmentation,[68] and linear MA.[69]

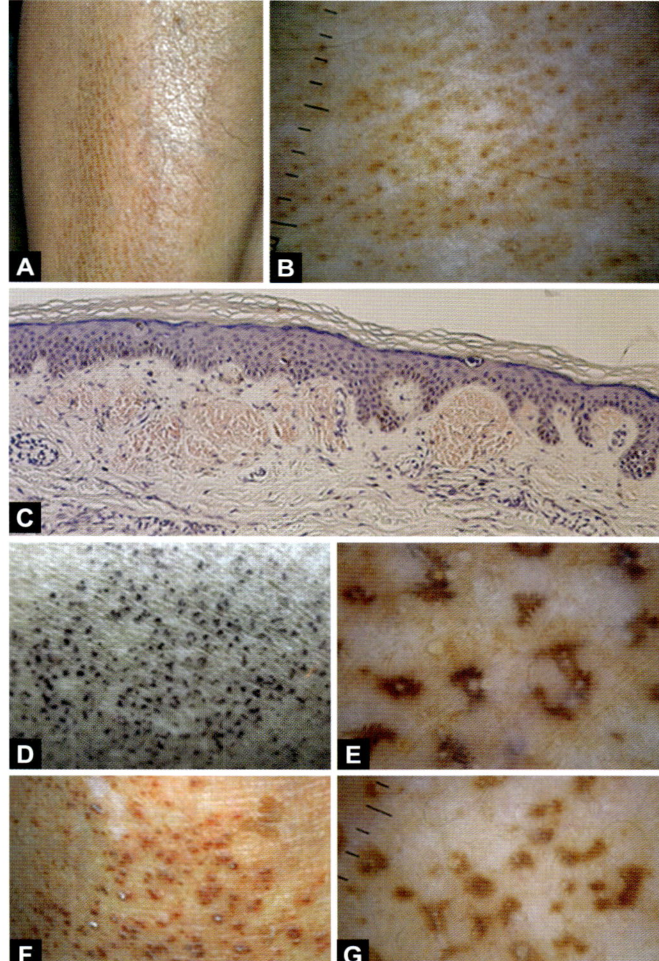

Figs 3A to G: Three cases of macular amyloidosis. Patient 1: (A) multiple rippled brownish macules on lower leg. (B) The dermoscopic findings reveal multiple uniform small central hubs with brown fine streaks radiating from the center. The color of the central hubs is brown. (C) The pathology demonstrates basket-weave orthokeratosis, basal hyperpigmentation, pigment incontinence, and amyloid deposition in the upper dermis. Patient 2: (D) clinical picture. (E) The dermoscopic pattern shows a venation like extension of pigmentation from each white central hub. Patient 3: (F) clinical picture. (G) For each macule, the dermoscopic picture demonstrates a non-circular thick pedal projection with a smooth border extending from a white central hub. (*Source:* Chuang YY, Lee DD, Lin CS, et al. Characteristic dermoscopic features of primary cutaneous amyloidosis: a study of 35 cases. BJD. 2012;167:548-54. © 2012 British Association of Dermatologists)

Anosacral amyloidosis is a rare form of cutaneous amyloidosis which presents as pruritic, well demarcated, brownish patches fanning out in lines from the anus to the sacral region and is more common in men.[70]

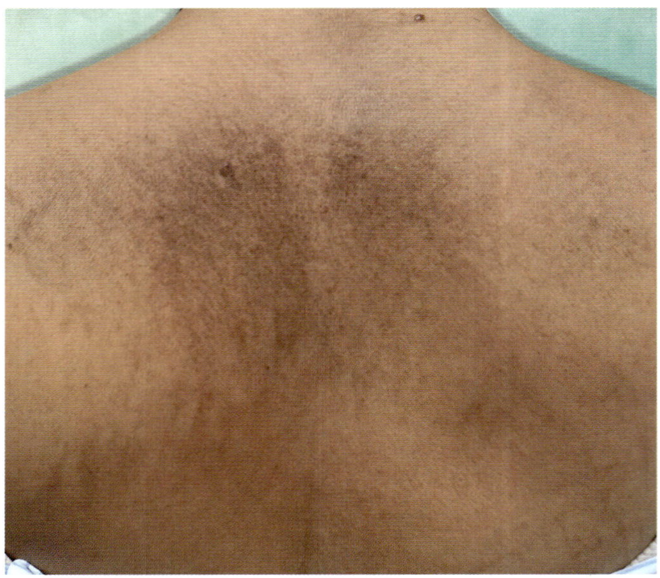

Fig. 4: Macular amyloidosis showing characteristic reticulate pigmentation with involvement of interscapular area

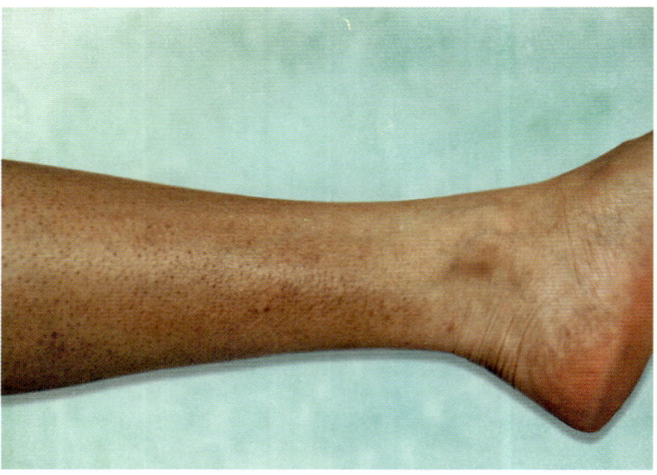

Fig. 5: Macular amyloidosis involving lower legs

Amyloidosis cutis dyschromica is another rare variant with hyperpigmented and hypopigmented xerotic lesions in sun-exposed skin. It is a congenital disorder with hypersensitivity to ultraviolet B (UVB) radiation, with possible DNA repair defects.[71]

The differential diagnosis of MA includes post-inflammatory hyperpigmentation, frictional melanosis, resolving lichen planus, neurodermatitis and the reticulate hyperpigmentation of neck in atopics (dirty neck).[72,73]

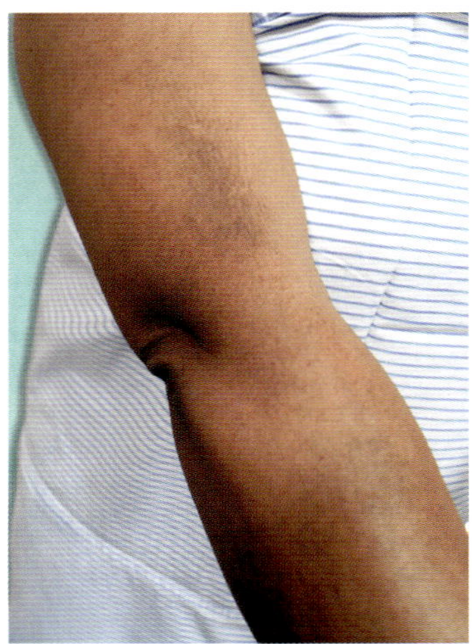

Fig. 6: Macular amyloidosis involving extensor aspect of arms

TREATMENT

Macular amyloidosis not only poses an important aesthetic concern but also many times causes intractable pruritus. The treatment of this condition is challenging and many times disappointing.[50] Various therapeutic modalities have been employed with variable success **(Table 2)**. Most of the treatments are directed toward relief of pruritus, and others to remove the amyloid deposits in the papillary dermis.

The management of this difficult problem involves first of all identifying and dealing with any underlying etiological factors, like atopic dermatitis, insulin resistance or autoimmune conditions. Avoidance of scratching and/or friction is of utmost importance. Sun protection measures should be instituted.

Antihistamines and topical steroids with or without occlusion are used to treat mild cases.[50] However, they provide temporary relief from pruritus, which soon relapses.

Topical application of 50–100% dimethyl sulfoxide has been shown to be efficacious in a few studies with disappearance of pruritus and reduction in pigmentation. The mechanism of action is not clear but is proposed to be degranulation and depletion of mast cells, and breaking the vicious "pruritus-amyloid deposition-pruritus" cycle. Histologically, there is no disappearance of amyloid deposits in the papillary dermis.[9,74,75] On the contrary, other authors reported only partial and transient results.[76]

There have been isolated reports of the beneficial effect of tretinoin,[77] etretinate[78] or acitretin[79] therapy in a proportion of patients. However, the condition relapses on discontinuation of treatment.[77] Topical tocoretinate,[80] transcutaneous electrical nerve stimulation[81] and UVB therapy[82] have been tried in a few cases with limited success.

Oral colchicine has been found to be useful with almost complete disappearance of pruritus as well as significant

Table 2: Management of macular amyloidosis		
Treatment of associated conditions	*Relief of pruritus*	*Removal of amyloid*
• Avoidance of friction • Atopy • Insulin resistance • Autoimmune conditions	• Sedating antihistamines • Topical corticosteroids • Calcipotriol • Ultraviolet B irradiation • Transcutaneous electrical nerve stimulation • Topical dimethyl sulfoxide • Topical tocoretinate • Etretinate or acitretin • Oral colchicine • Anti-interleukin-31 receptor therapy	• QS-Nd:YAG laser, either 532 nm or 1064 nm • Fractional photothermolysis • Antiamyloid antibodies (experimental)

Abbreviation: QS-Nd:YAG, quality-switched neodymium-doped yttrium aluminum garnet

reduction in the intensity of pigmentation in 3–4 months of therapy, without any reported relapse after 3 months of follow up.[72,83]

Anti-IL-31 therapy, which acts by reducing the pruritus, is in experimental stage.[84]

The quality-switched neodymium-doped yttrium aluminum garnet (QS-Nd:YAG) laser (532 nm and 1064 nm), being an ultra-short pulsed laser, helps by targeting the melanin debris of upper dermis seen in MA. In a study by Ostovari et al. 90% of patients with MA demonstrated more than 50% reduction in their pigmentation with the QS-Nd:YAG laser.[85]

Fractional photothermolysis creates microthermal lesions that allow transport and extrusion of dermal content through a compromised DE junction. It has been proposed that by this nonablative laser-induced transport mechanism the amyloid deposits as well as melanophages can get eliminated transepidermally through the channels created by the laser.[86] On a similar note, significant improvement has been reported in LA with fractional ablative 2940 nm Erbium:YAG laser.[87] In the author's personal experience, nonablative 1550 nm fiber laser produced significant reduction in the pigmentation of MA in two patients which was maintained at 6 months follow-up (unpublished data, 2012). However, no histological confirmation of reduction of amyloid was done. Larger controlled studies are required to further establish the efficacy of this promising treatment modality.

Recent understandings of the underlying mechanisms of amyloid deposition provide new concepts for inhibition of protein aggregation and its proinflammatory and cytotoxic effects. The main therapeutic approaches include: small compounds that inhibit aggregation, immunotherapy (antibody therapy and vaccination), and compounds that interfere with amyloid-cell or amyloid-protein interactions or responses thereof.[27]

Experiments in animal models for Alzheimer's disease have shown that immunotherapy against amyloidogenic proteins is a promising novel approach in the treatment of protein misfolding diseases.[88] Conformational antibodies directed against amyloid, to facilitate antibody-mediated clearance of amyloid deposits in the skin by direct intradermal injection are being researched on a mouse model.[89]

CONCLUSION

The etiology and pathogenesis of MA remains obscure. Thus, there is a need for further studies based on the direction provided by research in other well studied protein folding diseases, like Alzheimer's disease. This will help in discovering simple and effective treatments, and means of prevention of this common, yet challenging disorder.

REFERENCES

1. Glenner GG. Amyloid deposits and amyloidosis. The beta-fibrilloses (first of two parts). N Eng J Med. 1980;302(23):1283-92.
2. Botelho MG, Lupi O. Protein folding and cutaneous diseases. Int J Dermatol. 2008;47(12):1225-33.
3. Kibbi AG, Rubeiz NG, Zaynoun ST, et al. Primary localized cutaneous amyloidosis. Int J Dermatol. 1992;31(2):95-8.
4. Breathnach SM. Amyloid and amyloidosis. J Am Acad Dermatol. 1988;18(1 Pt 1):1-16.
5. Fernandez-Flores A. Cutaneous amyloidosis: a concept review. Am J Dermatopathol. 2012;34(1):1-17.
6. Palitz LL, Peck S. Amyloidosis cutis: a macular variant. AMA Arch Derm Syphilol. 1952;65(4):451-7.
7. Tan T. Epidemiology of primary cutaneous amyloidoses in southeast Asia. Clin Dermatol. 1990;8(2):20-4.

8. Ollague W, Ollague J, Ferretti H. Epidemiology of primary cutaneous amyloidoses in South America. Clin Dermatol. 1990;8(2):25-9.
9. Krishna A, Nath B, Dhir GG, et al. Study on epidemiology of cutaneous amyloidosis in northern India and effectiveness of dimethylsulphoxide in cutaneous amyloidosis. Indian Dermatol Online J. 2012;3(3):182-6.
10. Looi L M. Primary localised cutaneous amyloidosis in Malaysians. Australas J Dermatol. 1991;32(1):39-44.
11. Djuanda A, Wiryadi BE, Sularsito SA, et al. The epidemiology of cutaneous amyloidosis in Jakarta (Indonesia). Ann Acad Med Singapore. 1988;17(4):536-40.
12. al-Ratrout JT, Satti MB. Primary localized cutaneous amyloidosis: a clinicopathologic study from Saudi Arabia. Int J Dermatol. 1997;36(6):428-34.
13. Eswaramoorthy V, Kaur I, Das A, et al. Macular amyloidosis: etiological factors. J Dermatol. 1999;26(5):305-10.
14. Rasi A, Khatami A, Javaheri SM. Macular amyloidosis: an assessment of prevalence, sex, and age. Int J Dermatol. 2004;43(12):898-9.
15. Black MM, Jones EW. Macular amyloidosis: a study of 21 cases with special reference to the role of the epidermis in its histogenesis. Br J Dermatol. 1971;84(3):199-209.
16. Hashimoto K. Progress on cutaneous amyloidoses. J Invest Dermatol. 1984;82(1):1-3.
17. Schepis C, Siragusa M, Gagliardi ME, et al. Primary macular amyloidosis: an ultrastructural approach to diagnosis. Ultrastruct Pathol. 1999;23(5):279-84.
18. Kurban AK, Malak JA, Afifi AK, et al. Primary localized macular cutaneous amyloidosis: histochemistry and electron microscopy. Br J Dermatol. 1971;85(1):52-60.
19. Mukai H, Kanzaki T, Nishiyama S. Sulfhydryl and disulfide staining in amyloids of skin-limited and systemic amyloidoses. J Invest Dermatol. 1984;82(1):4-8.
20. Masu S, Hosokawa M, Seiji M. Amyloid in localized cutaneous amyloidosis: immunofluorescence studies with anti-keratin antiserum especially concerning the difference between systemic and localized cutaneous amyloidosis. Acta Derm Venereol. 1981;61(5):381-4.
21. Hashimoto K, Kobayashi H. Histogenesis of amyloid in the skin. Am J Dermatopathol. 1980;2(2):165-71.
22. Hashimoto K, Kumakiri M. Colloid-amyloid bodies in PUVA-treated human psoriatic patients. J Invest Dermatol. 1979;72(2):70-80.
23. Kobayashi H, Hashimoto K. Amyloidogenesis in organ-limited cutaneous amyloidosis: an antigenic identity between epidermal keratin and skin amyloid. J Invest Dermatol. 1983;80(1):66-72.
24. Eto H, Hashimoto K, Kobayashi H, et al. Differential staining of cytoid bodies and skin-limited amyloids with monoclonal anti-keratin antibodies. Am J Pathol. 1984;116(3):473-81.
25. Yanagihara M, Mori S. Histogenesis of macular amyloidosis. Nihon Hifuka Gakkai Zasshi. 1982;92(8):851-9.
26. Clos AL, Lasagna-Reeves CA, Kelly B, et al. Role of oligomers in the amyloidogenesis of primary cutaneous amyloidosis. J Am Acad Dermatol. 2011;65(5):1023-31.
27. Herczenik E, Gebbink MF. Molecular and cellular aspects of protein misfolding and disease. FASEB J. 2008;22(7): 2115-33.
28. Ghiso J, Frangione B. Amyloidosis and Alzheimer's disease. Adv Drug Deliv Rev. 2002;54(12):1539-51.
29. Bucciantini M, Calloni G, Chiti F, et al. Prefibrillar amyloid protein aggregates share common features of cytotoxicity. J Biol Chem. 2004;279(30):31374-82.
30. Merlini G, Bellotti V. Molecular mechanisms of amyloidosis. N Engl J Med. 2003;349(6):583-96.
31. Wong C, Lin C. Friction amyloidosis. Int J Dermatol. 1988;27(5):302-7.
32. Onuma L, Vega M, Arenas R, et al. Friction amyloidosis. Int J Dermatol. 1994;33(1):74.
33. Somani VK, Hari S, Sita VN, et al. Nylon friction dermatitis: A distinct subset of macular amyloidosis. Indian J Dermatol Venereol Leprol. 1995;61(3):145-7.
34. Siragusa M, Ferri R, Cavallari V, et al. Friction melanosis, friction amyloidosis, macular amyloidosis, towel melanosis: many names for the same clinical entity. Eur J Dermatol. 2001;11(6):545-8.
35. Hashimoto K, Ito K, Kumakiri M, et al. Nylon brush macular amyloidosis. Arch Dermatol. 1987;123(5):633-7.
36. Goulden V, Highet AS, Shamy HK. Notalgia paraesthetica—report of an association with macular amyloidosis. Clin Exp Dermatol. 1994;19(4):346-9.
37. Peña-Penabad MC, Garcia-Silva J, Armijo M. Notalgia paresthetica and macular amyloidosis: cause-effect relationship? Clin Exp Dermatol. 1995;20(3):279.
38. Wong CK. Cutaneous amyloidoses. Int J Dermatol. 1987;26(5):273-7.
39. Shanon J. Cutaneous amyloidosis associated with atopic disorders. Dermatologica. 1970;141(4):297-302.
40. Lee DD, Huang CK, Ko PC, et al. Association of primary cutaneous amyloidosis with atopic dermatitis: a nationwide population-based study in Taiwan. Br J Dermatol. 2011;164(1):148-53.
41. Hartshorne ST. Familial primary cutaneous amyloidosis in a South African family. Clin Exp Dermatol. 1999;24(6):438-42.
42. Verga U, Fugazzola L, Cambiaghi S, et al. Frequent association between MEN 2A and cutaneous lichen amyloidosis. Clin Endocrinol (Oxf). 2003;59(2):156-61.
43. Arita K, South AP, Hans-Filho G, et al. Oncostatin M receptor-beta mutations underlie familial primary localized cutaneous amyloidosis. Am J Hum Genet. 2008;82(1): 73-80.
44. Babilas P, Fiebig BS, Aslanidis C, et al. Identification of an oncostatin M receptor mutation associated with familial primary cutaneous amyloidosis. Br J Dermatol. 2009;161(4):944-7.

45. Dahdah MJ, Kurban M, Kibbi AG, et al. Primary localized cutaneous amyloidosis: a sign of immune dysregulation? Int J Dermatol. 2009;48(4):419-21.
46. Ogiyama Y, Hayashi Y, Kou C, et al. Cutaneous amyloidosis in patients with progressive systemic sclerosis. Cutis. 1996;57(1):28-32.
47. Chanoki M, Suzuki S, Hayashi Y, et al. Progressive systemic sclerosis associated with cutaneous amyloidosis. Int J Dermatol. 1994;33(9):648-9.
48. Azon-Masoliver A. Widespread primary localized cutaneous amyloidosis (macular form) associated with systemic sclerosis. Br J Dermatol. 1995;132(1):163-5.
49. Danielsen L, Christensen HE, Wanstrup J. Cutaneous amyloidosis. Classification, pathogenesis and relation to "collagen disease". Acta Pathol Microbiol Scand A. 1970;78(3):335-44.
50. Metabolic and nutritional disorders. In: Burns T, Breathnach S, Cox N, Griffiths C (Eds). Rook's Text Book of Dermatology, 7th edn. United States: Blackwell Publishing; 2004.
51. Tafarel JR, Lemos LB, Oliveira PM, et al. Cutaneous amyloidosis associated with primary biliary cirrhosis. Eur J Gastroenterol Hepatol. 2007;19(7):603-5.
52. Fujiwara K, Kono T, Ishii M, et al. Primary localized cutaneous amyloidosis associated with autoimmune cholangitis. Int J Dermatol. 2000;39(10):768-71.
53. Chang YT, Liu HN, Wong CK, et al. Detection of Epstein-Barr virus in primary cutaneous amyloidosis. Br J Dermatol. 1997;136(6):823-6.
54. Bitel CL, Feng Y, Souayah N, et al. Increased expression and local accumulation of the prion protein, Alzheimer Aβ peptides, superoxide dismutase 1, and nitric oxide synthases 1 & 2 in muscle in a rabbit model of diabetes. BMC Physiol. 2010;10:18.
55. Li WM. Histopathology of primary cutaneous amyloidosis and systemic amyloidosis. Clin Dermatol. 1990;8(2):30-5.
56. Maize J, Maize Jr J, Metcalf J. Metabolic diseases of the Skin. In: Elder David E, Elenitsas R, Johnson, Bernett L, Murphy (Eds). Lever's Histopathology of the Skin, 9th edn. Philadelphia: Lippincott Williams and Wilkins; 2005. pp. 436-41.
57. MacDonald DM, Black MM, Ramnarain N. Immunofluorescence studies in primary localized cutaneous amyloidosis. Br J Dermatol. 1996;96:635-41.
58. Chuang YY, Lee DD, Lin CS, et al. Characteristic dermoscopic features of primary cutaneous amyloidosis: a study of 35 cases. Br J Dermatol. 2012;167(3):548-54.
59. Shanon J, Sagher F. Interscapular cutaneous amyloidosis. Arch Dermatol. 1970;102(2):195-8.
60. Tanigaki T, Hata S, Kitano Y, et al. Unusual pigmentation on the skin over trunk bones and extremities. Dermatologica. 1985;170(5):235-9.
61. Habermann MC, Montenegro MR. Primary cutaneous amyloidosis: clinical, laboratorial and histopathological study of 25 cases. Identification of gammaglobulins and C3 in the lesions by immunofluorescence. Dermatologica. 1980;160(4):240-8.
62. Bedi TR, Datta BN. Diffuse biphasic cutaneous amyloidosis. Dermatologica. 1979;158(6):433-7.
63. Brownstein MH, Hashimoto K, Greenwald G. Biphasic amyloidosis: link between macular and lichenoid forms. Br J Dermatol. 1973;88(1):25-9.
64. Wong CK, Lee JY. Macular amyloidosis with widespread diffuse pigmentation. Br J Dermatol. 1996;135(1):135-8.
65. Black MM, Maibach HI. Macular amyloidosis simulating naevoid hyperpigmentation. Br J Dermatol. 1974;90(4):461-4.
66. Serna-Pérez MJ, Vázquez-Doval FJ, Idoate M, et al. Extensive macular amyloidosis associated with poikiloderma. Int J Dermatol. 1992;31(4):277-8.
67. Wu JJ, Su YN, Hsiao CH, et al. Macular amyloidosis presenting in an incontinentia pigmenti-like pattern with subepidermal blister formation. J Eur Acad Dermatol Venereol. 2008;22(5):635-7.
68. Van den Berg WH, Starink TM. Macular amyloidosis, presenting as periocular hyperpigmentation. Clin Exp Dermatol. 1983;8(2):195-7.
69. Abbas O, Ugent S, Borirak K, et al. Linear macular amyloidosis. J Eur Acad Dermatol Venereol. 2009;23(12):1446-8.
70. Wang WJ, Huang CY, Chang YT, et al. Anosacral cutaneous amyloidosis: a study of 10 Chinese cases. Br J Dermatol. 2000;143:1266-9.
71. Moriwaki S, Nishigori C, Horiguchi Y, et al. Amyloidosis cutis dyschromica. DNA repair reduction in the cellular response to UV light. Arch Dermatol. 1992;128(7):966-70.
72. Shah MP, Padhiar B, Karia U, et al. Primary cutaneous amyloidosis. Indian J Dermatol Venereol Leprol. 1997;63(2):105-6.
73. Hughes BR, Cunliffe WJ. Rippled hyperpigmentation resembling macular amyloidosis—a feature of atopic eczema. Clin Exp Dermatol. 1990;15(5):380-1.
74. Ozkaya-Bayazit E, Baykal C, Kavak A. Local DMSO treatment of macular and popular amyloidosis. Hautarzt. 1997;48(1):31-7.
75. Ozkaya-Bayazit E, Kavak A, Güngör H, et al. Intermittent use of topical dimethyl sulfoxide in macular and papular amyloidosis. Int J Dermatol. 1998;37(12):949-54.
76. Pandhi R, Kaur I, Kumar B. Lack of effect of dimethylsulphoxide in cutaneous amyloidosis. J Dermatolog Treat. 2002;13(1):11-4.
77. Rados J, Marinović Kulisić S, Lipozencić J, et al. Macular amyloidosis: a case report. Acta Dermatovenerol Croat. 2008;16(3):138-41.
78. Marschalko M, Daroczy J, Soos G. Etretinate for the treatment of lichen amyloidosis. Arch Dermato. 1998;11:574-7.

79. Hernandez-Nunez A, Dauden E, Moreno de Vega MJ, et al. Widespread biphasic amyloidosis: response to acitretin. Clin Exp Dermatol. 2001;26(3):256-9.
80. Terao M, Nishida K, Murota H, et al. Clinical effect of tocoretinate on lichen and macular amyloidosis. J Dermatol. 2011;38(2):179-84.
81. Yüksek J, Sezer E, Aksu M, et al. Transcutaneous electrical nerve stimulation for reduction of pruritus in macular amyloidosis and lichen simplex. J Dermatol. 2011;38(6):546-52.
82. Hudson LD. Macular amyloidosis: treatment with ultraviolet B. Cutis. 1986;38(1):61-2.
83. Chakravarty K, Chanda M. Role of colchicine in primary localised cutaneous amyloidosis. Indian J Dermatol Venereol Leprol. 1995;61(5):268-9.
84. Tanaka A, Arita K, Lai-Cheong JE, et al. New insight into mechanisms of pruritus from molecular studies on familial primary localized cutaneous amyloidosis. Br J Dermatol. 2009;161(6):1217-24.
85. Ostovari N, Mohtasham N, Oadras M, et al. 532-nm and 1064-nm Q-switched Nd:YAG laser therapy for reduction of pigmentation in macular amyloidosis patches. J Eur Acad Dermatol Venereol. 2008;22(4):442-6.
86. Hantash BM, Bedi VP, Sudireddy V, et al. Laser-induced transepidermal elimination of dermal content by fractional photothermolysis. J Biomed Opt. 2006;11(4): 041115.
87. Anitha B, Mysore V. Lichen Amyloidosis: Novel Treatment with Fractional Ablative 2,940 nm Erbium: YAG Laser Treatment. J Cutan Aesthet Surg. 2012;5(2):141-3.
88. Solomon B. Clinical immunologic approaches for the treatment of Alzheimer's disease. Expert Opin Investig Drugs. 2007;16(6):819-28.
89. Clos AL, Lasagna-Reeves CA, Wagner R, et al. Therapeutic removal of amyloid deposits in cutaneous amyloidosis by localised intra-lesional injections of anti-amyloid antibodies. Exp Dermatol. 2010;19(10):904-11.

52

Lichen Planus Pigmentosus

M Sendhil Kumaran, Amrinder Jit Kanwar

Key Features

- Lichen planus pigmentosus is an uncommon variant of lichen planus manifesting as brown colored to violaceous discrete macules which coalesces in due course to form large patches.
- Although a few risk factors have been hypothesized, its exact etiopathogenesis is still elusive.
- Till date no specific treatment exists for lichen planus pigmentosus.

INTRODUCTION

Lichen planus pigmentosus (LPP) is a unique variant of lichen planus (LP), clinically characterized by the insidious onset of discrete dark-brown macules appearing over sun-exposed areas and flexural folds with or without the association of pruritus in these lesions. It is liable that the earliest mention on this condition was by Gougerot in 1934.[1] He referred to the pigmented lesions in patients with LP in which the initial inflammatory phase was nominal. He termed it as "lichen invisible pigmentogene" meaning invisible pigmented LP. Subsequently, Shima[2] in 1956 demonstrated a similar condition from Japan and named it as "lichen pigmentosus". In Indian literature the first mention of LPP was made by Desai in 1956 who gave a descriptive term as "lichen planus pigmentosus sine lichen".[3] The first detailed description of LPP was delivered by Bhutani et al.[4] in 1974. LPP is frequently encountered in Indians, but subsequently it has been described among other racial and ethnic populations like Latin Americans, Middle East, Koreans and Japanese.[5,6]

Various pigmentary disorders with features identical to LPP have been described under various headings like ashy dermatosis[7] and erythema dyschromicum perstans (EDP).[8] Bhutani et al.[4] and later Kanwar et al.[9] delineated the various clinico-histopathological features of LPP. Vega et al.[10] in 1992 claimed that EDP and LPP are two distinct entities and put forward many clinical and histopathological differences between the two.

EPIDEMIOLOGY

Lichen planus pigmentosus has been described in up to 4.1% of the patients attending pigmentary clinic services at a tertiary center in India.[9] The male to female ratio varies from 1:1.2 in India[9] to 1.75: 1 in Kuwait.[11] The peak age of onset is usually between the third and fourth decades of life with males having an earlier onset by a decade. Few studies indicate a slight female preponderance.[9]

PATHOGENESIS

The exact pathogenesis of LPP still remains elusive. Based on various histopathologic alterations, LPP probably represents a type of lichenoid tissue reaction to an unknown antigen or stimulus. Since LPP demonstrates histopathological features identical to LP, the pathogenesis of LPP could be similar to that of LP. Both CD4+ and CD8+ T cells, accumulate in the dermis. While CD8+ T cells infiltrate the epidermis, in LP lesions. It has been hypothesized that CD8+ cytotoxic T cells recognize an unknown antigen associated with the major histocompatibility complex class I on keratinocytes present in the lesions and cause lysis.[12-14] Infiltrating CD8+ T cells, as well as keratinocytes, express a variety of different chemokines like interferon-γ (IFN-γ), tumor necrosis factor-α (TNF-α), interleukin-6 (IL-6) and lymphocyte function associated antigen-1 (LFA-1). Apoptosis of kertinocytes may be caused by various factors like granzyme B and bone morphogenetic protein-4 (BMP-4).[15,16] Kashima et al. revealed that, in LPP, the cytotoxic keratinocyte injury was less widespread and not as intense when compared with classic LP.[5] The pigmentation of

LPP is dermal resulting from damage to basal cells as well as disruption of the normal mechanism of transfer of melanin from the melanocytes to the keratinocytes. This results in pigmentary incontinence and collection of the pigment in dermal melanophages. Due to the "Tyndall effect" this pigmentation can present in various shades of color.

RISK FACTORS

The exact risk factors involved in the development of LPP is obscure, however, use of mustard oil and amla oil for body massage and hair dressing have been recognized as a risk factor for the development of LPP in India. Mustard oil has been experimentally shown to contain a chemical named allyl isothiocynate which is a potent photosensitizer, and hence could possibly play a role in the development of LPP.

Use of henna or hair dye for months to years has also been described in about 20% of patients.[9] However, no definite correlation could be established between its use and disease onset or aggravation. In a significant proportion of patients (17.8%) increased sun exposure has been observed as a risk factor.[9]

Earlier, Pinkus had commented on probable role environmental pollutants either as contactants, inhaled or ingested by a predisposed individual could cause the individual to present in this peculiar pattern of pigmentation.[17]

CLINICAL FEATURES

In early stages the lesions appear as small, discrete, ill-defined, dark-brown to grayish colored, oval to round macules, **(Figs 1A and B)**, which later becomes confluent to form large patches of hyperpigmentation. The pigmentation throughout the lesions is more or less uniform in a given patient. The color in LPP differs from brownish-black to slate-gray. The clinical presentation of hyperpigmentation can be in 4 different patterns like; diffuse, reticular, blotchy and perifollicular. [9]

The diffuse form is the commonly exhibited variant of hyperpigmentation.[9,11] Face and neck are first to be involved (commonly)[9,11] among which, the preauricular region (including the temples) and forehead, are predominantly the site of first onset and are involved in almost all patients. Subsequently, the pigmentation spreads to involve the upper limbs, upper part of the back and trunk. Lesions are often bilaterally symmetrical in distribution and predominant over the sun exposed sites. The term "lichen planus pigmentosus inversus" is often used when the lesions predominate over flexures, i.e. the axillae, groin and inframammary areas. Linear lesions occurring along Blaschko's lines have also been described.[18] Apart from this there are isolated case reports of LPP appearing in a zosteriform pattern. **Table 1** summarizes the various clinical patterns.

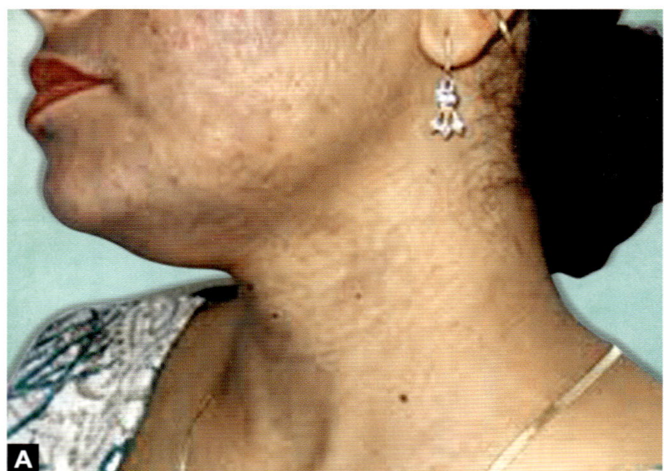

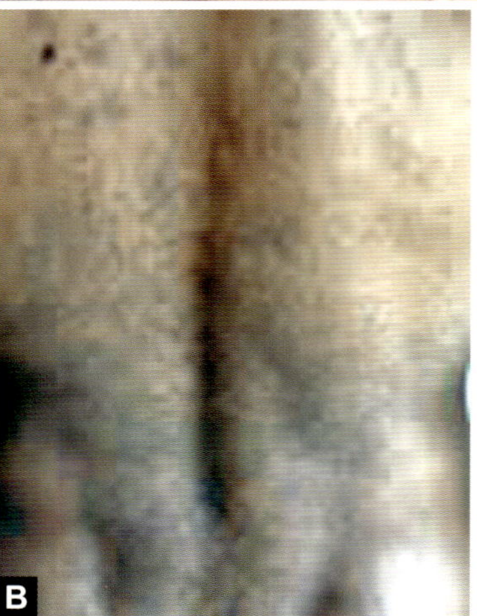

Figs 1A and B: (A) Vilaceous macules over cheeks, upper neck; (B) Small discrete violaceous macules over lower back. (*Source:* Dr Uma Nahar Saikia, Additional Professor, Department of Pathology, PGIMER, Chandigarh, India)

Table 1: Clinical patterns of LPP

Configuration	Classic, linear, zosteriform
Morphology	Diffuse, reticular, blotchy, perifollicular
Site	Flexural (inverse), linear, mucosal

Abbreviation: LPP; lichen planus pigmentosus

The disease has an insidious onset and runs a chronic course. It is generally asymptomatic, but mild pruritus and burning sensation has been seen in about one-third of patients suffering from LPP. The patients continue to develop newer lesions as old ones enlarge gradually at the periphery along with increase in the intensity of color.

Bhutani et al.[1] and Vega et al.[10] have described lesions of classic LP occurring in 11 out of 40 (27%) and 1 out of

11 (9%) of their study cohort respectively, either accompanying, preceding or following lesions of LPP. Mucosal involvement can occur in form of diffuse and speckled pigmentation in up to 3–4% of patients.[9,11]

INVESTIGATIONS

Histopathology

Histopathology shows vacuolar degeneration of the basal layer in the epidermis. In the dermis, a perivascular lymphohistiocytic infiltrate and the presence of melanophages may be seen, **(Figs 2A and B)**. Mutairi et al.[11] described two main histological patterns in LPP that may represent the two ends of the continuous histological spectrum of the disease. The first pattern was seen in recently developed lesions. In this the epidermal changes were primarily characterized by marked basal cell vacuolar degeneration, frequent keratinocyte apoptosis and mild changes of epidermal thickness. In the dermis, there was a predominant band-like lymphohistiocytic inflammatory infiltrate, along with scattered melanophages and mild to moderate melanin incontinence. In the other pattern, the epidermal changes were few predominantly consisting of focal or absent vacuolar degeneration, fewer apoptotic keratinocytes and atrophy of the epidermis with compact hyperkeratosis, in the dermis there was superficial mild perivascular lymphohistiocytic inflammatory infiltrate with dense melanin incontinence and frequent melanophages both perivascularly and interstitially. This pattern was mostly seen in older lesions. However, most of the patients had overlapping of the two patterns, with prominence of one of the patterns.

Among other investigations, evaluation for anti-HCV antibody may be required, particularly in HCV endemic regions.

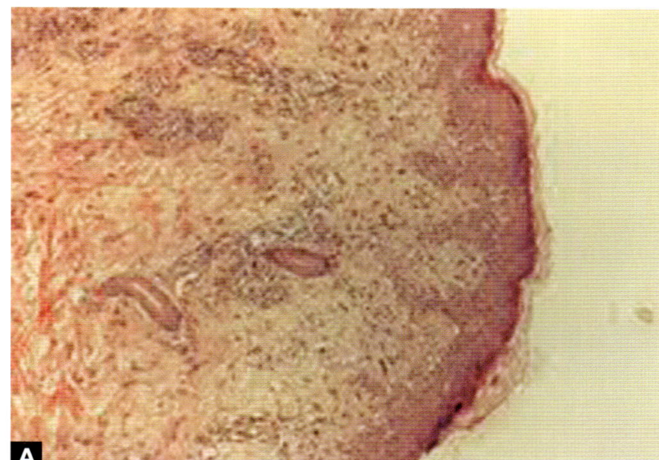

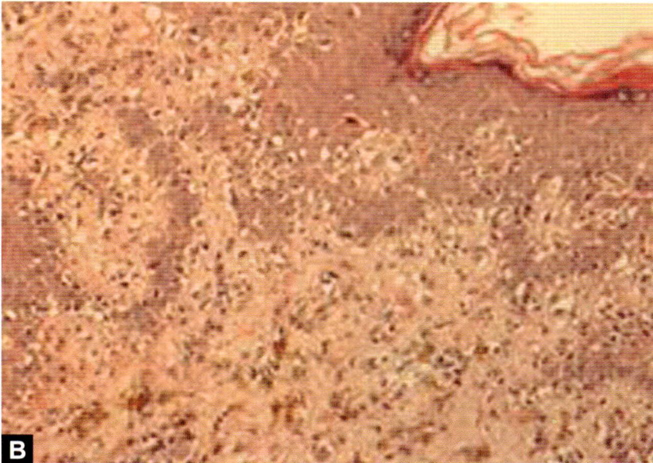

Figs 2A and B: (A) Microphotograph showing mild hypergranulosis with basal cell degeneration along with perivascular lymphocytic inflammation and melanin incontinence in the dermis. H&E x 10X; (B) Higher magnification showing basal degeneration and Civatte bodies. H&E x 20X. (*Source:* Dr Uma Nahar Saikia, Additional Professor, Department of Pathology, PGIMER, Chandigarh, India)

Associations with Lichen Planus Pigmentosus

Like in classic LP, association with hepatitis C virus (HCV) has been demonstrated in many case reports. In a study from Kuwait, 60% of patients with LPP were serologically positive for HCV.[11] Rarely LPP has been shown to present in association with acrokeratosis of Bazex,[19] nephrotic syndrome,[20] frontal fibrosing alopecia,[21] and therapy with gold.[22]

Differential Diagnosis

The differentials that should be considered while diagnosing LPP include EDP (ashy dermatosis of Ramirez), Reihl's melanosis, Addison's disease and exogenous ochronosis.

Erythema dyschromicum perstans is the most common differential diagnosis of LPP which is clinically characterized by blue-gray hyperpigmented macules with variable shape and size. Whether it is a variant of LPP or a separate entity, has been inconclusive. Bhutani, in 1986, in a letter titled in Shakesperian style "Ashy dermatosis or Lichen planus pigmentosis: What is in a name?" emphasized that these two entities were the same.[23] This letter was written in sheer disgust as a result of the apathy shown by various authors to the nomenclature (LPP) suggested by him. He pointed out that ashy dermatosis was a macular variant of LP, hence the term LPP as coined by him was more suitable than ashy dermatosis to describe this disorder of hyperpigmentation.

The credit for clarifying the not so logical status of these two entities goes to Vega et al. who in 1992 emphatically pointed out the difference between LPP and ashy dermatosis.[10,24] Vega et al. analyzed the clinical and histopathological characteristics of patients with LPP (n = 11) and ashy dermatosis (n = 20). They found significant clinical differences between the two dermatoses. Vega et al. concluded that although there were histopathological similarities between the 2 entities, there were significant clinical differences between LPP and ashy dermatosis. There are subtle clinical features which differentiate EDP from LPP, which has been summarized in **Tables 2 and 3**.

Reihl's melanosis may pose diagnostic problems in differentiation from LPP, **Table 4** delineates various subtle differences between LPP and Reihl's melanosis.

In Addison's disease, the pigmentation is most pronounced on the light exposed areas, flexures, palmar and plantar creases, areas subjected to repeated friction, nipples and genitalia and mucous membranes.

Exogenous ochronosis, a rare complication of hydroquinine, develops after prolonged use of high concentrations of the drug. It presents with diffuse pigmentation, which under high magnification shows tiny, sooty blue macules in a reticulate pattern. Lesions are usually present in the hydroquinone treated photo-exposed areas like cheeks, forehead and temporal and periorbital skin.

TREATMENT

There are no established treatments yet for LPP. Bhutani et al.[25] found that repeated courses of large doses of vitamin A resulted in improvement in few patients. Topical corticosteroids and topical calcineurin inhibitors (TCIs) along with photoprotection are probably the first line of treatment. But the response to topical steroids has been variable. Ohshima et al.[26] described a case of LPP inversus which responded well to treatment with mometasone ointment for 9 months.

Munox-Perez et al.[27] described a slight lightening of the lesion by treatment with oral deflazacort, initiated at 45 mg daily and gradually tapered to 6 mg daily over a period of 2 months. TCIs have also been found to be useful in treatment of LPP. In a study by Mutairi et al.[11] treatment with topical tacrolimus, for 16 weeks resulted in improvement in pigmentation in 7 of 13 (53.8%) patients.

Q-switched Nd:YAG laser in combination with topical tacrolimus resulted in complete clearance in one patient,[28] 1064-nm Q-switched neodymium:yttrium-aluminium-garnet

Table 2: Clinical differences between ashy dermatosis and LPP

	Ashy dermatosis	*LPP*
• Sex	F>M	M = F
• Age	3rd and 4th decades	Childhood to old age
• Etiology	Unknown ?mustard oil (consumption/application), henna application, fragrances, sun exposure,[9] HCV11	Unknown ?climatic, alimentary (ammonium nitrate ingestion), and occupational factors.[10]
• Reticulate pattern	–	+/–
• Distribution	Symmetrical	Non-characteristic
• Areas affected	Trunk, neck, face, upper limbs	Sun-exposed and flexural areas
• Pruritus	–	+/–
• Course	Chronic, insidious	Chronic, relapses and remissions

Abbreviations: F; females, M; males, HCV; hepatitis C virus

Table 3: Histopathological differences between ashy dermatosis and LPP

	Ashy dermatosis	*LPP*
• Epidermal thinning	+	–
• Hyperkeratosis/hypergranulosis	–	+
• Basal cell vacuolization	+	–
• Colloid bodies	+/–	+/–
• Lichenoid infiltrate	–	+/–
• Incontinence of pigment and melanophages	+	+
• Scarce/absent cellular infiltrate	+/–	–

Abbreviation: LPP; lichen planus pigmentosus

Table 4: Differences between Riehl's melanosis and LPP

	Riehl's melanosis	*LPP*
• *Clinical features*		
– Shape	Bizarre shaped, reticular, diffuse pigmentation	Small oval macules coalescing to form diffuse sheets of pigmentation
– Hue	Dark-brown predominantly	Bluish-black generally
– Site of predilection	Mainly face, often around neck	Face, neck, extremities, trunk
• *Histopathology*		
– Hypergranulosis	Usually absent	Usually present
– Spongiosis	Usually present	Usually absent
– Band like infiltration in upper dermis	Absent	May be present
– Causative agents	A variety of cosmetic allergens	Unknown; cosmetics may precipitate lesions
– Effect of allergen control	Dramatic	No significant effect

Abbreviation: LPP; lichen planus pigmentosus

laser (1.8 J/cm^2) was done every 3 weeks. Six weeks later, the lesions were much lighter and 4 months later, the lesions had cleared without a scar with no evidence of recurrence on 6 months of follow-up.

COURSE OF DISEASE

Usually, the course of LPP is chronic and persistent. Treatments are less effective for LPP than for classical LP.

CONCLUSION

Lichen planus pigmentosus is a resistant disorder of hyperpigmentation with obscure etiopathogenesis and resistant to most of the available therapies. More studies are required in future to clearly delineate its etiology thus helping in development of an ideal treatment modality.

REFERENCES

1. Gougerot H. Lichen atypiques ou invisibles pigmentogenes reveles par des pigmentations. Bull Scoc Fr Dermatol Syph. 1935;42:792-4.
2. Shima T. Supplementative study of lichen pigmentosus. Jpn J Dermatol. 1956;66:353.
3. Desai SC, Marquis L. Lichen planus: Clinical study of 67 cases with results of penicillin therapy. Indian J Dermatol Venereol. 1956;21:31-48.
4. Bhutani LK, Bedi TR, Pandhi RK, et al. Lichen planus pigmentosus. Dermatologica. 1974;149(1):43-50.
5. Kashima A, Tajiri A, Yamashita A, et al. Two Japanese cases of lichen planus pigmentosus-inversus. Int J Dermatol. 2007;46(7):740-2.
6. Hong S, Shin JH, Kang HY. Two cases of lichen planus pigmentosus presenting with a linear pattern. J Korean Med Sci. 2004;19(1):152-4.
7. Ramirez O, Lopez Lino DG. Current status of ashy dermatosis. Synonym—erythema dyschromicum perstans. Med Cutan Ibero Lat Am. 1984;12(1):11-8.
8. Convit J, Kerdel-Vegas F, Rodriguez G. Erythema dyschromicum perstans. A hitherto undescribed skin disease. J Invest Dermatol. 1961; 36: 457-62.
9. Kanwar AJ, Dogra S, Handa S, et al. A study of 124 Indian patients with lichen planus pigmentosus. Clin Exp Dermatol. 2003;28(5):481-5.
10. Vega ME, Waxtein L, Arenas R, et al. Ashy dermatosis and lichen planus pigmentosus: a clinicopathologic study of 31 cases. Int J Dermatol. 1992; 31: 90-4.
11. Al-Mutairi N, El-Khalawany M. Clinicopathological characteristics of lichen planus pigmentosus and its response to tacrolimus ointment: an open label, non-randomized, prospective study. J Eur Acad Dermatol Venereol. 2010;24(5):535-40.
12. Fayyazi A, Schweyer S, Soruri A, et al. T lymphocytes and altered keratinocytes express interferon-γ and interleukin 6 in lichen planus. Arch Dermatol Res. 1999;291(9):485-90.
13. Sugerman PB, Satterwhite K, Bigby M. Autocytotoxic T-cell clones in lichen planus. Br J Dermatol. 2000;142(3): 449–56.
14. Kawamura E, Nakamura S, Sasaki M, et al. Accumulation of oligoclonal T cells in the infiltrating lymphocytes in oral lichen planus. J Oral Pathol Med. 2003;32(5):282-9.
15. Ammar M, Mokni M, Boubaker S, et al. Involvement of granzyme B and granulysin in the cytotoxic response in lichen planus. J Cutan Pathol. 2008;35(7):630-4.
16. Kim SG, Chae CH, Cho BO, et al. Apoptosis of oral epithelial cells in oral lichen planus caused by upregulation of BMP-4. J Oral Pathol Med. 2006;35(1):37-45.

17. Pinkus H. Lichenoid tissue reactions. A speculative review of the clinical spectrum of epidermal basal cell damage with special reference to erythema dyschromicum perstans. Arch Dermatol. 1973;107(6):840-6.
18. Vachiramon V, Suchonwanit P, Thadanipon K. Bilateral linear lichen planus pigmentosus associated with hepatitis C virus infection. Case Rep Dermatol. 2010;2(3): 169-72.
19. Sassolas B, Zagnoli A, Leroy JP, et al. Lichen planus pigmentosus associated with acrokeratosis of Bazex. Clin Exp Dermatol. 1994;19(1):70-3.
20. Mancuso G, Berdondini RM. Coexistence of lichen planus pigmentosus and minimal change nephrotic syndrome. Eur J Dermatol. 2009;19(4):389-90.
21. Dlova NC. Frontal fibrosing alopecia and lichen planus pigmentosus: is there a link? Br J Dermatol. 2013;168(2): 439-42.
22. Ingber A, Weissmann-Katzenelson V, David M, et al. Lichen planus and lichen planus pigmentosus following gold therapy—case reports and review of the literature. Z Hautkr. 1986;61(5):315-9.
23. Bhutani LK. Ashy dermatosis or lichen planus pigmentosus: What is in a name? Arch Dermatol. 1986;122(2):133.
24. Vega ME, Waxtein L, Arenas R, et al. Ashy dermatosis versus lichen planus pigmentosus: a controversial matter. Int J Dermatol. 1992;31(2):87-8.
25. Bhutani LK, George M, Bhate SM. Vitamin A in the treatment of lichen planus pigmentosus. Br J Dermatol. 1979; 100(4):473-4.
26. Ohshima N, Shirai A, Saito I, et al. Lichen planus pigmentosus inversus occurring extensively in multiple intertriginous areas. J Dermatol. 2012;39(4):412-4.
27. Munoz-Perez MA, Camacho F. Pigmented and reticulated plaques of folds. A case of lichen planus pigmentosus-inversus? Eur J Dermatol. 2002;12(3):282.
28. Kim JE, Won CH, Chang S, et al. Linear lichen planus pigmentosus of the forehead treated by neodymium:yttrium-aluminum-garnet laser and topical tacrolimus. J Dermatol. 2012;39(2):189-91.

53

Maturational Hyperpigmentation

Sidharth Sonthalia, Rashmi Sarkar

Key Features

Maturational hyperpigmentation is a common, albeit under-reported hyperpigmentary dermatosis, especially in Indians:

- The epidemiology, clinical features, probable pathogenesis and potential therapeutic options have been discussed based on the authors' observations from 35 Indian patients with this condition.
- The significance of maturational hyperpigmentation as a cutaneous marker of insulin resistance and its association with comorbid conditions like hypertension, diabetes or pre-diabetes, hyperlipidemia and coronary artery disease are discussed.

INTRODUCTION

The diagnosis of a hyperpigmentary disorder in "skin of color" can be quite a challenge, due to difficult demarcation of lesions and overlapping morphological features of some pigmentary conditions. However, with plethora of studies devoted to this aspect, certain well-defined diagnostic features, both clinical and histopathological are now considered standard for diagnosis of some of these hyperpigmentary conditions.[1] Though cosmetic concerns often prevail over medical with respect to hyperpigmentation in the Indian subcontinent, many hyperpigmentary disorders also act as cutaneous markers of an underlying systemic problem, e.g. acanthosis nigricans as a marker of insulin resistance.[2]

A relatively new entity characterized by a typical pattern of facial hyperpigmentation, called maturational hyperpigmentation (MH) has been recently described by Dr A Melvin Alexander.[3] This condition, hitherto described only once in the Black population, is encountered in Indians too. However, it finds no mention in indexed journals till date and in this chapter we review the characteristic features and systemic implications of MH based on experience in our patients. It seems to be an under-diagnosed hyperpigmentary disorder, possibly due to lack of recognition by dermatologists owing to paucity of literature.

HISTORICAL ASPECTS

The term "maturational hyperpigmentation" was first coined and described by Dr A Melvin Alexander, a dermatologist from Baltimore who first noticed a peculiar facial pigmentation in his own brother and seven more individuals, all Blacks with age ranging from 26 years to 66 years.[3] He described it as dark-brown to black pigmentation localized over the malar and zygomatic areas will blurry ill-defined borders, gradually merging with the surrounding normal skin.[3] The other commonalities that he noticed in this peculiar disorder were adult onset, relative lack of symptoms, bilateral lesions being more common, patients being overweight, lack of preceding trauma and any significant history of allergic disorders, and a negative family history. As per Dr Alexander, role of ultraviolet radiation was also considered insignificant in the pathogenesis. Melanocyte proliferation in the basal cell layer of the epidermis with increased number of melanocytes but minimal dermal inflammation were the most common findings on histopathology.[3] In a larger follow-up study conducted with his co-investigator Dr Sloane consisting of 20 patients (16 females and 4 males), Dr Alexander observed that 17 patients (85%) showed a correlation between their preferred sleeping side and the side that exhibited the condition most prominently. Laboratory tests conducted on 14 subjects revealed hyperglycemia in 50%, and hyperinsulinemia in 36% with low levels of alpha melanocyte-stimulating hormone in six out of seven (86%) patients tested for it. They suggested MH to be a cutaneous marker for diabetes or pre-diabetes and emphasized upon the need to further explore certain unexplained features of MH like its predominance in overweight/obese adult patients with dark skin, its similarity with acanthosis nigricans, exact pathogenesis including the role of physical pressure or friction and treatment options.[4]

INDIAN SCENARIO

Hitherto considered to be an uncommon condition predominantly affecting the adult Black population, MH seems to be a relatively common hyperpigmentary dermatosis, especially in Indians. In our practice, we have encountered more than 40 adult patients within the past 2 years itself, suggesting that the condition is not uncommon in Indians. Dermatologists' and physicians' unawareness of this entity leading to under-diagnosis or misdiagnosis (most commonly as facial acanthosis nigricans), and patients' reluctance to seek a dermatology opinion seem to be the most likely reasons for under-reporting.

After conducting an extensive medical literature search, we found that currently there is no publication about this condition in any indexed journal. Thus, in this chapter, we are describing the demography, salient clinical and histological features and potential therapeutic options for this curious pigmentary dermatosis, based on our observations of patients with MH in the past 2 years. From July 2011 till July 2013, we identified 35 patients with MH, of the total 6,240 new patients presenting to us giving an incidence of 0.56%. Patients were labeled as cases of MH, based on the presence of characteristic pattern of facial pigmentation originally described by Dr Alexander. Patient evaluation consisted of detailed history including the duration, presence of any preceding dermatoses or trauma, symptomatology, sun-exposure, and correlation of pigmentation with the preferred sleeping side. Medical and family history of diabetes, hyperlipidemia, and hypertension were taken and patient's body mass index (BMI) was calculated. Cutaneous examination included evaluation of the location, extent, laterality, color and texture of the pigmented lesions. Laboratory investigations including blood sugar levels (fasting and postprandial), fasting serum insulin, and lipid profile were done for all, but facial skin biopsy for histopathology was conducted only in 7 patients who consented for the procedure. Based on our assessment of all these parameters, we observed the following characteristics of MH in Indian patients:

- It is primarily seen in adults and elderly with a mean age of 52.4 years (range: 37–68 years). In contrast to the Black population where MH is more common in females, males clearly outnumber females in Indians (68.5% versus 31.5%) with a slightly higher mean age of presentation in males. The duration of lesions was highly variable (3 months to 5 years) with an average of 15 months, with longer duration in patients more than 60 years of age.
- Most patients do not have history of preceding skin disease or trauma. Around a quarter of patients (mostly females) had melasma and/or freckles, of which 50% gave history of using hydroquinone based creams for a duration ranging from 6 months to 1 year, with no chronological relation with the appearance of lesions of MH. Similarly, use of over-the-counter moisturizing and fairness creams was common (40% patients) but unrelated with the onset of MH.
- Except for visible pigmentation, lesions of MH are asymptomatic with only 8% complaining of mild burning sensation on sweating. Majority of male patients seem to be unconcerned about the cosmetic appearance due to MH, whereas approximately 45% of female patients were bothered about it.
- There is a significant correlation between the side that exhibits the condition most prominently and the preferred sleeping side (noticed by 69% patients), suggesting role of pressure or friction in its pathogenesis.
- The role of sun-exposure in the pathogenesis of MH is unclear. Around 70% patients with MH gave history of never or only occasionally having used a sunscreen and 43% gave history of mild to moderate sun-exposure on a daily basis. However, in a tropical country like India, sun-exposure of general population is fairly common and regular use of sun-screens is not *in vogue*. Thus the net sun-exposure sustained by MH patients needs to be compared against an age and sex-matched control group to clearly establish its role in the pathogenesis of MH.
- Clinically, all patients have a typical dark-brown to black pigmentation over the face with blurry ill-defined borders, fading off gradually into the surrounding normal skin **(Fig. 1)**. Zygomatic area is predominantly involved (63%) followed by malar area (14%) and rarely the forehead **(Fig. 2)**. Confluent lesions involving zygomatic as well as malar areas were observed in 20% cases. The texture was rough and uneven in majority of patients (71%).
- Comorbid medical conditions like hypertension, diabetes, hyperlipidemia, and coronary heart disease were known to be present in 60%, 26%, 20%, and 8.6% patients respectively.
- Family history of MH-like pigmentation was given by 20% patients, though only 5% of them could be confirmed on examination. Others have either a different conditions like melasma, Reihl's melanosis or could not be brought for examination.
- As per BMI, more than 50% were found to be overweight.
- Abnormalities in blood sugar levels (30%), fasting insulin levels (60%) and lipid profile (70%) were detected in a significant number of cases, which included patients

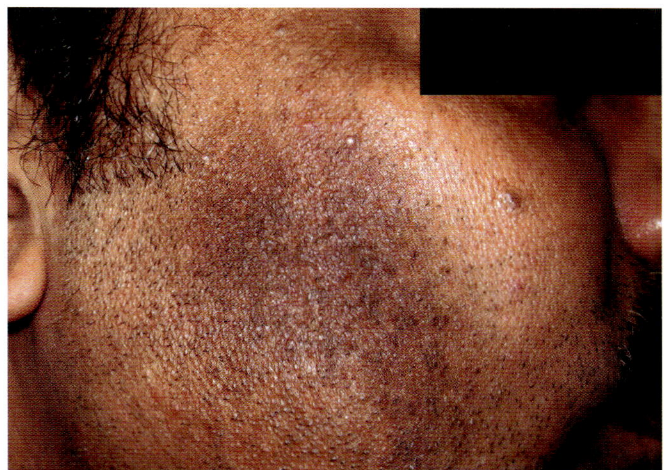

Fig. 1: Dark-brown pigmentation with a rough texture over the zygomatic region of the face with blurry ill-defined borders fading off gradually into the surrounding normal skin in a 43-year-old Indian man

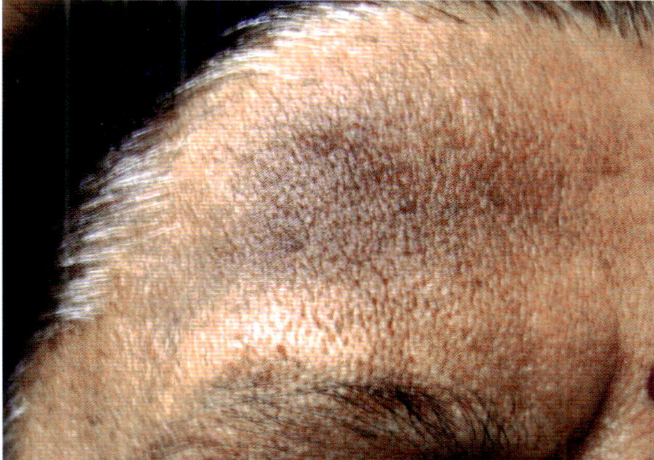

Fig. 2: Localized dark-brown pigmentation with relatively smoother texture over the forehead of a 50-year-old Indian lady

who were unaware about the co-existing comorbid conditions.

HISTOPATHOLOGY

Histopathology from biopsies taken from 7 patients revealed mild to moderate melanocyte proliferation in the basal cell layer of the epidermis, only mild or absent inflammation in the dermis with only mild papillomatosis in 2 cases.

DIFFERENTIAL DIAGNOSIS

Some conditions are relatively easily ruled out like melasma, post-inflammatory hyperpigmentation and lichen planus pigmentosus. Acanthosis nigricans shares many morphological features and associations, therefore, it should be ruled out with careful history and examination of other parts like the neck and axillae. Macular amyloidosis afflicts the face uncommonly, but should be considered in an odd case. Others include exogenous ochronosis, and other facial hypermelanosis. The *typical localization of lesions, gray to light brown color with ill-defined margins and merging with the surrounding skin and the rough texture* are clues to clinical diagnosis.

CONCLUSION

This first Indian study targeted toward elucidating the probable pathogenetic associations for this condition has revealed interesting findings.

Our results show the following points:

- Maturational hyperpigmentation primarily arises in the 4th or 5th decade in Indians and males outnumber females.
- It is mostly bilateral with gray to brown color and rough texture with ill-defined margins and involves the zygomatic area the most. Though asymptomatic, some perceive mild itching on exposure to sweat.
- Correlation between the preferred sleeping side and involved side in bilateral cases is quite apparent, a finding reported by Dr Alexander (94% in 20 patients)[3] as well, suggesting the role of sleeping pressure in worsening the condition.
- It seems to be a cutaneous indicator of current or impending insulin resistance and associated complications like lipid derangements and ischemic heart disease. Hyperglycemia (30% versus 35%) and hyperinsulinism (63% versus 50%) in both studies reinforces this fact.
- Overweight and frank obesity in more than 50% of subjects in our study and substantial percentage in study by Dr Alexander further suggests that presence of MH may be a useful marker for diabetes or pre-diabetes.

FUTURE APPROACH

The findings of Dr Alexander and our pilot study raises interesting questions:[3]

- What is the reason of predilection of MH in overweight/obese adult males and females, especially in skin of color?
- What is the similarity between MH and acanthosis nigricans as their morphological appearance and

association with diabetes and hyperlipidemia is similar! Are they two sides of the same coin?

- What might be the best cosmetic treatment for this condition? In our opinion, use of sun-screens, precautions to prevent pressure on that area, chemical peels, dermabrasion or microdermabrasion and fractional lasers may be effective. The treatment approach for this condition would hopefully be available in some time.

Maturational hyperpigmentation remains a mysterious condition for the skin of color. There is a need for larger prospective trials for evaluating the pathogenetic associations of MH, ultra-structural evaluation from biopsy samples and randomized double-blind studies to find an efficacious treatment for this condition. Awareness of this entity for each dermatologist is important due to the potential of early detection of lipid/glycemic abnormalities to ensure timely intervention.

REFERENCES

1. Grimes PE. Management of hyperpigmentation in darker racial ethnic groups. Semin Cutan Med Surg. 2009;28(2):77-85.
2. Alexander M. Investigating unusual facial hyperpigmentation in darker skin 2006. [online] Dermatology Times. Available from: http://dermatologytimes.modernmedicine.com/dermatology-times/news/clinical/dermatology/investigating-unusual-facial-hyperpigmentation-darker-sk. [Accessed, October, 2013]
3. Hilton L. Doctor studies 'maturational hyperpigmentation' (2006). [online] Dermatology Times. Available from: http://dermatologytimes.modernmedicine.com/dermatology-times/news/clinical/dermatology/doctor-studies-maturational-hyperpigmentation. [Accessed, October, 2013].

Index

Page numbers followed by *f* refer to figure, *t* refer to table and *b* refer to box.

C

T

U

V

W

X

Y

Z